Therapy of Parkinson's Disease

NEUROLOGICAL DISEASE AND THERAPY

Advisory Board

Additional Volumes in Preparation

Therapy of Parkinson's Disease

Third Edition, Revised and Expanded

edited by

Rajesh Pahwa
Kelly E. Lyons
University of Kansas Medical Center
Kansas City, Kansas, U.S.A.

William C. Koller
Mount Sinai School of Medicine
New York, New York, U.S.A.

MARCEL DEKKER, INC. NEW YORK · BASEL

The second edition was edited by William C. Koller and George Paulson (1994).

Library of Congress Cataloging-in-Publication Data
A catalog record for this book is available from the Library of Congress.

ISBN: 0-8247-5455-7

This book is printed on acid-free paper.

Headquarters
Marcel Dekker, Inc.,
270 Madison Avenue, New York, NY 10016, U.S.A.
tel: 212-696-9000; fax: 212-685-4540

Distribution and Customer Service
Marcel Dekker, Inc.,
Cimarron Road, Monticello, New York 12701, U.S.A.
tel: 800-228-1160; fax: 845-796-1772

Eastern Hemisphere Distribution
Marcel Dekker AG,
Hutgasse 4, Postfach 812, CH-4001 Basel, Switzerland
tel: 41-61-260-6300; fax: 41-61-260-6333

World Wide Web
http://www.dekker.com

The publisher offers discounts on this book when ordered in bulk quantities. For more information, write to Special Sales/Professional Marketing at the headquarters address above.

Foreword

There is perhaps no field in neurology in which therapy is advancing at such a rapid pace as Parkinson's disease. Parkinson's disease is an age-related neurodegenerative disorder that affects approximately one million persons in the United States. With the aging of the population it is anticipated that over the coming decades this number will triple or quadruple. Pathologically, Parkinson's disease is characterized by degeneration of dopamine neurons in the substantia nigra pars compacta and a corresponding loss of striatal dopamine. Modern therapy is based primarily on a dopamine replacement strategy using the precursor levodopa or a dopamine agonist. Such treatments, however, suffer limitations that include motor complications in as many as 80% of levodopa-treated patients, the development of features that do not respond to dopaminergic therapies (e.g., freezing, postural instability, and dementia), and inexorable progression that occurs despite symptomatic treatment. Thus, despite the best of modern treatment, many Parkinson's disease patients continue to suffer unacceptable levels of disability. This has prompted an intensive search for more effective treatment approaches that provide better symptomatic control, avoid or reverse motor complications, and slow or prevent disease progression.

This book represents a thorough and complete review of the different treatment approaches to Parkinson's disease. Chapters are devoted to a discussion of the strengths and weaknesses of each of the current therapies including levodopa, the dopamine agonists, and COMT inhibitors. Chapters are also provided on each of the different surgical approaches that are currently being used in the treatment of Parkinson's disease patients. Finally, there are reviews of more experimental treatments that offer hope for the future, including new pharmacological approaches, transplantation, stem cells, and trophic factors. The nonmotor aspects of Parkinson's disease have not been ignored and similar attention is paid to the important issues of diet, speech, and physical therapy in the management of Parkinson's disease patients.

The text is designed for neurologists with an interest in the therapeutics of Parkinson's disease. The authors are leaders in their fields. Chapters are concise, well written, and thoughtful. This text represents the third volume in a series that was originally begun by Drs. William Koller and George Paulson and is the most thorough and up to date in this series. For those with an interest in Parkinson's disease this book will be an important addition to their library. It illustrates how far we have come in our approach to Parkinson's disease management, and yet how far we still have to go. Clinicians, researchers, and patients alike, however, should take comfort in the fact that each of these treatments has evolved based on an understanding of underlying scientific principles. Such rationally based therapies provide hope that with ongoing research greater therapeutic gains are still to come.

C. Warren Olanow, M.D. F.R.C.P.C.
Professor and Chairman
Department of Neurology
Mount Sinai School of Medicine
New York, New York, U.S.A.

Preface

Parkinson's disease is a neurodegenerative condition for which the management can be difficult, especially in advanced stages. Our knowledge of Parkinson's disease treatment has increased tremendously in recent years. New medications have been approved, many medications and other treatment options are under investigation, and we have a better understanding of the use of surgical procedures in Parkinson's disease. However, there continue to be many issues related to the long-term management of Parkinson's disease and treatment continues to be a challenge.

We hope that this updated edition will continue to serve as a reference source for those seeking answers to the many questions related to the management of Parkinson's disease. Since the second edition, there has been a tremendous increase in our knowledge that makes this edition relevant and timely. This volume begins with a review of the history of medical and surgical therapy for Parkinson's disease. Clinical and imaging techniques used for assessment are also discussed. Detailed reviews of the use of and issues related to currently available medical treatments for Parkinson's disease, including levodopa, dopamine agonists, COMT inhibitors, anticholinergics, MAO-B inhibitors, and amantadine, as well as a review of surgical treatments including thalamotomy, pallidotomy, subthalamotomy, deep brain stimulation of the thalamus, globus pallidus, and subthalamic nucleus, are included. Other treatment options such as ECT, gamma knife, and transcranial magnetic stimulation are also discussed. Several chapters are devoted to the management of nonmotor symptoms of Parkinson's disease and include a discussion of the associated problems and treatment options related to autonomic nervous system dysfunction, sleep, dementia, psychosis, and depression. A review of dietary issues, speech therapy, physical therapy, and occupational therapy is also included. Finally, the current status of investigational treatments including new medications, transplantation, trophic factors, and stem cell therapy is reviewed. We feel that this book is a valuable resource to all physicians and health care professionals involved in the treatment of Parkinson's disease.

We thank all the authors for their time and commitment in preparing scholarly reviews of the various aspects of the treatment of Parkinson's disease. We also thank Jinnie Kim, Barbara Mathieu, and other Marcel Dekker, Inc., staff who assisted in the preparation of this book.

Rajesh Pahwa
Kelly E. Lyons
William C. Koller

Contents

Deep Brain Stimulation

Other Treatment Options

Therapy for Nonmotor Symptoms

Nonmedical Management

Investigational Therapies

Contributors

L. Alvarez, M.D. Neurological Service, Centro de Restauración Neurologica, Havana, Cuba

J. Arbizu, M.D., Ph.D. Neurological Service, Department of Neuroscience, Universidad de Navarra, Pamplona, Spain

Susan M. Baser, M.D. Associate Professor of Neurology, Drexel University School of Medicine, and Medical Director, Spasticity and Movement Disorders Center at Allegheny General Hospital, Pittsburgh, Pennsylvania, U.S.A.

Stephan Behrens, M.D. Associate Director, Clinical Development CNS, Schwarz Biosciences, Monheim, Germany

Kailash P. Bhatia, M.D., D.M., F.R.C.P. Senior Lecturer and Consultant Neurologist, Department of Clinical Neurology, Institute of Neurology, University College London, London, England

Nicholas M. Boulis, M.D. Center for Neurological Restoration, Department of Neurosurgery, Cleveland Clinic Foundation, Cleveland, Ohio, U.S.A.

Laura S. Boylan, M.D. Department of Neurology, Columbia-Presbyterian Medical Center and New York University, New York, New York, U.S.A.

Maria Bozi, M.D. Department of Clinical Neurology, Institute of Neurology, University College London, London, England

Helen Bronte-Stewart, M.D. Stanford Comprehensive Movement Disorders Center, Stanford University Medical Center, Stanford, California, U.S.A.

Kathryn A. Chung, M.D.   Fellow, Department of Neurology, Oregon Health and Science University, Portland, Oregon, U.S.A.

Ruth Djaldetti, M.D.   Department of Neurology, Rabin Medical Center, Tel Aviv University, Tel Aviv, Israel

Roger C. Duvoisin, M.D.   William Dow Lovett Professor Emeritus, Department of Neurology, University of Medicine and Dentistry of New Jersey–Robert Wood Johnson Medical School, New Brunswick, New Jersey, U.S.A.

Lawrence Elmer, M.D.   Associate Professor, Department of Neurology, Medical College of Ohio, Toledo, Ohio, U.S.A.

Raymond Faber, M.D.   Professor, Departments of Psychiatry and Neurology, University of Texas Health Science Center at San Antonio and South Texas Veterans Health Care Center, San Antonio, Texas, U.S.A.

Hubert H. Fernandez, M.D.[*]   Assistant Professor and Director, Department of Clinical Neuroscience, Parkinson Day Program, Memorial Hospital of Rhode Island, and Brown University School of Medicine, Providence, Rhode Island, U.S.A.

Cynthia Fox, Ph.D., CCC-SLP   National Center for Voice and Speech, Denver, Colorado, U.S.A.

Steven J. Frucht, M.D.   Assistant Professor of Neurology, Neurological Institute, Columbia University, New York, New York, U.S.A.

Nestor Galvez-Jimenez, M.D., F.A.C.P., F.A.H.A.   Associate Professor, Cleveland Clinic Florida, Weston, Florida, U.S.A.

Stephen Gancher, M.D.[†]   Adjunct Associate Professor, Department of Neurology, Oregon Health Sciences University, Portland, Oregon, U.S.A.

Don M. Gash, Ph.D.   Professor and Chair, Department of Anatomy and Neurobiology, University of Kentucky, Chandler Medical Center, Lexington, Kentucky, U.S.A.

Greg A. Gerhardt, Ph.D.   Professor, Departments of Anatomy and Neurobiology, and Neurology, Director, Morris K. Udall Parkinson's Disease Research Center of Excellence, and Director, Center for Sensor Technology (CenSeT), University of Kentucky, Chandler Medical Center, Lexington, Kentucky, U.S.A.

---

[*]*Current affiliation*: Director, Clinical Trials for Movement Disorders, Department of Neurology, College of Medicine, McKnight Brain Institute at University of Florida, Gainesville, Florida, U.S.A.
[†]*Current affiliation*: Staff Neurologist, Northwest Permanente, Portland, Oregon, U.S.A.

Oscar S. Gershanik, M.D. Professor and Chair, Department of Neurology, Centro Neurológico-Hospital Francés, and Director, Laboratory of Experimental Parkinsonism, Instituto de Investigaciones Farmacológicas, Buenos Aires, Argentina

Robert E. Gross, M.D., Ph.D. Assistant Professor, Department of Neurological Surgery, Emory University School of Medicine, Atlanta, Georgia, U.S.A.

Tanya Gurevich, M.D. Department of Neurology, Tel Aviv Sourasky Medical Center, Sackler School of Medicine, Tel Aviv University, Ramat-Aviv, Israel

J. Guridi, M.D., Ph.D. Neurological Service, Neuroscience Department, Universidad de Navarra, Pamplona, Spain

Maurice R. Hanson, M.D. Staff, Department of Neurology, Cleveland Clinic Naples, Naples, Florida, U.S.A.

Robert A. Hauser, M.D. Director and Professor of Neurology, Pharmacology, and Experimental Therapeutics, Parkinson's Disease and Movement Disorders Center, University of South Florida, Tampa, Florida, U.S.A.

Jaimie M. Henderson, M.D. Associate Staff, Department of Neurosurgery, Cleveland Clinic Foundation, Cleveland, Ohio, U.S.A.

Kathrynne E. Holden, M.S., R.D. Consultant, National Parkinson Foundation, Springfield, Missouri, U.S.A.

Drew S. Kern, M.S. Research Associate, Movement Disorders Center, Colorado Neurological Institute, Englewood, Colorado, U.S.A.

Amos D. Korczyn, M.D. Professor, Department of Neurology, Tel Aviv Sourasky Medical Center, Sackler School of Medicine, Tel Aviv University, Ramat-Aviv, Israel

Jaime Kulisevsky, M.D. Chief, Movement Disorders Unit, Department of Neurology, Autonomous University of Barcelona, Barcelona, Spain

Rajeev Kumar, M.D., F.R.C.P.C. Director, Functional Neurosurgery Program, Movement Disorders Center, Colorado Neurological Institute, Englewood, Colorado, U.S.A.

Elizabeth A. Letsch, Ph.D. Senior Fellow, Department of Neurology, University of Washington School of Medicine, Seattle, Washington, U.S.A.

Peter A. LeWitt, M.D. Professor of Neurology and Psychiatry, William Beaumont Hospital Research Institute and Clinical Neuroscience Center, Wayne State University School of Medicine, Southfield, Michigan, U.S.A.

G. Lopez-Flores, M.D. Neurological Service, Centro de Restauración Neurologica, Havana, Cuba

Kelly E. Lyons, Ph.D. Research Associate Professor of Neurology and Director of Research, Parkinson's Disease and Movement Disorder Center, University of Kansas Medical Center, Kansas City, Kansas, U.S.A.

R. Macias, M.D., Ph.D. Neurological Service, Centro de Rèstauración Neurologica, Havana, Cuba

M. Manrique, M.D., Ph.D. Neurological Service, Department of Neuroscience, Universidad de Navarra, Pamplona, Spain

Margery H. Mark, M.D. Associate Professor, Department of Neurology, University of Medicine and Dentistry of New Jersey–Robert Wood Johnson Medical School, New Brunswick, New Jersey, U.S.A.

W. R. Wayne Martin, M.D. Henri M. Toupin Professor of Neurological Sciences, Division of Neurology, Department of Medicine, University of Alberta, Edmonton, Alberta, Canada

Katherine M. Martinez, P.T., M.A., N.C.S. Research Physical Therapist and Adjunct Clinical Instructor, Department of Physical Therapy and Human Movement Sciences, Feinberg School of Medicine, Northwestern University, Chicago, Illinois, U.S.A.

Eldad Melamed, M.D. Department of Neurology, Rabin Medical Center, Tel Aviv University, Tel Aviv, Israel

Thorkild V. Norregaard, M.D. Assistant Professor, Department of Surgery, Harvard Medical School, and Division of Neurosurgery, Beth Israel Deaconess Medical Center, Boston, Massachusetts, U.S.A.

John G. Nutt, M.D. Professor, Department of Neurology, Oregon Health and Science University, Portland, Oregon, U.S.A.

J. A. Obeso, M.D., Ph.D. Neurological Service, Department of Neuroscience, Universidad de Navarra, Pamplona, Spain

Fabienne Ory, M.D. Assistant Professor, Department of Neurology, Toulouse University Hospital, Toulouse, France

Rajesh Pahwa, M.D. Associate Professor of Neurology and Director, Parkinson's Disease and Movement Disorder Center, University of Kansas Medical Center, Kansas City, Kansas, U.S.A.

Joel S. Perlmutter, M.D. Elliott H. Stein Family Professor of Neurology, Departments of Neurology, Radiology, Neurobiology, and Physical Therapy, Washington University School of Medicine, St. Louis, Missouri, U.S.A.

Seth L. Pullman, M.D. Associate Professor, Columbia-Presbyterian Medical Center and New York University, New York, New York, U.S.A.

José Martin Rabey, M.D.   Professor, Department of Neurology, Assaf Harofeh Medical Center and Tel Aviv University, Zerifin, Israel

Alejandro A. Rabinstein, M.D.   Assistant Professor, Department of Neurology, University of Miami School of Medicine, Miami, Florida, U.S.A.

Lorraine Olson Ramig, Ph.D., CCC-SLP   Professor, Department of Speech, Language, Hearing Sciences, University of Colorado–Boulder, and Senior Scientist, National Center for Voice and Speech, Denver, Colorado, U.S.A.

Olivier Rascol, M.D., Ph.D.   Professor, Laboratoire de Pharmacologie Médicale et Clinique, Faculté de Medicine, Clinical Investigation Centre and INSERM U455, Toulouse, France

Ali R. Rezai, M.D.   Associate Staff, Department of Neurosurgery, Cleveland Clinic Foundation, Cleveland, Ohio, U.S.A.

Winthrop S. Risk II, M.D.   Fellow, Department of Neurology, University of Iowa Hospitals and Clinics, Iowa City, Iowa, U.S.A.

Robert L. Rodnitzky, M.D.   Professor, Department of Neurology, University of Iowa Hospitals and Clinics, Iowa City, Iowa, U.S.A.

M. C. Rodríguez-Oroz, M.D., Ph.D.   Neurological Service, Neuroscience Department, Universidad de Navarra, Pamplona, Spain

Mark W. Rogers, Ph.D., P.T.   Associate Professor and Director of Research, Department of Physical Therapy and Human Movement Sciences, and Associate Professor of Physical Medicine and Rehabilitation, Feinberg School of Medicine, Northwestern University, Chicago, Illinois, U.S.A.

Joshua M. Rosenow, M.D.[*]   Fellow, Department of Neurosurgery, Cleveland Clinic Foundation, Cleveland, Ohio, U.S.A.

Pedro García Ruiz, M.D., Ph.D.   Assistant Neurologist, Department of Neurology, Facultad de Medicina, Universidad Autónoma de Madrid, Madrid, Spain

Pradeep K. Sahota, M.D.   Associate Professor and Chair, Department of Neurology, and Director, Sleep Disorders Center, University of Missouri Health Care, Columbia, Missouri, U.S.A.

Shimon Sapir, Ph.D., CC-SLP   Associate Professor, Department of Communication Sciences and Disorders, Faculty of Social Welfare and Health Studies, University of

---

[*]*Current affiliation*: Assistant Professor, Department of Neurosurgery, Northwestern University, Chicago, Illinois, U.S.A.

Haifa, Haifa, Israel, and Research Associate, National Center for Voice and Speech, Denver, Colorado, U.S.A.

Alba Serrano, Ph.D. Department of Neurology, Facultad de Medicina, Universidad Autónoma de Madrid, Madrid, Spain

Kapil D. Sethi, M.D. Professor, Department of Neurology, and Director, Movement Disorders Clinic, Medical College of Georgia, Augusta, Georgia, U.S.A.

Leslie Shinobu, M.D., Ph.D. Assistant in Neurology and Instructor, Parkinson's Disease Movement Disorders Center, Massachusetts General Hospital and Harvard Medical School, Boston, Massachusetts, U.S.A.

Lisa M. Shulman, M.D. Associate Professor of Neurology, Codirector of the Maryland Parkinson's Disease and Movement Disorders Center, and the Rosalyn Newman Distinguished Scholar in Parkinson's Disease, University of Maryland School of Medicine, Baltimore, Maryland, U.S.A.

Clifford W. Shults, M.D. Professor, Department of Neurosciences, University of California, San Diego, School of Medicine, La Jolla, and VA San Diego Healthcare System, San Diego, California, U.S.A.

Tanya Simuni, M.D. Director, Parkinson's Disease and Movement Disorders Center, Department of Neurology, Feinberg School of Medicine, Northwestern University, Chicago, Illinois, U.S.A.

Debbie K. Song, M.D. Department of Neurosurgery, University of Michigan, Ann Arbor, Michigan, U.S.A.

Fabrizio Stocchi, M.D., Ph.D. Institute of Neuroscience, "Neuromed," Pozzilli (IS), Italy

Daniel Tarsy, M.D. Associate Professor, Department of Neurology, Harvard Medical School and Beth Israel Deaconess Medical Center, Boston, Massachusetts, U.S.A.

Eduardo Tolosa, M.D. Chief, Neurology Services, Hospital Clinic, University of Barcelona, Barcelona, Spain

Alexander I. Tröster, Ph.D. Associate Professor, Department of Neurology, University of North Carolina School of Medicine, Chapel Hill, North Carolina, U.S.A.

Paul J. Tuite, M.D. Assistant Professor, Department of Neurology, University of Minnesota, Minneapolis, Minnesota, U.S.A.

William J. Weiner, M.D. Professor, Department of Neurology, University of Maryland School of Medicine, Baltimore, Maryland, U.S.A.

Brian A. Weisenberg Research Assistant, Department of Neurology, University of Minnesota, Minneapolis, Minnesota, U.S.A.

Justo Garcia de Yébenes, M.D., Ph.D. Professor and Chair, Department of Neurology, Facultad de Medicina, Universidad Autónoma de Madrid, Madrid, Spain

Theresa A. Zesiewicz, M.D. Associate Professor of Neurology, Parkinson's Disease and Movement Disorders Center, University of South Florida, Tampa, Florida, U.S.A.

Therapy of Parkinson's Disease

1

History of the Medical Therapy of Parkinson's Disease

Margery H. Mark and Roger C. Duvoisin

University of Medicine and Dentistry of New Jersey—Robert Wood Johnson Medical School, New Brunswick, New Jersey, U.S.A.

I. THE BEGINNING: JAMES PARKINSON

James Parkinson wrote in his historic *Essay on the Shaking Palsy*, published in 1817 (1), that there was "sufficient reason for hoping that some remedial process may ere long be discovered, by which, at least, the progress of the disease may be stopped ... although the removing of the effects already produced, might be hardly to be expected." Until such a remedy was discovered, however, he could only propose bleeding, vesicatories, and purging the bowels, albeit not with great enthusiasm. Specifically, he recommended "bleeding from the upper part of the back of the neck ... after which vesicatories should be applied to the same part and a purulent discharge obtained by appropriate use of Sabine Liniment."

Parkinson does not seem to have been optimistic about the value of such therapy. He emphasized "the long period to which the disease may be extended," noting that the festinating gait may not develop "until the disease has existed ten or twelve years, or more" and then opined that "as slow as is the progress of the disease, so slow in all probability must be the period of the return to health." Patients would "seldom"persevere so long in such treatment, and so he concluded that "in most cases" all that could be accomplished would be to check its further progress.

We should not be too severe with Parkinson on this point, for even today we tend to speak of the therapy of Parkinson's disease (PD) with undue optimism, glossing over the fact that our best therapies are merely palliative. Contrary to Parkinson's expectations, no treatment has yet been capable of stopping or slowing the progress of PD.

Interestingly, Parkinson considered the use of "internal medicines" to be "scarcely warrantable." He also thought that tonic medicines and a "highly nutritious diet" would yield little benefit. Although he expressed skepticism as to the possible value of purging, he cited an anecdotal description of a patient whose complaints of "numbness and prickling

1

with a feeling of weakness in both arms, accompanied ... at times by a slight trembling of the hands" were "entirely removed" by moderate doses of calomel and Epsom salts administered to empty the bowels.

The modern reader should grant Parkinson credit for avoiding the allopathic excesses of his contemporaries, who might have prescribed large doses of toxic preparations of mercury, arsenic, or antimony, and applaud his skepticism about the value of purging. Yet we cannot avoid observing that the "removing of the effects already produced," i.e., the relief of symptoms, is precisely what is regularly achieved today by the use of "internal medicines" such as levodopa.

II. THE SOLANACEOUS ALKALOIDS

A half century elapsed before any effective therapy was recognized. In a three-part review published in 1861–1862, Charcot and Vulpian (2) observed that therapy was "powerless against the progress of the disease." A few years later, Charcot's student Ordenstein reported in his doctoral thesis of 1867 (3) that a preparation of hyoscine temporarily calmed the tremor to some extent. Charcot, in his Salpétrière Lectures, collected and edited by Bourneville (4), stated that he had found strychnine, ergot products from rye and belladonna, and opium of no effect. He mentions, however, that several patients felt improved on hyoscyamine; he judged the effect "simply palliative." Bourneville (4) remarks that hypodermic injections of potassium arsenate had been tried on Charcot's patients without any satisfactory result. Camphor bromide had also been tried with only transient amelioration of "certain symptoms."

Peterson, in his account of paralysis agitans prepared for M. Allen Starr's textbook *Familiar Forms of Nervous Disease*, published in 1890 (5), listed various remedies that had been tried. His list included, in addition to the belladonna alkaloids, veratrum, ergot, strychnine, opium, coniine, curare, gelsemium, and many others. Gowers (6) also recommended Indian hemp. Peterson (5) stated that only the belladonna alkaloids were of any use. Scattered accounts of the effects of belladonna alkaloids in individual patients appeared in the medical literature of the late nineteenth century, although no systematic clinical trials were described. Therapeutic recommendations offered in many review articles and medical textbooks of the period indicate awareness of the limited palliative effects of hyoscine, hyoscyamus, tincture of belladonna, datura stramonium, and other related alkaloid preparations.

In retrospect, it seems significant that virtually all known medicinal preparations of botanical origin had been tested in the treatment of parkinsonism, but that only the belladonna alkaloids received enduring and widespread recognition for their modest palliative effects entirely on the basis of empirical observation in the absence of any knowledge of their anticholinergic properties.

III. POSTENCEPHALITIC PARKINSONISM

The epidemics of encephalitis lethargica in the years 1916–1926 gave rise to a large population of patients presenting a distinctive parkinsonian syndrome accompanied by other extrapyramidal features, plus ocular and bulbar palsies, oculogyric crisis, and behavioral disorders (7). Initially regarded as chronic encephalitis and later as postencephalitic parkinsonism, the condition was for many years more prevalent than

PD. During the 1930s it accounted for two thirds of the parkinsonian patients seen in neurological clinics (8).

Again, a wide range of treatments was tried. An extensive review is provided in the third report of the Matheson Encephalitis Commision (9). Although drugs such as nicotine, curare, and bulbocapnine were tried, the most effective treatment again proved to be the use of the belladonna alkaloids and extracts of *Atropa belladonna* root (10). Postencephalitic patients benefited more from such treatment than did patients with PD. They tolerated very large doses, and various regimens using high doses were developed. Römer's high-dose atropine treatment is an example (11). Doses as high as 20 mg three times daily were employed. Not only the extrapyramidal motor syndrome, but the tics, behavioral abnormalities, and oculogyric crises typical of the postencephalitic syndrome were often markedly relieved. With such high doses, combinations of central and peripheral atropinic toxicity were commonly encountered. Pilocarpine was employed to counteract blurring of vision and dryness of the mouth.

A crude white wine extract of *Atropa belladonna* root prepared by the Bulgarian herbalist Ivan Raeff received widespread acclaim in the 1920s and came to be known as the "Bulgarian treatment." An interesting account of this preparation is given by von Witzleben (10) in his 1942 monograph on the treatment of postencephalitic parkinsonism. The main alkaloids identified in belladonna root were hyoscyamine, scopolamine, atropine, and belladonine. Belladonna grown in Bulgaria was held to be more potent than plants grown elsewhere, but the reason for this was never established. A standardized preparation of extracts of Bulgarian belladonna developed by von Witzleben was marketed in Europe in the 1930s under the name "Bulgakur." Various wine extracts of Bulgarian belladonna and belladonna marketed under names such as "Bellabulgara," "Bulgadonna," and "Vinobel" were widely employed in the United States in the 1940s (12,13). Another mixture of belladonna alkaloids in tablet form named "Rabellon" was also widely prescribed in the 1940s and early 1950s. The first edition of Merritt's *Textbook of Neurology* published in 1955 (14) described the dosages and manner of administration of these now-forgotten preparations of the natural alkaloids.

Although the alkaloid preparations are no longer prescribed for parkinsonism, hyoscyamine HBr, marketed under the name *Cystospaz*, is commonly used by urologists to inhibit urinary urgency caused by the detrusor hyperreflexia (13). PD patients receiving this agent for this indication may experience some beneficial effect on their extrapyramidal motor symptoms, but sometimes also some central anticholinergic toxicity. Few physicians prescribing this medication are likely to be aware that it was once commonly employed in the treatment of parkinsonism.

IV. THE SYNTHETIC ANTICHOLINERGICS

The products of nature were largely superseded in the 1950s by a series of synthetic anticholinergic agents. Medicinal chemists pursued several approaches to developing synthetic agents, which they hoped would be more effective antispasmodics than the belladonna alkaloids and produce fewer anticholinergic side effects. Numerous analogs of atropine were derived by modifying the acidic moiety of the molecule. One of these, benztropine (Cogentin), is the diphenyl ether of tropanol. It is the most potent of the synthetic anticholinergics, being effective in doses of 0.5–1 mg orally (14). It is less potent than atropine but does not differ from it in any clinically significant way. It is still marketed as an antiparkinsonian agent. Perhaps the first synthetic to be tried in parkinsonism was the drug caramiphen (Parparnit), introduced in 1946 (15). It is no longer produced, but some of its analogs [e.g., benactyzine (Suavitil)], were used for many years as antispasmodics in gastrointestinal disorders.

A series of piperidine compounds structurally unrelated to atropine developed by Denton et al. (16) in the 1940s was found by Cunningham et al. (17) to have significant antiacetylcholine activity. The first of these to be introduced into clinical practice as an antiparkinsonian agent, trihexyphenidyl (Artane) (18,19), became during the 1950s the most widely used antiparkinsonian agent and is still used today as an adjuvant to levodopa therapy. Additional analogs of this series were developed in rapid succession. A number were studied in clinical trials in PD patients, and three of these—cycrimine (Pagitane), procyclidine (Kemadrin), and biperiden (Akineton)—were widely used in clinical practice to treat parkinsonism. Strikingly similar to trihexyphenidyl in chemical structure, they were equipotent and clinically indistinguishable.

The antihistamine diphenhydramine (Benadryl) was found empirically to have some antiparkinsonian activity (20,21). Two congeners, orphenadrine (Disipal) (22,23) and chlorphenoxamine (Phenoxene), (24,25) were later developed and employed primarily as antiparkinsonian agents. These were generally employed as adjuvants to the more potent anticholinergics. Many other antihistamines appeared to be equally effective but did not receive recognition as antiparkinsonian agents (23).

The first group of phenothiazine derivatives introduced into clinical practice—fenethazine, promethazine (Phenergan), diethazine (Diparcol), and ethopropazine (Parsidol)—were also found to have some clinically useful antiparkinsonian activity (24–26). Like atropine, they possessed significant anticholinergic, antihistaminic, sedative, and local anesthetic properties. Only diethazine and ethopropazine were marketed specifically as antiparkinsonian agents. The former was withdrawn because of reports of cases of agranulocytosis, and ethopropazine is no longer available in the United States, but remains available in Canada and Europe. Although in large doses of 200–300 mg per day it could serve as the primary drug in the treatment of parkinsonism, it was generally used as an adjuvant in much smaller doses and was available in 10, 50, and 100 mg tablets (27).

These earlier phenothiazine drugs differ from the major tranquilizers chiefly in the greater length of the aliphatic chain connecting the tricyclic phenothiazine structure to the nitrogen atom of the amine moiety. Increasing this chain to a three-carbon propyl group reduced the antihistaminic and anticholinergic properties but conferred the novel property of causing tranquilization without sedation. The first of this series of phenothiazine derivatives introduced into clinical practice, chlorpromazine, was soon found to induce various extrapyramidal reactions including, notably, parkinsonism and acute dystonia. For this reason, Delay and Deniker termed this new class of drugs "*neuroleptics*"(28). The then astonishing observation that a "chemical" parkinsonism could be induced by chlorpromazine and also by an entirely different agent, reserpine, aroused hope that a biochemical understanding of parkinsonism would soon be achieved (29). A chemical pathology of parkinsonism that led to a revolution in its therapy was indeed realized within the following decade.

Although their efficacy was confirmed in many clinical trials, the selection of the synthetic drugs that comprised the antiparkinson armamentarium of the 1950s and 1960s was based on empirical observation, as had been the recognition of the palliative effects of the belladonna alkaloids in the late nineteenth century and not on a rational understanding of their *modus operandi*. Nor was it ever documented that the synthetics were in any way superior to the belladonna alkaloids. Physicians during the 1950s believed that some agents were more effective against tremor, while others were more effective against rigidity. They commonly used combinations of these agents in individualized regimens tailored to each patient. This approach justified the use of a number of similar agents with identical pharmacological profiles.

Recognition of the role of acetylcholine in nervous system function, first in the peripheral autonomic nervous system and subsequently in the central nervous system, led Feldberg (30), an early pioneer of neuropharmacology, to suggest that the clinical efficacy of atropine and scopolamine in parkinsonism was due to a "central atropine-acetylcholine antagonism." This suggestion was strengthened by the observation that the clinical efficacy of the various antiparkinson drugs, including the antihistamines, correlated well with their antiacetylcholine activity as measured on the isolated guinea pig ileum (31), their capacity to block the central toxic effects of physostigmine in mice (32), and the ability of the cholinomimetics tremorine and oxotremorine (33,34) to block electroencephalographic arousal induced by cholinergic agents (35).

Feldberg's suggestion was confirmed in human patients by the demonstration that physostigmine exacerbated the clinical manifestations of parkinsonism and cancelled the antiparkinson effects of previously administered benztropine (36). A therapeutic effect could be restored by further doses of benztropine. These observations indicated that the motor symptoms of parkinsonism reflected overactivity of central cholinergic systems and were consistent with the hypothesis that loss of a normally inhibitory dopamine input to the striatum resulted in disinhibition of the rich striatal cholinergic neuronal system. Thus, there was a seesaw relationship between dopamine and acetylcholine neurotransmitter systems in the striatum. Both inhibition of acetylcholine and replenishment of dopamine could restore more normal function.

Thus, for over a century, from the first observation of the palliative effect of hyoscine in 1867 to the introduction of levodopa in 1970, anticholinergic agents were the mainstay of the medicinal treatment of parkinsonism. The side effects were those to be expected from any centrally active anticholinergic agent. The psychotoxicity was remarkably high; as many as 50% of patients over age 65 experienced hallucinosis (37,38). The beneficial effects were modest at best—a reasonable estimate is a 25% reduction in the severity of symptoms.

V. AMANTADINE

The serendipitous observation by Schwab et al. (39) in 1969 that a PD patient given amantadine as prophylaxis against the flu experienced symptomatic benefit led to clinical trials that confirmed the initial observations (40–42). The drug was soon widely used even though U.S. Food and Drug Administration (FDA) approval was not granted until 1971. It had a novel side effect not previously encountered in PD patients—the development of a cyanotic mottling of the skin of the legs and forearms termed *livedo reticularis*, often accompanied by ankle and pretibial edema (43). Initial alarm over this phenomenon subsided as further studies uncovered no untoward consequences.

There was some mystery as to the mechanism of amantadine's efficacy. Although many of its side effects were typical of anticholinergics, it did not inhibit acetylcholine on the guinea pig ileum, block the vasodepressor response to acetylcholine in dogs, or antagonize tremor induced by oxotremorine—the major bioassays employed at the time to identify anticholinergic activity (44). In animal studies it exhibited dopamine-releasing properties in the periphery and inhibited dopamine reuptake activity in vitro (45,46). It was thus suggested that these actions explained the limited usefulness of amantadine in treating parkinsonism. Snyder et al. (47), however, had shown that all the synthetic anticholinergics employed as antiparkinson agents inhibited dopamine uptake in vitro, whereas atropine, a more potent antiparkinson drug, did not. Moreover, Delwaide et al. (48) showed that the much more potent dopamine uptake inhibitor mazindol had no effect in Parkinson's patients. Despite these inconsistencies, the suggestion was widely and uncritically accepted. Pharmacological studies through the early 1990s suggested that the actions of amantadine include an indirect anticholinergic action. Amantadine was found by Albuquerque et al. (49) to suppress ionic conductance of the acetylcholine receptor in denervated mammalian muscle. Lupp et al. (50) and Stoof et al. (51) showed that amantadine inhibited N-methyl-D-aspartate (NMDA)–evoked acetylcholine release in the rabbit caudate nucleus. Moreover, Stoof et al. (51) showed that this occurred at concentrations that did not affect release of dopamine. A report that physostigmine had reversed intoxication due to massive overdosage with amantadine taken with suicidal intent indicates that the drug indeed has powerful central anticholinergic effects (52).

More recently, amantadine's mechanism of action has been found to be an inhibitor of glutamatergic NMDA receptors (53). Of more clinical relevance, this drug has experienced a new awakening as a treatment for dopa-induced dyskinesias; several small studies have demonstrated objective reduction in dyskinesias at doses of 200–400 mg daily, with no loss of motor function (53).

VI. LEVODOPA

A. Levodopa: A Natural Compound

Levodopa is a naturally occurring compound, and preparation of this modified amino acid from bean extraction was long favored over the synthetic method because it did not yield the D-isomer of dopa (54). The major source for early synthetic manufacture was vanillin; it was estimated that world consumption of vanillin grew 10% annually, reaching 8 million pounds in 1969 (54). Levodopa is found in a variety of plant species, mostly from *Macuna*, a genus of tropical or twining bean plants. It makes up about 5% of the velvet bean (*Macuna deeringiana*), first analyzed in 1920 (55). Five other species of *Macuna* also contain levodopa; the best known are *Macuna urens*, or the Florida bean, and *Macuna pruriens,* or cowhage (also called cowage, cowitch, or cowhedge plant). Levodopa was first isolated from the latter in 1937 (56,57). *Macuna holtonii*, a coarse vinyl plant from Guatemala, contains the highest amount of levodopa of all the *Macuna* seeds. Melanin-pigmented plants, besides the velvet bean, also contain levodopa, e.g., *Vicia angustifolia*, *Astragalus cicer*, *Lupinus polyphyllus*, and *Baptisia australis* (58). Notably, bananas (genus *Musa*) have melanin pigmentation, but contain dopamine, not levodopa, and cannot be used therapeutically in PD (58). The best known bean and a commercial source of levodopa, the broad bean, also known as the fava bean or *Vicia faba*, was the first from which levodopa was isolated in 1913 (59). Duvoisin calculated over 30 years ago that "if broad beans contain 50 gm/kg of levodopa, then 0.1 kg would yield about 5 gm of levodopa; about 1/4 pound per day would yield an adequate dose of levodopa, and thus one could give patients one bowl of broad beans per day to treat PD."

B. Dopamine in PD

The levodopa story begins in 1951, when dopamine in human brain, and especially in caudate, was described by Raab and Gigee (60), although they called it "encephalin"; they also showed that levodopa alone was able to increase its concentration. Because they did not relate their work to dopamine per se, it was soon forgotten (61,62). More directly, the tale of dopamine and levodopa in PD formally begins in 1957 (63–65), with the discovery of dopamine in whole brain homogenates of mammals and was confirmed by Carlsson and coworkers the following year (66). Also beginning in 1957, a series of pharmacological studies on brain dopamine were reported. Carlsson and colleagues first reported the reversal of reserpine-induced catalepsy in rodents by levodopa (67); this reserpine-antagonist effect of levodopa was later confirmed in humans by Degkwitz et al. (68). In 1959, Bertler and Rosengren (69) in dogs and Sano et al. (70) in humans demonstrated that dopamine was largely confined to the striatum. Bertler and Rosengren (69) concluded that their "results favor the assumption that dopamine is concerned with the function of the corpus striatum and thus with the control of motor function ... supported by the fact that ... reserpine produces motor hypoactivity and may cause various components of Parkinson's syndrome" and "excess of dopamine in brain produced by administration of DOPA is accompanied by motor hyperactivity." Thus, these findings were the trigger that led other investigators, notably Hornykiewicz and colleagues, to examine the role of dopamine in PD (63). The following year, Ehringer and Hornykiewicz (71) published their findings of a profound depletion of striatal dopamine in patients with PD. A "chemical pathology" had now been defined for this disorder (72).

Later work demonstrating that dopamine was concentrated in striatal terminals of neurons in the pars compacta of the substantia nigra in rats (73,74) and unilateral nigral lesions resulting in ipsilateral striatal dopamine loss in monkeys (75,76) confirmed that parkinsonism was a pathophysiological state of dysfunction of the nigrostriatal dopaminergic system. As Hornykiewicz (77) suggested, PD could now be defined as a syndrome of striatal dopamine deficiency.

C. Levodopa in the Treatment of PD: 1961–1967

The foundation of the pharmacological research in PD led both Carlsson (78) and Hornykiewicz (63) to conclude that perhaps parkinsonian patients could be treated with levodopa, the chemical precursor of dopamine that would cross the blood-brain barrier. Hornykiewicz and Walther Birkmayer injected 50–150 mg of levodopa solution into parkinsonian subjects and reported a striking "abolition or substantial relief of akinesia" and improvement in all motor activities (63,79). The dopa effect appeared soon after injection, reached a peak between 2 and 3 hours, and diminished by 24 hours. Side effects of diaphoresis and vomiting occurred with the higher doses and if injection was too rapid.

The same year, McGeer et al. (80) used diphenhydramine and DL-dopa to treat drug-induced parkinsonism secondary to reserpine and phenothiazines. They used doses of dopa of 4–22 gm, but only 4 of 22 patients experienced mild improvement, whereas the diphenhydramine was more effective. Their patients were also treated with 100–420 mg/day of pyridoxine (vitamin B_6) in an attempt to enhance conversion of dopa to dopamine, as pyridoxine is a cofactor for dopa decarboxylase. This may have been partially responsible for dopa's failure in that, although not known at that time, pyridoxine blocks the effects of levodopa (81).

The following year, Barbeau and coworkers (82) administered orally both D- and L-dopa to a small number of PD patients. They used doses of 100–200 mg of dopa and reported at least 50% improvement in rigidity with levodopa, beginning 30 minutes after ingestion and lasting about 2–2.5 hours. These investigators then undertook long-term administration of levodopa, finding the best results with 50 mg doses, six times daily, with procyclidine three times daily.

Between 1963 and 1966, at least 12 studies were undertaken to evaluate the effects of dopa on PD (83–94). Few trials were performed with placebo controls or in a blind fashion. Friedhoff et al. (83) in 1963 administered an intravenous infusion of levodopa in six patients at a dose of 2.5 mg/kg body weight. On other days, they were given placebo infusions of sodium lactate, and the results were judged by examiners who did not know which preparation the patients were receiving. The patients were also blind to drug. They reported a "favorable" reduction in rigidity but not tremor, with relief subsiding after several hours. Greer and Williams (84), on the other hand, could not demonstrate any change with 1 g of DL-dopa in two patients. Gerstenbrand et al. (85) studied the effects of levodopa in 30 PD patients. About half the patients received intravenous injections of 100–150 mg, and 20 patients received oral doses of 100–200 mg. They reported a marked improvement in akinesia, mild improvement in rigidity, and no change in tremor in a small number of patients on oral mediciation: 6 had no change, and 9 had only slight improvement. Intravenous therapy gave good results for 11 patients, but the rest had little or no improvement. In 1964, Hirschmann and Mayer (86) gave 10 patients 25–50 mg of intravenous levodopa and reported "total remission or pronounced diminution of akinesia" with the larger dose. The effect began within one-half hour and peaked at 2–3 hours. Umbach and Bauman (87) examined 30 patients with intravenous levodopa in dose ranges of 100–150 mg, with 20 patients exhibiting reduced akinesia for 3–12 hours. Umbach and Tzavellas (88) used 50 mg of levodopa plus 20 mg of propylhexedrine in 35 patients and reported a better response than with either drug alone. The response lasted for 3–4 days, instead of the hours seen with levodopa infusions alone. Bruno and Bruno (89) injected levodopa in doses of 1–2 mg/kg and recorded a "marked improvement" lasting a few hours. Placebo injections in three subjects showed no response. Less impressed with levodopa were Pazzagli and Amadal (90), who gave nine patients 60–120 mg of levodopa intravenously, and another patient 1.2 g orally. They found a modest effect in 2 patients, a slight response in 4, and no effect in 4. Rinaldi and coworkers agreed (91); in 10 patients they found no change with 50 mg of intramuscular dopa or 300 mg of oral dopa.

Other investigators were also skeptical of levodopa. In a placebo-controlled trial, McGeer and Zeldewicz (92) treated 10 patients with oral doses of 1–5 g of DL-dopa daily and intravenous doses of 200–500 mg. Subjective improvement was found in 5 patients, but objective results were seen in only 2 patients on oral medication, both receiving the highest dose; in one, the improvement was maintained on placebo. One other patient had some response to intravenous D- and DL-dopa but none to oral drug. Another patient with "arteriosclerotic parkinsonism" was maintained for 2 years on 3 g of DL-dopa without any untoward effects. Improvements in all cases were mild. Side effects were consistent—primarily nausea and lightheadedness. Nausea occurred in half the patients at 1–2.5 g, and in all patients on 5 g of dopa daily. They concluded that dopa was not a useful treatment for PD. It should also be noted, however, that they, like many others, were still administering pyridoxine concomitantly, which may have contributed to dopa's lack of efficacy (81).

Three years after their initial observations, Birkmayer and Hornykiewicz (93), reviewing over 200 cases of parkinsonism they had treated with levodopa, dampened their early enthusiasm for the drug, finding that only about half their patients had any sort of "dopa effect." Further, if their anticholinergic medications were withdrawn, levodopa was no longer effective. About 20% of patients had some improvement in akinesia, and 30% had no response at all.

A double-blind trial was conducted by Fehling (94) in 1966. She administered intravenous levodopa in doses of 1.5 mg/kg to 27 patients one day and a saline placebo the second day. Two patients reported improvement after levodopa, two after placebo, and one after both. There were no differences in response at all between levodopa and placebo, except that nine patients had nausea on levodopa. In 1968, another double-blind trial was reported by Rinne and Sonninen (95), who examined similar doses of intravenous levodopa with similar results.

Thus, by the mid-1960s, many investigators were not convinced that levodopa would have much of a role in the treatment of PD. Duvoisin, in a review of therapies for PD current to 1965, wrote (96) that "a number of investigators, repeating a pattern that is all too familiar in the history of the treatment of parkinsonism, have studied the use of DOPA but have either been unable to confirm the described response to DOPA or have noted only an occasional and transient effect. Despite enthusiastic claims of therapeutic benefit, no evidence has been presented that the DOPA effect is in any way specific or that it differs from the effect of other sympathomimetic amines." Bertler and Rosengren (97), who first described the presence of dopamine in the mammalian striatum, stated that "the effect of L-dopa is too complex to permit a conclusion about disturbances of the striatal dopaminergic system in PD." Hornykiewicz (63) notes that "the reserved tone of the discussion in Bertler and Rosengren's 1966 overview very faithfully reflects the then-prevailing mood on the part of the majority of the catecholamine researchers."

D. High-Dose Levodopa Therapy: 1967–1970

The turning point, and the foundation for the modern treatment of PD, came in 1967 with the report of Cotzias et al. (98) These investigators administered a racemic mixture of DL-dopa (because of the "great expense" of the L-compounds) orally to 16 patients, but the difference in their study was that they used doses of 3–16 g daily. Half the patients had "complete, sustained disappearance or marked amelioration of their individual manifestations of Parkinsonism." Two others had "sustained improvement," but "significant degrees of either tremor or rigidity remained." Four patients were unimproved; one became worse. Gradual increases in the dose of dopa (by 0.2 g) prevented the side effects of nausea, faintness, and vomiting seen with larger incremental dose increases (0.5 g/dose). Improvement occurred in two of eight cases at doses under 12 g daily, whereas it occurred in all but one of the eight at doses of 12 g or more. Also, dyskinetic movements were noted in three patients who had dosages of 9, 12, and 16 g daily.

This study demonstrated that dopa had pronounced central effects with high dosages, which could not be achieved with other "sympathomimetic amines" (96) because of serious cardiovascular manifestations. It also showed, for the first time, the side effects of abnormal involuntary movements as a consequence of increased striatal dopaminergic transmission.

In the next 3 years, numerous reports by a large number of investigators (99–106) confirmed the findings of Cotzias et al.'s 1967 study (98). Many reported single- or double-blind trials (99–104), and others reported their open-label experience (105,106). Uniformly, approximately 80% of patients among all the trials demonstrated significant improvement. The introduction of high-dose oral levodopa during these years constituted nothing less than a therapeutic revolution. The "dopa effect" far exceeded the benefits of the anticholinergics. A marked reversal of the motor signs and symptoms of parkinsonism was achieved in a considerable proportion of patients, even in those afflicted for many years and in advanced stages of the disease. Reports in the news media generated enormous interest, and for a time the few clinics able to provide the new treatment were overwhelmed by large numbers of patients seeking the miraculous new treatment.

Although levodopa appeared to be a rational therapy based on a specific knowledge of pathology, albeit primarily a chemical pathology, it was quite surprising, indeed counterintuitive to many, that merely feeding patients a simple amino acid precursor of a central nervous system neurotransmitter could have such dramatic therapeutic effects. The nerve cells normally containing that neurotransmitter had presumably degenerated and the synaptic organization of the basal ganglia had consequently been permanently altered. How then could such a therapeutic strategy work? There was no precedent for such a result.

For the skeptics, such profound benefits also had their down side, and a symposium in 1969 (107) enumerated the side effects and limitations of chronic levodopa therapy. Motor fluctuations, the on-off effect, and dyskinesias were all noted by several investigators at the meeting, despite such short-term experience with levodopa.

In recent years, the skeptics have continued to cavil, and controversy has flared over whether levodopa is toxic to or protective of dopaminergic neurons. The first double-blind study to evaluate levodopa's effect on the natural history of PD was completed in 2002 (108), 35 years after the initial report of Cotzias and colleagues (98). The Earlier vs. Later Levodopa study (ELLDOPA) (108) demonstrated at the end of 40 weeks of treatment significant, sustained improvement in patients on all doses of levodopa. Thus, levodopa continues to maintain its position as the primary treatment for PD.

VII. PERIPHERAL DOPA DECARBOXYLASE INHIBITORS

It took almost no time for those treating PD to search for and find a solution to the problem of the very large oral doses needed to make levodopa effective. In 1969 Birkmayer (109) discussed the evolution of his team's use of a dopa decarboxylase inhibitor, Ro 4-4602 (N-DL-seryl-N-[2,3,4-trihydroxybenzyl]-hydrazine), which they first used in 1964 for treating hypertension, affective disorders, and, in particular, chorea. They found that it made chorea worse; consequently, they used it in combination with levodopa and found that the "effect of the combined treatment is more pronounced and lasts longer than that of the dopa alone." Their work was confirmed by a number of investigators, among them Tissot and colleagues (110) and Siegfried (111), also using Ro 4-4602. They further found that the effective oral doses of levodopa could be reduced dramatically, by 6–10 times, and side effects of nausea, vomiting, and hypotension became rare.

Another extracerebral dopa decarboxylase inhibitor, MK-486, or L-alpha-methyldopa hydrazine, was also studied. In 1971, Yahr et al. (112) in an open study and Calne et al. (113) in a double-blind trial found that the new drug allowed for a 75% reduction in levodopa dose. Gastrointestinal side effects were considerably reduced. They noted, however, similar antiparkinsonian effects and no change in dyskinesias. Cotzias and coworkers (99) reported in 1969 the concomitant use of the racemic mixture of alpha-methyldopa hydrazine (MK-485) in three patients, with similar findings.

As postulated by Yahr et al. (112), by selectively inhibiting the conversion of dopa to dopamine in peripheral tissues but not in brain, dopa's peripheral utilization is reduced, thus decreasing peripheral side effects and allowing for much smaller and longer-lasting oral doses of levodopa. Another advantage of the decarboxylase inhibitors was the protection against pyridoxine's enhancement of the decarboxylation of levodopa (81,113,114). Many subsequent open-label (115–117) and double-blind trials (118) of Ro 4-4602, later called benserazide, and open (119) and double-blind studies (120–122) of MK-486, or carbidopa, supported the early findings. Little difference was found between benserazide and carbidopa, each in combination with levodopa (123), and marketed as Madopar® and Sinemet®, respectively. They form the mainstay of the current treatment of PD worldwide.

VIII. DOPAMINE AGONISTS

A. Apomorphine

The first direct-acting dopamine agonist used to treat PD, apomorphine, a weak tertiary catecholamine, was used in 1951 by Schwab and colleagues (124). Its antiparkinson effect was good but short-lived. Apomorphine was used as an emetic, but over the next 20 years it was generally forgotten as investigators concentrated on levodopa. In 1970, however, Cotzias et al. (125) reexamined apomorphine injections in a placebo-controlled trial. Small doses of the drug effectively duplicated their results with levodopa, although the duraton was less than 2 hours. These results were soon repeated by others (126). Cotzias's group then examined the oral administration of apomorphine (127) but found the excessively high doses nephrotoxic. They then studied N-propylnoraporphine (NPA) as an adjunct to levodopa, which allowed them to use higher oral doses and avoid serious side effects (127–129). Although their results were favorable, NPA fell by the wayside with the emergence of newer agonists. In 1979, Corsini et al. (130) reexamined apomorphine injections, successfully combining it for the first time with domperidone to counteract the side effects of nausea and sedation. Apomorphine was subsequently ignored for nearly 2 decades, but it has seen a reemergence of late in treating severe motor fluctuations in PD, not only with intravenous (131) and subcutaneous (132) injections, but also with intranasal (133) and sublingual (134) preparations.

B. Piribedil

In 1971, Corrodi et al. (135), testing new dopaminergic compounds, found that 7-[2″-pyrimidyl]-4-piperonyl-piperazine (ET 495) was a potent dopamine receptor–stimulating agent in rats. The attraction of an orally administered dopamine agonist was great, as apomorphine could only be used parenterally. Clinical trials (136–139) were undertaken with the new drug, called piribedil. It was found to be modestly effective as an antiparkinsonian treatment, primarily improving tremor. It was best used as an adjuvant to levodopa. Nevertheless, side effects, particularly dyskinesias and psychotoxicity, and its relatively minor antiparkinsonian effects limited its usefulness (140), and the drug was not developed further.

C. Bromocriptine and Beyond

Corrodi and colleagues (141) kept up the search for more potent, longer-lasting, safer, and more effective agonists. In 1973 they found an ergot derivative, CB 154, to have similar actions to apomorphine in the rat. Clinical trials of the drug, bromocriptine, were begun, and initial reports of patients, both on levodopa (142–144) and dopa-naive (144,145), were favorable. Fairly high doses, on average 40–50 mg/day, were used. In some long-term studies (146,147) bromocriptine was helpful in reducing motor fluctuations and allowed some patients to eliminate levodopa, but other investigators (148) did not find it as useful as levodopa. It caused similar side effects as levodopa, and in combination with levodopa potentiated abnormal involuntary movements, but in de novo patients it did not cause dyskinesias (148). Bromocriptine (Parlodel®) became the first approved oral dopamine agonist used as adjuvant therapy with levodopa.

During initial trials with bromocriptine, another ergot dopamine agonist, lergotrile mesylate, was tested in PD patients (149–151). At low doses (mean 11 mg) it was, like piribedil, modestly effective, and then mostly for tremor (149). At doses of 52 mg/day, improvements in all features of parkinsonism as well as motor fluctuations were noted (151). In spite of its antiparkinsonian efficacy, hepatotoxicity was a major problem, and the drug was discontinued (152). Newer agonists such as lisuride (Dopergin®) (153,154) and pergolide (Permax®) (154) began testing in the late 1970s, and ushered in the era of the continuing search for a safer, better agonist, resulting in approval of two nonergot agonists, pramipexole (Mirapex®) and ropinirole (Requip®) (155), in the 1990s. The future looks not just to safer, more effective drugs, but transdermal delivery to offer more continuous dopaminergic stimulation (156).

IX. MONOAMINE OXIDASE INHIBITORS

Monoamine oxidase (MAO) is one of the enzymes of catecholamine catabolism. MAO inhibitors prevent the breakdown of dopamine at the receptor and may prolong the antiparkinson effect of levodopa. The first MAO inhibitors used with levodopa were the standard antidepressant drugs, including isocarboxazid, tranylcypromine, nialamide, pargyline, and clorgyline.

In 1962, based on the concept of decreasing dopamine catabolism, Birkmayer and Hornykiewicz (157) first used a MAO inhibitor (isocarboxazid) as pretreatment for levodopa to prolong the dopa effect. Cardiovascular side effects limited the pursuit of such a combination. Yet most of the early levodopa studies either added or pretreated with a MAO inhibitor. Some found no further benefit and an increase in side effects (82,87). One thought pretreatment enhanced the beneficial effect on parkinsonism but also increased side effects (85), another felt there was more improvement with the combination of MAO inhibitor and levodopa (89), while yet another claimed that a MAO inhibitor alone (pargyline) was more effective than levodopa (91).

By 1970, however, it was shown that the combination of traditional MAO inhibitors and levodopa could potentially be dangerous because of significant pressor responses (158). The addition of a dopa decarboxylase inhibitor helped (159) but was not protective enough to warrant further use of these drugs together.

The MAO story began to change, however, when it was shown that there existed two types of MAO, A and B (160). It was later demonstrated that dopamine is metabolized preferentially by the B type (161,162). A MAO-B–selective inhibitor would be of value to use as an adjunctive medication in PD while avoiding the dangerous pressor effect of the MAO-A inhibitors. L-Deprenyl (selegiline)(Eldepryl® or Jumex®) was developed and used with levodopa in initial trials; at doses of up to 10 mg it was helpful in controlling motor fluctuations (162–165). These drugs became the center of great interest and controversy, centered around the issue of neuroprotection. To date, this issue remains unresolved (166).

X. CATECHOL-*O*-METHYLTRANSFERASE INHIBITORS

Catechol-*O*-methyltransferase (COMT), like MAO, is a catabolic enzyme of dopamine and the other catecholamines. The era of COMT inhibitors in the treatment of PD began recently with the approval of entacapone (Comtan®) and tolcapone (Tasmar®) (167), yet an early COMT inhibitor was tested in 1971. By that time, evidence had amassed that *O*-methylation of dopa and dopamine could render them ineffective, and a new drug, GPA 1714 (*N*-butyl gallate), was found to inhibit COMT both in vitro and in vivo. Ericsson (168) conducted a trial in 10 PD patients on optimal levodopa treatment with up to 750 mg of GPA 1714. No adverse effects were noted, and improvements in all features of parkinsonism, dyskinesias, nausea, and hypotension were all demonstrated. GPA 1714 was most beneficial as adjunct to levodopa. This was the only published trial of this drug. Subsequent investigation showed no symptomatic effects, cardiovascular toxicity was noted and the drug was withdrawn.

XI. OTHER DRUGS

A plethora of drugs have been tried in the treatment of PD over the years. These have included strychnine, harmaline, and the analeptic phenylenetetrazol (Metrazol) (169). Amphetamines had long been touted as helpful in PD. In an early levodopa study, Umbach and Tzavellas (88) demonstrated prolonged improvement when levodopa was combined with 20 mg of propylhexedrine. Umbach (170), in a subsequent report, found that propylhexedrine or methyl amphetamine (methedrine) gave a "somewhat smaller" response than levodopa alone and again recommended use of levodopa and an amphetamine in combination. Dextroamphetamine, methamphetamine, and methylphenidate have all been recommended (27,169). In 1971, it was noted (169) that their antiparkinsonian effects have "been generally disappointing, but an occasional patient may derive some benefit." They seem to have been of more use in combating the somnolence in postencephalitic parkinsonism (169).

Alpha-methyldopa (Aldomet)(AMD) was used in combination with levodopa since it acted as a dopa decarboxylase inhibitor (171–174). Early results showed improvement in parkinsonism. Since AMD crosses the blood-brain barrier, it also acts as an inhibitor of brain dopa decarboxylase (27). AMD has been shown to induce (175) or exacerbate (176) parkinsonism, and it is no longer considered a viable adjunctive medication in PD.

Long before the levodopa era, Constable and Doshay (177) undertook a study to treat 98 patients with parkinsonism with Rauwolfia compounds. They used doses of reserpine up to 4.0 mg/day. Not surprisingly, the patients did not do very well. They reported that, "aside from an improvement in spirit, well-being, and mild tremor in a third of the cases, there was little impact on the more severe extraneous symptoms of Parkinsonism. In the face of marked agitation, excitement, insomnia, and advanced tremor, Rauwolfia was almost entirely without effect, even when doses of reserpine, as high as 2.0 or 4.0 mg per day, were employed."

Only during the last 20–30 years has our understanding of the pathophysiology, biochemistry, and pharmacology of PD allowed us to choose and design treatment options based on rational therapeutic strategies. Most recent findings in pathogenetic mechanisms (178) are directing new therapies toward neuroprotective strategies (179–182). These developments have dramatically changed our approaches to neurodegenerative diseases.

REFERENCES

1. Parkinson J. An Essay on the Shaking Palsy. London: Sharewood, Neely & Jones, 1817.
2. Charcot JM, Vulpian A. De la paralysie agitante. Gaz Hebdom Med Chirurg 1861; 8:765–767, 816–820; 1862; 9:24–59.
3. Ordenstein L. Sur la Paralysie Agitante et le Sclerose en Plaques Generalisees. Paris: Martinet, 1867.
4. Charcot JM. Leçons sur les Maladies du Systéme nerveux Faites a la Salpétrière. 4th ed. Paris: Delahaye et Le Crosnier, 1880:155–188.
5. Peterson F. Paralysis agitans. Starr MA, ed. Familiar Forms of Nervous Disease. New York: Columbia University Press, 1890.
6. Gowers WR. A Manual of Diseases of the Nervous System. 2nd ed. Philadelphia: Blakiston, 1893: 636–657.
7. Duvoisin RC, Yahr MD. Encephalitis and parkinsonism. Arch Neurol 1965; 12:227–239.
8. Dimsdale H. Changes in the Parkinson syndrome in the twentieth century. Q J Med 1946; 15: 155–170.
9. Rappleye WC, Emerson H, Park WH, et al. Epidemic Encephalitis, Etiology, Epidemiology, Treatment. Third Report by the Matheson Encephalitis Commission. New York: Columbia University Press, 1939:48–82.
10. von Witzleben HD. Methods of Treatment in Postencephalitic Parkinsonism. New York: Grune & Stratton, 1942:91–131.
11. Römer C. Die Behandlung der post-enzephalitischen Parkinsonismus mit hohen Atropindosen. Münch Med Wschrft 1933; 80:819.
12. Price JC, Merritt HH. The treatment of parkinsonism: results obtained with wine of Bulgarian belladonna and alkaloids of U.S P. belladonna. JAMA 1941; 117:335–337.
13. Fabing HD, Zeligs MA. Treatment of the post-encephalitic parkinsonism syndrome with desiccated white wine extract of U.S.P. belladonna root. JAMA 1941; 117:332–334.
14. Merritt HH. Textbook of Neurology. Philadelphia: Lea & Febiger, 1955:425–441.
15. Schwab RS, Leigh D. Parparnit in the treatment of Parkinson's disease. JAMA 1949; 139:629–634.
16. Denton JJ, Schedl HP, Neier WR, Lawson VA. Antispasmodics IV. Morpholinyl and piperidyl tertiary alcohols. J Am Chem Soc 1949; 71:2048–2055.
17. Cunningham RW, Harned BK, Clark MC, et al. Pharmacology of 3-(N-piperidyl)-1-phenyl-1-cyclohexyl-1-propanalol (Artane) and related compounds. J Pharm Exp Ther 1949; 95:151–165.
18. Doshay LJ, Constable K, Fromer S. Preliminary study of a new anti-parkinson agent. Neurology 1952; 2:233–243.
19. Doshay LJ, Constable K, Zier A. Five year follow-up of treatment with trihexyphenidyl (Artane). JAMA 1954; 154:1334–1336.
20. Budnitz J. The use of Benadryl in Parkinson's disease. New Eng J Med 1948; 238:874–875.
21. Ryan GMS, Wood JS. Benadryl in the treatment of parkinsonism. Results in 40 cases. Lancet 1949; 1:258.
22. Gillhespy RO, Ratcliffe AH. Treatment of parkinsonism with a new compound (B.S. 5930). Br Med J 1955; 2:352–355.
23. Doshay LJ, Constable K. Treatment of paralysis agitans with orphenadrine (Disipal): results in one hundred seventy six cases. JAMA 1957; 163:1352–1357.
24. Doshay LJ, Constable K. Treatment of paralysis agitans with chlorphenoxamine hydrochloride. JAMA 1959; 170:37–41.
25. Uldall PR, Walton JN, Newell DJ. Chlorphenoxamine hydrochloride in parkinsonism. Br Med J 1961; 1:1649–1652.

26. Doshay LJ, Constable K, Agate FJ. Ethopropazine (Parsidol) hydrochloride in treatment of paralysis agitans. JAMA 1956; 160:348–351.
27. Yahr MD, Duvoisin RC. Drug therapy of parkinsonism. N Engl J Med 1972; 287:20–24.
28. Delay J, Deniker P, Ropert R. Syndromes neurologiques provoques par les neurolepticques. Rev Neurol 1959; 100:771–773.
29. Merritt HH. Paralysis agitans [editorial]. J Chronic Dis 1956; 3:654–657.
30. Feldberg W. Present views on the mode of action of acetylcholine in the central nervous system. Physiol Rev 1945; 25:596–642.
31. Ahmed A, Marshall PB. Relationship between anti-acetylcholine and anti-tremor activity in antiparkinsonian and related drugs. Br J Pharmacol 1962; 18:247–254.
32. Faucon G, Lavarenne J, Collard M. Mis en évidence de l'activité antiparkinsonienne au moyen du tremblement ésérinique. Therapie 1965; 20:137–147.
33. Everett GM, Blockus LE, Sheppard IM. Tremor induced by tremorine and its antagonism by antiparkinson drugs. Science 1956; 124:79.
34. Cho AK, Haslett WL, Jenden DJ. The identification of an active metabolite of tremorine. Biochem Biophys 1961; 2:276–279.
35. Himwich HE. An analysis of the activating system including its use for screening antiparkinson drugs. Yale J Biol Med 1955; 28:308–319.
36. Duvoisin RC. Cholinergic-anticholinergic antagonism in parkinsonism. Arch Neurol 1967; 17: 124–136.
37. Porteous HB, Ross DN. Mental symptoms in parkinsonism following benzhexol hydrochloride therapy. Br Med J 1956; 2:138.
38. Duvoisin RC, Yahr MD. Behavioral abnormalities occurring in parkinsonism during treatment with levodopa. Malitz SL-Dopa and behavior. New York: Raven Press, 1972:57–72.
39. Schwab RS, England AC Jr, Poskanzer DC, Young RR. Amantadine in the treatment of Parkinson's disease. JAMA 1969; 208:1168–1170.
40. Dallos V, Heathfield K, Stone P, Allen FAD. Use of amantadine in Parkinson's disease: results of a double blind trial. Br Med J 1970; 4:24–26.
41. Parkes JD, Zilkha DK, Calver DM, et al. Controlled trial of amantadine hydrochloride in Parkinson's disease. Lancet 1970; 1:259–262.
42. Fahn S, Isgreen WP. Long term evaluation of amantadine and levodopa combination in parkinsonism by double-blind crossover analysis. Neurology 1975; 25:695–700.
43. Shaly N, Weeth JB, Mercier D. Livedo reticularis in patients with parkinsonism receiving amantadine. JAMA 1970; 212:1522–1523.
44. Vernier VG, Harmon JB, Stump JM, Lynes TE, Marvel JP, Smith DH. The toxicologic and pharmacologic properties of amantadine hydrochloride. Toxicol Appl Pharmacol 1969; 15:642–645.
45. Grelak RP, Clark R, Stump JM, Vernier VF. Amantadine-dopamine interaction: possible mode of action in parkinsonism. Science 1970; 169:203–204.
46. von Voigtlander PF, Moore KE. Dopamine release from the brain in vivo by amantadine. Science 1971; 174:408–410.
47. Coyle JT, Snyder SH. Antiparkinson drugs: Inhibition of dopamine uptake in the corpus striatum as a possible mechanism of action. Science 1969; 166:899–901.
48. Delwaide PJ, Martinelli P, Schoenen J. Mazindol in the treatment of Parkinson's disease. Arch Neurol 1983; 40:788–790.
49. Albuquerque EX, Eldefrawi AT, Eldefrawi ME, Mansour NA, Tsai, M-C. Amantadine: neuromuscular blockade by suppression of ionic conductance of the acetylcholine receptor. Science 1978; 199:788–790.
50. Lupp A, Lucking CH, Koch R, Jackisch R, Feuerstein TJ. Inhibitory effects of the antiparkinsonian drugs memantine and amantadine on N-methyl-D-aspartate-evoked acetylcholine release in the rabbit caudate nucleus in vitro. J Pharmacol Exp Ther 1992; 263: 717–724.
51. Stoof JC, Booij J, Drukarch B, Wolters EC. The anti-parkinson drug amantadine inhibits the N-methyl-D-aspartic acid-evoked release of acetylcholine in a non-competitive way. Eur J Pharmacol 1992; 213:439–443.
52. Casey DE. Amantadine intoxication reversed by physostigmine [lett]. N Engl J Med 1978; 298:516.
53. Blanchet PJ, Metman LV, Chase TN. Renaissance of amantadine in the treatment of Parkinson's disease. Adv Neurol 2001; 91:251–257.53.
54. Anonymous. L-dopa: Which way to a winner? Chem Week 1970; Oct 1.
55. Miller ER. Dihydroxyphenylalanine, a constituent of the velvet bean. J Biol Chem 1920; 44: 481–486.

56. Damodaran M, Ramaswamy R. Isolation of L-dopa from the seeds of *Macuna pruriens*. Biochemistry 1937; 31:2149–2151.
57. Manyam BV. Paralysis agitans and levodopa in "ayurveda": ancient Indian medical treatise. Mov Disord 1990; 5:47–48.
58. Andrews RS, Pridham JB. Melanins from dopa-containing plants. Phytochemistry 1967; 6:13–18.
59. Guggenheim M. Dioxyphenylalanin, eine neue Aminosäure aus Vicia faba. Z Physiol Chem 1913; 88:276–284.
60. Raab W, Gigee W. Concentration and distribution of "encephalin" in the brain of humans and animals. Proc Soc Exp Biol Med 1951; 76:97–100.
61. Hornykiewicz O. Historical aspects and frontiers of Parkinson's disease research. Adv Exp Med Biol 1976; 90:1–9.
62. Fahn S. History of parkinsonism. Mov Disord 1989; 4(suppl 1):S2–S10.
63. Hornykiewicz O. From dopamine to Parkinson's disease: a personal research record. Samson F, Adelman G, eds. The Neurosciences: Paths of Discovery, II. Boston: Birkhäuser, 1992:125–146.
64. Montagu KA. Catechol compounds in rat tissues and in brains of different animals. Nature 1957; 180:244–245.
65. Weil-Malherbe H, Bone AD. Intracellular distribution of catecholamines in the brain. Nature 1957; 180:1050–1051.
66. Carlsson A, Lindqvist M, Magnusson T, Waldeck B. On the presence of 3-hydroxytyramine in brain. Science 1958; 127:471.
67. Carlsson A, Lindqvist M, Magnussson T. 3,4-Dihydroxyphenylalanine and 5-hydroxytryptophan as reserpine antagonists. Nature 1957; 180:1200.
68. Degkwitz R, Frowen R, Kulenkampff C, Mohs U. Über die Wirkungen des L-DOPA beim Menschen und deren Beeinflussung durch Reserpin, Chlorpromazin, Ipronizzid und vitamin B$_6$. Klin Wochenschr 1960; 38:120–123.
69. Bertler A, Rosengren E. Occurrence and distribution of dopamine in brain and other tissues. Experientia 1959; 15:10–11.
70. Sano I, Gamo T, Kakimoto Y, Taniguchi K, Takesada M, Nishinuma K. Distribution of catechol compounds in human brain. Biochem Biophys Acta 1959; 32:586–587.
71. Ehringer H, Hornykiewicz O. Veteilung von Noradrenalin und Dopamin (3-Hydroxytyramin) im Gehirn des Menschen und ihr Verhalten bei Erkrankungen des extrapyramidalen Systems. Klin Wochenschr 1960; 38:1236–1239.
72. Duvoisin RC. History of parkinsonism. Pharmacol Ther 1987; 32:1–17.
73. Andén NE, Carlsson A, Dahlstrom A, et al. Demonstration and mapping out of nigro-neostriatal dopamine neurons. Life Sci 1964; 3:523–530.
74. Andén NE, Dahlstrom A, Fuxe K, Larsson K. Further evidence for the presence of nigro-striatal dopamine neurons in the rat. Am J Anat 1965; 116:329–333.
75. Poirier LJ, Sourkes TL. Influence of the substantia nigra on the catecholamine content of the striatum. Brain 1965; 88:181–192.
76. Goldstein M, Anagnoste B, Owen S, Battista AF. The effects of ventromedial biosynthesis of catecholamines in the striatum. Life Sci 1966; 5:2171–2176.
77. Hornykiewicz O. Parkinson's disease: from brain homogenates to treatment. Fed Proc Fed Am Soc Exp Biol 1973; 32:183–190.
78. Carlsson A. The occurence, distribution, and physiological role of catecholamines in the nervous system. Pharmacol Rev 1959; 11:490–493.
79. Birkmayer W, Hornykiewicz O. Der L-3,4-Dioxyphenylalanin (= DOPA)—Effekt bei der Parkinson-Akinese. Wien Klin Wochenschr 1961; 73:787–788.
80. McGeer PL, Boulding JE, Gibson WC, Foulkes RG. Drug-induced extrapyramidal reactions. Treatment with diphenhydramine hydrochloride and dihydroxyphenylalanine. JAMA 1961; 177:665–670.
81. Duvoisin RC, Yahr MD, Coté LJ. Pyridoxine reversal of L-dopa effect in parkinsonism. Trans Am Neurol Assoc 1969; 94:81–84.
82. Barbeau A, Sourkes TL, Murphy GF. Les catécholamines dans la maladie de Parkinson. De Ajuriaguerra J, ed. Monoamines et Système Nerveux Central. Paris: Masson, 1962: 925–927.
83. Friedhoff AJ, Hekimian L, Alpert M. Dihydroxyphenylalanine in extrapyramidal disease. JAMA 1963; 184:285–286.
84. Greer M, Williams CM. Dopamine metabolism in Parkinson's disease. Neurology 1963; 13:73–76.
85. Gerstenbrand F, Patiesky K, Prosenz P. Erfahrungen mit L-dopa in der therapie die parkinsonismus. Psychiatr Neurol 1963; 146:246–261.

86. Hirschmann J, Mayer K. Neue Wege zur Beeinflussung extrapyramidalmotorischer Störungen. Arzneimittel forschung 1964; 4:599–601.

87. Umbach W, Baumann D. Die wirkamkeit von L-dopa bei Parkinsonpatienten mit und ohne stereotaktischen Hirneingriff. Arch Psychiatr Nervenkr 1964; 205:281–292.

88. Umbach W, Tzavellas O. Zur Behandlung akinetischer Begleitsymptome beim Parkinson-syndrom. Deutsche Med Wschr 1965; 90:1941–1944.

89. Bruno A, Bruno SC. Effetti della L-3,34-diidrossifenilalanina (L-dopa) nei pazienti parkinsoniani. Riv Sper Fren 1966; 90:39–50.

90. Pazzagli A, Amaducci L. La sperimentazione clinica del dopa nelle sindromi parkinsoniane. Riv Neurobiol 1966; 12:138–145.

91. Rinaldi F, Margherita G, De Divitiis E. Effetti della somministrazione di DOPA a pazienti parkinsoniani pretrattati con inibitore delle monoaminossidasi. Ann Freniatr Sci Affini 1965; 78:105–113.

92. McGeer PL, Zeldowicz LR. Administration of dihydroxyphenylalanine to parkinsonian patients. Can Med Assoc J 1964; 90:463–466.

93. Birkmayer W, Hornykiewicz O. Weitere experimentelle untersuchungen über beim Parkinson-syndrom und reserpin-parkinsonismus. Arch Psychiatr Zeitschr Neurol 1964; 206:367–381.

94. Fehling C. Treatment of Parkinson's syndrome with L-dopa, a double-blind study. Acta Neurol Scand 1966; 43:367–372.

95. Rinne UK, Sonninen V. A double-blind study of L-dopa treatment in Parkinson's disease. Eur Neurol 1968; 1:180–191.

96. Duvoisin RC. A review of drug therapy in parkinsonism. Bull NY Acad Med 1965; 41:898–910.

97. Bertler A, Rosengren E. Possible role of brain dopamine. Pharmacol Rev 1966; 18:769–773.

98. Cotzias GC, Van Woert MH, Schiffer LM. Aromatic amino acids and modification of parkinsonism. N Engl J Med 1967; 276:374–379.

99. Cotzias GC, Papavasiliou PS, Gellene R. Modification of Parkinson's disease—chronic treatment with L-dopa. N Engl J Med 1969; 280:337–345.

100. Cotzias GC, Papavasiliou PS, Gellene R. L-Dopa in Parkinson's disease [lett]. N Engl J Med 1969; 281:272.

101. Yahr MD, Duvoisin RC, Schear MJ, Barrett RE, Hoehn MM. Treatment of parkinsonism with levodopa. Arch Neurol 1969; 21:343–354.

102. Godwin-Austen RB, Tomlinson EB, Frears CC, Kok HWL. Effects of L-dopa in Parkinson's disease. Lancet 1969; 2:165–168.

103. Calne DB, Spiers ASD, Stern GM, Laurence DR, Armitage P. L-Dopa in idiopathic parkinsonism. Lancet 1969; 2:973–976.

104. McDowell FH, Lee JE, Sweet R, Swift T, Ogsbury S, Kessler J. The treatment of Parkinson's disease with dihydroxyphenylalanine. Ann Intern Med 1970; 72:19–25.

105. Paulson GW, Wiederholt WC, Allen JN, Shuttleworth EC, Friedman HM. The use of L-dopa in parkinsonism. Ohio State Med J 1969; 65:995–999.

106. Barbeau A. L-Dopa therapy in Parkinson's disease: a critical review of nine years' experience. Can Med Assoc J 1969; 101:59–68.

107. Barbeau A, McDowell FH, eds. L-Dopa and Parkinsonism. Philadelphia: FA Davis, 1970.

108. Fahn S, Parkinson's Study Group. Results of the ELLDOPA (Earlier vs. Later Levodopa) study. Mov Disord 2002; 17(suppl 5):S13–S14.

109. Birkmayer W. Clinical effects of L-dopa plus Ro 4–4602. Barbeau A, McDowell FH, eds. L-Dopa and Parkinsonism. Philadelphia: FA Davis, 1970:53–54.

110. Tissot R, Gaillard J-M, Guggisberg M, Gauthier G, de Ajuriaguerra J. Thérapeutique du syndrome de Parkinson par la L-dopa "per os" associée a un inhibiteur de la décarboxylase (Ro IV 46.02). Presse Méd 1969; 77:619–622.

111. Siegfried J. Deux ans d'expérience avec la L-DOPA associée à un inhibiteur de la décarboxylase. Rev Neurol 1970; 122:243–248.

112. Yahr MD, Duvoisin RC, Mendoza MR, Schear MJ, Barrett RE. Modification of L-dopa therapy of parkinsonism by alpha-methyldopa hydrazine (MK-486). Trans Am Neurol Assoc 1971; 96:55–58.

113. Calne DB, Reid JL, Vakil SD, et al. Idiopathic parkinsonism treated with an extracerebral decarboxylase inhibitor in combination with levodopa. Br Med J 1971; 3:729–732.

114. Klawans HL, Ringel SP, Shenker DM. Failure of vitamin B_6 to reverse the L-dopa effect in patients on a dopa decarboxylase inhibitor. J Neurol Neurosurg Psychiatry 1971; 34:682–686.

115. Dupont E, Hansen E, Melsen S, Pakkenberg H, Holm P. Treatment of parkinsonism with a combination of levodopa and the decarboxylase inhibitor Ro 4–4602 (a comparison with levodopa treatment alone). Acta Neurol Scand Suppl 1972; 51:115–117.

116. Holmsen R, Kvan L, Presthus J, Thoresen GB. Treatment of parkinsonism with a compound of L-dopa (Larodopa(R)) and a decarboxylase inhibitor (Ro 4–4602). Acta Neurol Scand Suppl 1972; 51:121–122.

117. Miller EM, Wiener L. Ro 4–4602 and levodopa in the treatment of parkinsonism. Neurology 1974; 24:482–486.

118. Rinne UK, Birket-Smith E, Dupont E, et al. Levodopa alone and in combination with a peripheral decarboxylase inhibitor benserazide (Madopar®) in the treatment of Parkinson's disease. J Neurol 1975; 211:1–9.

119. Marsden CD, Barry PE, Parkes JD, Zilkha KJ. Treatment of Parkinson's disease with levodopa combined with L-alpha-methyldopahydrazine, an inhibitor of extracerebral DOPA decarboxylase. J Neurol Neurosurg Psychiatry 1973; 36:10–14.

120. Schwartz AM, Olanow CW, Spencer A. A double-blind controlled study of MK-486 in Parkinson's disease. Trans Am Neurol Assoc 1973; 98:301–303.

121. Markham CH, Diamond SG, Treciokas LJ. Carbidopa in Parkinson's disease and in nausea and vomiting of levodopa. Arch Neurol 1974; 31:128–133.

122. Lieberman A, Goodgold A, Jonas S, Leibowitz M. Comparison of dopa decarboxylase inhibitor (carbidopa) combined with levodopa and levodopa alone in Parkinson's disease. Neurology 1975; 25:911–916.

123. Korten JJ, Keyser A, Joosten EMG, Gabreëls FJM. Madopar versus Sinemet. A clinical study on their effectiveness. Eur Neurol 1975; 13:65–71.

124. Schwab RS, Amador LV, Lettvin JY. Apomorphine in Parkinson's disease. Trans Am Neurol Assoc 1951; 76:251–253.

125. Cotzias GC, Papavasiliou PS, Fehling C, Kaufman B, Mena I. Similarities between neurologic effects of L-dopa and of apomorphine. N Engl J Med 1970; 282:31–33.

126. Braham J, Sarova-Pinhas I, Goldhammer Y. Apomorphine in parkinsonian tremor. Br Med J 1970; 3:768.

127. Cotzias GC, Papavasiliou PS, Tolosa E, Bell-Midura MA, Ginos JZ. Aporphines in Parkinson's disease. Trans Am Neurol Assoc 1975; 100:178–181.

128. Cotzias GC, Papavasiliou PS, Tolosa ES, Mendez JS, Bell-Midura M. Treatment of Parkinson's disease with aporphines. N Engl J Med 1976:567–572.

129. Papavasiliou PS, Cotzias GC, Rosal VLF, Miller ST. Treatment of parkinsonism with N-n-propyl norapomorphine and levodopa (with or without carbidopa). Arch Neurol 1978; 35:787–791.

130. Corsini GU, Del Zompo M, Gessa GL, Mangoni A. Therapeutic efficacy of apomorphine combined with an extracerebral inhibitor of dopamine receptors in Parkinson's disease. Lancet 1979; 1: 954–956.

131. Manson AJ, Hanagasi H, Turner K, et al. Intravenous apomorphine therapy in Parkinson's disease: clinical and pharmacokinetic observations. Brain 2001; 124:331–340.

132. Pietz K, Hagell P, Odin P. Subcutaneous apomorphine in late stage Parkinson's disease: a long term follow up. J Neurol Neurosurg Psychiatry 1998; 65:709–716.

133. Dewey RB Jr, Maraganore DM, Ahlskog JE, Matsumoto JY. A double-blind, placebo-controlled study of intranasal apomorphine spray as a rescue agent for off-states in Parkinson's disease. Mov Disord 1998; 13:782–787.

134. Ondo W, Hunter C, Almaguer M, Gancher S, Jankovic J. Efficacy and tolerability of a novel sublingual apomorphine preparation in patients with fluctuating Parkinson's disease. Clin Neuropharmacol 1999; 22:1–4.

135. Corrodi H, Fuxe K, Ungerstedt U. Evidence for a new type of dopamine receptor stimulating agent. J Pharm Pharmacol 1971; 23:989–991.

136. Vakil SD, Calne DB, Reid JL, Seymour CA. Pyrimidyl-piperonyl-piperazine (ET 495) in parkinsonism. Adv Neurol 1973; 3:121–125.

137. Chase TN, Woods AC, Glaubiger GA. Parkinson disease treated with a suspected dopamine receptor agonist. Arch Neurol 1974; 30:383–386.

138. Sweet RD, Wasterlain C, McDowell FH. Piribedil—an oral dopamine agonist for treatment of Parkinson's disease. Trans Am Neurol Assoc 1974; 100:258–260.

139. Fiegenson JS, Sweet RD, McDowell FH. Piribedil: its synergistic effect in multidrug regimens for parkinsonism. Neurology 1976; 26:430–433.

140. Lieberman AN, Shopsin B, Le Brun Y, Boal D, Zolfaghari M. Studies on piribedil in parkinsonism. Adv Neurol 1975; 9:399–407.

141. Corrodi H, Fuxe K, Hökfelt T, Lidbrink P, Ungerstedt U. Effect of ergot drugs on central catecholamine neurons: evidence for a stimulation of central dopamine neurons. J Pharm Pharmacol 1973; 25:409–412.

142. Calne DB, Teychenne PF, Claveria LE, Eastman R, Greenacre JK, Petrie A. Bromocriptine in parkinsonism. Br Med J 1974; 4:442–444.
143. Calne DB, Teychenne PF, Leigh PN, Bamji AN, Greenacre JK. Treatment of parkinsonism with bromocriptine. Lancet 1974; 2:1355–1356.
144. Galea Debono A, Donaldson I, Marsden CD, Parkes JD. Bromocriptine in parkinsonism. Lancet 1975; 2:987–988.
145. Lees AJ, Shaw KM, Stern GM. Bromocriptine in parkinsonism. Lancet 1975; 2:709–710.
146. Calne DB, Plotkin C, Williams AC, Nutt JG, Neophytides A, Teychenne PF. Long-term treatment of parkinsonism with bromocriptine. Lancet 1978; 1:735–738.
147. Lieberman AN, Kupersmith M, Gopinathan G, Estey E, Goodgold A, Goldstein M. Bromocriptine in Parkinson disease: Further studies. Neurology 1979; 29:363–369.
148. Shaw KM, Lees AJ, Stern GM. Bromocriptine in parkinsonism. Lancet 1978; 1:1255.
149. Lieberman A, Miyamoto T, Battista AF, Goldstein M. Studies on the antiparkinsonian efficacy of lergotrile. Neurology 1975; 25:459–462.
150. Klawans HL, Weiner WJ, Nausieda PA, Volkman P, Goetz C, Lupton MD. The effect of lergotrile in Parkinson disease [abstr]. Neurology 1977; 27:390.
151. Lieberman A, Estey E, Kupersmith M, Gopinathan G, Goldstein M. Treatment of Parkinson's disease with lergotrile mesylate. JAMA 1977; 238:2380–2382.
152. Lieberman AN, Gopinathan G, Estey E, Kupersmith M, Goodgold A, Goldstein M. Lergotrile in Parkinson disease: Further studies. Neurology 1979; 29:267–272.
153. Schachter M, Blackstock J, Dick JPR, George RJD, Marsden CD, Parkes JD. Lisuride in Parkinson's disease. Lancet 1979; 2:1129.
154. Lieberman AN, Leibowitz M, Neophytides A, et al. Pergolide and lisuride for Parkinson's disease. Lancet 1979; 2:1129–1130.
155. Hobson DE, Pourcher E, Martin WR. Ropinirole and pramipexole, the new agonists. Can J Neurol Sci 1999; 26(Suppl 2):S27–33.
156. Metman LV, Gillespie M, Farmer C, et al. Continuous transdermal dopaminergic stimulation in advanced Parkinson's disease. Clin Neuropharmacol 2001; 24:163–169.
157. Birkmayer W, Hornykiewicz O. Der L-Dioxyphenylalanin (=L-DOPA)—Effekt beim Parkinson-Syndrom des Menschen: zur Pathogenese und Behandlung der Parkinson-Akinese. Arch Psychiatr Nervenkr 1962; 203:560–574.
158. Hunter KR, Boakes AJ, Laurence DR, Stern GM. Monoamine oxidase inhibitors and L-dopa. Br Med J 1970; 3:388.
159. Teychenne PF, Calne DB, Lewis PJ, Findley LJ. Interactions of levodopa with inhibitors of monoamine oxidase and L-aromatic amino acid decarboxylase. Clin Pharmacol Ther 1975; 18:273–277.
160. Johnston JP. Some observations upon a new inhibitor of monoamine oxidase in brain tissue. Biochem Pharmacol 1968; 17:1285–1297.
161. Glover V, Sandler M, Owen F, Riley GJ. Dopamine is a monoamine oxidase-B substrate in man. Nature 1977; 265:80–81.
162. Riederer P, Jellinger K, Danielczyk W, et al. Combination treatment with selective monoamine oxidase inhibitors and dopaminergic agonists in Parkinson's disease: biochemical and clinical observations. Adv Neurol 1983; 37:159–176.
163. Birkmayer W, Riederer P, Youdim MBH, Linauer W. The potentiation of the anti akinetic effect after L-dopa treatment by an inhibitor of MAO-B, deprenil. J Neural Trans 1975; 36:303–326.
164. Birkmayer W, Riederer P, Ambrozi L, Youdim MBH. Implications of combined treatment with "Madopar" and L-deprenil in Parkinson's disease. Lancet 1977; 1:439–443.
165. Lees AJ, Shaw KM, Kohout LJ, et al. Deprenyl in Parkinson's disease. Lancet 1977; 2:791–795.
166. Shoulson I, Oakes D, Fahn S, et al. Impact of sustained deprenyl (selegiline) in levodopa-treated Parkinson's disease: a randomized placebo-controlled extension of the deprenyl and tocopherol antioxidative therapy of parkinsonism trial. Ann Neurol 2002; 51:604–612.
167. Factor SA, Molho ES, Feustel PJ, Brown DL, Evans SM. Long-term comparative experience with tolcapone and entacapone in advanced Parkinson's disease. Clin Neuropharmacol 2001; 24:295–299.
168. Ericsson AD. Potentiation of the L-dopa effect in man by the use of catechol-O-methyltransferase inhibitors. J Neurol Sci 1971; 14:193–197.
169. Duvoisin RC, Yahr MD. Drugs used in the treatment of parkinsonism. In: DiPalma JR ed. Drill's Pharmacology in Medicine. 4th ed. New York: McGraw-Hill Inc, 1971:318–323.
170. Umbach W. Different effects of drugs before and after stereotaxic operation. Confin Neurol 1966; 27:258–261.

171. Sweet RD, Lee JE, McDowell F. Alpha-methyldopa as an adjunct to levodopa treatment of Parkinson's disease. Trans Am Neurol Assoc 1971; 96:59–65.
172. Fermaglich J, O'Doherty DS. Synergism of levodopa by alpha methyldopa. Trans Am Neurol Assoc 1971; 96:231–234.
173. Fermaglich J, Chase TN. Methyldopa or methyldopahydrazine as levodopa synergists. Lancet 1973; 1:1261–1262.
174. Mones RJ. Evaluation of alpha methyl dopa and alpha methyl dopa hydrazine with L-dopa therapy. NY State J Med 1974; 74:47–51.
175. Strang RR. Parkinsonism occurring during methyldopa therapy. Can Med Assoc J 1966; 95: 928–929.
176. Rosenblum AM, Montgomery EB. Exacerbation of parkinsonism by methyldopa [lett]. JAMA 1980; 244:2727–2728.
177. Constable K, Doshay LJ. Rauwolfia compounds in the treatment of parkinsonism. J Am Med Wom Assoc 1956; 11:165–168.
178. Mouradian MM. Recent advances in the genetics and pathogenesis of Parkinson disease. Neurology 2002; 58:179–185.
179. Shults C. Effects of coenzyme Q10 in early Parkinson's disease, evidence for slowing of the functional decline (the QE2 study). Mov Disord 2002; 17(suppl 5):S14.
180. Guo X, Dawson VL, Dawson TM. Neuroimmunophilin ligands exert neuroregeneration and neuroprotection in midbrain dopaminergic neurons. Eur J Neurosci 2001; 13:1683–1693.
181. Saporito MS, Hudkins RL, Maroney AC. Discovery of CEP-1347/KT-7515, an inhibitor of the JNK/SAPK pathway for the treatment of neurodegenerative diseases. Prog Med Chem 2002; 40:23–62.
182. Hashimoto M, Hsu LJ, Rockenstein E, Takenouchi T, Mallory M, Masliah E. alpha-Synuclein protects against oxidative stress via inactivation of the c-Jun N-terminal kinase stress-signaling pathway in neuronal cells. J Biol Chem 2002; 277:11465–11472.

2

History of Surgery for Parkinson's Disease

Helen Bronte-Stewart

Stanford University Medical Center, Stanford, California, U.S.A.

I. INTRODUCTION

Neurosurgical treatment of parkinsonism has been attempted for over a century. The first era (1890–1940) was stimulated by the lack of useful medical therapy but suffered from high rates of morbidity and mortality. The second era (1940–1970) was enhanced by the development of stereotactical neurosurgical techniques, which enabled the neurosurgeon to reach basal ganglia targets without the morbidity of a direct approach. This era was eclipsed by the advent of levodopa and dopamine agonist medical therapy. The third era (1990–1999) was a return to neurosurgical treatment due to the emergence of a model of basal ganglia circuitry, which gave scientific rationale to basal ganglia ablation, and by the adverse effects of long-term medical therapy. The current era of deep brain stimulation (DBS) emerged from advances in technology and allowed for bilateral intervention, which increased morbidity with ablative treatment. Advances in neurobiology are paving the way to a future era when surgical therapy will be based on restorative or cellular replacement strategies rather than on the modulation of basal ganglia circuitry. This chapter will chronicle the history, current status, and future of surgery for Parkinson's disease (PD).

II. THE PAST

A. Surgery for Hyperkinesis (1890–1970)

From Horsley's first report in 1890 to the 1940s, surgery for movement disorders consisted of attempts to lesion the pyramidal system (1–4). These ranged from excision of the pyramidal tract in the upper cervical cord to extirpation of cortical areas 4 and 6. The procedures resulted in resolution of tremor with side effects of contralateral hemiparesis, hypalgesia, hypothermia, and seizures. Mortality rates were so high that in 1951 Mackay expressed his opinion of surgery for parkinsonism and hyperkinesis (5): "the surgical relief of extrapyramidal hyperkinesis seems to boil down to the artificial production of

21

paralysis. The risk of post-operative seizures constitutes another disadvantage. On the whole surgery has little application to this vast field." This served as the epitaph for surgery on the pyramidal tract as a treatment for hyperkinesis.

Surgical treatment for PD continued during the 1940s. The shift from pyramidal targets to targets in the basal ganglia was initiated by Meyers and Guiot (6,7). Advances in neurosurgical techniques led to improved outcomes. In 1952 Spiegel et al. (8) published the first technique paper for performing stereotactic neurosurgical procedures in humans. Other important developments in the 1950s included the introduction of intraoperative temporary lesions to determine the optimal site for the final permanent lesion. These included intrapallidal injections of procaine (9) and high-frequency electro-stimulation, which led to the current technology of DBS (7,10).

The most effective targets were found to be the internal segment of the globus pallidus (GPi), its efferent pathways, namely the ansa lenticularis, and the ventrolateral region of the thalamus (6,8,11,12). Ventrolateral thalamotomy for the treatment of tremor and rigidity became the most commonly chosen target for PD, with reports of successful outcomes in 70–90% of patients (13–19). A comparison of thalamic with pallidal lesions in 408 cases (20) demonstrated that thalamotomy was superior to pallidotomy for alleviating tremor but that pallidotomy was superior for alleviating rigidity.

The exact sites within the thalamus and pallidum varied, and this may have accounted for the variability in outcome. In 1960, Svennilson (21) summarized a study of pallidotomy in 81 patients with PD. In the first 30 patients Leksell varied the lesion site in the GPi. In the next 30 patients he varied the lesion size, and in the final 21 patients he confined the lesion to the posterolateral segment of the GPi, which yielded the best results. The importance of lesion location was confirmed from autopsy studies, showing that lesions confined to the GPi or to the basal part of the ventrolateral thalamus were associated with abolition of tremor (13).

Surgical complications reported in the 1960s and 1970s revealed significant improvements compared to the 1950s. Mortality rates fell to less than 2%, and all complication rates fell as the number of procedures performed increased (14,15,20,22). However, unilateral thalamotomies were shown to cause serious and often permanent complications, such as dysarthria, dysphagia, and disequilibrium, in 9–23% of patients with PD or essential tremor (ET) and in 16–41% of patients with multiple sclerosis (MS). Bilateral thalamotomies carried an even higher risk, which virtually eliminated their use in the treatment of PD or bilateral tremor by the late 1970s (23,24).

These early studies created the foundation for subsequent surgical protocols. For instance, patient selection criteria were developed. Criteria used today to optimize outcome from surgical procedures developed from experiences during the previous surgical era; namely, the importance of patient selection, lesion location, macrostimulation, and the reduction of morbidity and mortality associated with the procedure in proportion to the experience of the neurosurgeon.

Surgical therapy lost its dominance in the 1960s, 1970s, and 1980s largely due to the discovery of levodopa and dopamine agonists. In addition, criticisms of the surgical literature also led to a decrease in the use of neurosurgical approaches. Studies were open label and retrospective, and the outcomes were largely descriptive and subjective. A notable exception was Svennilson's study (21), which became the foundation for the reemergence of pallidotomy to treat PD. Clinical rating scales had not been developed, which made it hard to compare outcomes across studies.

III. THE REEMERGENCE OF ABLATIVE PROCEDURES

A. Parkinson's Disease and Tremor

By the 1990s it was apparent that dopaminergic medication, in combination with advancing disease, resulted in motor complications that became as disabling as the cardinal signs of PD. By this time there had been significant advances in neuroimaging techniques such as computed tomography (CT) and magnetic resonance imaging (MRI), which allowed visual identification of the nuclei of the basal ganglia. This, along with advances in stereotactic technique, allowed more precise anatomical targeting.

The development of animal models of PD, using striatal 6-hydroxydopamine (6-OHDA) and 1-methyl-4-phenyl-1,2,3,6-tetrahydropyridine (MPTP) lesions, had accelerated basic research in PD. A model of basal ganglia circuitry, with anatomical, neurotransmitter, and functional properties, had emerged, which provided a stronger scientific rationale for surgical interventions in the basal ganglia for PD. Physiological recordings in primates revealed that the anatomical site for sensorimotor processing of the primate internal pallidum was in its posteroventral aspect (25,26). This explained the success Leksell had found empirically by placing lesions in the posteroventral GPi (21). In addition, the anterodorsal aspects of GPi were found to be involved with associative and cognitive function (27), explaining the less successful results of the past, where lesions were placed in more anterior regions. Thus, it appeared that improvement in motor abnormalities in PD were linked with lesions confined to the sensorimotor regions of the target nucleus.

B. Basal Ganglia Pathophysiology in Parkinson's Disease

An anatomical and physiological framework had now developed for the surgical treatment of PD. The hypothesis was to interrupt the abnormal signals emerging from GPi. This was such a major advance in the understanding of PD that a brief description of the circuit model of basal ganglia dysfunction in PD is important to include in the historical development of surgical treatment.

The basal ganglia comprise several functionally distinct circuits that are components of a network connecting cortical and subcortical structures important in the control of movement and posture (Fig. 1). The main output nuclei of the basal ganglia are the GPi and the substantia nigra pars reticularis (SNr), which send gamma-aminobutyric acid (GABA)–mediated inhibitory efferents to pallidal receiving areas of the motor thalamus. Within the basal ganglia, information flows from the input (striatum) to output (GPi and SNr) nuclei through anatomically and neurochemically distinct projections, termed the "direct" and "indirect" pathways. The direct pathway, from the striatum to GPi, is mediated by GABA/substance P. The indirect pathway runs from the striatum to GPi, via the external pallidum (GPe) and the subthalamic nucleus (STN), and is mediated by GABA/enkephalin.

The STN is an important nucleus in the functional organization of the basal ganglia (26,28). The STN receives excitatory inputs from motor and premotor cortex and exerts a powerful excitatory effect on its target nuclei, GPi , GPe, SNr, SNc (pars compacta), and the pedunculopontine nucleus (PPN) (28–32). The dopaminergic pathway from the SNc innervates medium spiny neurons within the matrisomes of the striatum (33) and appears to modulate the activity of the two striato-pallidal pathways differentially by activation of different dopamine receptors. Thus, dopamine appears to facilitate transmission

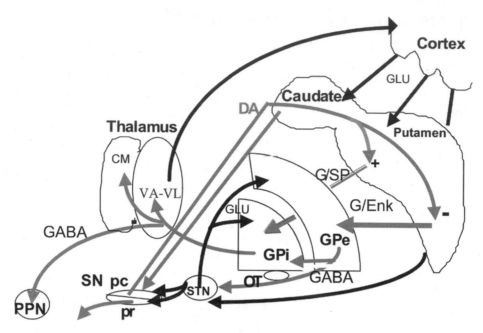

Figure 1 Schematic diagram of the main neuroanatomical pathways of the basal ganglia. The cortical output is excitatory to striatum and STN; the striatal, GPe, and GPi output is inhibitory; the STN and thalamic output is excitatory. The nigrostriatal pathway (from SNpc) is dopaminergic. CM, central median; DA, dopamine; G/Enk, GABA/enkephalin; G/SP, GABA/substance P; GABA, gamma-aminobutyric acid; GPe, globus pallidus externa; GPi, globus pallidus interna; Glu, glutamate; OT, optic tract; PPN, pedunculopontine nucleus; SN_{pr}, substantia nigra pars reticulata; SN_{pc}, substantia nigra pars compacta; STN, subthalamic nucleus; VA-VL, ventral anterior/ventral lateral.

over the "direct" pathway (via D1 receptors) and to inhibit transmission over the "indirect" pathway (via D2 receptors).

Loss of dopaminergic neurons in the SNc results in the appearance of the classical signs of PD (Fig. 2). Dopamine depletion in the striatum is proposed to lead to a reduction in the activity of the direct pathway and an increase in the activity of the indirect pathway (dashed and thicker lines in Fig. 2, respectively). The net result would be an excessive increase in neuronal activity in GPi and STN, which in turn would lead to over inhibition of thalamocortical and brainstem projections. Experimental studies have supported the model. Mean discharge rates are increased and firing patterns are more irregular in both STN and GPi in MPTP treated primates (26,32,34–37) and in patients with PD (38,39). Experimental results in MPTP monkeys have shown that increased firing rates in both GPi and STN occur prior to the onset of symptoms (40).

Inactivation of these structures, either reversibly (DBS) or irreversibly [radiofrequency (RF) lesions, ibotenic acid], leads to amelioration of tremor, rigidity, and bradykinesia. This has been demonstrated in both the primate model of PD (34,41–43) and patients with idiopathic PD (44–46).

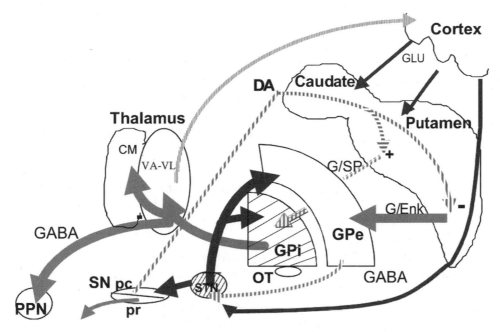

Figure 2 Changes in the basal ganglia pathways in Parkinson's disease. The dashed lines represent downregulated pathways, and the thicker lines represent upregulated pathways. The resulting increased neuronal activity in STN and GPi is represented by shading of each nucleus. CM, central median; DA, dopamine; G/Enk, GABA/enkephalin; G/SP, GABA/substance P; GABA, gamma-aminobutyric acid; GPe, globus pallidus externa; GPi, globus pallidus interna; Glu, glutamate; OT, optic tract; PPN, pedunculopontine nucleus; SN_{pr}, substantia nigra pars reticulata; SN_{pc}, substantia nigra pars compacta; STN, subthalamic nucleus; VA-VL, ventral anterior/ventral lateral.

C. Unilateral Posteroventral Pallidotomy for the Treatment of Parkinson's Disease

In 1992 Laitinen reported a 92% improvement in rigidity and hypokinesia and an 81% improvement in tremor in 38 patients after unilateral posteroventral pallidotomy (PVP) (48). Unilateral PVP was shown to be effective for control of all the cardinal symptoms of PD (46,49–59). The magnitude of benefit for motor improvement in the medication "off" state ranged from 17 to 40% using the Unified Parkinson's Disease Rating Scale (UPDRS) Motor subscore (59). The benefit was mainly on the contralateral side. Out of 24 studies reporting pallidotomy outcomes, 12 included postural control (45,46,49,51–58, 60). Only one of 12 studies reported no early improvement in postural control (56). Although the other studies reported early improvements, only two saw long-term benefit of unilateral pallidotomy on postural control (57,60).

Unilateral pallidotomy did not significantly improve motor performance in the medication on state but improved contralateral levodopa-induced dyskinesias up to 90%. The benefit of pallidotomy for tremor, rigidity, and dyskinesias has been reported to last over 5 years in some patients (57,58,61), albeit declining over time. However, on medication UPDRS scores declined over time as expected in PD patients treated only with medication (58).

Patients with advanced PD have bilateral and axial symptoms. However, the high incidence of complications reported in the thalamotomy literature lent caution to the use of bilateral pallidotomies in PD. Case series of bilateral pallidotomy with small numbers of patients showed further improvement in motor scores but largely confirmed the potential of similar side effects to those seen with bilateral thalamotomy (48,62,63). By the mid-1990s interest in unilateral pallidotomy was waning due to varied outcomes, varied lesion locations, and the limitation of its use for patients with bilateral disease. New dopamine agonists were becoming available and the technology of DBS was emerging.

IV. THE PRESENT

A. Emergence of Deep Brain Stimulation as an Alternative to Ablative Procedures

Electrical stimulation of brain structures has been used in neurophysiological research for many years. Stimulation usually results in excitation of neurons, axons, or fibers. For instance, low-frequency stimulation of the pyramidal tract will result in a muscle twitch, whereas higher frequency will result in continuous contractions or tetany. In the 1950s Hassler and Guiot used high-frequency trains of electrical pulses as a sham lesion prior to electrocoagulation of the thalamus and pallidum (7,10). This high-frequency train resulted in improvement of parkinsonian signs and produced the same effect as the lesion. It became the standard technique for testing the effects of the lesion prior to irreversible electrocoagulation in both thalamotomies and pallidotomies.

In 1987 Benabid and Pollak began to treat tremor using unilateral chronic high-frequency stimulation (DBS) of the ventral intermediate nucleus (VIM) of the thalamus with a quadripolar stimulating depth electrode and an implantable pulse generator (IPG) (Medtronic Inc., Minneapolis, MN) (64). They reported total or almost complete suppression of tremor in over 38 out of 43 thalami stimulated (26 patients with PD and 6 with ET), which was maintained for up to 29 months. Adverse effects were related to stimulation intensity and were reversible. They most typically included transient paraesthesias, limb dystonia, and cerebellar dysmetria. Bilateral thalamic DBS or DBS plus contralateral thalamotomy was associated with mild dysarthria and disequilibrium in five out of 18 cases.

Subsequently, numerous studies have demonstrated that DBS of the VIM of the thalamus is a safe and efficacious treatment for ET and the tremor seen in PD, MS, and traumatic central nervous system (CNS) lesions (65–74). Schuurman et al. found that DBS and thalamotomy were equally effective for the control of tremor but that thalamic DBS was associated with fewer adverse effects and a greater functional improvement than thalamotomy. Bilateral thalamic DBS afforded greater improvement in appendicular and midline tremor without as high an incidence of the adverse effects as had been seen with bilateral thalamotomies (75).

B. Deep Brain Stimulation for Parkinson's Disease

In 1994 Benabid and colleagues implanted a DBS electrode in the STN of a 51-year-old PD patient and reported instant relief of rigidity and akinesia in the contralateral limbs (76). Overall, studies of bilateral STN DBS for the treatment of PD have reported an average of 36–70% improvement in UPDRS Motor and a 30–70% improvement in activities of daily living (ADL) subscores from bilateral DBS (without medication) at 6 months (77–84). Studies of bilateral GPi DBS have also shown benefit, although the improvement in motor scores from bilateral GPi DBS is generally lower than that reported for STN

DBS (77,78,80,85–87). DBS has the added advantage that the stimulation parameters can be adjusted over time to optimize the clinical benefit while minimizing side effects. The operative risks involved with DBS are similar to those seen with ablative procedures and are reported at 5% or lower depending on the study and center (77,82). DBS has additional risks seen with implanted hardware, namely lead breakage, erosion of leads and/or the extension wire and postoperative infection. A recent report showed an incidence of hardware complications in 20 of 79 patients followed for a mean duration of 33 months following bilateral DBS (88). Seven out of 12 cases of lead erosion and/or infection occurred over one year after surgery.

The DBS electrode could be considered a "brain pacemaker," which requires programming, similar to a cardiac pacemaker. DBS programming can be viewed as a form of "electro-medicine" where electrode polarity, stimulation parameters, and intensity can be adjusted over time in a similar fashion to pharmacological drug and dose manipulation. In the case of STN DBS, neurostimulation mimics the effect of medication in most motor functions and patients reduce their medication by 30–100% (77–79,81). In contrast, large reductions in medication are not usually seen with GPi DBS (77,78). The reason for this is unknown, except that microdialysis studies in animals have shown that STN stimulation increases striatal levels of dopamine metabolites, whereas GPi stimulation does not (89).

The clinical effect of DBS appears to be similar to that of a lesion but may have a different mechanism of action. Following the pathophysiological circuitry model, it was assumed initially that DBS must somehow be "silencing" the overactive neurons in GPi and STN. However, it has been shown that a beneficial effect is only produced with frequencies higher than 100 Hz (12,45,90,91). This, plus the finding that pulse widths as low as 60 µs are effective, has led to new interpretations of the mechanism of action of DBS. From analysis of the characteristics of intensity-pulse width curves, Rizzone et al. suggested that the therapeutic effects of STN DBS are most likely affected by activation of fibers (90). Assuming an inhibitory effect, he speculated that the mechanism was due to activation of inhibitory fibers afferent to the STN (90). This is in agreement with other studies on the effect of DBS of the STN for tremor and of GPi (92,93). The side effects of paraesthesias, dystonia, and or dysarthria from STN DBS and visual field deficits and dysarthria from GPi DBS are most sensitive to voltage increments and thus to increasing the volume of stimulation to include structures such as the medial lemniscus and/or pyramidal tract (STN) and optic tract and/or pyramidal tract (GPi). These appear to be due to their inactivation (34), although this has not been proved. Vitek has shown that STN DBS in parkinsonian primates increases firing rates in GPi, which is presumed to result from excitation of STN output (Fig. 1) (93a). He and others have suggested that the therapeutic effect of DBS may therefore lie in its ability to drive the downstream (irregularly firing) neurons in GPi and/or thalamus at more regular frequencies, thus restoring encodable information transfer (93a,93b).

C. Summary of the Current Era of Surgical Procedures to Treat Parkinson's Disease

From studies performed since 1991, the preferred surgical technique for treating the symptoms of PD has become DBS of the STN or GPi. There is a lower incidence of adverse effects of bilateral DBS compared to bilateral ablative procedures. DBS is reversible and adaptable such that parameters can be manipulated over time to meet the needs of the patient's symptoms. Most patients with STN DBS reduce their doses of medication over time and report a more predictable amount and quality of on time. In addition, the reversibility of DBS means that future therapies would remain a viable treatment option, which otherwise might be rendered ineffective as a result of an ablative lesion. DBS compared to ablative therapy is associated with a higher incidence of infection and hardware problems, such as lead breakage. DBS is more expensive and requires proximity to a center experienced in the complex programming required for DBS. DBS is regarded as adjunctive therapy to medication for a select group of patients who have maintained a good medication response despite concurrent dyskinesias and motor fluctuations, and who are not cognitively impaired.

V. THE FUTURE

A. Fetal Mesencephalic Tissue Transplantation

Experimental transplantation of dopamine-producing neurons has been studied in animal models of PD for the last three decades. Basic research revealed some general guidelines for dopaminergic neuronal replacement strategies (94). Transplants from older animals did not survive and grow compared to those from fetal preparations. Grafts were best prepared as cellular suspensions rather than lumps of tissue. Survival improved if growth factors were transplanted with the cellular suspension. Outgrowth of neurites from grafts was short enough that the site of transplantation was critical; the graft should be close to the site of the denervated nigrostriatal terminals. With these developments, Sladek and others demonstrated survival of the graft and neuritic outgrowth that formed appropriate dopaminergic synapses with the host striatum (95). Success was reported with transplantation of adult adrenal tissue to the lateral ventricle in two PD patients. Overall success was transient, rare, and may have been a placebo effect, and morbidity was high.

Small clinical trials using intrastriatal fetal dopaminergic tissue transplantation (97–116) reported clinical benefit that persisted for several years with evidence from [18]fluoro-dopa (^{18}F-Dopa) positron emission tomography (PET) of graft survival. This led to the first NIH-funded double-blind placebo-controlled trial of fetal mesencephalic transplantation for advanced PD (117). Forty patients with PD were randomized to receive either embryonic mesencephalic tissue delivered to bilateral putamen or placebo via a sham procedure, where the needles did not penetrate the dura. After one year the placebo group was given the option to undergo implantation and the groups were then followed in an open-label fashion. There was no difference between placebo versus grafted patients on patient global rating scales. However, ^{18}F-Dopa PET scans showed increased uptake around the graft site (114). Autopsy studies in two patients revealed extensive neuritic outgrowth that extended across the full width of the putamen 3 years posttransplantation. The patients were initially separated based on age: younger or older than 60 years. In the younger group there were significant improvements in rigidity and bradykinesia but not in freezing or motor fluctuations, and gait scores worsened. The older group showed no significant improvement.

More adverse events that were not associated with the surgery occurred in the operated group. Five of 33 patients developed disabling dyskinesias off medication. Three of these patients were later successfully treated with GPi DBS. The 5 patients showed significantly greater increases in ^{18}F-Dopa uptake in the putamen postoperatively compared to 12 age-matched transplant recipients, who did not develop "off-dyskinesias" (118). The relatively increased uptake was seen in posterodorsal regions of the putamen where uptake was low preoperatively, but also in more ventral zones where uptake had been preserved preoperatively. The authors suggest that unbalanced increases in dopaminergic uptake can lead to off dyskinesias posttransplantation. A separate study of 14 patients from other fetal mesencephalon transplantation series who had postoperative "off-dyskinesias" did not show any correlation with increased uptake in ^{18}F-Dopa PET, although no mention was made as to whether measurement of uptake in ^{18}F-Dopa was made in different regions of the putamen (119).

Problems with controlling graft rejection (for allogenic transplanted tissue), dopamine production, survivability of fetal tissue, and the availability of such tissue in the United States have hampered the transition of fetal mesencephalic transplantation from an experimental procedure to accepted clinical practice.

B. Stem Cell Transplantation

The brain had been regarded as an organ that did not renew itself; the maximum number of neurons were thought to be present at birth and attenuated over the lifetime of the organism. Reports have shown that the adult brain also contains undifferentiated cells capable of self-renewal, proliferation, and differentiation into neurons or glia (120–122). These are the criteria required to define a stem cell and as such are defined as neural stem cells. Furthermore, the use of specific growth factors has allowed proliferation of neural stem cells into multipotent progenitor cells and further to neurons and glia (123). Indeed, dopaminergic neurons have been generated from cultures of human fetal mesencephalic stem cells using mitogens [epidermal growth factor (EGF), and fibroblast growth factor-2 (FGF-2)] and differentiation stimulators of interleukins and glial cell line–derived neurotrophic factor (GDNF) (124–126). These techniques have the potential to provide an unlimited supply of progenitor cells, which if expanded and differentiated into dopaminergic neurons in a controlled fashion may provide a more plentiful and standardized source of replacement dopamine.

Adult neuronal stem cells have been shown to be present in parts of the brain such as the subventricular zone and forebrain of rodents (127–129). These cells can be induced to proliferate, differentiate, and migrate to an area of neuronal injury (such as the striatum) if injury is combined with infusions of growth factors (130,131). Techniques to turn on endogenous neurogenesis are being investigated, but again may need careful study to avoid the problems encountered in uncontrolled proliferation.

Neuronal stem cell therapy may advance the treatment of many neurodegenerative diseases such as PD (132). However, stem cell therapy still faces the hurdles facing fetal tissue transplantation before clinical trials can begin. More refined protocols are needed to protect the embryonic stem (ES) cells after transplantation using a combination of antioxidant, antiexcitotoxic, antiapoptotic, and trophic strategies and thus improve urvival. The basic neurobiology of growth factors and a better understanding of the topography of the striatum are needed to determine the best site of placement of the ES cells to optimize functional connectivity. Better strategies are needed to control differentiation and proliferation and to improve the survival of grafted cells.

C. Alternative Sources of Cells

It is unclear whether the cells used for grafting need to be neuronal, i.e., exhibit impulse dependent release of dopamine. Other cells, that can secrete dopamine or L-dopa have been investigated such as adrenal chromaffin cells (133,134), glomus cells from the carotid body (135), and engineered cells (136–138). So far these have poor survivability and limited functional responses. Other animal experiments have shown that implants of dopamine-releasing polymers (139,140) or encapsulated PC-12 cells (141,142), which produce dopamine or L-dopa, can act as mini-pumps that can tonically activate dopamine receptors. Similar to the insulin pumps used for diabetes, intracerebral application of a continuous source of dopamine may in the future be a more efficacious therapy than oral boluses of dopamine or levodopa.

D. Gene Transfer Techniques

Gene transfer techniques have been used to replace dopamine in the striatum and also to introduce enzymes involved in dopamine synthesis, and/or potential neuroprotective molecules, such as growth factors, that may either prevent dopaminergic cells from dying or stimulate functional regeneration in the damaged nigrostriatal system. The application of key enzymes has had some early but no prolonged benefit (143,144) in the rat model partly due to their instability in noncatecholaminergic cells.

Growth factors, such as brain-derived neurotrophic factor (BDNF) and GDNF, when applied intracerebrally, have been shown to improve tissue transplant survival with potent effects on dopamine nigral neurons. Methods to administer growth factors have used either lentiviral or adenoviral vectors (145–148) or engineered fibroblast cell lines (149–151). Kordower et al. showed that lentiviral delivery of GDNF into both the striatum and the nigra of parkinsonian primates resulted in extensive GDNF expression with both anterograde and retrograde transport, reversal of motor deficits, and prevention of further nigrostriatal degeneration (152). However, a previous attempt to apply GDNF to a PD patient was unsuccessful (153). This was largely due to an ineffective delivery method through the ventricles and serves to emphasize the need for careful scientific study into the neurobiology of growth factors in PD, the appropriate delivery method, and optimal target site for trophic factors and other potential restorative therapies before clinical studies commence.

REFERENCES

1. Horsley V. The function of the so-called motor area of the brain. Br Med J 1909; 21:125–132.
2. Putnam T. Relief from unilateral paralysis agitans by section of the lateral pyramidal tract. Arch Neurol Psychiatry 1938; 40:1049.
3. Klemme R. Surgical treatment of dystonia, paralysis agitans and athetosis. Arch Neurol Psychiatry 1940; 44:926.
4. Bucy P, Case J. Surgical relief of tremor at rest. Ann Surg 1945; 122:933–941.
5. Mackay R. Yearbook of Neurology, Psychiatry and Neurosurgery (Introduction). Neurology 1952:7–8.
6. Meyers R. Surgical experiments in the therapy of certain 'extrapyramidal' diseases: A current evaluation. Acta Psychiat Neurol Scand 1951; (suppl 67):1–42.
7. Guiot G. Le traitement des syndromes parkinsoniens par la destruction du pallidum interne. Neurochirurgia (Stuttg) 1958; 1:94–98.
8. Spiegel E, Wycis H, Freed H. Stereoencephalotomy: thalamotomy and related procedures. J Am Med Assoc 1952; 148:446–451.
9. Cooper I. Intracerebral injection of Procaine into the globus pallidus in hyperkinetic disorders. Science 1954; 119:417–418.
10. Hassler R, Riechert T, Mundinger F, Umbach W, Ganglberger J. Physiological observations in stereotaxic operations in extrapyramidal motor disturbances. Brain 1960; 83:337–350.
11. Cooper I. Surgical alleviation of Parkinsonism: effects of occlusion of the anterior choroidal artery. J Am Geriat Soc 1954; 11:691–717.

12. Hassler R, Riechert T. Indikationen und Lokalisationsmethode der gezielten Hirnoperationen. Nervenartz 1954; 25:441–447.
13. Krayenbuhl H, Wyss O, Yasargil M. Bilateral thalamotomy and pallidotomy as treatment for bilateral parkinsonism. J Neurosurg 1961; 18:428–444.
14. Cooper I. Parkinsonism. Its Medical and Surgical Therapy. Springfield, IL: Charles C. Thomas, 1961.
15. Cooper I. Surgical treatment of parkinsonism. Ann Rev Med 1965; 16:309–330.
16. Bertrand C, Martiniz N. Experimental and clinical surgery in dyskinetic disease. Confin Neurol 1962; 22:375–382.
17. Broager B. The surgical treatment of parkinsonism. Acta Neurol Scand 1963; 39(suppl 4): 181–187.
18. Gillingham F, Kalyanaraman S, Donaldson A. Bilateral stereotaxic lesions in the management of parkinsonism and the dyskinesias. Br Med J 1964; ii:656–659.
19. Tasker R. Tremor of parkinsonism and stereotactic thalamotomy [editorial]. Mayo Clin Proc 1987; 62:736–739.
20. Mundinger F, Riechert T. Ergebnisse der stereotaktischen Hirnoperationen bei extrapyramidalen Bewegungsstorungen auf Grund postoperativer und Langzeituntersuchungen. Dtsch Z Nervenheilk 1961; 182:542–576.
21. Svennilson E, Torvik A, Lowe R, Leksell L. Treatment of parkinsonism by stereotactic thermolesions in the pallidal region. Acta Psychiatr Scand 1960; 35:358–377.
22. Riechert T. Long term follow-up of results of stereotaxic treatment in extrapyramidal disorders. Confin Neurol (Basel) 1962; 22:356–363.
23. Matsumoto K, Asano T, Baba T, Miyamoto T, Ohmoto T. Long-term follow-up results of bilateral thalamotomy for parkinsonism. Appl Neurophysiol 1976; 39:257–260.
24. Selby G. Stereotactic surgery for the relief of Parkinson's. J Neurol Sci 1967; 5(2):315–342.
25. DeLong MR, Crutcher MD, Georgopoulos AP. Primate globus pallidus and subthalamic nucleus: functional organization. J Neurophysiol 1985; 53(2):530–543.
26. DeLong M. Primate models of movement disorders of basal ganglia origin. Trends Neurosci 1990; 13(7):281–285.
27. Mega MS, Cummings JL. Frontal-subcortical circuits and neuropsychiatric disorders. J Neuropsychiatry 1994; 6:358–370.
28. Feger I, Hassani OK, Mouroux M. The subthalamic nucleus and its connections. New electrophysiological and pharmacological data. Adv Neurol 1997; 74:31–43.
29. Hammond C, Deniau J, Rizk A, Feger J. Electrophysiological demonstration of an excitatory subthalamonigral pathway in the rat. Brain Res 1978; 151(2):235–244.
30. Kita H, Kitai S. Intracellular study of rat globus pallidus neurons: membrane properties and responses to neostriatal, subthalamic and nigral stimulation. Brain Res 1991; 564(2):296–305.
31. Robledo P, Feger J. Excitatory influence of rat subthalamic nucleus to substantia nigra pars reticulata and the pallidal complex: electrophysiological data. Brain Res 1990; 518(1–2):47–54.
32. Wichmann T, Bergman H, DeLong M. The primate subthalamic nucleus. I. Functional properties in intact animals. J Neurophysiol 1994; 72(2):494–506.
33. Bouyer J, Joh T, Pickel V. Ultrastructural localization of tyrosine hydroxylase in rat nucleus accumbens. J Compar Neurol 1984; 227(1):92–103.
34. Bergman H, Wichmann T, DeLong M. Reversal of experimental parkinsonism by lesions of the subthalamic nucleus. Science 1990; 249(4975):1436–1438.
35. Bergman H, Wichmann T, Karmon B, DeLong M. The primate subthalamic nucleus. II. Neuronal activity in the MPTP model of parkinsonism. J Neurophysiol 1994; 72(2):507–520.
36. Filion M, Tremblay L. Abnormal spontaneous activity of globus pallidus neurons in monkeys with MPTP-induced parkinsonism. Brain Res 1991; 547(1):142–151.
37. Miller W, DeLong M. Altered Tonic Activity of Neurons in the Globus Pallidus and Subthalamic Nucleus in the Primate MPTP Model of Parkinsonism. New York: Plenum Press, 1987.
38. Vitek J, Bakay RA, Hashimoto T, et al. Microelectrode-guided pallidotomy: technical approach and its application in medically intractable Parkinson's disease. J Neurosurg 1998; 88(6):1027–1043.
39. Lozano A, Hutchison W, Kiss Z, Tasker R, Davis K, Dostrovsky J. Methods for microelectrode-guided posteroventral pallidotomy. J Neurosurg 1996; 84(2):192–202.
40. Bezard E, Boraud T, Bioulae B, Gross C. Presymptomatic revelation of experimental parkinsonism. Neuro Report 1997; 8:435–438.
41. Aziz T, Peggs D, Sambrook M, Crossman A. Lesion of the subthalamic nucleus for the alleviation of 1-methyl-4-phenyl-1,2,3,6-tetrahydropyridine (MPTP)-induced parkinsonism in the primate. Mov Disord 1991; 6(4):288–292.

42. Aziz T, Peggs D, Agarwal E, Sambrook M, Crossman A. Subthalamic nucleotomy alleviates parkinsonism in the 1-methyl-4-phenyl-1,2,3,6-tetrahydropyridine (MPTP)-exposed primate. Br J Neurosurg 1992; 6(6):288–292.

43. Benazzouz A, Gross C, Fegar J, Boraud T, Bioulac B. Reversal of rigidity and improvement in motor performance by subthalamic high-frequency stimulation in MPTP-treated monkeys. Eur J Neurosci 1993; 5(4):382–389.

44. Limousin P, Pollak P, Benazzouz A, et al. Effect of parkinsonian signs and symptoms of bilateral subthalamic nucleus stimulation. Lancet 1995; 345(8942):91–95.

45. Baron MS, Vitek JL, Bakay RA, et al. Treatment of advanced Parkinson's disease by posterior GPi pallidotomy: 1-year results of a pilot study. Ann Neurol 1996; 40(3):355–366.

46. Lozano A, Hutchison W, Dostrovsky J. Microelectrode monitoring of cortical and subcortical structures during stereotactic surgery. Acta Neurochir 1995; 64(suppl):30–34.

47. Laitinen L. Leksell's posteroventral pallidotomy in the treatment of parkinson's disease. J Neurosurg 1992; 76(1):53–61.

48. Lang AE, Duff J, Saint-Cyr JA, et al. Posteroventral medial pallidotomy in Parkinson's disease. J Neurol 1999; 246(suppl 2):II/28–II/41.

49. Dogali M, Fazzine E, Kolodny E, et al. Stereotactic ventral pallidotomy for Parkinson's disease. Neurology 1995; 45:753–761.

50. Fazzini E, Dogali M, Sterio D, Eidelberg D, Beric A. Stereotactic pallidotomy for Parkinson's disease: a long-term follow-up of unilateral pallidotomy. Neurology 1997; 48:1273–1277.

51. Iacono R, RR L, Ulloth J, Shima F. Postero-ventral pallidotomy in Parkinson's disease. J Clin Neurosci 1995; 2:140–145.

52. Johansson F, Malm J, Nordh E, Hariz M. Usefulness of pallidotomy in advanced Parkinson's disease. J Neurol Neurosurg Psychiatry 1997; 62:125–132.

53. Kishore A, Turnbull IM, Snow BJ, et al. Efficacy, stability and predictors of outcome of pallidotomy for Parkinson's disease. Six-month follow-up with additional 1-year observations. Brain 1997; 120:729–737.

54. Masterman D, DeSalles A, Baloh RW, et al. Motor, cognitive, and behavioral performance following unilateral ventroposterior pallidotomy for Parkinson disease. Arch Neurol 1998; 55: 1201–1208.

55. Samuel M, Caputo E, Brooks DJ, et al. A study of medial pallidotomy for Parkinson's disease: clinical outcome, MRI location and complications. Brain 1998; 121:59–75.

56. Melnick M, Dowling G, Aminoff M, Barbaro N. Effect of pallidotomy on postural control and motor function in Parkinson disease. Arch Neurol 1999; 56:1361–1365.

57. Baron MS, Vitek JL, Bakay RA, et al. Treatment of advanced Parkinson's disease by unilateral posterior GPi pallidotomy: 4-year results of a pilot study. Mov Disord 2000; 15:230–237.

58. Fine J, Duff J, Chen R, Hutchison W, Lozano A, Lang A. Long term follow-up of unilateral pallidotomy in advanced Parkinson's disease. N Engl J Med 2000; 342(23):1708–1714.

59. Fahn S, Elton RL, Members of the UPDRS Development Committee. Unified Parkinson's Disease Rating Scale. In: Fahn S, Marsden CD, Calne D, Goldstein N, eds. Recent Developments in Parkinson's Disease. Vol. 2. Florham Park, NJ: Macmillan Healthcare Information, 1987:153–163.

60. Bronte-Stewart HM, Minn AY, Rodrigues K, Buckley EL, Nashner LM. Postural instability in idiopathic Parkinson's disease: the role of medication and unilateral pallidotomy. Brain 2002; 125(pt 9):2100–2114.

61. Vitek J, Bakay R, DeLong M. Microelectrode-guided pallidotomy for medically intractable Parkinson's disease. Adv Neurol 1997; 74:183–198.

62. Schuurman P, De Bie R, Speelman J, Bosch D. Bilateral posteroventral pallidotomy in advanced Parkinson's disease in three patients. Mov Disord 1997; 12:752–755.

63. Scott R, Gregory R, Hines N, et al. Neuropsychological, neurological and functional outcome following pallidotomy for Parkinson's disease—a consecutive series of eight simultaneous bilateral and twelve unilateral procedures. Brain 1998; 121:659–675.

64. Benabid AL, Pollak P, Gervason C, et al. Long-term suppression of tremor by chronic stimulation of the ventral intermediate thalamic nucleus. Lancet 1991; 337:403–406.

65. Koller W, Pahwa R, Busenbark K, et al. High-frequency unilateral thalamic stimulation in the treatment of essential and parkinsonian tremor. Ann Neurol 1997; 42:292–299.

66. Benabid AL, Pollak P, Gao D, et al. Chronic electrical stimulation of the ventralis intermedius nucleus of the thalamus as a treatment of movement disorders. J Neurosurg 1996; 84:203–214.

67. Blond S, Caparros-Lefebvre D, Parker F, et al. Control of tremor and involuntary movement disorders by chronic stereotactic stimulation of the ventral intermediate thalamic nucleus. J Neurosurg 1992; 77:62–68.

68. Geny C, Nguyen JP, Pollin B, et al. Improvement of severe postural cerebellar tremor in multiple sclerosis by chronic thalamic stimulation. Mov Disord 1996; 11:489–494.

69. Hubble J, Busenbark K, Wilkinson S, Penn R, Lyons K, Koller W. Deep brain stimulation for essential tremor. Neurology 1996; 46:1150–1153.

70. Ondo W, Jankovic J, Schwartz K, Almaguer M, Simpson R. Unilateral thalamic deep brain stimulation for refractory essential tremor and Parkinson's disease tremor. Neurol 1998; 51: 1063–1069.

71. Pollak P, Benabid A, Gervason C, Hoffmann D, Seigneuret E, Perret J. Long-term effects of chronic stimulation of the ventral intermediate thalamic nucleus in different types of tremor. Adv Neurol 1993; 60:408–413.

72. Siegfried J, Lippitz B. Chronic electrical stimulation of the VL-VPL complex and of the pallidum in the treatment of movement disorders: personal experience since 1982. Stereotact Funct Neurosurg 1994; 62:71–75.

73. Tasker RR, Munz M, Junn FS, et al. Deep brain stimulation and thalamotomy for tremor compared. Acta Neurochir Suppl (Wien) 1997; 68:49–53.

74. Schuurman PR, Bosch DA, Bossuyt PM, et al. A comparison of continuous thalamic stimulation and thalamotomy for suppression of severe tremor. N Engl J Med 2000; 342:461–468.

75. Ondo W, Almaguer M, Jankovic J, Simpson R. Thalamic deep brain stimulation. Arch Neurol Psychiatry 2001; 58:218–222.

76. Benabid AL, Pollak P, Gross C, et al. Acute and long-term effects of subthalamic nucleus stimulation in Parkinson's disease. Stereotact Funct Neurosurg 1994; 62(1–4):76–84.

77. Obeso J, Olanow C, Rodriguez-Oroz M, Krack P, Kumar R, Lang A. Deep-brain stimulation of the subthalamic nucleus or the pars interna of the globus pallidus in Parkinson's disease. N Engl J Med 2001; 345:956 963.

78. Volkmann J, Allert N, Voges J, Weiss P, Freund H-J, Sturm V. Safety and efficacy of pallidal or subthalamic nucleus stimulation in advanced PD. Neurology 2001; 56:548–551.

79. Moro E, Scerrati M, Romito L, Roselli R, Tonali P, Albanese A. Chronic subthalamic nucleus stimulation reduces medication requirements in Parkinson's disease. Neurology 1999; 53(1): 85–90.

80. Burchiel K, Anderson V, Favre J, Hammerstad J. Comparison of pallidal and subthalamic nucleus deep brain stimulation for advanced Parkinson's disease: results of a randomized, blinded pilot study. Neurosurgery 1999; 45(6):1375–1382.

81. Kumar R, Lozano AM, Kim YJ, et al. Double-blind evaluation of subthalamic nucleus deep brain stimulation in advanced Parkinson's disease. Neurology 1998; 51(3):850–855.

82. Limousin P, Krack P, Pollak P, et al. Electrical stimulation of the subthalamic nucleus in advanced Parkinson's disease. N Engl J Med 1998; 339(16):1105–1111.

83. Alegret M, Junque C, Valldeoriola F, et al. Effects of bilateral subthalamic stimulation on cognitive function in Parkinson's disease. Arch Neurol 2001; 58(8):1223–1227.

84. Bronte-Stewart H, Hill B, McGuire K, Minn A, Courtney T, Heit G. Superior outcomes of bilateral STN DBS in IPD attributed to precise intraoperative localization techniques. Neurology 2001; 56(suppl 3):A279.

85. Krack P, Poepping M, Weinert D, Schrader B, Deuschl G. Thalamic, pallidal, or subthalamic surgery for Parkinson's disease. J Neurol 2000; 247(suppl 2):II/122–134.

86. Kumar R, Lozano A, Montgomery E, Lang A. Pallidotomy and deep brain stimulation of the pallidum and subthalamic nucleus in advanced Parkinson's disease. Mov Disord 1998; 13(suppl 1): 73–82.

87. Brown R, Dowsey PL, Brown P, et al. Impact of deep brain stimulation on upper limb akinesia in Parkinson's disease. Ann Neurol 1999; 45(4):473–488.

88. Oh MY, Abosch A, Kim SH, Lang AE, Lozano AM. Long-term hardware-related complications of deep brain stimulation. Neurosurgery 2002; 50(6):1268–1274.

89. Meissner W, Harnack D, Paul G, et al. Neurosci Lett 2002; 328:105–108.

90. Rizzone M, Lanotte M, Bergamasco B, et al. Deep brain stimulation of the subthalamic nucleus in Parkinson's disease: effects of variation in stimulation parameters. J Neurol Neurosurg Psychiatry 2001; 71:215–219.

91. Moro E, Esselink RJA, Xie J, Hommel M, Benabid AL, Pollak P. The impact on Parkinson's disease of electrical parameter settings in STN stimulation. Neurology 2002; 59:706–713.

92. Ashby P, Kim YJ, Kumar R, Lang AE, Lozano AM. Neurophysiological effects of stimulation through electrodes in the human subthalamic nucleus. Brain 1999; 122:1919–1931.

93. Ashby P, Wu YR, Levy R, Tasker R, Dostrovosky JO. Does stimulation of the GPi control dyskinesia by activating inhibitory axons? Neurology 2000; 54(suppl 3):A284.

93a. Vitek JL. Mechanisms of deep brain stimulation: excitation or inhibition. Mov Disord 2002; 17(suppl 3):S69–S72.

93b. Montgomery EJ, Baker K. Mechanisms of deep brain stimulation and future technical developments. Neurol Res 2000; 22:259–266.

94. Bjorklund A, Stenevi AU, Schmidt RH, Dunnet SB, Gage FH. Intracerebral grafting of neuronal cell suspensions, II. Survival and growth of nigral cell suspensions implanted into different brain sites. Acta Physiol Scand 1983; (suppl 522):9–18.

95. Sladek JR, Collier TJ, Elsworth JD, Taylor JR, Roth RH, Redmond DE. Can graft-derived neurotrophic activity be used to direct axonal outgrowth of grafted dopamine neurons for circuit reconstruction in primates? Exp Neurol 1993; 124:134–139.

96. Madrazo I, Drucker-Colin R, Diaz V, Martinez-Mata J, Torres C, Becerril JJ. Open microsurgical autograft of adrenal medulla to the right caudate nucleus in two patients with intractable Parkinson's disease. N Engl J Med 1987; 316(14):831–834.

97. Freed CR, Breeze RE, Rosenberg NL, et al. Transplantation of human fetal dopamine cells for Parkinson's disease: results at 1 year. Arch Neurol 1990; 47:505–512.

98. Lindvall O, Brundin P, Widner H, et al. Grafts of fetal dopamine neurons survive and improve motor function in Parkinson's disease. Science 1990; 247:574–577.

99. Freed CR, Breeze RE, Rosenberg NL, et al. Survival of implanted fetal dopamine cells and neurologic improvement 12 to 46 months after transplantation for Parkinson's disease. N Engl J Med 1992; 327:1549–1555.

100. Freed CR, Breeze RE, Rosenberg NL, et al. Survival of implanted fetal dopamine cells and neurologic improvement 12 to 46 months after transplantation for Parkinson's disease. N Engl J Med 1992; 327:1549–1555.

101. Breeze RE, Wells TH Jr., Freed CR. Implantation of fetal tissue for the management of Parkinson's disease: a technical note. Neurosurgery 1995; 36:1044–1047.

102. Freed CR, Breeze RE, Rosenberg NL, Schneck SA. Embryonic dopamine cell implants as a treatment for the second phase of Parkinson's disease: replacing failed nerve terminals. Adv Neurol 1992; 60:721–728.

103. Spencer DD, Robbins RJ, Naftolin F, et al. Unilateral transplantation of human fetal mesencephalic tissue into the caudate nucleus of patients with Parkinson's disease. N Engl J Med 1992; 327:1541–1548.

104. Widner H, Tetrud J, Rehncrona S, et al. Bilateral fetal mesencephalic grafting in two patients with parkinsonism induced by 1-methyl-4-phenyl-1,2,3,6-tetrahydropyridine (MPTP). N Engl J Med 1992; 327:1556–1563.

105. Lindvall O, Sawle G, Widner H, et al. Evidence for long-term survival and function of dopaminergic grafts in progressive Parkinson's disease. Ann Neurol 1994; 35:172–180.

106. Freed CR, Breeze RE, Schneck SA, Bakay RAE, Ansari AA. Fetal neural transplantation for Parkinson's disease. In: Rich RR, ed. Clinical Immunology: Principles and Practice. St Louis: Mosby-Year Book, 1995:1677–1687.

107. Ansari AA, Mayne A, Freed CR, et al. Lack of detectable systemic humoral/cellular allogeneic response in human and nonhuman primate recipients of embryonic mesencephalic allografts for the therapy of Parkinson's disease. Transplant Proc 1995; 27:1401–1405.

108. Freeman TB, Olanow CW, Hauser RA, et al. Bilateral fetal nigral transplantation into the post-commissural putamen in Parkinson's disease. Ann Neurol 1995; 38:379–388.

109. Kordower JH, Freeman TB, Snow BJ, et al. Neuropathological evidence of graft survival and striatal reinnervation after the transplantation of fetal mesencephalic tissue in a patient with Parkinson's disease. N Engl J Med 1995; 332:1118–1124.

110. Peschanski M, Defer G, N'Guyen JP, et al. Bilateral motor improvement and alteration of L-dopa effect in two patients with Parkinson's disease following intrastriatal transplantation of foetal ventral mesencephalon. Brain 1994; 117:487–99.

111. Defer GL, Geny C, Ricolfi F, et al. Long-term outcome of unilaterally transplanted parkinsonian patients. I. Clinical approach. Brain 1996; 119:41–50.

112. Kopyov OV, Jacques D, Lieberman A, Duma CM, Rogers RL. Clinical study of fetal mesencephalic intracerebral transplants for the treatment of Parkinson's disease. Cell Transplant 1996; 5:327–337.

113. Freed CR, Breeze RE, Leehey MA, et al. Ten years' experience with fetal neurotransplantation in patients with advanced Parkinson's disease (abstr). Soc Neurosci 1998; 24:559.

114. Wenning G, Odin P, Morrish P, et al. Short- and long-term survival and function of unilateral intrastriatal dopaminergic grafts in Parkinson's disease. Ann Neurol 1997; 42:95–107.

115. Hauser RA, Freeman TB, Snow BJ, et al. Long-term evaluation of bilateral fetal nigral transplantation in Parkinson disease. Arch Neurol 1999; 56:179–187.

116. Piccini P, Brooks DJ, Bjorklund A, et al. Dopamine release from nigral transplants visualized in vivo in a Parkinson's patient. Nat Neurosci 1999; 12:1137–1140.
117. Freed CR, Greene PE, Breeze RE, et al. Transplantation of embryonic dopamine neurons for severe Parkinson's disease. N Engl J Med 2001; 344:710–719.
118. Ma Y, Feigin A, Dhawan V, et al. Dyskinesia after fetal cell transplantation for parkinsonism: a PET study. Ann Neurol 2002; 52(5):628–634.
119. Hagell P, Piccini P, Bjorklund A, et al. Dyskinesias following neural transplantation in Parkinson's disease. Nat Neurosci 2002; 5:627–628.
120. Shihabuddin LS, Palmer TD, Gage FH. The search for neural progenitor cells: prospects for the therapy of neurodegenerative disease. Mol Med Today 1999; 5:474–480.
121. Gage FH, Kempermann G, Palmer TD, Peterson DA, Ray J. Multipotent progenitor cells in the adult dentate gyrus. J Neurobiol 1998; 36:246–266.
122. Fisher LJ. Neural precursor cells: applications for the study and repair of the central nervous system. Neurobiol Dis 1997; 4:1–22.
123. Palmer TD, Ray J, Gage FH. FGF-2-responsive neuronal progenitors reside in proliferative and quiescent regions of the adult rodent brain. Mol Cell Neurosci 1995; 6:474–486.
124. Kim JH, Auerbach JM, Rodriguez-Gomez JA, et al. Dopamine neurons derived from embryonic stem cells function in an animal model of Parkinson's disease. Nature 2002; 418: 50–56.
125. Storch A, Paul G, Csete M, et al. Long-term proliferation and dopaminergic differentiation of human mesencephalic neural precursor cells. Exp Neurol 2001; 170(2):317–325.
126. Sawamoto K, Nakao N, Kakishita K, et al. Generation of dopaminergic neurons in the adult brain from mesencephalic precursor cells labeled with a nestin-GFP transgene. J Neurosci 2001; 21(11): 3895–3903.
127. Lois C, Alvarez-Buylla A. Proliferating subventricular zone cells in the adult mammalian forebrain can differentiate into neurons and glia. Proc Natl Acad Sci 1993; 90:2074–2077.
128. Johansson C, Momma S, Clarke D, Risling M, Lendahl U, Frisen J. Identification of a neural stem cell in the adult mammalian central nervous system. Cell 1999; 96(1):25–34.
129. Clarke DL, Johansson CB, Wilbertz J, et al. Generalized potential of adult neural stem cells. Science 2000; 288:1660–1663.
130. Fallon J, Reid S, Kinyamu R, et al. In vivo induction of massive proliferation, directed migration, and differentiation of neural cells in the adult mammalian brain. Proc Natl Acad Sci 2000; 97(26):14686–14691.
131. Nakatomi H, Kuriu T, Okabe S, et al. Regeneration of hippocampal pyramidal neurons after ischemic brain injury by recruitment of endogenous neural progenitors. Cell 2002; 110:429–441.
132. Holden C. Stem cells. $2.2 million for cells to fight Parkinson's. Science 2001; 293(5537):1966.
133. Brundin P, Duan W, Sauer H. Functional Neural Transplantation. New York: Raven, 1994.
134. Goetz CG, Stebbins GT, Klawans HL, et al. United Parkinson Foundation Neurotransplantation Registry on adrenal medullary transplants: presurgical, and 1-year and 2-year follow up. Neurology 1991; 41:1719–1722.
135. Espejo E, Montoro R, Armengol J, Lopez-Barneo J. Cellular and functional recovery of parkinsonian rats after intrastriatal transplantation of carotid body cell aggregates. Neuron 1998; 20:197–206.
136. Fisher L, Jinnah H, Kale L, Higgins G, Gage F. Survival and function of intrastriatally grafted primary fibroblasts genetically modified to produce l-DOPA. Neuron 1991; 6:371–380.
137. Lundberg C, Horellou P, Mallet J, Bjorklund A. Generation of DOPA-producing astrocytes by retroviral transduction of the human tyrosine hydroxylase gene: in vitro characterisation and in vivo effects in the rat Parkinson model. Exp Neurol 1996; 139:39–53.
138. Anton R, Kordower JH, Maidment NT, et al. Neural-targeted gene therapy for rodent and primate hemiparkinsonism. Exp Neurol 1994; 127:207–218.
139. Winn SR, Wahlberg L, Tresco PA, Aebischer P. An encapsulated dopamine-releasing polymer alleviates experimental parkinsonism in rats. Exp Neurol 1989; 105:244–250.
140. Becker JB, Robinson TE, Barton P, Sintov A, Siden R, Levy RJ. Sustained behavioral recovery from unilateral nigrostriatal damage produced by the controlled release of dopamine from a silicone polymer pellet placed into the denervated striatum. Brain Res 1990; 508:60–64.
141. Aebischer P, Goddard M, Signore A, Timpson R. Functional recovery in hemiparkinsonian primates transplanted with polymer-encapsulated PC12 cells. Exp Neurol 1994; 126:151–158.
142. Emerich DF, McDermott PE, Krueger PM, Frydel B, Sanberg PR, Winn SR. Polymer-encapsulated PC12 cells promote recovery of motor function in aged rats. Exp Neurol 1993; 122:37–47.

143. Raymon H, Thode S, Gage F. Application of ex vivo gene therapy in the treatment of Parkinson's disease. Exp Neurol 1997; 144:82–91.

144. Kang U. Potential of gene therapy for Parkinson's disease: neurobiologic issues and new developments in gene transfer methodologies. Mov Disord 1998; 13:59–72.

145. Choi-Lundberg DL, Lin Q, Chang YN, et al. Dopaminergic neurons protected from degeneration by GDNF gene therapy. Science 1997; 275:838–841.

146. Mandel R, Spratt S, Snyder R, Leff S. Midbrain injection of recombinant adenoassociated virus encoding rat glial cell line-derived neurotrophic factor protects nigral neurons in a progressive 6-hydroxydopamine-induced degeneration model of Parkinson's disease in rats. Proc Natl Acad Sci 1997; 94:14083–14088.

147. Bilang-Bleuel A, Revah F, Colin P, et al. Intrastriatal injection of an adenoviral vector expressing glial-cell-line-derived neurotrophic factor prevents dopaminergic neuron degeneration and behavioral impairment in a rat model of Parkinson's disease. Proc Natl Acad Sci 1997; 94: 8818–8823.

148. Choi-Lundberg DL, Lin Q, Schallert T, et al. Behavioral and cellular protection of rat dopaminergic neurons by an adenoviral vector encoding glial cell line-derived neurotrophic factor. Exp Neurol 1998; 154:261–275.

149. Frim DM, Uhler TA, Galpern WR, Beal MF, Breakefield XO, Isacson O. Implanted fibroblasts genetically engineered to produce brain-derived neurotrophic factor prevent 1-methyl-4-phenylpyridinium toxicity to dopaminergic neurons in the rat. Proc Natl Acad Sci 1994; 91:5104–5108.

150. Levivier M, Przedborski S, Bencsics C, Kang U. Intrastriatal implantation of fibroblasts genetically engineered to produce brain-derived neutrophic factor prevents degeneration of dopaminergic neurons in a rat model of Parkinson's disease. J Neurosci 1995; 15:7810–7820.

151. Tseng J, Baetge E, Zurn A, Aebischer P. GDNF reduces drug-induced rotational behavior after medial forebrain bundle transection by a mechanism not involving striatal dopamine. J Neurosci 1997; 17:325–333.

152. Kordower JH, Emborg M, Bloch J, et al. Neurodegeneration prevented by lentiviral vector delivery of GDNF in primate models of Parkinson's disease. Science 2000; 290:767–773.

153. Kordower JH, Palfi S, Chen EY, et al. Clinicopathological findings following intraventricular glial-derived neurotrophic factor treatment in a patient with Parkinson's disease. Ann Neurol 1999; 46(3):419–424.

3

Clinical Assessments

Steven J. Frucht

Columbia University, New York, New York, U.S.A.

The last decade has witnessed great strides in understanding the etiology and progression of Parkinson's disease (PD). Despite these advances, the diagnosis of PD remains clinical, and this will remain so for the foreseeable future. Most patients with PD have no known family members with parkinsonism, making screening for identified PD genes a difficult and low-yield proposition. Single photon emission computed tomography (SPECT) and positron emission tomography (PET) scanning are very sensitive to nigrostriatal damage, but their cost precludes their routine application. Unless a sensitive and specific peripheral biological marker for PD is discovered, neurologists will continue to rely on clinical symptoms and signs for diagnosis and follow-up.

This chapter reviews the clinical assessment of the PD patient. The first part describes how clinical symptoms and signs are used to evaluate patients in the office. Afterwards there is a review of the most commonly used PD rating scales, including those that measure ancillary motor features and nonmotor manifestations of the disease. Quality-of-life measures and outcome ratings will also be considered.

I. INITIAL CLINICAL ASSESSMENT

Although PD is the most common cause of parkinsonism, other etiologies should be considered when evaluating a patient. A careful history usually reveals drug-induced parkinsonism. Once excluded, the three most common diagnoses that mimic PD are multiple system atrophy (MSA), progressive supranuclear palsy (PSP), and cortiocobasal ganglionic degeneration (CBGD). These disorders are grouped under the rubric of "Parkinson-plus" conditions.

PSP typically presents with early falls, slow vertical saccades, and prominent axial rigidity with relatively preserved appendicular mobility. CBGD may take myriad forms, most commonly a rigid, dystonically postured limb that is stiff and useless. Myoclonus, alien limb phenomena, apraxia, and higher cortical sensory deficits may be seen to varying degrees. MSA includes three disorders: striatonigral degeneration (atremulous parkinsonism, which is typically poorly responsive to levodopa), Shy-Drager syndrome (autonomic failure), and olivopontocerebellar atrophy (prominent vermian cerebellar dysfunction). Of these, patients with striatonigral degeneration are the closest mimics of PD.

Several recent studies illustrate that it can be difficult even for the most experienced examiner to differentiate PD from Parkinson-plus syndromes. Hughes and colleagues examined 100 consecutive cases clinically diagnosed as PD in which postmortem tissue was available at the U.K. PD Society Brain Research Center (1). Ninety cases fulfilled pathological criteria for PD, and of the other 10 the most common diagnosis at postmortem was MSA. The authors concluded that even applying rigorous diagnostic criteria for PD, the maximum clinical diagnostic accuracy would be 90%. Results from the DATATOP study (a trial of selegiline and/or vitamin E in early PD) yielded similar results. Of 800 patients diagnosed with PD and enrolled in the trial, 65 patients (8.1%) were later found to have an alternate diagnosis (2). These patients were more bradykinetic, and had more postural impairment and less prominent tremor. They were also less likely to present with tremor and more likely to complain of early falls or gait difficulty.

Symptoms and signs can help guide the examiner in distinguishing PD from its mimics. A robust response to levodopa is the best evidence that a patient has PD—virtually 95% of patients with pathologically confirmed PD respond. Patients with PSP seldom benefit from levodopa, and the improvement is subtle at best. However, as many as one third of MSA patients may initially benefit from levodopa, and the response can be quite dramatic. In practice, MSA is the Parkinson-plus disorder most difficult to distinguish from PD, particularly the striatonigral variant of MSA. Wenning et al. analyzed the clinical presentations of 100 consecutive cases of pathologically confirmed PD, comparing them to 38 cases of MSA (3). The best predictors of a diagnosis of MSA were age of symptom onset ≤55 years, absence of early tremor, asymmetry of exam, early balance impairment, poor initial response to levodopa, and absence of hallucinations from dopaminergic medications. Even so, as many as 10% of patients predicted to have PD will ultimately have MSA.

Gelb and colleagues reviewed the cardinal clinical symptoms and signs of PD and proposed diagnostic criteria for the disorder (4). PD is usually asymmetrical, and in general the side that is involved first remains more severe throughout the course of the illness. Although asymmetry cannot distinguish PD from PSP or MSA, the latter two disorders are more likely to be symmetrical. CBGD usually presents with a markedly asymmetrical exam. A characteristic rest tremor of 3–4 Hz frequency is very common in PD (present in over 75% of patients), but tremor in some PD patients may be faster than 3 Hz, may occur predominantly with action, and may change during the course of the illness. Tremor is extremely uncommon in PSP, and while patients with CBGD may appear to have tremor, careful examination usually reveals that these movements are myoclonic. As many as one third of MSA patients may display tremor during their illness, and the tremor may precisely mimic that of PD. In contrast to tremor, bradykinesia and rigidity are not useful in distinguishing PD from its mimics. Postural instability is much more useful, as it is much more common in Parkinson-plus disorders, particularly PSP.

Guidelines for the clinical diagnosis of PD (Tables 1 and 2) are useful for clinical trial design and also for predicting patients' clinical course. In their classic paper, Hoehn and Yahr noted that patients with prominent tremor early in their illness have slower disease progression (5). Zetusky and colleagues confirmed this observation in the post-levodopa era (6). So-called "tremor-predominant" patients encounter less motor impairment and

Table 1 Diagnostic Clinical Features

Group A features: characteristic of Parkinson's disease
  Resting tremor
  Bradykinesia
  Rigidity
  Asymmetrical onset

Group B features: suggestive of alternative diagnoses
  Prominent postural instability in the first 3 years
  Freezing in the first 3 years
  Hallucinations unrelated to medications in the first 3 years
  Dementia preceding motor symptoms in the first year
  Supranuclear gaze palsy
  Severe symptomatic dysautonomia unrelated to medications
  Secondary cause of parkinsonism

Source: Adapted from Ref. 4.

have better-preserved cognition relative to other PD patients (7). In contrast, patients who present with postural instability and gait impairment ("PIGD" group) are more likely to dement, and their motor performance deteriorates more rapidly (6). These clinical features should guide the clinician to treat PIGD patients more aggressively so as to intervene before falls occur.

Table 2 Proposed Diagnostic Criteria for Parkinson's Disease

Possible Parkinson's disease
  At least two of the four features in Group A are present, one of which is tremor or bradykinesia
                                                   and
either   None of the features in Group B are present
or   Symptoms have been present for less than 3 years, and no features of Group B are present
                                                   and
either   Substantial, sustained response to levodopa or dopamine agonist
or   Patient has not had an adequate trial of levodopa or dopamine agonist

Probable Parkinson's disease
  At least three of the four features in Group A are present
                                                   and
  None of the features in Group B are present (disease duration of 3 years)
                                                   and
  Substantial, sustained response to levodopa or dopamine agonist

Definite Parkinson's disease
  All criteria for **Possible Parkinson's disease** are met
                                                   and
  Autopsy confirmation of diagnosis by histopathology

Source: Adapted from Ref. 4.

II. CLINICAL RATING SCALES FOR PD

A. Primary Rating Scales

In 1987 the Unified Parkinson's Disease Rating Scale (UPDRS) was developed to present a common, uniform tool for evaluating PD patients (8). Although other rating scales preceded it, the UPDRS is by far the most widely used and accepted clinical rating scale for PD. A copy of the UPDRS appears at the conclusion of this chapter.

The UPDRS consists of six sections: Part I—mentation, behavior, and mood; Part II—activities of daily living; Part III—motor examination; Part IV—complications of therapy; Part V—modified Hoehn and Yahr staging; Part VI—Schwab and England Activities of Daily Living scale. Parts I, II and VI require the patient or their caregiver to select answers to questions about performance. Part III documents the clinical examination including speech, facial expression, tremor, rigidity, bradykinesia, posture, gait, and postural stability. Dyskinesias, on/off phenomena, sleep disturbance, and symptomatic orthostasis are recorded in Part IV. Patients may be rated by the examiner in either the on or the off state for all parts of the scale. Items are scored on a 5-point system, with 0 representing normal and 4 severe impairment.

Can PD patients reliably assess their limitations? Brown and colleagues surveyed 66 PD patients using a detailed Activities of Daily Living (ADL) questionnaire (9). Patients rated themselves, and a relative performed the same ratings independently. These ratings were compared to a physician's direct assessment of the patient performing many of the tasks included in the questionnaire. Patient-rated and relative-rated ADLs were highly correlated, and neither the patient's nor the relative's level of depression affected the ratings. Patients with cognitive impairment tended to modestly underestimate their disability compared to physician ratings. Louis and colleagues measured the ability of nondemented PD patients to reliably self-administer the historical sections (parts I and II) of the UPDRS (10). Thirty PD patients completed these sections before their visit with the neurologist, at which time the sections were administered again. Concordance between patient and neurologist ratings was excellent, with highest reliability for questions about salivation, swallowing, and dressing and lowest reliability for memory, hallucinations, and hygiene. These two studies illustrate that PD patients are capable of reliably estimating their disability in performing daily tasks in their home environment.

The validity and reliability of the UPDRS have been carefully studied. Martinez-Martin and colleagues assessed the validity of the UPDRS by analyzing ratings from six independent evaluations of 40 PD patients. Interobserver reliability was excellent, with the exception of items 17 (sensory complaints), 19 (facial expression), 21 (action or postural tremor), and 31 (body bradykinesia) (11). Richards and colleagues also assessed the interrater reliability of the UPDRS by having two neurologists simultaneously examine 24 PD patients (12). Interrater reliability was excellent, with the exception of speech (item 18) and facial expression (item 19).

Martinez-Martin and colleagues performed a factor analysis of the UPDRS revealing six primary factors: mobility of the extremities, gait, functional ability, tremor, communication, and bradykinesia. Tremor was the one factor that did not correlate with other measures, whereas all other factors were highly correlated (11). Stebbins and Goetz (13) investigated the factor structure of the UPDRS in 294 consecutive PD patients examined in the on state and also identified six factors: gait, rest tremor, rigidity, bradykinesia (right and left), and postural tremor. Again, neither rest nor postural tremor was associated with other measures of disability as measured by Hoehn and Yahr stage, Schwab and England

ADL, or UPDRS total score. These findings agree with the clinical observation that the severity of tremor correlates poorly with other elements of parkinsonian disability.

One of the advantages of the UPDRS is that it is easy to use and nonphysician personnel can administer it reliably. A teaching tape is available that documents scoring (14). Bennett and colleagues measured the ability of three nurse clinicians to administer the UPDRS (15). After extensive training, three nurses examined 75 subjects at two intervals separated by 3 weeks. Agreement between nurses and the expert neurologist was high, and there was good short-term stability of ratings of individual elements of the scale.

Mitchell and colleagues examined the pattern of use and clinimetric properties of randomized drug trials for PD published between 1966 and 1998 (16). The UPDRS was the most commonly used scale, and from 1994 to 1998 nearly 70% of trials adopted the UPDRS as an endpoint. In a recent systematic review of rating scales for disability in PD, Ramaker et al. reached a similar conclusion (17), although they stressed the limitations in the UPDRS activities of daily living section and the redundant nature of the scale. Nevertheless, there is widespread agreement that for both medical and surgical (18) trials of PD, the UPDRS is the preferred clinical rating scale.

The UPDRS is so widely accepted that it is unlikely to be replaced; however, there have been efforts to simplify and amend the scale. Van Hilten and colleagues removed five items from part II (salivation, falling, freezing, tremor and sensory symptoms) and also reduced part III to eight items with no loss of reliability (19). They developed the Short Parkinson Evaluation Scale (SPES), an abbreviated form of the UPDRS. Rabey and colleagues examined 117 PD patients using the UPDRS and the SPES, showing that the two scales were comparable (20). In a follow-up study they compared the two scales in 23 patients before and after receiving levodopa, again showing good concordance (21). The SPES's main advantage is that it is shorter and therefore quicker to use. However, it is unlikely that the SPES will gain widespread acceptance, because most movement disorder specialists are familiar with the UPDRS and many large clinical trials have already employed it.

There are several unanticipated benefits of the UPDRS. The scale not only provides a means by which to measure functional performance and medication response, but also provides a fair measure of the severity of the pathological lesion in PD. Vingerhoets et al. studied 35 PD patients using a modified version of the UPDRS, the Purdue pegboard test (a measure of bradykinesia), and ^{18}F-6-fluorodopa PET scanning (22). Fluorodopa uptake in the putamen correlated with the UPDRS score, particularly the bradykinesia subscale. The highest correlation was seen between PET scanning and Purdue pegboard scores, while tremor scores showed no significant correlation with the scans. This suggests that the best single clinical test of nigrostriatal dysfunction is an off bradykinesia score.

The UPDRS also provides a measure of the placebo response. Goetz and colleagues analyzed the placebo arm of the DATATOP study (23), defining a placebo response as a reduction in UPDRS motor scores of 50% or a change of two or more points on at least two different items on the motor scale of the UPDRS. Of the patients in the placebo arm, 17% experienced a placebo effect as defined by these parameters. The UPDRS was sensitive enough to measure the placebo effect, and placebo effects occurred in all parkinsonian clinical domains.

B. Ancillary Motor Scales

The UPDRS is less than ideal at measuring specific motor features of PD. Ancillary motor scales and techniques have been designed to assess three elements of the PD motor exam—gait, bradykinesia, and dyskinesias. Measurement of rigidity is highly subjective, and while it can be quantified (24,25), these measurements are unlikely to be used by clinicians.

Gait impairment is one of the four cardinal features of parkinsonism, and impairment in walking may be the most important clinical deficit due to its impact on patient autonomy. Physicians vary greatly in their ability to rate gait impairment. Further, gait parameters do not correlate well with other measures of PD disability. Vieregge and colleagues examined gait parameters in 17 PD patients and compared them to 33 healthy age-matched controls (26). Stride length, cadence, and gait velocity were significantly reduced in PD patients relative to controls. Stride length correlated with bradykinesia scores, and gait velocity correlated with both bradykinesia and axial motor scores. Total UPDRS motor scores did not correlate with any component of stride data. O'Sullivan and colleagues measured the influence of levodopa on gait parameters in 15 PD patients using a portable gait analysis system (27). Significant increases in gait velocity and stride length were seen when patients were treated with levodopa, but these changes did not correlate with improvements in UPDRS scores.

Gait and balance impairment are of critical importance in PD because of the need to prevent falls. Smithson and colleagues examined 10 PD patients with a history of falls, 10 PD patients with no history of falls, and 10 normal controls, recording performance on steady stance, tandem stance, single-limb stance, functional reach, and pull test. PD patients who fell were able to maintain steady stance, yet were significantly less able to maintain tandem and single limb stance. They also were less able to recover on pull test (28). Bloem and colleagues prospectively studied 59 patients with moderate PD and 55 controls, documenting falls over a 6-month period. One in 4 patients had recurrent falls, and these were most commonly "center of mass" falls triggered by turning, standing up and bending forward. The best clinical predictors of falls were a history of prior falls, disease severity, and an abnormal Romberg test. Surprisingly, the pull test did not adequately predict falls (29).

Inability to initiate movement (akinesia), reduction in amplitude of movement (hypokinesia), and slowing of movement execution (bradykinesia) are the cardinal elements of the motor deficit of PD (30). Bradykinesia correlates well with movement time and, to a lesser extent, with reaction time in motor control testing paradigms (31). These measurements are sensitive but impractical to apply to large numbers of patients. A similarly intensive approach was applied by Van Hilten and colleagues using an activity monitor continuously worn on the wrist to quantify motor performance in 64 patients with PD and 104 controls (32). Objective evidence of slowness correlated poorly with UPDRS measurements, suggesting that the UPDRS may not adequately reflect patients' functional performance at home.

Giovannoni and colleagues developed a simpler and more practical method for measuring bradykinesia, the BRAIN TEST (bradykinesia akinesia incoordination test) (33). This test uses a standard personal computer keyboard and measures the ability of patients to alternatively strike target keys with their index finger. Objective measures of bradykinesia correlated well with motor scores on the UPDRS, and this test's great advantage is its portability and ease of use. Other tests that are even simpler include the Purdue pegboard (in which patients are asked to transfer pegs from a rack into appropriate holes) and a tapping test (in which patients tap a contact board with a pencil as quickly as possible). Muller and colleagues examined 157 previously untreated PD patients (34) and demonstrated that both tests correlated well with parts II and III of the UPDRS; of the two, the pegboard was superior.

Dyskinesias are notoriously difficult to rate for several reasons. Patients are often unaware of dyskinesias, or they may confuse dyskinesias with tremor. Dyskinesias vary with the timing and dosing of levodopa, limiting the ability of neurologists to rate them in a brief office visit. Items 32 and 33 of the UPDRS ask patients to rate the duration and severity of their dyskinesias and are thus dependent on patient recall. To address these concerns, Goetz and colleagues assessed the reliability of a dyskinesia rating scale in 40 patients with PD, by videotaping patients and asking neurologists to rate patients' dyskinesias by severity and type (35); inter- and intra-rater reliability was high. Patients can be trained to recognize dyskinesias using an instructive videotape, and this training is retained over time (36). Hagell and Widner proposed a new rating scale for dyskinesias, the Clinical Dyskinesia Rating Scale (CDRS) (37). The CDRS scores the severity of hyperkinesias and dystonia in the face, neck, trunk, and left and right upper and lower extremity using a 5-point scale (0–4). Using a similar videotape review protocol, inter- and intra-rater agreement were excellent. Hauser and colleagues proposed a simpler means for rating dyskinesias using a home diary filled out by the patient at 30-minute intervals throughout the day (38). Patients were able to distinguish between four clinical states: off, on without dyskinesias, on with nontroublesome dyskinesias, and on with troublesome dyskinesias (those that interfere with function or cause meaningful discomfort). A more quantitative measure of dyskinesias is provided by an approach used by Manson and colleagues (39). They used an ambulatory monitor worn on the shoulder to continuously record dyskinesias, showing that measurements correlated well with videotape recordings and standard rating scale measures.

C. Nonmotor Measures

Nonmotor manifestations of PD are extremely common and remarkably varied. Rating scales have been applied to olfaction, depression, sialorrhea, and swallowing. Hawkes and colleagues measured olfactory dysfunction in PD using the University of Pennsylvania Smell Identification test (40) demonstrating significant deficits in 70–90% of patients, including those with early PD. Specific odors (pizza and wintergreen) were selectively misidentified. Depression is extremely common in PD and almost certainly under-recognized. Various clinical rating scales for depression are available, including the Beck Depression Inventory, Hamilton, and Montgomery-Asberg scales. Leentjens and colleagues screened 53 nondemented PD patients using the Beck Depression Inventory and a structured clinical interview (41). The Beck scale was not able to distinguish depressed from nondepressed patients with a single cut-off score. In a related study, the same group examined 63 nondemented PD patients using the Hamilton and Montgomery-Asberg scales, with greater success in delineating depressed patients (42).

Sialorrhea is a vexing problem for up to 70% of PD patients, and standard treatments using anticholinergic agents are rarely satisfactory (43). Pal and colleagues treated PD patients using botulinum toxin A injected directly into the parotid gland (43). They measured saliva production using patient ratings and objective assessments using dental rolls placed inside the mouth. A similar study performed by Friedman and Potulska (44) also showed that the treatment was effective and well tolerated.

Swallowing disturbances are extremely common in PD. Nilsson et al. assessed 75 PD patients using a quantitative measure of swallowing—the Repetitive Oral Suction Swallow (ROSS) test (45). This objective test measures suction pressure, suction time, and bolus volume during a single swallow, as well as performance during forced repetitive swallows. Although patients rarely complained of swallowing difficulty, abnormalities on the ROSS test were seen in 58, 93, 91 and 94% of patients in Hoehn and Yahr stages 1–4, respectively. Mari and colleagues asked which clinical features best predict patients who are at risk for aspiration (46). A history of coughing on swallowing, combined with coughing during or up to one minute after completion of swallowing a 3 oz cup of water, reliably predicted swallowing abnormalities seen on videofluroscopy.

III. QUALITY-OF-LIFE AND OUTCOME MEASURES

Increased attention has been paid to the impact of chronic neurological disease on health-related quality of life. Karlsen et al. studied 111 PD patients over a 4-year period using the Nottingham health profile questionnaire (47). Patients reported a decrease in physical mobility over time, but also increased distress from pain, social isolation, and emotional stress. Schrag and colleagues studied 124 patients with PD using the European Quality of Life questionnaire, the PD Questionnaire-39, and the Medical Outcome Study Short Form (48), demonstrating similar impairments in mobility, self-care, activities of daily living, physical and social functioning, cognition, communication, pain, and emotional well-being. Patient-completed quality-of-life assessments may be filled out in the office or by telephone questionnaire with no significant loss of validity (49).

Several attempts have been made to measure PD patients' perception of their health status. The Parkinson's Disease Questionnaire (PDQ-39) is a 39-item written tool that measures eight dimensions of health, including mobility, ADL, emotional well-being, stigma, social support, cognition, communication, and body discomfort (50). One hundred and forty six PD patients were examined using the questionnaire and the UPDRS, and scores were highly correlated (50). A similar scale, the Parkinson's Disease Activities of Daily Living Scale (PADLS), was developed and tested in 132 PD patients with similar results (51). The PDQ-39 and PADLS are simple and easy to use, although they are probably too time-consuming to use in routine clinical practice.

Increased attention is also being directed at outcome measures in chronic neurological disorders. These are particularly relevant to PD, given the prolonged disease course and the tendency for many patients to require 24-hour care late in the illness. Aarsland and colleagues measured the rate and predictors of nursing home placement in 178 PD patients (52) and found that older age, functional impairment, dementia, and especially hallucinations were independent predictors of admission to a nursing home. Among PD patients already in nursing homes, the 3-year mortality rate is 50% (53), with increased mortality among patients who are older, white, male, more cognitively impaired, or who develop pneumonia or congestive heart failure.

IV. PRACTICAL GUIDELINES FOR USING RATING SCALES

In this chapter, the most commonly used clinical rating scales are reviewed. These scales are typically applied in clinical trials of investigational treatments for PD. The UPDRS is a powerful, simple, and elegant rating tool for following PD patients. It should be used in the routine care of PD patients, asking patients to fill out the first two sections prior to meeting with the doctor to save time.

The UPDRS motor scores allow the physician to assess the impact of therapeutic interventions and also to measure the clinical progression of disease in a simple and practical manner. Ancillary motor and nonmotor scales can also be useful in clinical practice.

THE UNIFIED PARKINSON DISEASE RATING SCALE (UPDRS)

I. Mentation, Behavior, and Mood

1. Intellectual Impairment
   0 = None
   1 = Mild. Consistent forgetfulness with partial recollection of events and no other difficulties.
   2 = Moderate memory loss, with disorientation and moderate difficulty handling complex problems. Mild but definite impairment of function at home with need of occasional prompting.
   3 = Severe memory loss with disorientation for time and often to place. Severe impairment in handling problems.
   4 = Severe memory loss with orientation preserved to person only. Unable to make judgements or solve problems. Requires much help with personal care. Cannot be left alone at all.

2. Thought Disorder
   0 = None
   1 = Vivid dreaming.
   2 = "Benign" hallucinations with insight retained.
   3 = Occasional to frequent hallucinations or delusions; without insight; could interfere with daily activities.
   4 = Persistent hallucinations, delusions, or florid psychosis. Not able to care for self.

3. Depression
   0 = Not present
   1 = Periods of sadness or guilt greater than normal, never sustained for days or weeks.
   2 = Sustained depression (1 week or more).
   3 = Sustained depression with vegetative symptoms (insomnia, anorexia, weight loss, loss of interest).
   4 = Sustained depression with vegetative symptoms and suicidal thoughts or intent.

4. Motivation/Initiative
   0 = Normal
   1 = Less assertive than usual; more passive.
   2 = Loss of initiative or disinterest in elective (non-routine) activities.
   3 = Loss of initiative or disinterest in day-to-day (routine) activities.
   4 = Withdrawn, complete loss of motivation.

II. Activities of Daily Living (Determine for ON and OFF medications)

5. Speech
   0 = Normal
   1 = Mildly affected. No difficulty being understood.
   2 = Moderately affected. Sometimes asked to repeat statements.
   3 = Severely affected. Frequently asked to repeat statements.
   4 = Unintelligible most of the time.

6. Salivation
   0 = Normal
   1 = Slight but definite excess of saliva in mouth; may have nighttime drooling.
   2 = Moderately excessive saliva; may have minimal drooling.
   3 = Marked excess of saliva with some drooling.
   4 = Marked drooling, requires constant tissue or handkerchief.

7. Swallowing
   0 = Normal
   1 = Rare choking.
   2 = Ocassional choking.
   3 = Requires soft food.
   4 = Requires NG tube or gastrostomy feeding.

8. Handwriting
   0 = Normal
   1 = Slightly slow or small.
   2 = Moderately slow or small; all words are legible.

3 = Severely affected; not all words are legible.

4 = The majority of words are not legible.

9. Cutting food and handling utensils

   0 = Normal

   1 = Somewhat slow and clumsy, but no help needed.

   2 = Can cut most foods, although clumsy and slow; some help needed.

   3 = Food must be cut by someone, but can still feed slowly.

   4 = Needs to be fed.

10. Dressing

   0 = Normal

   1 = Somewhat slow, but no help needed.

   2 = Occasional assistance with buttoning, getting arms in sleeves.

   3 = Considerable help required, but can do some things alone.

   4 = Helpless.

11. Hygiene

   0 = Normal

   1 = Somewhat slow, but no help needed.

   2 = Needs help to shower or bathe; or very slow in hygienic care.

   3 = Requires assistance for washing, brushing teeth, combing hair, going to bathroom.

   4 = Foley catheter or other mechanical aids.

12. Turning in bed and adjusting bed clothes

   0 = Normal

   1 = Somewhat slow and clumsy, but no help needed.

   2 = Can turn alone or adjust sheets, but with great difficulty.

   3 = Can initiate, but not turn or adjust sheets alone.

   4 = Helpless.

13. Falling (unrelated to freezing)

   0 = None

   1 = Rare falling.

   2 = Occasionally falls, less than once per day.

   3 = Falls an average of once daily.

   4 = Falls more than once daily.

14. Freezing when walking

   0 = None

   1 = Rare freezing when walking; may have start-hesitation.

   2 = Occasional freezing when walking.

   3 = Frequent freezing. Occasionally falls from freezing.

   4 = Frequent falls from freezing.

15. Walking

   0 = Normal

   1 = Mild difficulty. May not swing arms or may tend to drag leg.

   2 = Moderate difficulty, but requires little or no assistance.

   3 = Severe disturbance of walking, requiring assistance.

   4 = Cannot walk at all, even with assistance.

16. Tremor (*score right and left side separately*)

   0 = Absent

   1 = Slight and infrequently present.

   2 = Moderate; bothersome to patient.

   3 = Severe; interface with many activities.

   4 = Marked, interferes with most activities.

17. Sensory complaints related to parkinsonism

   0 = None

   1 = Occasionally has numbness, tingling, or mild aching.

   2 = Frequently has numbness, tingling or aching; not distressing.

   3 = Frequent painful sensations.

   4 = Excruciating pain.

III. Motor Examination

18. Speech
    0 = Normal
    1 = Slight loss of expression, diction and/or volume.
    2 = Monotone, slurred but understandable; moderately impaired.
    3 = Marked impairment, difficult to understand.
    4 = Unintelligible.
19. Facial expression
    0 = Normal
    1 = Minimal hypomimia, could be normal "poker face".
    2 = Slight but definitely abnormal diminution of facial expression.
    3 = Moderate hypomimia; lips parted some of the time.
    4 = Masked or fixed facies with severe or complete loss of facial expression; lips parted 1/4 inch or more.
20. Tremor at rest (*score face, lip and chin; right upper; left upper; right lower; left lower*)
    0 = Absent
    1 = Slight and infrequently present.
    2 = Mild in amplitude and persistent or moderate in amplitude, but only intermittently present.
    3 = Moderate in amplitude and present most of the time.
    4 = Marked in amplitude and present most of the time.
21. Action or postural tremor of hands (*score right and left separately*)
    0 = Absent
    1 = Slight; present with action.
    2 = Moderate in amplitude, present with action.
    3 = Moderate in amplitude with posture holding as well as action.
    4 = Marked in amplitude; interferes with feeding.
22. Rigidity (*Judged on passive movement of major joints relaxed in sitting position. Cogwheeling to be ignored. Score neck; right upper; left upper; right lower; left lower*)
    0 = Absent
    1 = Slight or detectable only when activated by mirror or other movements.
    2 = Mild to moderate.
    3 = Marked, but full range of motion easily achieved.
    4 = Severe, range of motion achieved with difficulty.
23. Finger taps (*tap thumb with index finger in rapid succession, with widest amplitude possible, score each hand separately*)
    0 = Normal
    1 = Mild slowing and/or reduction in amplitude.
    2 = Moderately impaired. Definite and early fatiguing. May have occasional arrests in movement.
    3 = Severely impaired. Frequent hesitating in initiating movement or arrests in ongoing movement.
    4 = Can barely perform the task.
24. Hand movements (*Patient opens and closes hands in rapid succession with widest amplitude possible, score each hand separately*)
    0 = Normal
    1 = Mild slowing and/or reduction in amplitude.
    2 = Moderately impaired. Definite and early fatiguing. May have occasional arrests in movement.
    3 = Severely impaired. Frequent hesitation in initiating movement or arrests in ongoing movement.
    4 = Can barely perform the task.
25. Rapid alternating movements of hands (*Pronation/supination movements of hands, vertically or horizontally, with as large an amplitude as possible, both hands simultaneously but score each hand separately*)
    0 = Normal
    1 = Mild slowing and/or reduction in amplitude.
    2 = Moderately impaired. Definite and early fatiguing. May have occasional arrests in movement.
    3 = Severely impaired. Frequent hesitation in initiating movement or arrests in ongoing movement.
    4 = Can barely perform the task.
26. Leg agility with knee bent (*Patient taps heel on ground in rapid succession, picking up entire foot. Amplitude should be about 3 inches, score each leg separately*)

0 = Normal
1 = Mild slowing and/or reduction in amplitude.
2 = Moderately impaired. Definite and early fatiguing. May have occasional arrests in movement.
3 = Severely impaired. Frequent hesitation in initiating movement or arrests in ongoing movement.
4 = Can barely perform the task.

27. Arising from chair (*Patient attempts to arise from straight backed chair with arms folded across chest*)
    0 = Normal
    1 = Slow; or may need more than one attempt.
    2 = Pushes self up from arms of seat.
    3 = Tends to fall back and may have to try more than one time, but can get up without help.
    4 = Unable to rise without help.

28. Posture
    0 = Normal erect
    1 = Not quite erect, slightly stooped posture; could be normal for older person.
    2 = Moderately stooped posture, definitely abnormal; can be slightly leaning to one side.
    3 = Severely stooped posture with kyphosis; can be moderately leaning to one side.
    4 = Marked flexion with extreme abnormality of posture.

29. Gait
    0 = Normal
    1 = Walks slowly, may shuffle with short steps but no festination or propulsion.
    2 = Walks with difficulty, but requires little or no assistance; may have some festination, short steps, or propulsion.
    3 = Severe disturbance of gait, requiring assistance.
    4 = Cannot walk at all, even with assistance.

30. Postural stability (*Response to sudden posterior displacement produced by pull on shoulders while patient erect with eyes open and feet slightly apart. Patient is prepared*)
    0 = Normal
    1 = Retropulsion, but recovers unaided.
    2 = Absence of postural response; would fall if not caught by examiner.
    3 = Very unstable, tends to loss balance spontaneously.
    4 = Unable to stand without assistance.

31. Body bradykinesia and hypokinesia (*Combining slowness, hesitancy, decreased arm swing, small amplitude, and poverty of movement in general*)
    0 = None
    1 = Minimal slowness, giving movement a deliberate character; could be normal for some persons. Possibly reduced amplitude.
    2 = Mild degree of slowness and poverty of movement which is definitely abnormal. Alternatively, some reduced amplitude.
    3 = Moderate slowness, poverty or small amplitude of movement.
    4 = Marked slowness, poverty or small amplitude of movement.

IV. Complications of Therapy

A. Dyskinesias

32. Duration: *What proportion of the waking day are dyskinesias present? Historical information*
    0 = None
    1 = 1%–25% of day.
    2 = 26%–50% of day.
    3 = 51%–75% of day.
    4 = 76%–100% of day.

33. Disability: *How disabling are the dyskinesias? Historical information; may be modified by office examination*
    0 = Not disabling.
    1 = Mildly disabling.
    2 = Moderately disabling.
    3 = Severely disabling.
    4 = Completely disabling.

34. Painful dyskinesias: *How painful are the dyskinesias?*
    0 = No painful dyskinesias
    1 = Slight
    2 = Moderate
    3 = Severe
    4 = Marked
35. Presence of early morning dystonia: *Historical information*
    0 = No
    1 = Yes

B. Clinical Fluctuations

36. Are any "off" periods predictable as to timing after a dose of medications?
    0 = No
    1 = Yes
37. Are any "off" periods unpredictable as to timing after a dose of medication?
    0 = No
    1 = Yes
38. Do any of the "off" periods come on suddenly, e.g. over a few seconds?
    0 = No
    1 = Yes
39. What proportion of the waking day is the patient "off" on average?
    0 = None
    1 = 1%–25% of day.
    2 = 26%–50% of day.
    3 = 51%–75% of day.
    4 = 76%–100% of day.

C. Other Complications

40. Does the patient have anorexia, nausea, or vomiting?
    0 – No
    1 = Yes
41. Does the patient have any sleep disturbances, e.g. insomnia or hypersomnolence?
    0 = No
    1 = Yes
42. Does the patient have symptomatic orthostasis?
    0 = No
    1 = Yes

V. Modified Hoehn and Yahr Staging

Stage 0   = No signs of disease
Stage 1   = Unilateral disease
Stage 1.5 = Unilateral plus axial involvement
Stage 2   = Bilateral disease, without impairment of balance
Stage 2.5 = Mild bilateral disease, with recovery on pull test
Stage 3   = Mild to moderate bilateral disease; some postural instability; physically independent
Stage 4   = Severe disability; still able to walk or stand unassisted
Stage 5   = Wheelchair bound or bedridden unless aided

VI. Schwab and England Activities of Daily Living Scale

100% - Completely independent. Able to do all chores without slowness, difficulty or impairment. Essentially normal. Unaware of any difficulty.
 90% - Completely independent. Able to do all chores with some degree of slowness, difficulty and impairment. Might take twice as long. Beginning to be aware of difficulty.

80% - Completely independent in most chores. Takes twice as long. Conscious of difficulty and slowness.

70% - Not completely independent. More difficulty with some chores. Three to four times as long in some. Must spend a large part of the day with chores.

60% - Some dependency. Can do most chores, but exceedingly slowly and with much effort. Errors; some impossible.

50% - More dependent. Help with half, slower, etc. Difficulty with everything.

40% - Very dependent. Can assist with all chores, but few alone.

30% - With effort, now and then does a few chores alone or begins alone. Much help needed.

20% - Nothing alone. Can be a slight help with some chores. Severe invalid.

10% - Totally dependent, helpless. Complete invalid.

0% - Vegetative functions such as swallowing, bladder and bowel functions are not functioning. Bedridden.

REFERENCES

1. Hughes AJ, Daniel SE, Lees AJ. Improved accuracy of clinical diagnosis of Lewy body Parkinson's disease. Neurology 2001; 57:1497–1499.
2. Jankovic J, Rajput AH, McDermott MP, Perl D. The evolution of diagnosis in early Parkinson's disease. Arch Neurol 2000; 57:369–372.
3. Wenning GK, Ben-Shlomo Y, Hughes A, Daniel SE, Lees A, Quinn NP. What clinical features are most useful to distinguish definite multiple system atrophy from Parkinson's disease. J Neurol Neurosurg Psychiatry 2000; 68:434–440.
4. Gelb DJ, Oliver E, Gilman S. Diagnostic criteria for Parkinson disease. Arch Neurol 1999; 56:33–39.
5. Hoehn MM, Yahr MD. Parkinsonism: onset, progression and mortality. Neurology 1967; 17: 427–442.
6. Zetusky WJ, Jankovic J, Pirozzolo FJ. The heterogeneity of Parkinson's disease. Neurology 1985; 35:522–526.
7. Hershey LA, Feldman BJ, Kim KY, Commichau C, Lichter DG. Tremor at onset. Predictor of cognitive and motor outcome in Parkinson's disease. Arch Neurol 1991; 48:1049–1051.
8. Fahn S, Elton RL, and the members of the UPDRS Development Committee. The Unified Parkinson's disease Scale. In: Fahn S, Marsden CD, Calne DB, Goldstein M, eds. Recent Developments in Parkinson's Disease. Vol. 2. Florham Park, NJ: Macmillan Healthcare Information, 1987:153–163, 293–304.
9. Brown RG, MacCarthy B, Jahanshahi M, Marsden CD. Accuracy of self-reported disability in patients with parkinsonism. Arch Neurol 1989; 46:955–959.
10. Louis ED, Lynch T, Marder K, Fahn S. Reliability of patient completion of the historical section of the Unified Parkinson's Disease Rating Scale. Mov Disord 1996; 11:185–192.
11. Martinez-Martin P, Gil-Nagel A, Morlan Gracia L, Balseiro Gomez J, Martinez-Sarries J, Bermejo F and the cooperative multicentric group. Unified Parkinson's Disease Rating Scale characteristics and structure. Mov Disord 1994; 9:76–83.
12. Richards M, Marder K, Cote L, Mayeux R. Interrater reliability of the Unified Parkinson's Disease Rating Scale motor examination. Mov Disord 1994; 9:89–91.
13. Stebbins GT, Goetz CG. Factor structure of the Unified Parkinson's Disease Rating Scale: motor examination section. Mov Disord 1998; 13:633–636.
14. Goetz CG, Stebbins GT, Chmura TA, Fahn S, Klawans HL, Marsden CD. Mov Disord 1995; 10:263–266.
15. Bennett DA, Shannon KM, Beckett LA, Goetz CG, Wilson RS. Metric properties of nurses' ratings of parkinsonian signs with a modified Unified Parkinson's Disease Rating Scale. Neurology 1997; 49:1580–1587.
16. Mitchell SL, Harper DW, Lau A, Bhalla R. Patterns of outcome measurement in Parkinson's disease clinical trials. Neuroepidemiology 2000; 19:100–108.
17. Ramaker C, Marinus J, Stiggelbout AM, van Hilten BJ. Systematic evaluation of rating scales for impairment and disability in Parkinson's disease. Mov Disord 2002; 17:867–876.
18. Defer G, Widner H, Marie R, Remy P, Levivier M. Core assessment program for surgical interventional therapies in Parkinson's disease (CAPSIT-PD). Mov Disord 1999; 14:572–584.
19. van Hilten JJ, van der Zwan AD, Zwinderman AH, Roos RAC. Rating impairment and disability in Parkinson disease: evaluation of the Unified Parkinson's Disease Rating Scale. Mov Disord 1994; 9:84–88.
20. Rabey JM, Bass H, Bonuccelli U, Brooks D, Klotz P, Korczyn AD, Kraus P, Martinez-Martin P, Morrish P, van Sauten W, van Hilten B. Evaluation of the Short Parkinson's Evaluation Scale:

a new friendly scale for the evaluation of Parkinson's disease in clinical drug trials. Clin Neuropharmacol 1997; 20:322–337.

21. Rabey JM, Klein C, Molochnikov A, Van Hilten B, Krauss P, Bonuccelli U. Comparison of the Unified Parkinson's Disease Rating Scale and the Short Parkinson's Evaluation Scale in patients with Parkinson's disease after levodopa loading. Clin Neuropharmacol 2002; 25:83–88.

22. Vingerhoets FJG, Schulzer M, Calne DB, Snow BJ. Which clinical sign of Parkinson's disease best reflects the nigrostriatal lesion? Ann Neurol 1997; 41:58–64.

23. Goetz CG, Leurgans S, Raman R and the Parkinson Study Group. Placebo-associated improvements in motor function: comparison of subjective and objective sections of the UPDRS in early Parkinson's disease. Mov Disord 2002; 17:283–288..

24. Prochazka A, Bennett DJ, Stephens MJ, Patrick SK, Sears-Duru R, Roberts T, Jhamandas JH. Measurement of rigidity in Parkinson's disease. Mov Disord 1997; 12:24–32.

25. Fung VSC, Burne JA, Morris JGL. Objective quantification of resting and activated parkinsonian rigidity: a comparison of angular impulse and work scores. Mov Disord 2000; 15:48–55.

26. Vieregge P, Stolze H, Klein C, Heberlein I. Gait quantitation in Parkinson's disease—locomotor disability and correlation to clinical rating scales. J Neural Transm 1997; 104:237–248.

27. O'Sullivan JD, Said CM, Dillon LC, Hoffman M, Hughes AJ. Gait analysis in patients with Parkinson's disease and motor fluctuations: influence of levodopa and comparison with other measures of motor function. Mov Disord 1998; 13:900–906.

28. Smithson F, Morris M, Iansek R. Performance on clinical tests of balance in Parkinson's disease. 1998; 78:577–592.

29. Bloem BR, Grimbergen YAM, Cramer M, Willemsen M, Zwinderman AH. Prospective assessment of falls in Parkinson's disease. J Neurol 2001; 248:950–958.

30. van Hilten JJ, Hoff JI, Middelkoop HAM, Roos RAC. The clinimetrics of hypokinesia in Parkinson's disease: subjective versus objective assessment. J Neurol Transm [P-D Sect] 1994; 8:117–121.

31. Zappia M, Montesanti R, Colao R, Quattrone A. Usefulness of movement time in assessment of Parkinson's disease. J Neurol 1994; 241:543–550.

32. van Hilten JJ, Hooglan G, van der Velde EA, van Dijk JG, Kerkhof GA, Roos RAC. Quantitative assessment of parkinsonian patients by continuous wrist activity monitoring. Clin Neuropharmacol 1993; 16:36–45.

33. Giovannoni G, van Schalkwyk J, Fritz VU, Lees AJ. Bradykinesia akinesia incoorination test (BRAIN TEST): an objective computerized assessment of upper limb motor function. J Neurol Neurosurg Psychiatry 1999; 67:624–629.

34. Muller T, Schafer S, Kuhn W, Przuntek H. Correlation between tapping and inserting of pegs in Parkinson's disease. Can J Neurol Sci 2000; 27:311–315.

35. Goetz CG, Stebbins GT, Shale HM, Lang AE, Chernik DA, Chmura TA, Ahlskog JE, Dorflinger EE. Utility of an objective dyskinesia rating scale for Parkinson's disease: inter- and intrarater reliability assessment. Mov Disord 1994; 9:390–394.

36. Goetz CG, Stebbins GT, Blasucci LM, Grobman MS. Efficacy of a patient-training videotape on motor fluctuations for on-off diaries in Parkinson's disease. Mov Disord 1997; 12:1039–1041.

37. Hagell P, Widner H. Clinical rating of dyskinesias in Parkinson's disease: use and reliability of a new rating scale. Mov Disord 1999; 14:448–455.

38. Hauser RA, Friedlander J, Zesiewicz TA, Adler CH, Seeberger LC, O'Brien CF, Molho ES, Factor SA. A home diary to assess functional status in patients with Parkinson's disease with motor fluctuations and dyskinesia. Clin Neuropharmacol 2000; 23:75–81.

39. Manson AJ, Brown P, O'Sullivan JD, Asselman P, Buckwell D, Lees AJ. An ambulatory dyskinesia monitor. J Neurol Neurosurg Psychiatry 2000; 68:196–201.

40. Hawkes CH, Shephard BC, Daniel SE. Olfactory dysfunction in Parkinson's disease. J Neurol Neurosurg Psychiatry 1997; 62:436–446.

41. Leentjens AF, Verhey FR, Luijckx G, Troost J. The validity of the Beck depression inventory as a screening and diagnostic instrument for depression in patients with Parkinson's disease. Mov Disord 2000; 15:1221–1224.

42. Leentjens AF, Verhey FR, Lousberg R, Spitsbergen H, Wilmink FW. The validity of the Hamilton and Montgomery-Asberg depression rating scales as screening and diagnostic tools for depression in Parkinson's disease. Int J Geriatr Psychiatry 2000; 15:644–649.

43. Pal PK, Calne DB, Calne S, Tsui JKC. Botulinum toxin A as a treatment for drooling saliva in PD. Neurology 2000; 54:244–247.

44. Friedman A, Potulska A. Quantitative assessment of parkinsonian sialorrhea and results of treatment with botulinum toxin. Parkinsonism Rel Disord 2001; 7:329–332.

45.   Nilsson H, Ekberg O, Olsson R, Hindfelt B. Quantitative assessment of oral and pharyngeal function in Parkinson's disease. Dysphagia 1996; 11:144–150.
46.   Mari F, Matei M, Ceravolo MG, Pisani A, Montesi A, Provinciali L. Predictive value of clinical indices in detecting aspiration in patients with neurological disorders. J Neurol Neurosurg Psychiatry 1997; 63:456–460.
47.   Karlsen KH, Tandberg E, Arsland D, Larsen JP. Health related quality of life in Parkinson's disease: a prospective longitudinal study. J Neurol Neurosurg Psychiatry 2000; 69:584–589.
48.   Schrag A, Jahanshahi M, Quinn N. How does Parkinson's disease affect quality of life? A comparison with quality of life in the general population. Mov Disord 2000; 15:1112–1118.
49.   Damiano AM, McGrath MM, Willian MK, Snyder CF, LeWitt PA, Reyes PF, Richter RR, Means ED. Evaluation of a measurement strategy for Parkinson's disease: assessing patient health-related quality of life. Qual Life Res 2000; 9:87–100.
50.   Jenkinson C, Fitzpatrick R, Peto V, Greenhall R, Hyman N. The Parkinson's Disease Questionnaire (PDQ-39): development and validation of a Parkinson's disease summary index score. Age Aging 1997; 26:353–357.
51.   Hobson JP, Edwards NI, Meara RJ. The Parkinson's Disease Activities of Daily Living Scale: a new simple and brief subjective measure of disability in Parkinson's disease. Clin Rehab 2001; 15:241–246.
52.   Aarsland D, Larsen JP, Tandberg E, Laake K. Predictors of nursing home placement in Parkinson's disease: a population-based, prospective study. J Am Geriatr Soc 2000; 48:938–942.
53.   Fernandez HH, Lapane KL. Predictors of mortality among nursing home residents with a diagnosis of Parkinson's disease. Med Sci Monit 2002; 8:241–246.

4

Magnetic Resonance Imaging and Positron Emission Tomography Investigations

Joel S. Perlmutter

Washington University School of Medicine, St. Louis, Missouri, U.S.A.

W. R. Wayne Martin

University of Alberta, Edmonton, Alberta, Canada

I. INTRODUCTION

Parkinson's disease (PD) is a progressive disorder that produces tremor, slowness, rigidity, and postural instability. Pathologically there is selective neuronal loss in the substantia nigra with the presence of intraneuronal inclusions (Lewy bodies) containing abnormal deposition of alpha-synuclein, reduced nigrostriatal neuronal projections, and subsequent striatal dopamine deficiency (1). Symptomatic treatment focuses on replacing striatal dopamine; however, no treatment has been proven to slow or halt progression of the disease (2,3). Further, the etiology remains unknown, with ongoing controversy about the role of genetics versus environment (4–8). Other neurodegenerative diseases, like progressive supranuclear palsy (PSP) and multiple system atrophy (MSA), directly damage striatum and may also cause bradykinesia, rigidity, and postural instability. Until recently, these diseases were distinguished from idiopathic PD by subtle clinical features, response to levodopa, or postmortem findings (9).

Many advances in neuroimaging in the last several years have been applied to the study of parkinsonism. In this chapter we will review magnetic resonance (MR)–based and positron emission tomography (PET)–based imaging studies and how they have helped to reveal new insights into the pathophysiology and mechanisms of treatment of PD. Further, we will emphasize potential clinical applications, including attempts at developing diagnostic evaluations.

II. MAGNETIC RESONANCE IMAGING AND SPECTROSCOPY

MR imaging and spectroscopy rely primarily on the interplay between external magnetic fields and the resonant frequency of water protons in tissue. Most imaging is based on the fact that hydrogen nuclei are the most abundant nuclei in biological tissues, although images could in theory be made using other nuclei (e.g., phosphorus). Image contrast depends on the specific imaging parameters utilized, but usually represents a complex function of proton density, longitudinal (spin-lattice) relaxation time (T1), and transverse (spin-spin) relaxation time (T2) of protons in tissue. Magnetic field inhomogeneities induced by tissue attributes modify the apparent T2 and have an important effect on image contrast, termed $T2^*$.

A.   Conventional Magnetic Resonance Imaging

T1-weighted images tend to display superior gray-white matter differentiation compared with images obtained with T2-weighted sequences and allow the head of the caudate nucleus and the lenticular nucleus to be delineated clearly. They do not, however, allow the lenticular nucleus to be subdivided into its two major components. In contrast, T2-weighted images allow this nucleus to be subdivided into the globus pallidus and putamen, with the former structure displaying reduced signal intensity as compared to the latter. This differentiation becomes increasingly evident through the first three decades of life. The pallidal signal then remains relatively constant until the sixth or seventh decade, after which the signal attenuation becomes more prominent. Similar areas of reduced signal are seen in the midbrain (red nucleus and substantia nigra), the dentate nucleus, and, to a lesser extent, the putamen.

The low signal regions seen on T2-weighted images correlate with sites of ferric ion accumulation as determined in vitro by Perls' Prussian blue stain. Tissue iron decreases T2 relaxation times through the $T2^*$ effect, i.e., a local inhomogeneity in the magnetic field that dephases proton spin, resulting in signal loss. This iron susceptibility effect is best seen on heavily T2-weighted images obtained with high field (1.5 tesla) MR systems (10,11). It is important to note that gradient echo sequences are much more sensitive to iron-induced susceptibility changes than are the fast spin echo sequences that have become the routine method for producing T2-weighted images in many clinical centers.

In the early days of clinical MR, the anatomical detail evident in images of the midbrain led investigators to evaluate the potential utility of this technology in PD. As noted above, T2-weighted images demonstrate a prominent low signal area in the red nucleus and the substantia nigra pars reticulata, structures that are separated by the substantia nigra pars compacta. A narrowing or smudging of this high signal zone separating the red nucleus and the pars reticulata has been reported in PD, consistent with the well-established prominent pathological involvement in this area (12,13).

Although the demonstration of these midbrain changes may ultimately be of diagnostic value in PD, conventional clinical MR techniques are not sufficiently sensitive at present to detect these changes routinely. Nigral changes in PD may be detected in population studies, but technical factors such as slice thickness, partial volume averaging, and positioning make it difficult to conclusively define nigral abnormalities in individual patients. The field of MR, however, is evolving rapidly, and the development of new methods, such as that described by Hutchinson and Raff (14) using a combination of inversion recovery pulse sequences with image segmentation, shows promise for increasing the sensitivity to the degenerative nigral changes of PD. These investigators reported structural changes in the nigra, even in the earliest stages of symptomatic PD, with this combination of sequences. Hu et al. (15) reported that nigral changes on inversion recovery sequences in PD correlate with measures of striatal dopaminergic function using [^{18}F]fluorodopa PET.

Abnormalities in other neurodegenerative parkinsonian disorders have been reported with conventional MR imaging. In PSP, atrophy of the midbrain with a dilated cerebral aqueduct and enlarged perimesencephalic cisterns has been reported (16). There may be increased signal in periaqueductal regions, coincident with the neuropathological finding of gliosis in these regions. The diameter of the midbrain is significantly decreased in PSP and is normal in PD (17). Dubinsky and Jankovic (18) have reported that as many as 33% of patients with a clinical presentation of PSP have multiple infarcts on MR. In corticobasal ganglionic degeneration, T2-weighted images have been reported to show decreased signal intensity in the lenticular nucleus, ventricular enlargement, and asymmetrical cortical atrophy (19).

MRI may be useful in differentiating MSA from PD (20–23). The most frequently reported abnormality has been a low signal in the putamen on T2-weighted images, more prominent than that seen in normal subjects. Lang and coworkers (24) reported a "slit-like void" in the putamen on T2-weighted images (and to a lesser degree on T1-weighted images) in patients with striatonigral degeneration (SND), which they suggest is highly characteristic of this disorder. In their study, the MRI changes correlated with the extent of neuronal loss and gliosis and with the pattern of iron deposition evident at autopsy. These authors and others (25) also reported the presence of a high signal rim on the lateral border of the putamen on T2-weighted images in SND. Putamenal atrophy has been reported to correlate with the severity of parkinsonian symptoms (23). Kraft et al. (26) suggested that the combination of dorsolateral putamenal low signal with a high signal lateral rim is highly specific for MSA, whereas putamenal low signal alone does not exclude a diagnosis of PD. Cerebellar and brainstem atrophy has been reported in patients with parkinsonian and cerebellar subtypes of MSA (27,28).

B. Quantitative Estimation of Regional Brain Iron

The brain has a very high iron content, particularly in the basal ganglia. Elevated iron levels are evident in various neurodegenerative disorders, including PD where increased iron in the substantia nigra has been reported (29,30). Extended x-ray absorption fine structure experiments have shown that ferritin is the only storage protein detectable in both control and parkinsonian brain, with increased iron loading of ferritin in PD (31).

Ferritin in aqueous solution strongly affects transverse relaxation times, but these changes are much less prominent in tissue. T2 relaxation times were reduced in substantia nigra, caudate, and putamen in PD patients as compared to healthy controls (32), but these decreases were small, and there was substantial overlap between groups. Vymazel et al. (33) reported a trend toward T2 shortening in the substantia nigra in PD. Others have also observed an imperfect correlation between T2 values and quantitative assays of iron and ferritin (34). The lack of a more substantial difference is not surprising since regional iron content is only one of several determinants of transverse relaxation times in tissue.

Methods have been developed to estimate iron content directly with MR. Bartzokis et al. (35) utilized the influence of the external magnetic field strength on ferritin-induced T2 changes to derive an index of regional tissue ferritin levels. Others have exploited the ability of paramagnetic substances such as iron to create local magnetic field inhomogeneities that alter transverse relaxation times in the brain (36,37). A strong direct relationship between age and both putamen and caudate iron content measured with this methodology has been reported (38). This age-related increase may increase the probability of free-radical formation in the striatum, thereby representing a "risk factor" for the development of PD in which nigrostriatal neurons may be affected by increased oxidative stress. Significantly increased iron content in the putamen and pallidum in PD and a correlation with the severity of clinical symptomatology with more severely affected patients having a higher iron content in these structures has also been reported (39,40).

C. Magnetic Resonance Spectroscopy

Magnetic resonance spectroscopy (MRS) provides a noninvasive method to quantify metabolite concentrations in the brain. This technique is based on the general principle that the resonant frequency of a specific metabolite depends on its chemical environment. Clinical MRS studies have concentrated primarily on metabolites visible with proton (^{1}H) spectroscopy and measured in single, localized tissue volumes in the brain. These metabolites consist primarily of N-acetyl aspartate (NAA), creatine/phosphocreatine (Cr), and choline. NAA is contained almost exclusively within neurons (41) and is therefore a marker of neuronal loss or dysfunction. Several studies utilizing ^{1}H MRS in PD have been reported (42). In general, no significant changes have been observed (43,44). Ellis and coworkers (45), however, while reporting no significant difference in the NAA/Cr ratio in levodopa-treated patients, did observe a reduced NAA/Cr ratio in drug-naïve PD patients compared with both a treated PD group and a normal control group. These authors suggested that the reduced ratio in PD may reflect a functional abnormality of striatal neurons, which can be reversed with levodopa treatment.

In contrast to the apparent lack of significant changes in PD, there does appear to be a significant reduction in basal ganglia NAA concentration in MSA. Davie et al. (46) reported a significant reduction in absolute levels of NAA in the lentiform nucleus, particularly in patients with SND, suggesting that the spectroscopic measurement of NAA levels may provide a clinically useful technique to help differentiate MSA from PD. In spite of these observations, however, a systematic review of striatal spectroscopy in parkinsonian syndromes concluded that results are sufficiently heterogeneous to preclude the use of spectroscopy in differential diagnosis at the present time (47).

In conclusion, the technology and quality of MR imaging and spectroscopy continues to evolve rapidly, allowing investigators to define new features to differentiate the parkinsonian syndromes. While the clinical utility of these modalities is limited at present, new developments can be expected to expand our knowledge of these disorders. Novel pulse sequences may provide new information regarding the pathology of these conditions, while improved spectroscopic techniques will enhance our ability to study energy metabolism and other metabolite changes. Lastly, although not considered in the present review, functional MR imaging shows great promise in evaluating the role of the basal ganglia in motor control and cognition, both in normal individuals and in those with PD and related disorders.

III. POSITRON EMISSION TOMOGRAPHY

PET provides an in vivo measure of brain function and has been a useful tool for investigation of the pathophysiology and therapy of PD. This technique, depending upon the type of radiopharmaceutical, experimental design, method of data collection, and data analysis, can be used to measure different aspects of cerebral function. The following section will focus on studies relating to PD that illustrate the utility of different types of PET-based measurements including regional pathophysiology, physiologic and pharmacological activation, radioligand binding, and assessment of presynaptic nigrostriatal neurons.

A. Regional Pathophysiology

PET permits measurements of regional cerebral blood flow or metabolism either at rest or during activation. In general, blood flow and metabolism reflect neuronal activity (48), but it is important to note that increased flow or metabolism may accompany either increased excitation or inhibition, since both may cost energy to maintain or change membrane gradients (49,50). Thus, a PET-measured blood flow response could indicate a change of input (increased or decreased) to that region or alterations in local interneuronal activity (51). Under pathological conditions, changes in flow may not coincide with changes in local metabolism or neuronal activity (52).

Regional PET measurements have been used to identify sites of abnormal function in diseases such as PD. Abnormalities of local flow or metabolism found in basal ganglia in patients with PD reflect the known striatal dopamine deficiency, but PET studies have found other functional abnormalities in other brain regions involved not only with motor control but also with cognitive functions (53–59). Application of sophisticated statistical techniques to determine the pattern of regional glucose metabolism permits differentiation of idiopathic PD patients from normals and those with SND (60).

B. Physiological and Pharmacological Activation

Comparisons of PET scans collected before and during physiological activation permit identification of brain responses or dysfunction not found in the resting state alone. Such activation studies can be a powerful way to determine which regions of the normal brain are associated with a stimulus and to determine the functional consequences of neurological disorders, such as PD.

Statistical challenges can complicate analysis of activation studies, since this typically involves large numbers of regional comparisons potentially leading to false-positive responses or Type 1 errors. Several sophisticated techniques that differ in the degree of conservatism with which they approach the problem of multiple comparisons have been used. The hypothesis generation, hypothesis-testing approach is designed to minimize Type 1 errors and ensure that each finding is reliable (61,62), but this strategy may have limited sensitivity for detection of low-level responses. Alternatives include the widely used Statistical Parametric Mapping analysis software (SPM99) (63) that examines the entire data set for voxels and clusters of voxels that have significant group or condition effects or interactions, using a multiple comparison correction. A more elaborate approach called the Scaled Subprofile Model developed by Moeller et al. (64) and applied by Eidelberg et al. determines the regional metabolic covariation patterns for groups of patients or controls (60,65). This covariance pattern can be applied to each subject and a value generated that indicates how well the covariance pattern fits the individual and whether or not two groups differ in how closely they fit the pattern. However, this method does not provide information on the actual activity levels of different regions. Thus, the results and conclusions of a given blood flow study will in part depend upon the statistical procedures used to analyze it.

Activation paradigms have been applied to the study of PD. Some studies have attempted to use behavioral activation of the sensorimotor system with motor control tasks (66,67): imagined motor tasks (68,69), sensory paradigms (70), or certain cognitive systems (e.g., working memory) (71). Interpretation of some studies may be hampered by differences in task performance between PD and controls, making it difficult to determine whether brain activation differs due to the disease state or to the performance state. In other words, if PD patients are slower than controls on a motor activation task and their pattern of brain activity is different from controls during the task, it may reflect the fact that the brain operates differently when movement is slowed, rather than a fundamental difference due to the disease. One solution to this problem is to use tasks that PD patients are not impaired on or to make the tasks equivalently difficult for the two groups (e.g., speed up or degrade the stimuli for controls).

Pharmacological activation provides another means for investigation of relevant brain pathways. For PD, this has mostly involved studies of responses to dopaminergic challenges using PET. The utility of pharmacological activation has been demonstrated in animal studies starting with ex vivo autoradiography in rat models of parkinsonism that revealed new insights into the functional anatomy of dopamine D1- and D2-influenced basal ganglia pathways (72–77). These types of studies have been extended to nonhuman primates using PET which have demonstrated the specificity and sensitivity of this approach and identified the relationship among functional pathways mediated by D2, D1-like, and D3-preferring dopamine agonists (72,78–80).

PET pharmacological activation has been used to investigate dopa-induced dyskinesias (DID) (81). Treatment with levodopa, a precursor of dopamine, initially ameliorates the clinical symptoms of PD including stiffness, slowness, and resting tremor. However, chronic levodopa treatment can produce severe involuntary movements, limiting treatment. Pallidotomy, placement of a surgical lesion in the internal segment of the globus pallidus (GPi), reduces DID. Because this result is inconsistent with current theories of both basal ganglia function and DID, the brain's response to levodopa was investigated. A dose of levodopa that produced clinical benefit without inducing DID was used to examine the brain response to levodopa without the confounding effect of differences in motor behavior. Patients with DID had a significantly greater response in ventrolateral thalamus, and this response was associated with decreased activity in primary motor cortex. These findings provide a testable physiological explanation for the clinical efficacy of pallidotomy and demonstrate a fundamental change in how the brain responds to levodopa after chronic treatment.

Activation studies also have been used to identify changes in brain function associated with physiological tasks produced by surgical interventions such as pallidotomy (82), subthalamotomy (83), deep brain stimulation of the pallidum (84,85), and stimulation of the subthalamic nucleus (86). The mechanism of action of deep brain stimulation has been examined using PET. Stimulation of the ventral intermediate nucleus of the thalamus increased blood flow in the supplementary motor area, a direct target of this thalamic region, suggesting that deep brain stimulation drives efferent axons (87).

Others have determined the effects of levodopa upon physiological activation tasks to identify changes in patterns of regional metabolic covariance that is typical for PD (88), drug-mediated pathways important for activities such as working memory (89), and changes in responses to motor tasks (90). Agonist-mediated pharmacological activation studies may be more sensitive to detection of changes in a pathway than direct measurement of specific receptors, but it is possible that responses are influenced by co-modulators, tone of other transmitter systems, etc. Although pharmacological activation may be a sensitive test, it may have limited specificity. Subsequent investigation of receptors or markers of presynaptic nigrostriatal neurons may be necessary to identify the specific causes of the altered response to a drug.

C. Radioligand Binding

Noninvasive PET measurement of radioligand binding is a powerful tool for in vivo study of neuropharmacology. A variety of radioligands have been developed for the study of different brain receptors by PET (91), but this review will focus on the dopaminergic system. These radioligands are generally labeled with carbon-11 (^{11}C)($t_{1/2} = 20$ min) or fluorine-18 (^{18}F) ($t_{1/2} = 110$ min), isotopes that can be produced in curie quantities by in-house medical cyclotrons. The shorter half-life of ^{11}C limits its utility to radioligands that require relatively short imaging times after injection into the subject, but has the potential advantage of allowing repeat studies within the same imaging session, as well as a lower absorbed radiation burden. Fluorine-18 is useful as a label for radioligands that require longer imaging sequences and has the potential advantage of greater laboratory convenience due to its longer half-life.

Application to parkinsonism revealed that striatal D2-like radioligand binding was either elevated, unchanged, or reduced, suggesting that a variety of methodological differences across studies produced such discrepancies (92–96). These discrepancies may be explained by a time-dependent change in D2 receptors in nonhuman primates after induction of a nigrostriatal lesion (97–99). This latter finding provided new insights into the relationship between striatal dopamine deficiency and the clinical manifestations of either parkinsonism or dystonia. In fact, a PET study in patients with primary dystonia revealed a reduction in radioligand binding in the putamen (100) as in a previous animal study. Subsequent genetic studies have now confirmed that childhood-onset primary dystonia may be associated with a specific genetic defect in the DYT1 gene that codes for a protein torsin A, which is expressed in the pars compacta of the substantia nigra, a key source of dopaminergic neurons projecting to the putamen (101).

Radioligand with only moderate affinity for D2-like receptors, like [^{11}C]raclopride, are displaceable by endogenous dopamine (102). Therefore, changes in synaptic dopamine concentrations alter binding of radioligand to D2-like receptors due to competition, and binding of [^{11}C]raclopride as measured by PET is inversely related to the synaptic concentrations of dopamine. Using this technique, multiple investigators have demonstrated that a variety of drugs alter synaptic dopamine (103–108). This approach has revealed that physiological activity such as flexing an ankle releases dopamine in the contralateral putamen more in normals than in people with PD (109). Combining administration of amphetamine with PET measures of [^{11}C]raclopride may also provide a measure of endogenous dopamine release. This approach has been used to demonstrate increased dopamine release associated with persisting benefit from fetal cell transplantation in a patient with PD (110).

D. Measurement of Presynaptic Nigrostriatal Neurons

Since it is well known that degeneration of nigrostriatal neurons underlies PD, measurement of these presynaptic neurons is a goal of many PET studies. Garnett et al. (111) first reported the preferential accumulation of radioactivity in normal human striata after administration of the dopa analog [^{18}F]fluorodopa (FD), which crosses the blood-brain barrier (BBB) and is decarboxylated to [^{18}F]fluorodopamine, a charged molecule which is trapped extravascularly in a manner similar to levodopa. Normally, presynaptic terminals of nigrostriatal dopaminergic neurons contain most of the striatal decarboxylase activity. Thus FD PET presumably reflects dopaminergic innervation. However, as presynaptic neurons degenerate, a greater portion of residual decarboxylase activity resides in other compartments (112). Nevertheless, [^{18}F]fluorodopamine accumulation likely reflects decarboxylase activity, which may indirectly reflect, in part, residual nigrostriatal neurons (113,114).

The potential clinical utility of FD was promising as PET images clearly revealed decreased striatal accumulation in people with PD (65,115–117). Other radiotracers have been used to label other components of presynaptic nigrostriatal neurons. These other tracers can be divided into those that bind to presynaptic dopamine uptake sites or vesicular transport sites or, like FD, reflect dopa decarboxylase activity. Each of these has been demonstrated to have reduced striatal uptake in either people with PD or in animal models of parkinsonism (118–121); with differing degrees of correlation to various motor manifestations or in vitro measures of nigrostriatal function (122–124).

One key question is whether PET imaging can be used as a diagnostic test to supplement clinical diagnosis. A diagnostic test requires high specificity and high sensitivity with a high positive predictive value. Such investigations have not been done for PET and PD. There are several studies that begin to address specificity. Low striatal FD uptake may distinguish PD from normals (125–128) or those with dopa-responsive dystonia (129), but other presynaptic tracers may also provide similar information (130–132) or distinguish PD from essential tremor (133). Specificity is a greater problem. FD uptake alone does not separate PD from patients with MSA (134,135), Machado-Joseph disease (136), or spinocerebellar ataxia with parkinsonism (137), but relatively small studies suggest that combining FD with other tracers such as measures of dopamine receptors or fluorodeoxyglucose (FDG) may improve the ability to distinguish PD from MSA or PSP (138,139). Markers of the dopamine transporter system also provide some distinction between these different parkinsonian groups (140). Potentially, PET may be able to distinguish underlying idiopathic PD in people with exposure to dopamine receptor–blocking drugs since those patients with low FD uptake may be more likely to have long-lasting or progressive parkinsonism after cessation of the offending drug compared to those with normal FD uptake (141).

Despite the questionable specificity of PET measures of nigrostriatal neurons to distinguish PD from other parkinsonian conditions, there are still several potential uses of these PET markers. Presymptomatic diagnosis of PD could be an important clinical and research tool. Asymptomatic patients exposed to 1-methyl-4-phenyl-1,2,3,6-tetra-hydropyridine (MPTP) had intermediate values of striatal FD uptake compared to PD and normals (115). Monkeys treated with low doses of MPTP that did not produce parkinsonian signs had decreased striatal uptake (142). Other studies have reported that some unaffected monozygotic twins and nontwin relatives of PD patients had abnormally low striatal FD uptake (143–146) or in asymptomatic family members that have a parkin gene mutation (147). These latter studies emphasize the importance of a potential identification of an endophenotype for genetics research.

PET may also provide an objective measure of disease progression in PD (125, 148–149), which can be particularly useful for assessing changes in rate of progression with a variety of interventions. For example, several groups have attempted to use either FD PET or other markers of presynaptic neurons to examine disease progression in early PD patients treated with either ropinirole or pramipexole (150–152). From a neuroimaging perspective, there are important caveats that must be considered for proper interpretation of these studies. First, it is important to determine whether the intervention acutely alters the uptake of tracer. For example, dopamine agonists may alter release of presynaptic dopamine (153), which could alter uptake of selective imaging markers. Some studies have demonstrated differential effects of short-term exposure to levodopa compared to a dopamine agonist (in this case pramipexole) on dopamine transport markers (154). It is not clear whether other dopamine agonists may have a similar effect (155), but such data emphasize that this is an important issue for interpretation of such studies.

PET also has been used to monitor the efficacy of fetal dopamine cell implantation into striatum of patients with PD. In two patients who had unilateral implantation into caudate and putamen, there was little improvement after 5–6 months and no increased uptake of FD (156). Another patient who also had unilateral implantation of fetal mesencephalic dopamine neurons into the putamen had clinical improvement beginning at 5 weeks, and his clinical condition stabilized about 3 months after surgery (157). FD PET in that subject demonstrated an increased uptake of FD 5 months after transplant. Two of seven patients that had bilateral fetal tissue transplantation had FD PET before and as long as 33 months after surgery (158). In one patient, the uptake of FD in the posterior putamen increased. The other patient had no increase in FD uptake 9 months posttransplantation. Bilateral fetal tissue implants into the caudate and putamen in two MPTP-induced parkinsonian patients produced no change 5–6 months postoperatively but a marked increase by 12–13 months, paralleling clinical improvement (159). Two other PD patients that had fetal mesencephalic tissue transplanted unilaterally into the putamen had gradual clinical improvement beginning 6 and 12 weeks later and reaching a maximum at 4–5 months post-operatively (160). FD PET demonstrated increased uptake at the operative site that continued to increase after there was no further clinical improvement (161). Results from a blinded clinical trial of fetal transplant demonstrated that those under 60 years had benefit, whereas those older than 60 did not; yet, FD PET demonstrated that both groups had equally improved striatal uptake after transplantation (162). Furthermore, in that same study two patients had come to autopsy. Each had marked asymmetry of immunostaining of tyrosine hydroxylase (a marker of dopaminergic neurons), but symmetrically increased uptake of FD after transplantation (163). Interestingly, one study found that FD uptake was higher in patients who have developed markedly increased dyskinesias (which may indicate excessive dopamine activity) after transplantation (164), whereas another group found no relationship of dyskinesias to degree of increased FD uptake (165). These clinical/PET discrepancies raise questions about specificity of interpretation of the FD PET findings for these studies.

Most investigators assume that increased accumulation of FD reflects functioning grafts with either increased decarboxylase activity or increased neuronal storage capacity. The following supports this position: (a) there is no change in the BBB to gadolinium MR imaging, (b) the delayed time-course of the increased FD uptake and the clinical improvement coincide, and (c) animal experiments demonstrate intact BBB. However, other data suggest that the BBB may not be intact. First, gadolinium is a large molecule and may not indicate relevant changes in BBB to smaller molecules like FD. Second, increased accumulation of [^{18}Ga]EDTA at the surgical site where FD uptake also increased in patients 6 weeks after adrenal medullary implants suggests an impairment of the BBB (166). Third, increased FD accumulation may occur at a surgical cavitation in an MPTP-treated monkey that did not have tissue transplantation (167). Fourth, studies in rats provide clues that the BBB may change after transplantation. For example, progressive angiogenesis develops in the thalamus after transplantation of dissociated fetal cells (168). Although the permeability of these vessels may be normal to large particles or molecules, like India ink and peroxidase, the surface area of the vessels in the region of the transplant increases, which could increase passage of tracer molecules like FD. These data suggest that increased accumulation of FD may indicate changes in tracer uptake not due to functioning graft tissue. It is important to consider that postmortem studies of PD patients who had fetal transplants with postoperative increased FD uptake have had viable, functioning transplanted neurons (163,169). Therefore, there may be an important role for FD PET in the evaluation of these procedures.

FD has been used to investigate the clinical response to levodopa. Leenders et al. (170) compared mildly to severely affected PD patients with rapid clinical fluctuations in response to individual doses of levodopa. Severely affected patients had the greatest decrease in uptake ratio compared to normals, and mild patients had intermediate values. The authors suggested that ratios directly reflect striatal storage capacity of dopamine, and the marked decrease in severely affected patients causes rapid, symptomatic fluctuations to oral levodopa. Alterations in tracer delivery, differential effects from variable length of time patients stopped levodopa prior to study, and changes in metabolism of FD are potential alternate explanations for their findings.

Some patients have less benefit from oral levodopa if taken at mealtimes. Nutt et al. (171) found that large neutral amino acids caused an increase in symptoms in patients treated with continuous intravenous infusions of levodopa. To investigate the mechanism of this observation, Leenders et al. (172) found that intravenous amino acid loading caused a marked decrease in striatal uptake of [^{18}F] activity in a normal volunteer. These findings represent the first direct evidence in humans for competition between levodopa and other amino acids for striatal uptake.

IV. CONCLUDING REMARKS

MRI and PET are expensive technologies that permit noninvasive evaluation of brain structure and function. As such, they can potentially provide new insights into the pathophysiology of PD. Clinical efficacy must be demonstrated prior to routine clinical-application (173,174). However, these neuroimaging modalities have provided exciting new insights into the pathophysiology and treatment of PD. They also hold promise for providing objective measures needed for developing new treatments to alter the progression of this devastating disease.

ACKNOWLEDGMENTS

Supported by: NIH grants NS39913 and NS41509, the Greater St. Louis Chapter of the American Parkinson Disease Association (APDA), APDA Advanced Center for PD Research at Washington University, the Ruth Kopolow Fund, and the Barnes-Jewish Hospital Foundation.

REFERENCES

1. Gibb WR. The pathology of parkinsonian disorders. In: Quinn NP, Jenner PG, eds. Disorders of Movement: Clinical, Pharmacological and Physiological Aspects. London: Academic Press, 1989:33–58.

2. Shoulson I. Experimental therapeutics of neurodegenerative disorders: unmet needs. Science 1998; 282:1072–1073.
3. Shults CW, Oakes D, Kieburtz K, Beal F, Haas R, Plumb S, Juncos JL, Nutt J, Shoulson I, Carter J, Kompoliti K, Perlmutter JS, Reich S, Stern M, Watts RL, Kurlan R, Molho E, Harrison M, Lew M, and the Parkinson Study Group. Effects of coenzyme Q10 in early Parkinson disease: evidence of slowing of the functional decline. Arch Neurol 2002; 59:1541–1550.
4. Duvoisin RC. Genetic and environmental factors in Parkinson's disease. Adv Neurol 1999; 80: 161–163.
5. Tanner CM, Ottman R, Goldman SM, Ellenberg J, Chan P, Mayeux R, Langston JW. Parkinson disease in twins: an etiologic study. JAMA 1999; 281:341–346.
6. Langston JW. Epidemiology versus genetics in Parkinson's disease: progress in resolving an age-old debate. Ann Neurol 1998; 44:S45–52.
7. De Michele G, Filla A, Volpe G, De Marco V, Gogliettino A, Ambrosio G, Marconi R, Castellano AE, Campanella G. Environmental and genetic risk factors in Parkinson's disease: a case-control study in southern Italy. Mov Disord 1996; 11:17–23.
8. Racette BA, McGee-Minnich L, Moerlein SM, Mink JW, Videen TO, Perlmutter JS. Welding related parkinsonism: clinical features, treatment and pathophysiology. Neurology 2001; 56:8–13.
9. Rajput AH, Pahwa R, Pahwa P, Rajput A. Prognostic significance of the onset mode in parkinsonism. Neurology 1993; 43:829–830.
10. Olanow CW. Magnetic resonance imaging in parkinsonism. Neurol Clin 1992; 10:405–420.
11. Rutledge JN, Hilal SK, Silver AJ, et al. Study of movement disorders and brain iron by MR. AJNR 1987; 8:397–411.
12. Duguid JR, De la Paz R, DeGroot J. Magnetic resonance imaging of the midbrain in Parkinson's disease. Ann Neurol 1986; 20:744–747.
13. Braffman BH, Grossman RI, Goldberg HI, et al. MR imaging of Parkinson disease with spin-echo and gradient-echo sequences. AJR Am J Roentgenol 1989; 152:159–165.
14. Hutchinson M, Raff U. Structural changes of the substantia nigra in Parkinson's disease as revealed by MR imaging. AJNR 2000; 21:697–701.
15. Hu MTM, White SJ, Herlihy AH, et al. A comparison of 18F-dopa PET and inversion recovery MRI in the diagnosis of Parkinson's disease. Neurology 2001; 56:1195–1200.
16. Savoiardo M, Strada L, Girotti F, et al. MR imaging in progressive supranuclear palsy and Shy-Drager syndrome. J Comput Assist Tomogr 1989; 13:555–560.
17. Warmuth-Metz M, Naumann M, Csotti I, Solymosi L. Measurement of the midbrain diameter on routine magnetic resonance imaging. Arch Neurol 2001; 58:1076–1079.
18. Dubinsky RM, Jankovic J. Progressive supranuclear palsy and a multi-infarct state. Neurology 1987; 37:570–576.
19. Hauser RA, Hauser RA, Murtaugh FR, Akhter K, Gold M, Olanow CW. Magnetic resonance imaging of corticobasal degeneration. J Neuroimaging 1996; 6:222–226.
20. Drayer BP, Olanow W, Burger P, et al. Parkinson plus syndrome: diagnosis using high field MR imaging of brain iron. Radiology 1986; 159:493–498.
21. Stern MB, Braffman BH, Skolnick BE, Hurtig HI, Grossman RI. Magnetic resonance imaging in Parkinson's disease and parkinsonian syndromes. Neurology 1989; 39:1524–1526.
22. Pastakia B, Polinsky R, Di Chiro G, Simmons JT, Brown R, Wener L. Multiple system atrophy (Shy-Drager syndrome): MR imaging. Radiology 1986; 159:499–502.
23. Wakai M, Kume A, Takahashi A, Ando T, Hashizume Y. A study of parkinsonism in multiple system atrophy: clinical and MRI correlation. Acta Neurol Scand 1994; 90:225–231.
24. Lang AE, Curran T, Provias J, Bergeron C. Striatonigral degeneration: iron deposition in putamen correlates with the slit-like void signal of magnetic resonance imaging. Can J Neurol Sci 1994; 21:311–318.
25. Konagaya M, Konagaya Y, Iida M. Clinical and magnetic resonance imaging study of extrapyramidal symptoms in multiple system atrophy. J Neurol Neurosurg Psychiatry 1994; 57:1528–1531.
26. Kraft E, Schwarz J, Trenkwalder C, Vogl T, Pfluger T, Oertel WH. The combination of hypointense and hyperintense signal changes on T2-weighted magnetic resonance imaging sequences: a specific marker of multiple system atrophy?. Arch Neurol 1999; 56:225–228.
27. Savoiardo M, Strada L, Girotti F, D'Incerti L, Sberna M, Soliveri P, Balzarini L. Olivoponto-cerebellar atrophy: MR diagnosis and relationship to multiple system atrophy. Radiology 1990; 174:693–696.

28. Schulz JB, Klockgether T, Petersen D, Jauch M, Muller-Schauenburg W, Spieker S, Voigt K, Dichgans J. Multiple system atrophy: natural history, MRI morphology, and dopamine receptor imaging with 123IBZM-SPECT. J Neurol Neurosurg Psychiatry 1994; 57:1047–1056.

29. Dexter DT, Wells FR, Lees AJ, Agid F, Agid Y, Jenner P, Marsden CD. Increased nigral iron content and alterations in other metal ions occurring in brain in Parkinson's disease. J Neurochem 1989; 52:1830–1836.

30. Sofic E, Riederer P, Heinsen H, Beckmann H, Reynolds GP, Hebenstreit G, Youdim MB. Increased iron (III) and total iron content in post mortem substantia niga of parkinsonian brain. J Neural Transm 1988; 74:199–205.

31. Griffiths PD, Dobson BR, Jones GR, Clarke DT. Iron in the basal ganglia in Parkinson's disease: an in vitro study using extended X-ray absorption fine structure and cryo-electron microscopy. Brain 1999; 122:667–673.

32. Antinoni A, Leenders KL, Meier D, Oertel WH, Boesiger P, Anliker M. T2 relaxation time in patients with Parkinson's disease. Neurology 1993; 43:697–700.

33. Vymazal J, Righini A, Brooks RA, Canesi M, Mariani C, Leonardi M, Pezzoli G. T1 and T2 in the brain of healthy subjects, patients with Parkinson disease, and patients with multiple system atrophy: relation to iron content. Radiology 1999; 211:489–495.

34. Chen JC, Hardy PA, Kucharczyk W, et al. MR of human postmortem brain tissue: correlative study between T2 and assays of iron and ferritin in Parkinson and Huntington disease. AJNR 1993; 14:275–281.

35. Bartzokis G, Aravagiri M, Oldendorf WH, Mintz J, Marder SR. Field dependent transverse relaxation rate increase may be a specific measure of tissue iron stores. Magn Reson Med 1993; 29:459–464.

36. Ordidge RJ, Gorell JM, Deniau JC, Knight RA, Helpern JA. Assessment of relative brain iron concentrations using T2-weighted and T2*-weighted MRI at 3 Tesla. Magn Reson Med 1994; 32:335–341.

37. Ye FQ, Martin WRW, Allen PS. Estimation of the brain iron in vivo by means of the interecho time dependence of image contrast. Magn Reson Med 1996; 36:153–158.

38. Martin WRW, Ye FQ, Allen PS. Increasing striatal iron content associated with normal aging. Mov Disord 1998; 13:281–286.

39. Bartzokis G, Cummings JL, Markham CH, Marmarelis PZ, Treciokas LJ, Tishler TA, Marder SR, Mintz J. MRI evaluation of brain iron in earlier- and later-onset Parkinson's disease and normal subjects. Magn Reson Imaging 1999; 2:213–222.

40. Ye FQ, Allen PS, Martin WRW. Basal ganglia iron content in Parkinson's disease measured with magnetic resonance. Mov Disord 1996; 11:243–249.

41. Unrejak J, Williams SR, Gadian DG, Noble M. Proton nuclear magnetic resonance spectroscopy unambiguously identifies different neural cell types. J Neurosci 1993; 13:981–989.

42. Davie C. The role of spectroscopy in parkinsonism. Mov Disord 1998; 13:2–4.

43. Holshauser BA, Komu M, Moller HE, et al. Localised proton NMR spectroscopy in the striatum of patients with idiopathic Parkinson's disease: a multicenter pilot study. Magn Reson Med 1995; 33:589–594.

44. Clarke CE, Lowry M, Horsman A. Unchanged basal ganglia N-acetylaspartate and glutamate in idiopathic Parkinson's disease measured by proton magnetic resonance spectroscopy. Mov Disord 1997; 12:297–301.

45. Ellis CM, Lemmens G, Williams SCR, Simmons A, Dawson J, Leigh PN, Chaudhuri KR. Changes in putamen N-acetylaspartate and choline ratios in untreated and levodopa treated Parkinson's disease: a proton magnetic resonance spectroscopy study. Neurology 1997; 49:438–444.

46. Davie CA, Wening G, Barker GJ, Tofts PS, Kendall BE, Quinn N, McDonald WI, Marsden CD, Miller DH. Differentiation of multiple system atrophy from idiopathic Parkinson's disease using proton magnetic resonance spectroscopy. Ann Neurol 1995; 37:204–210.

47. Clarke CE, Lowry M. Systematic review of proton magnetic resonance spectroscopy of the striatum in parkinsonian syndromes. Eur J Neurol 2001; 8:573–577.

48. Raichle ME. Circulatory and metabolic correlates of brain function in normal humans. In: Mountcastle VB, ed. Handbook of Physiology: The Nervous System V, Part 2. Bethesda MD: American Physiological Society, 1987:643–674.

49. Lauritzen M. Relationship of spikes, synaptic activity, and local changes of cerebral blood flow. J Cereb Blood Flow Metab 2001; 21:1367–1383.

50. Logothetis NK, Pauls J, Augath M, Trinath T, Oeltermann A. Neurophysiological investigation of the basis of the fMRI signal. Nature 2001; 412:150–157.

51. Jueptner M, Weiller C. Review: Does measurement of regional cerebral blood flow reflect synaptic activity? Implications for PET and fMRI. Neuroimage 1995; 2:148–156.
52. Perlmutter JS, Raichle ME. Pure hemidystonia with basal ganglion abnormalities on positron emission tomography. Ann Neurol 1984; 15:228–233.
53. Leenders KL, Wolfson L, Gibbs JM, Wise RJS, Causon R, Jones T, Legg NJ. The effects of l-dopa on regional cerebral blood flow and oxygen metabolism in patients with Parkinson's disease. Brain 1985; 108:171–191.
54. Martin WR, Stoessl AJ, Adam MJ, Ammann W, Bergstrom M, Harrop R, Laihinen A, Rogers JG, Ruth TJ, Sayre CI, et al. Positron emission tomography in Parkinson's disease: glucose and DOPA metabolism. Adv Neurol 1986; 45:95–98.
55. Perlmutter JS, Raichle ME. Regional blood flow in hemiparkinsonism. Neurology 1985; 35: 1127–1134.
56. Wolfson LI, Leenders KL, Brown LL, Jones T. Alterations of regional cerebral blood flow and oxygen metabolism in Parkinson's disease. Neurology 1985; 35:1399–1400.
57. Lozza C, Marie RM, Baron JC. The metabolic substrates of bradykinesia and tremor in uncomplicated Parkinson's disease. Neuroimage 2002; 17:688–699.
58. Mentis MJ, McIntosh AR, Perrine K, Dhawan V, Berlin B, Feigin A, Edwards C, Mattis P, Eidelberg D. Relationships among the metabolic patterns that correlate with mnemonic, visuospatial, and mood symptoms in Parkinson's disease. Am J Psychiatry 2002; 159:746–754.
59. Antonini A, Moeller JR, Nakamura T, Spetsieris P, Dhawan V, Eidelberg D. The metabolic anatomy of tremor in Parkinson's disease. Neurology 1998; 51:803–810.
60. Eidelberg D, Moeller J, Dhawan V, Spetsieris P, Takikawa S, Ishikawa T, Chaly T, Robeson W, Margouleff D, Przedborski S. The metabolic topography of parkinsonism. J Cereb Blood Flow Metab 1994; 14:783–801.
61. Burton H, Videen TO, Raichle ME. Tactile-vibration-activated in insular and parietal-opercular cortex studied with positron emission tomography: mapping the second somatosensory area in humans. Somatosensory and Motor Research 1993; 10:297–308.
62. Drevets WC, Burton H, Videen TO, Snyder AZ, Simpson JR, Raichle ME. Blood flow changes in human somatosensory cortex during anticipated stimulation. Nature 1995; 373:198–199.
63. Friston KJ, Holmes AP, Worsley KJ. How many subjects constitute a study?. Neuroimage 1999; 10:1–5.
64. Moeller JR, Strother SC, Sidtis JJ, Rottenberg DA. Scaled subprofile model: a statistical approach to the analysis of functional patterns in positron emission tomographic data. J Cereb Blood Flow Metab 1987; 7:649–658.
65. Eidelberg D, Moeller JR, Dhawan V, Sidtis JJ, Ginos JZ, Strother SC, Cedarbaum J, Greene P, Fahn S, Rottenberg DA. The metabolic anatomy of Parkinson's disease: complementary [^{18}F] fluorodeoxyglucose and [^{18}F]fluorodopa positron emission tomographic studies. Mov Disord 1990; 5:203–213.
66. Jenkins IH, Fernandez W, Playford ED, Lees AJ, Frackowiak RS, Passingham RE et al. Impaired activation of the supplementary motor area in Parkinson's disease is reversed when akinesia is treated with apomorphine. Ann Neurol 1992; 32:749–757.
67. Catalan MJ, Ishii K, Honda M, Samii A, Hallett M. A PET study of sequential finger movements of varying length in patients with Parkinson's disease. Brain 1999; 122:483–495.
68. Cunnington R, Egan GF, O'Sullivan JD, Hughes AJ, Bradshaw JL, Colebatch JG. Motor imagery in Parkinson's disease: a PET study. Mov Disord 2001; 16:849–857.
69. Samuel M, Ceballos-Baumann AO, Boecker H, Brooks DJ. Motor imagery in normal subjects and Parkinson's disease patients: an H215O PET study. Neuroreport 2001; 12:821–828.
70. Boecker H, Ceballos-Baumann A, Bartenstein P, Weindl A, Siebner HR, Fassbender T, Munz F, Schwaiger M, Conrad B. Sensory processing in Parkinson's and Huntington's disease: investigations with 3D H(2)(15)O-PET. Brain 1999; 122:1651–1665.
71. Owen AM, Doyon J, Dagher A, Sadikot A, Evans AC. Abnormal basal ganglia outflow in Parkinson's disease identified with PET. Implications for higher cortical functions. Brain 1998; 121: 949–965.
72. Black KJ, Gado MH, Perlmutter JS. PET measurement of dopamine D_2 receptor-mediated changes in striatopallidal function. J Neurosci 1997; 17:3168–3177.
73. Engber TM, Susel Z, Kuo S, Chase TN. Chronic levodopa treatment alters basal and dopamine agonist-stimulated cerebral glucose utilization. J Neurosci 1990; 10:3889–3895.
74. McCulloch J, Edvinsson L. Cerebral circulatory and metabolic effects of piribedil. Eur J Pharmacol 1980; 66:327–337.

75. McCulloch J, Kelly PA, Ford I. Effect of apomorphine on the relationship between local cerebral glucose utilization and local cerebral blood flow (with an appendix on its statistical analysis). J Cereb Blood Flow Metab 1982; 2:487–499.
76. Morelli M, Pontieri FE, Linfante I, Orzi F, Di Chiara G. Local cerebral glucose utilization after D1 receptor stimulation in 6-OHDA lesioned rats: effect of sensitization (priming) with a dopaminergic agonist. Synapse 1993; 13:264–269.
77. Trugman JM, Wooten GF. Selective D1 and D2 dopamine agonists differentially alter basal ganglia glucose utilization in rats with unilateral 6-hydroxydopamine substantia nigra lesions. J Neurosci 1987; 7:2927–2935.
78. Black KJ, Hershey T, Gado M, Perlmutter JS. A dopamine D1 agonist activates temporal lobe structures in primates. J Neurophysiol 2000; 84:549–557.
79. Hershey T, Black KJ, Carl JL, Perlmutter JS. Dopa-induced blood flow responses in non-human primates. Exp Neurol 2000; 166:342–349.
80. Black KJ, Hershey TA, Koller JM, Videen TO, Price JL, Perlmutter JS. Prefrontal and limbic effects of a D3-preferring dopamine agonist: a possible substrate for dopamine-related changes in mood and behavior. Proc Natl Acad Sci 2002; 99:17113–17118.
81. Hershey T, Black KJ, Stambuk MK, Carl JL, McGee-Minnich L, Perlmutter JS. Altered thalamic response to levodopa in Parkinson's disease patients with dopa-induced dyskinesias. Proc Natl Acad Sci 1998; 95:12016–12021.
82. Eidelberg D, Moeller JR, Ishikawa T, Dhawan V, Spetsieris P, Silbersweig D, Stern E, Woods RP, Fazzini E, Dogali M, Beric A. Regional metabolic correlates of surgical outcome following unilateral pallidotomy for Parkinson's disease. Ann Neurol 1996; 39:450–459.
83. Su PC, Ma Y, Fukuda M, Mentis MJ, Tseng HM, Yen RF, Liu HM, Moeller JR, Eidelberg D. Metabolic changes following subthalamotomy for advanced Parkinson's disease. Ann Neurol 2001; 50:514–520.
84. Fukuda M, Mentis M, Ghilardi MF, Dhawan V, Antonini A, Hammerstad J, Lozano AM, Lang A, Lyons K, Koller W, Ghez C, Eidelberg D. Functional correlates of pallidal stimulation for Parkinson's disease. Ann Neurol 2001; 49:155–164.
85. Fukuda M, Ghilardi MF, Carbon M, Dhawan V, Ma Y, Feigin A, Mentis MJ, Ghez C, Eidelberg D. Pallidal stimulation for parkinsonism: improved brain activation during sequence learning. Ann Neurol 2002; 52:144–152.
86. Schroeder U, Kuehler A, Haslinger B, Erhard P, Fogel W, Tronnier VM, Lange KW, Boecker H, Ceballos-Baumann AO. Subthalamic nucleus stimulation affects striato-anterior cingulate cortex circuit in a response conflict task: a PET study. Brain 2002; 125:1995–2004.
87. Perlmutter JS, Mink JW, Bastian AJ, Zackowski K, Hershey T, Miyawaki E, Koller W, Videen TO. Blood flow responses to deep brain stimulation of thalamus. Neurology 2002; 58:1388–1394.
88. Feigin A, Fukuda M, Dhawan V, Przedborski S, Jackson-Lewis V, Mentis MJ, Moeller JR, Eidelberg D. Metabolic correlates of levodopa response in Parkinson's disease. Neurology 2001; 57:2083–2088.
89. Cools R, Stefanova E, Barker RA, Robbins TW, Owen AM. Dopaminergic modulation of high-level cognition in Parkinson's disease: the role of the prefrontal cortex revealed by PET. Brain 2002; 125:584–594.
90. Feigin A, Ghilardi MF, Fukuda M, Mentis MJ, Dhawan V, Barnes A, Ghez CP, Eidelberg D. Effects of levodopa infusion on motor activation responses in Parkinson's disease. Neurology 2002; 59:220–226.
91. Frost JJ, Wagner HN Jr (eds). Quantitative Imaging. Neuroreceptors, Neurotransmitters and Enzymes. New York: Raven Press, 1990:51–192.
92. Perlmutter JS, Kilbourn MR, Raichle ME, Welch MJ. MPTP induced up-regulation of in vivo dopaminergic radioligand-receptor binding in man. Neurology 1987; 37:1575–1579.
93. Rinne JO, Laihinen A, Ruottinen H, Ruotsalainen U, Nagren K, Lehikoinen P, Oikonen V, Rinne UK. Increased density of dopamine D2 receptors in the putamen, but not in the caudate nucleus in early Parkinson's disease: a PET study with [11C]raclopride. J Neurol Sci 1995; 132:156–161.
94. Turjanski N, Lees AJ, Brooks DJ. In vivo studies on striatal dopamine D1 and D2 site binding in L-dopa-treated Parkinson's disease patients with and without dyskinesias. Neurology 1997; 49:717–723.
95. Antonini A, Schwarz J, Oertel WH, Pogarell O, Leenders KL. Long-term changes of striatal dopamine D2 receptors in patients with Parkinson's disease: a study with positron emission tomography and [11C]raclopride. Mov Disord 1997; 12:33–38.

96. Kaasinen V, Ruottinen HM, Nagren K, Lehikoinen P, Oikonen V, Rinne JO. Upregulation of putaminal dopamine D2 receptors in early Parkinson's disease: a comparative PET study with [11C] raclopride and [11C]N-methylspiperone. J Nucl Med 2000; 41:65–70.

97. Perlmutter JS, Tempel LW, Black KJ, Parkinson D, Todd RD. MPTP induces dystonia & parkinsonism: clues to the pathophysiology of dystonia. Neurology 1997; 49:1432–1438.

98. Todd RD, Carl J, Harmon S, O'Malley KL, Perlmutter JS. Dynamic changes in striatal dopamine D2 and D3 receptor protein and mRNA in response to MPTP denervation in baboons. J Neurosci 1996; 16:7776–7782.

99. Doudet DJ, Holden JE, Jivan S, McGeer E, Wyatt RJ. In vivo PET studies of the dopamine D2 receptors in rhesus monkeys with long-term MPTP-induced parkinsonism. Synapse 2000; 38:105–113.

100. Perlmutter JS, Stambuk MK, Markham J, Black KJ, McGee-Minnich L, Jankovic J, et al. Decreased [^{18}F]spiperone binding in putamen in idiopathic focal dystonia. J Neurosci 1997; 17:834–842.

101. Augood SJ, Penney JB Jr, Friberg IK, Breakefield XO, Young AB, Ozelius LJ, Standaert DG. Expression of the early-onset torsion dystonia gene (DYT1) in human brain. Ann Neurol 1998; 43:669–673.

102. Seeman P, Guan HC, Niznik HB. Endogenous dopamine loweres the dopamine D2 receptor density as measured by [^{3}H]raclopride: implications for positron emission tomography of the human brain. Synapse 1989; 3:96–98.

103. Antonini H, Schwarz J, Oertel WH, Beer HF, Madeja UD, Leenders KL. [^{11}C]Raclopride and positron emission tomography in previously untreated patients with Parkinson's disease: influence of L-dopa and lisuride on striatal dopamine D$_2$-receptors. Neurology 1994; 44:1325–1329.

104. Tedroff J, Pedersen M, Aquilonius S-M, Hartvig P, Jacobsson G, Långström B. Levodopa-induced changes in synaptic dopamine in patients with Parkinson's disease as measured by [^{11}C]raclopride displacement and PET. Neurology 1996; 46:1430–1436.

105. Breier A, Su T-P, Saunders R, Carson RE, Kolachana BS, de Bartolomeis A, Weinberger DR, Weisenfeld N, Malhotra AK, Eckelman WC, Pickar D. Schizophrenia is associated with elevated amphetamine-induced synaptic concentrations: evidence from a novel positron emission tomography method. Proc Natl Acad Sci USA 1997; 94:2569–2574.

106. Carson RE, Breier A, de Bartolomeis A, Saunders RC, Su TP, Schmall B, Der MG, Pickar D, Eckelman WC. Quantification of amphetamine-induced changes in [^{11}C]raclopride binding with continuous infusion, J Cereb Blood Flow Metab 1997; 17:437–447.

107. Dewey SL, Smith GS, Logan J, Brodie JD, Fowler JS, Wolf AP. Striatal binding of the PET ligand ^{11}C-raclopride is altered by drugs that modify synaptic drug levels. Synapse 1993; 13:350–356.

108. Schlaepfer TE, Pearlson GD, Wong DF, Marenco S, Dannals DF. PET Study of competition between intravenous cocaine and [^{11}C]raclopride at dopamine receptors in human subjects. Am J Psychiatry 1997; 154:1209–1213.

109. Ouchi Y, Yoshikawa E, Futatsubashi M, Okada H, Torizuka T, Sakamoto M. Effect of simple motor performance on regional dopamine release in the striatum in Parkinson disease patients and healthy subjects: a positron emission tomography study. J Cereb Blood Flow Metab 2002; 22:746–752.

110. Piccini P, Brooks DJ, Bjorklund A, Gunn RN, Grasby PM, Rimoldi O, Brundin P, Hagell P, Rehncrona S, Widner H, Lindvall O. Dopamine release from nigral transplants visualized in vivo in a Parkinson's patient. Nat Neurosci 1999; 2:1137–1140.

111. Garnett ES, Firnau G, Nahmias C. Dopamine visualised in the basal ganglia of living man. Nature 1983; 305:137–138.

112. Martin WRW, Perlmutter JS. Assessment of fetal tissue transplantation in Parkinson's disease: does PET play a role? Neurology 1994; 44:1777–1780.

113. Pate BD, Kawamata T, Yamada T, McGeer EG, Hewitt KA, Snow BJ, et al. Correlation of striatal fluorodopa uptake in the MPTP monkey with dopaminergic indices. Ann Neurol 1993; 34:331–338.

114. Snow BJ, Tooyama I, McGeer EG, Yamada T, Calne DB, Takahashi H, et al. Human positron emission tomographic [^{18}F]fluorodopa studies correlate with dopamine cell counts and levels. Ann Neurol 1993; 34:324–330.

115. Calne DB, Langston JW, Martin WRW, Stoessl AJ, Ruth TJ, Adam MJ, Pate BD, Schulzer M. Positron emission tomography after MPTP: observations relating to the cause of Parkinson's disease. Nature 1985; 317:246–248.

116. Hoshi H, Kuwabara H, Leger G, Cumming P, Guttman M, Gjedde A. 6-[18F]Fluoro-L-dopa metabolism in living human brain: a comparison of six analytical methods. J Cereb Blood Flow Metab 1993; 13:57–69.

117. Leenders KL, Salmon EP, Tyrrell P, Perani D, Brooks DJ, Sager H, Marsden CD, Frackowiak RS. The nigrostriatal dopaminergic system assessed in vivo by positron emission tomography in healthy volunteer subjects and patients with Parkinson's disease. Arch Neurol 1990; 47: 1290–1298.

118. Huang WS, Ma KH, Chou YH, Chen CY, Liu RS, Liu JC. 99mTc-TRODAT-1 SPECT in healthy and 6-OHDA lesioned parkinsonian monkeys: comparison with 18F-FDOPA PET. Nucl Med Commun 2003; 24:77–83.

119. De La Fuente-Fernandez R, Lim AS, Sossi V, Adam MJ, Ruth TJ, Calne DB, Stoessl AJ, Lee CS. Age and severity of nigrostriatal damage at onset of Parkinson's disease. Synapse 2003; 47: 152–158.

120. Ribeiro MJ, Vidailhet M, Loc'h C, Dupel C, Nguyen JP, Ponchant M, Dolle F, Peschanski M, Hantraye P, Cesaro P, Samson Y, Remy P. Dopaminergic function and dopamine transporter binding assessed with positron emission tomography in Parkinson disease. Arch Neurol 2002; 59:580–586.

121. Kazumata K, Dhawan V, Chaly T, Antonini A, Margouleff C, Belakhlef A, Neumeyer J, Eidelberg D. Dopamine transporter imaging with fluorine-18-FPCIT and PET. J Nucl Med 1998; 39:1521–1530.

122. Eberling JL, Pivirotto P, Bringas J, Bankiewicz KS. Tremor is associated with PET measures of nigrostriatal dopamine function in MPTP-lesioned monkeys. Exp Neurol 2000; 165:342–346.

123. Yee RE, Huang SC, Stout DB, Irwin I, Shoghi-Jadid K, Togaski DM, DeLanney LE, Langston JW, Satyamurthy N, Farahani KF, Phelps ME, Barrio JR. Nigrostriatal reduction of aromatic L-amino acid decarboxylase activity in MPTP-treated squirrel monkeys: in vivo and in vitro investigations. J Neurochem 2000; 74:1147–1157.

124. Broussolle E, Dentresangle C, Landais P, Garcia-Larrea L, Pollak P, Croisile B, Hibert O, Bonnefoi F, Galy G, Froment JC, Comar D. The relation of putamen and caudate nucleus 18F-Dopa uptake to motor and cognitive performances in Parkinson's disease. J Neurol Sci 1999; 166:141–151.

125. Morrish P, Rakshi J, Bailey D, Sawle G, Brooks D. Measuring the rate of progression and estimating the preclinical period of Parkinson's disease with [18F]dopa PET. J Neurol Neurosurg Psychiatry 1998; 64:314–319.

126. Ishikawa T, Dhawan V, Kazumata K, Chaly T, Mandel F, Neumeyer J, Margouleff C, Babchyck B, Zanzi I, Eidelberg D. Comparative nigrostriatal dopaminergic imaging with iodine-123-beta CIT-FP/SPECT and fluorine-18-FDOPA/PET. J Nucl Med 1996; 37:1760–1765.

127. Morrish PK, Sawle GV, Brooks DJ. Regional changes in [18F]dopa metabolism in the striatum in Parkinson's disease. Brain 1996; 119:2097–2103.

128. Sossi V, de La Fuente-Fernandez R, Holden JE, Doudet DJ, McKenzie J, Stoessl AJ, Ruth TJ. Increase in dopamine turnover occurs early in Parkinson's disease: evidence from a new modeling approach to PET 18 F-fluorodopa data. J Cereb Blood Flow Metab 2002; 22:232–239.

129. Snow BJ, Nygaard TG, Takahashi H, Calne DB. Positron emission tomographic studies of dopa-responsive dystonia and early-onset idiopathic parkinsonism. Ann Neurol 1993; 34:733–738.

130. Ma Y, Dhawan V, Mentis M, Chaly T, Spetsieris PG, Eidelberg D. Parametric mapping of [18F]FPCIT binding in early stage Parkinson's disease: a PET study. Synapse 2002; 45:125–133.

131. Frey KA, Koeppe RA, Kilbourn MR, Vander Borght TM, Albin RL, Gilman S, Kuhl DE. Presynaptic monoaminergic vesicles in Parkinson's disease and normal aging. Ann Neurol 1996; 40:873–884.

132. Rinne JO, Ruottinen H, Bergman J, Haaparanta M, Sonninen P, Solin O. Usefulness of a dopamine transporter PET ligand [(18)F]beta-CFT in assessing disability in Parkinson's disease. J Neurol Neurosurg Psychiatry 1999; 67:737–741.

133. Antonini A, Moresco RM, Gobbo C, De Notaris R, Panzacchi A, Barone P, Calzetti S, Negrotti A, Pezzoli G, Fazio F. The status of dopamine nerve terminals in Parkinson's disease and essential tremor: a PET study with the tracer [11-C]FE-CIT. Neurol Sci 2001; 22:47–48.

134. Antonini A, Leenders K, Vontobel P, Maguire R, Missimer J, Psylla M, Gunther I. Complementary PET studies of striatal neuronal function in the differential diagnosis between multiple system atrophy and Parkinson's disease. Brain 1997; 120:2187–2195.

135. Burn DJ, Sawle GV, Brooks DJ. Differential diagnosis of Parkinson's disease, multiple system atrophy, and Steele-Richardson-Olszewski syndrome: discriminant analysis of striatal 18F-dopa PET data. J Neurol Neurosurg Psychiatry 1994; 57:278–284.

136. Shinotoh H, Thiessen B, Snow B, Hashimoto S, MacLeod P, Silveira I, Rouleau GA, Schulzer M, Calne DB. Fluorodopa and raclopride PET analysis of patients with Machado-Joseph disease. Neurology 1997; 49:1133–1136.

137. Furtado S, Farrer M, Tsuboi Y, Klimek ML, de la Fuente-Fernandez R, Hussey J, Lockhart P, Calne DB, Suchowersky O, Stoessl AJ, Wszolek ZK. SCA-2 presenting as parkinsonism in an Alberta family: clinical, genetic, and PET findings. Neurology 2002; 59:1625–1627.
138. Kim YJ, Ichise M, Ballinger JR, Vines D, Erami SS, Tatschida T, Lang AE. Combination of dopamine transporter and D2 receptor SPECT in the diagnostic evaluation of PD, MSA, and PSP. Mov Disord 2002; 17:303–312.
139. Ghaemi M, Hilker R, Rudolf J, Sobesky J, Heiss WD. Differentiating multiple system atrophy from Parkinson's disease: contribution of striatal and midbrain MRI volumetry and multi-tracer PET imaging. J Neurol Neurosurg Psychiatry 2002; 73:517–523.
140. Booij J, Speelman JD, Horstink MW, Wolters EC. The clinical benefit of imaging striatal dopamine transporters with [123I]FP-CIT SPET in differentiating patients with presynaptic parkinsonism from those with other forms of parkinsonism. Eur J Nucl Med 2001; 28:266–272.
141. Burn DJ, Brooks DJ. Nigral dysfunction in drug-induced parkinsonism: an 18F-dopa PET study. Neurology 1993; 43:552–556.
142. Guttman M, Yong VW, Kim SU, Calne DB, Martin WR, Adam MJ, et al. Asymptomatic striatal dopamine depletion: PET scans in unilateral MPTP monkeys. Synapse 1988; 2:469–473.
143. Piccini P, Morrish P, Turjanski N, Sawle G, Burn D, Weeks R, Mark MH, Maraganore DM, Lees AJ, Brooks DJ. Dopaminergic function in familial Parkinson's disease: a clinical and 18F-dopa positron emission tomography study. Ann Neurol 1997; 41:222–229.
144. Burn DJ, Mark MH, Playford ED, Maraganore DM, Zimmerman TR, Jr., Duvoisin RC, et al. Parkinson's disease in twins studied with ^{18}F-dopa and positron emission tomography. Neurology 1992; 42:1894–1900.
145. Holthoff V, Vieregge P, Kessler J, Pietrzyk U, Herholz K, Bonner J, Wagner R, Wienhard K, Pawlik G, Heiss WD. Discordant twins with Parkinson's disease: positron emission tomography and early signs of impaired cognitive circuits. Ann Neurol 1994; 36:176–182.
146. Laihinen A, Ruottinen H, Rinne JO, Haaparanta M, Bergman J, Solin O, Koskenvuo M, Marttila R, Rinne UK. Risk for Parkinson's disease: twin studies for the detection of asymptomatic subjects using [18F]6-fluorodopa PET. J Neurol 2000; 247(suppl 2):II110–113.
147. Khan NL, Valente EM, Bentivoglio AR, Wood NW, Albanese A, Brooks DJ, Piccini P. Clinical and subclinical dopaminergic dysfunction in PARK6-linked parkinsonism: An 18F-dopa PET study. Ann Neurol 2002; 52:849–853.
148. Nurmi E, Ruottinen HM, Kaasinen V, Bergman J, Haaparanta M, Solin O, Rinne JO. Progression in Parkinson's disease: a positron emission tomography study with a dopamine transporter ligand [18F]CFT. Ann Neurol 2000; 47:804–808.
149. Nurmi E, Ruottinen HM, Bergman J, Haaparanta M, Solin O, Sonninen P, Rinne JO. Rate of progression in Parkinson's disease: a 6-[18F]fluoro-L-dopa PET study. Mov Disord 2001; 16:608–615.
150. Rakshi JS, Pavese N, Uema T, Ito K, Morrish PK, Bailey DL, Brooks DJ. A comparison of the progression of early Parkinson's disease in patients started on ropinirole or L-dopa: an (18)F-dopa PET study. J Neural Transm 2002; 109:1433–1443.
151. Parkinson Study Group. Pramipexole vs levodopa as initial treatment for Parkinson disease: A randomized controlled trial. Parkinson Study Group. JAMA 2000; 284:1931–1938.
152. Parkinson Study Group. Dopamine transporter brain imaging to assess the effects of pramipexole vs levodopa on Parkinson disease progression. JAMA 2002; 287:1653–61.
153. de La Fuente-Fernandez R, Lim AS, Sossi V, Holden JE, Calne DB, Ruth TJ, Stoessl AJ. Apomorphine-induced changes in synaptic dopamine levels: positron emission tomography evidence for presynaptic inhibition. J Cereb Blood Flow Metab 2001; 21:1151–1159.
154. Guttman M, Stewart D, Hussey D, Wilson A, Houle S, Kish S. Influence of L-dopa and pramipexole on striatal dopamine transporter in early PD. Neurology 2001; 56:1559–1564.
155. Ahlskog JE, Uitti RJ, O'Connor MK, Maraganore DM, Matsumoto JY, Stark KF, Turk MF, Burnett OL. The effect of dopamine agonist therapy on dopamine transporter imaging in Parkinson's disease. Mov Disord 1999; 14:940–946.
156. Lindvall O, Rehncrona S, Brundin P, Gustavii B, Astedt B, Widner H, Lindholm T, Bjorklund A, Leenders KL, Rothwell JC. Human fetal dopamine neurons grafted into the striatum in two patients with severe Parkinson's disease. Arch Neurol 1989; 46:615–631.
157. Lindvall O, Brundin P, Widner H, Rehncrona S, Gustavii B, Frackowiak R, Leenders KL, Sawle G, Rothwell JC, Marsden CD, et al. Grafts of fetal dopamine neurons survive and improve motor function in Parkinson's disease. Science. 1990; 247:574–577.
158. Freed CR, Breeze RE, Rosenberg NL, Schneck SA, Kriek E, Qi JX, Lone T, Zhang YB, Snyder JA, Wells TH. Survival of implanted fetal dopamine cells and neurologic improvement 12 to 46 months after transplantation for Parkinson's disease. N Engl J Med 1992; 327:1549–1555.

159. Widner H, Tetrud J, Rehncrona S, Snow B, Brundin P, Gustavii B, et al. Bilateral fetal mesencephalic grafting in two patients with parkinsonism induced by 1-methyl-4-phenyl-1,2,3, 6-tetrahydropyridine. N Engl J Med. 1992; 327:1556–1563.
160. Lindvall O, Widner H, Rehncrona S, Brundin P, Odin P, Gustavii B, Frackowiak R, Leenders KL, Sawle G, Rothwell JC, et al. Transplantation of fetal dopamine neurons in Parkinson's disease: one-year clinical and neurophysiological observations in two patients with putaminal implants. Ann Neurol. 1992; 31:155–165.
161. Sawle GV, Bloomfield PM, Bjorklund A, Brooks DJ, Brundin P, Leenders KL, Lindvall O, Marsden CD, Rehncrona S, Widner H, et al. Transplantation of fetal dopamine neurons in Parkinson's disease: PET [^{18}F]6-L-fluorodopa studies in two patients with putaminal implants. Ann Neurol. 1992; 31:166–173.
162. Nakamura T, Dhawan V, Chaly T, Fukuda M, Ma Y, Breeze R, Greene P, Fahn S, Freed C, Eidelberg D. Blinded positron emission tomography study of dopamine cell implantation for Parkinson's disease. Ann Neurol 2001; 50:181–187.
163. Freed CR, Greene PE, Breeze RE, Tsai WY, DuMouchel W, Kao R, Dillon S, Winfield H, Culver S, Trojanowski JQ, Eidelberg D, Fahn S. Transplantation of embryonic dopamine neurons for severe Parkinson's disease. N Engl J Med 2001; 344:710–719.
164. Ma Y, Feigin A, Dhawan V, Fukuda M, Shi Q, Greene P, Breeze R, Fahn S, Freed C, Eidelberg D. Dyskinesia after fetal cell transplantation for parkinsonism: a PET study. Ann Neurol 2002; 52: 628–634.
165. Hagell P, Piccini P, Bjorklund A, Brundin P, Rehncrona S, Widner H, Crabb L, Pavese N, Oertel WH, Quinn N, Brooks DJ, Lindvall O. Dyskinesias following neural transplantation in Parkinson's disease. Nat Neurosci 2002; 5:627–628.
166. Guttman M, Burns RS, Martin WR, Peppard RF, Adam MJ, Ruth TJ, et al. PET studies of parkinsonian patients treated with autologous adrenal implants. Can J Neurol Sci 1989; 16:305–309.
167. Miletich RS, Bankiewicz R, Plunkett R, et al. L-[^{18}F]6-fluorodopa PET images of catecholaminergic tissue implants in hemi-parkinsonian monkeys. Neurology 1988; 38:S145.
168. Dusart I, Nothias F, Roudier F, Besson JM, Peschanski M. Vascularization of fetal cell suspension grafts in the excitotoxically lesioned adult rat thalamus. Brain Res Dev Brain Res 1989; 48: 215–228.
169. Kordower JH, Freeman TB, Chen EY, Mufson EJ, Sanberg PR, Hauser RA, Snow B, Olanow CW. Fetal nigral grafts survive and mediate clinical benefit in a patient with Parkinson's disease. Mov Disord 1998; 13:383–393.
170. Leenders KL, Palmer AJ, Quinn N, Clark JC, Firnau G, Garnett ES. Brain dopamine metabolism in patients with Parkinson's disease measured with positron emission tomography. J Neurol Neurosurg Psychiatry 1986; 49:853–860.
171. Nutt JG, Woodward WR, Hammerstad JP, Carter JH, Anderson JL. The "on-off" phenomenon in Parkinson's disease: relations to levodopa absorption and transport. N Engl J Med 1984; 310: 483–487.
172. Leenders KL, Poewe WH, Palmer AJ, Brenton DP, Frackowiak RSJ. Inhibition of l-[^{18}F]fluoro-dopa uptake into human brain by amino acids demonstrated by positron emission tomography. Ann Neurol 1986; 20:258–262.
173. Kent DL, Larson EB. Magnetic resonance imaging of the brain and spine—Is clinical efficacy established after the first decade? Ann Int Med 1988; 108:402–424.
174. Chalmers TC. PET scans and technology assessment. JAMA 1988; 260:2713–2715.

5

Is Levodopa Toxic?

Ruth Djaldetti and Eldad Melamed

Tel Aviv University, Tel Aviv, Israel

I. INTRODUCTION

Parkinson's disease (PD) is a neurodegenerative disorder characterized mainly by a progressive loss of dopaminergic neurons of the substantia nigra pars compacta. The changes consist of gross and microscopic neuronal depigmentation, neuronal loss, extracellular melanin, and accumulation of iron and Lewy bodies in the remaining neurons (1). One of the major breakthroughs in the understanding of the pathophysiology of PD in the twentieth century was the discovery of a marked reduction in the neuro transmitter dopamine in the striatum of affected patients and the correlation between this loss and the clinical characteristics, i.e., rigidity, tremor, and bradykinesia. It is now recognized that a repertoire of other neurotransmitters (glutamate, noradrenaline, serotonin) is involved in the functional anatomy of the basal ganglia and might interact with or balance dopaminergic neurotransmission. Dopamine is synthesized in the brain from the amino acid L-tyrosine, which is converted to L-3,4-dihydroxyphenylalanine (L-dopa), the precursor of dopamine via the rate-limiting enzyme tyrosine hydroxylase. Dopamine is stored in vesicles and is transported by a carrier-mediated transport system against a concentration gradient. Under physiological conditions, dopamine is continuously released into the synaptic cleft and activates the postsynaptic receptors. It is returned to the dopaminergic terminals by a carrier-mediated reuptake system and sequestered in the synaptic vesicles for reuse. Dopamine is enzymatically inactivated by the action of mitochondrial monoamine oxidase (MAO) and catechol-O-methyl-transferase (COMT), which are localized primarily in glial cells.

Once the connection between a loss of dopamine and the clinical features of PD was established, a new era in the treatment of PD began. Because exogenous dopamine does not cross the blood-brain barrier (BBB), researchers turned to L-dopa, which is converted to dopamine when it reaches the striatum by the enzyme dopa decarboxylase, which is present in the surviving nigrostriatal terminals and in nondopaminergic cellular compartments. The early clinical trials showed that the administration of L-dopa combined with a dopa decarboxylase inhibitor to block the peripheral conversion of L-dopa to dopamine led to incredible improvement in parkinsonian symptoms. Debilitated patients could walk and move again, and life expectancy increased with less institutionalization and greater mobility. However, cumulative evidence from clinical and basic research indicated that after the initial "honeymoon" period when the response to treatment is smooth and reproducible, patients begin to show a lesser response, a response to individual doses ("wearing off"), an increased latency to turning on ("delayed on"), and no response to some doses, especially in the afternoon ("no on"). Involuntary choreic movements can appear, usually at the peak of the "on" period, but also at its beginning or end (2). These phenomena apparently emerge because of replacement of endogenous dopamine by L-dopa in a nonphysiological manner. Given orally, the drug floods not only the substantia nigra but the entire brain. Furthermore, as opposed to endogenous dopamine, which is stored in vesicles and released according to constant firing rates, the dopamine formed by exogenous L-dopa is not stored within vesicles but is spilled into the synapse as soon as it is generated.

Clinicians and researchers have therefore raised two major concerns with regard to chronic L-dopa treatment: (a) its possible toxicity to the remaining dopaminergic neurons, leading to accelerated disease progression, and (b) the possible relationship of this toxicity to the emergence of motor complications. In this chapter current models for investigating possible mechanisms of L-dopa toxicity are described and the current findings yielded so far are discussed.

II. CULTURE MODELS

Most culture studies of L-dopa and dopamine toxicity use the various cells involved in the metabolism of dopamine, namely, fetal mesencephalic cells, pheochromocytoma PC12 cells, sympathetic neurons, and neuroblastoma cell lines. Investigations involving cerebellar and fetal fibroblasts have also been reported. The effect of L-dopa on tissue culture has already been thoroughly reviewed by Fahn (3).

III. ANIMAL MODELS

Several experimental models of PD have been developed. One of the early ones involved the intranigral injection of 6-hydroxydopamine (6-OHDA), which kills dopaminergic neurons by the generation of free radicals. However, it does not lead to a progressive loss of neurons or to the formation of Lewy bodies, nor does it replicate the clinical symptoms of PD. Furthermore, the therapeutic assessment in this model is based on the rotation behavior of the animals, i.e., increased rotation contralateral to the injected side following apomorphine injection or increased ipsilateral rotation following amphetamine injection. Thereafter, researchers introduced a better model, 1-methyl-4-phenyl-1,2,3,6-tetrahydropyridine (MPTP) injection in mice and primates. This model was based on reports of clinical signs of PD in young drug addicts who injected a synthetic meperidine analogue contaminated by MPTP. MPTP is metabolized to an active toxic compound, 1-methyl-4-phenylpyridinium (MPP+), a polar molecule that can freely enter cells and cause progressive loss of dopaminergic neurons, probably by impairment of mitochondrial function, increased production of reactive oxygen species (ROS), and activation of factors responsible for programmed cell death (4). The studies showed that MPTP induced the clinical symptoms and some pathological features of PD. However, the model is limited by the acute and nonprogressive nature of cell death, without formation of inclusion bodies. The only model that generates Lewy body–like inclusions and produces progressive cell death is injection of the toxin rotenone. This toxin also kills dopaminergic neurons by oxidative stress. The major disadvantage of this model is the variability of susceptibility of the animal's response to the toxin.

The more recent genetic studies linking several gene mutations to the pathogenesis of neurodegenerative diseases created a new direction in animal research. Two of the best studied mutations are α-synuclein, which causes progressive loss of dopaminergic neurons in the substantia nigra (5), and Superoxide dismutase (SOD_1), which leads to clinical and pathological signs resembling those of amyotrophic lateral sclerosis (6). SOD_1 mutation might cause gradual and progressive loss of dopaminergic neurons in the substantia nigra of transgenic mice, with formation of cytoplasmic inclusions in this region (7).

IV. MECHANISMS OF L-DOPA TOXICITY

In general, the intracellular mechanisms of L-dopa toxicity include apoptosis (8–10), alterations in intracellular calcium content (11), and altered mitochondrial function (12). There is well-based evidence for the role of oxidative stress in the process of nigral degeneration in PD (13,14). Even under normal conditions, the nigra is exposed to oxidative stress during the metabolism of excessive amounts of dopamine. This action is converted by detoxifying enzymes, particularly glutathione peroxidase, which reduced the generation of ROS. In patients with PD, however, a combination of environmental and genetic factors may render the nigra more susceptible or reduce the capacity of the inactivating systems to handle the ROS and the deleterious consequences of L-dopa metabolism. Several mechanisms might be responsible for the toxic effect of dopamine and L-dopa on dopamine neurons:

1. The enzymatic oxidation of L-dopa to dopamine and its metabolism by monoamine oxidase B (MAO-B) produce hydrogen peroxide (H_2O_2), which is toxic. H_2O_2 can be converted by iron-mediated Fenton reactions to produce the more toxic radical (OH^-), which can induce oxidative damage. Exogenous L-dopa is rapidly metabolized to dopamine, thereby increasing its turnover. Therefore, excess H_2O_2 is formed, and this enhances the already notorious process of oxidative stress (15).

2. L-Dopa is oxidized to semiquinone and O-quinone derivatives on the route to melanin formation. These substances are toxic and may themselves be lethal to cells (16–18).

3. L-Dopa does not need to be metabolized to dopamine in order to exert toxicity. Studies have shown that dopamine is toxic to thymocytes, which have no dopamine reuptake systems. This indicates that auto-oxidation of L-Dopa results in toxicity (19–20). Moreover, L-Dopa toxicity is not prevented by SOD or catalase in rat mesencephalic cultures, indicating that H_2O_2 is not involved in the toxic effect (21). Auto-oxidation may generate a variety of free radicals, including superoxide and hydroxyl radicals.

4. L-Dopa and its damaging metabolites may kill cells by causing membranal lipid cell membrane peroxidation. They may also cause nuclear and mitochondrial DNA damage (22).

5. The disruption in dopamine disposition and metabolism may cause intracellular toxicity. This is supported by findings that upregulation of proteins involved in dopamine synthesis, vesicular sequestration, reuptake, and metabolism (vesicular monoamine transferase, MAO-A, and glutathione S-transferase) can protect against dopamine cytotoxicity (23).

V. IN VITRO STUDIES

Most of the in vitro studies of dopaminergic and dopaminergic-like cell cultures have demonstrated L-Dopa toxicity at concentrations of 100–250 μM for 1–5 days (9,21,24,25). The cells are less viable in the presence of both dopamine and L-Dopa (26,27), although dopamine is apparently more toxic than L-Dopa and the d-isomer of dopa (28). Indeed, many studies have used both agents to study the neuroprotective effect of antiparkinsonian medications (29–36). The cytotoxic effects of L-Dopa in cell cultures are believed to be due, in part, to oxidative stress and reversible by antioxidants. Other mechanisms, such as protein synthesis, glutamate toxicity, and apoptotic cell death, have also been postulated. Metal ions might also add to the toxic effect.Manganese was found to increase L-Dopa toxicity in PC-12 cells, presumably by enhancement of its auto-oxidation (37), and iron magnifies the oxidative stress and apoptosis caused by L-Dopa (13,38,39).

Under certain conditions L-Dopa can induce an opposite effect. The presence of glia cells in culture make L-Dopa neuroprotective. In one study L-Dopa at a concentration of 200 μM was toxic in glia-free cultures but had neurotrophic effects in catecholaminergic and dopaminergic cultures when astrocytes were added (40–42). There are a few explanations for this bidirectional activity: (a) glia cells contain high concentrations of catalase and glutathione peroxidase which detoxify H_2O_2. One astrocyte has the capacity to protect 20 neurons against the toxicity induced by 100 μM/L H_2O_2 (43); (b) glia cells produce neurotrophic factors and antioxidants, whereas astrocytes release trophic factors that enhance development, survival, neurite extension, and resistance to neurotoxins (44–47). They provide enzymatic protection, which enhances the protective mechanisms against free radical damage. The factors with the strongest protective action in culture are glia-derived neurotrophic factor (GDNF) and brain–derived neurotrophic factor (BDNF). The dose of L-Dopa may also play a role. At low concentrations (30–50 μM), L-Dopa can apparently increase the number and branching of dopamine processes (42) due to its intrinsic neurotrophic effect, perhaps via upregulation of enzymes that detoxify free radicals (48). Studies have shown that in the absence of serum and trophic factors, 3–30 μM of dopamine and L-Dopa enhanced survival of PC12 cells (49), whereas in higher concentrations they were toxic (26,36,50). The authors suggested that dopamine's protective effect remains unchanged after its uptake or is inhibited because it works outside of the cell to enhance cell survival. Its protective effect was also not blunted when L-Dopa metabolism to dopamine was inhibited, indicating that at low concentrations dopamine protects against cell death via elevation of the intracellular calcium concentration, followed by activation of mitogen-activating protein kinase.

This dose-dependent biphasic effect of L-Dopa warrants further explanation. In PD, exogenous L-Dopa is handled differently by the few surviving dopaminergic neurons, which undergo increased neurotransmitter metabolism, leading to an augmented rate of dopamine oxidation. As a result, oxidative stress is increased and disease progression accelerates. In this context, the administration of very high doses of L-Dopa causes a marked elevation in intracellular dopamine concentrations and of hydroxyl radical production. By contrast, low doses of L-Dopa might spare the surviving dopaminergic neurons. As there is no need for these cells to compromise for the loss of dopamine, the metabolic rate of dopamine and the amount of oxidative stress would be reduced.

VI. ANIMAL STUDIES

The evidence from animal models is rather conflicting. Several studies found that long-term treatment of intact rats and mice with L-dopa for long periods did not cause a loss of dopaminergic neurons (51–54). L-Dopa inhibited complex I activity, but this effect was reversible on drug withdrawal, and there was no permanent damage. In mice with 6-OHDA–induced partial or complete lesions and in the MPTP mouse model, a few studies showed a modest reduction in the number of dopaminergic neurons (55,56,57), but the majority reported no decrease in either the number of neurons or the amount of dopamine in the striatum (51,52,54,58). Apparently, like the situation in cell cultures, L-dopa can be either toxic or neuroprotective, depending on the dose, time of administration, and presence of other compounds. L-Dopa generates different properties according to the amount of ascorbate added to brain homogenates (22). Murer et al. (59), in the first study to demonstrate L-dopa's possible protective effect, found that chronic oral treatment with L-dopa did not change the counts of tyrosine hydroxylase (TH)–immunoreactive neurons in the substantia nigra in rats with 6-OHDA lesions or the amounts of dopamine transporter and vesicular monoamine transferase in the striatum. Surprisingly, the animals with moderate lesions showed partial recovery of dopaminergic markers, whereas in those with severe lesions L-dopa reversed the upregulation of D2 receptors, characteristic of a severe loss of dopamine in the striatum. Although these results could not be replicated in the MPTP mouse model (54), others reported some supportive evidence. L-Dopa was administered for one week to rats with 6-OHDA lesions, and an increase in dopamine uptake sites on the dopaminergic nerve terminals in the striatum was noted (60). Longer periods of treatment had the opposite effect. Rats with a partial lesion had a decreased number of TH-positive cells during the first weeks of treatment, but after chronic L-dopa treatment for several weeks, the number of neurons with a dopaminergic phenotype increased. Systemic L-dopa administration, either intraperitoneal or intrastriatal, did not increase the amount of free radical formation, even at high doses (61), and prior damage to the nigrostriatal system did not predispose the surviving neurons to increased production of free radicals.

The inconsistent effect of L-dopa may also be explained by the type of animal model used. L-Dopa treatment of mice prior to 6-OHDA lesion induction worsened the depletion of striatal dopamine, whereas treatment given before intraperitoneal injection of MPTP reduced the MPP+-induced depletion (62). In summary, on the basis of the large majority of studies, there is no evidence that L-dopa promotes cell death in intact animals or in animal models of PD.

VII. HUMAN STUDIES

It is still unclear whether studies in cultures and animal models are relevant to PD and if their results are applicable to the human brain. L-Dopa and dopamine interact with culture media and form H_2O_2 and semiquinones (63). This might explain the toxic in vitro effect of dopa and dopamine, and therefore there is no relevance to human studies. Moreover, the human body has the potential to adjust, counteract, and react differently to offensive mechanisms. Clearly there is no evidence of L-dopa toxicity in healthy people. Volunteers and patients who were mistakenly treated with L-dopa for many years did not develop parkinsonism or the motor complications characteristic of PD patients after chronic L-dopa treatment (64,65), and post mortem analysis of the brains did not reveal loss of dopaminergic neurons or accumulation of Lewy bodies (64). Probably the normal brain has defense mechanisms against the toxic effects of L-dopa. There was one exception: a patient treated for 25 years for dopa-responsive dystonia had some loss of dopa uptake on positron emission tomography (PET). Another argument against L-dopa toxicity is that it increases the life span of patients with PD by preventing immobility and recurrent infections (66). This was true especially when treatment was started early (67,68). Even within the same family, patients treated with L-dopa for a mean of 7 years had longer survival and slower disease progression than their untreated relatives (69). Nevertheless, some studies failed to find an association between chronic treatment with L-dopa and increased mortality (70,71). There was no structural difference between L-dopa–treated and untreated patients with PD in a postmortem study (72); however, the dopaminergic cells were not counted.

In vivo experiments are unfeasible in humans, but some have provided clues addressing this problem. The cerebrospinal fluid of patients with PD is toxic to mesencephalic cell cultures, but no significant difference in toxicity parameters has been found between untreated and L-dopa–treated patients (73). In addition, active axonal outgrowth was demonstrated in a fetal mesencephalic transplant in a patient with PD despite continuous dopaminergic treatment (74).

Recent clinical trials accompanied by PET and single photon emission computed tomography (SPECT) studies have evaluated the rate of disease progression in newly diagnosed patients with dopamine agonists or L-dopa. The rate of disease progression was slower in the dopamine agonist group (75,76). This could point either to a neuroprotective effect of the agonists or to a toxic effect of L-dopa. It may also explain the findings of a higher mortality rate in early PD patients treated with L-dopa compared to those treated with bromocriptine (77). This question warrants further study.

VIII. PRESENT STATUS

L-Dopa treatment of patients with PD, despite its simple pharmacological rationale, i.e., reestablishing dopamine to the striatum, raises complex issues, most of them still poorly understood. A consensus meeting held in Austria in January 2002 concluded that the motor complications of PD are related to both disease severity and the abnormal and pulsatile stimulation of the dopaminergic receptors due to the short half-life of L-dopa. Therefore, it is the mode of administration and not the molecule itself that is the cause of these complications. With regard to the issue of L-dopa toxicity, the main conclusions were that (a) in vitro studies have little relevance to PD patients, as the results are influenced by the experimental conditions which are different from the human brain, (b) animal studies have not proven any toxicity of the drug, and (c) in human patients, the progression of the disease is due to continued degeneration of dopaminergic and nondopaminergic neurons, and there is no evidence that L-dopa causes or accelerates neuronal death.

Future clinical and imaging studies need to be designed to comprehensively establish whether L-dopa is toxic or has any effect on disease progression. Meanwhile, treatment should be individually tailored, taking into account patient age, occupation, response to therapy, and side effects.

REFERENCES

1. Alvord EC, Forno LS, Kusske JA, Kauffman RJ, Rhodes JS, Goetowski CR. The pathology of parkinsonism: a comparison of degenerations in cerebral cortex and brainstem. Adv Neurol 1974; 5:175–193.
2. Fahn S. Fluctuations of disability in Parkinson's disease. Pathophysiological aspects. Marsdem CD, Fahn S, eds. Movement Disorders. London: Butterworth Scientific, 1984:123–145.
3. Fahn, S. Is levodopa toxic? Neurology 1996; 47(suppl 3):S184–S195.
4. Przedborski S, Vila M. MPTP: a review of its mechanism of toxicity. Clin Neurosci Res 2001; 1:407–418.
5. Perez-Sanchez F, Milan M, Farinas I. Animal models of α-Synuclein pathology. In: Tolosa E, Schulz JB, McKeith IG, Ferrer I, eds. Neurodegenerative Disorders Associated with α-Synuclein Pathology. Barcelona: Ars Medica, 2002:23–36.
6. Gurney ME, Pu H, Chiu AY, Dal Canto MC, Polchow CY, Alexander DD, Caliendo J, Hentati A, Kwon YW, Deng HX, et al. Motor neuron degeneration in mice that express a human Cu, Zn superoxide dismutase mutation. Science 1994; 264:1772–1775.
7. Kostic V, Gurney ME, Deng, HX, Siddique T, Epstein CJ, Przedborski S. Midbrain dopaminergic neuronal degeneration in a transgenic mouse model of familial amyotrophic lateral sclerosis. Ann Neurol 1997; 41:497–504.
8. Walkinshaw G, Waters CM. Induction of apoptosis in catecholaminergic PC12 cells by L-DOPA: implications of treatment of Parkinson's disease. J Clin Invest 1995; 95:2458–2464.
9. Ziv I, Melamed E, Nardi N, Luria D, Achiron A, Offen D, Barzilai A. Dopamine induces apoptosis-like cell death in cultured chick sympathetic neurons—a possible novel pathogenetic mechanism in Parkinson's disease. Neurosci Lett 1994; 170:136–140.
10. Zhang, J, Price JO, Graham DG, Montine TJ. Secondary excitotoxicity contributes to dopamine-induced apoptosis of dopaminergic neuronal cultures. Biochem Biophys Res Commun 1998; 248:812–816.
11. Isaacs KR, Wolpoe ME, Jacobowitz DM. Calretinin-immunoreactive dopaminergic neurons from embryonic rat mesencephalon are resistant to levodopa-induced neurotoxicity. Exp Neurol 1997; 46:25–32.
12. Przedborski S, Jackson-Lewis V, Muthane U, Jiang H, Ferreira M, Naini AB, Fahn S. Chronic levodopa administration alters cerebral mitochondrial respiratory chain activity. Ann Neurol 1993; 34:715–723.
13. Fahn S, Cohen G. The oxidant stress hypothesis in Parkinson's disease: evidence supporting it. Ann Neurol 1992; 32:804–812.
14. Jenner PG, Olanow CW. Pathological evidence for oxidative stress in Parkinson's disease and related degenerative disorders. In: Olanow CW, Jenner P, Youdim M, eds. Neurodegeneration and Neuroprotection in Parkinson's Disease. San Diego: Academic Press, 1996:23–45.
15. Ogawa N, Edamatsu R, Mizukawa K, Asanuma M, Kohno M, Mori A. Degeneration of dopamine neurons and free radicals: possible participation of levodopa. Adv Neurol 1993; 60:242–250.
16. Graham DG. Oxidative pathways to catecholamines in the genesis of neuromelanin and cytotoxic quinines. Mol Pharmcol 1978; 14:633–643.
17. Graham DG, Tiffany SM, Bell WR Jr, Gutknecht WF. Autooxidation versus covalent binding of quinones as the mechanism of toxicity of dopamine, 6-hydroxydopamine, and related compounds toward C1300 neuroblastoma cells in vitro. Mol Pharmacol 1978; 14:644–653.
18. Stokes AH, Hastings TG, Vrana KE. Cytotoxic and genotoxic potential of dopamine. J Neurosci Res 1999; 55:659–665.
19. Offen D, Ziv I, Sternin H, Melamed E, Hochman A. Prevention of dopamine-induced cell death by thiol oxidants: possible implications for treatment of Parkinson's disease. Exp Neurol 1996; 141:32–39.
20. Basma AN, Morris EJ, Niclas WJ, Gella HM. L-dopa cytotoxicity to PC 12 cells in culture is via its auto-oxidation. J Neurochem 1995; 64:825–832.
21. Mytilineou C, Han S-K, Cohen G. Toxic and protective effects of L-dopa on mesencephalic cell cultures. J Neurochem 1993; 61:1470–1478.
22. Li CL, Werner P, Cohen G. Lipid peroxidation in brain: interactions of L-dopa/dopamine with ascorbate and iron. Neurodegeneration 1995; 4:147–153.

23. Weingarten P, Zhou QY. Protection of intracellular dopamine cytotoxicity by dopamine disposition and metabolism factors. J Neurochem 2001; 77:776–785.
24. Michel PP, Hefti F. Toxicity of 6-hydroxydopamine and dopamine for dopaminergic neurons in culture. J Neurosci Res 1990; 26:428–435.
25. Pardo B, Mena MA, Casarejos MJ, Paino CL, De Yebenes JG. Toxic effects of L-dopa on mesencephalic cell cultures: protection with antioxidants. Brain Res 1995; 682:133–143.
26. Lai CT, Yu PH. Dopamine and L-beta-3,4-dihydroxyphenylalanine hydrochloride (L-DOPA)-induced cytotoxicity towards catecholaminergic neuroblastoma SH-SY5Y cells. Effects of oxidative stress and antioxidative factors. Biochem Pharmacol 1997; 53:363–372.
27. Nakao N, Nakai K, Itakura T. Metabolic inhibition enhances selective toxicity of L-DOPA toward mesencephalic dopamine neurons in vitro. Brain Res 1997; 777:202–209.
28. Alexander T, Sortwell CE, Sladek CD, Roth RH, Steece Collier K. Comparison of neurotoxicity following repeated administration of L-dopa and dopamine to embryonic mesencephalic dopamine neurons in cultures derived from Fisher 344 and Sprague-Dawley donors. Cell Transplant 1997; 6:309–315.
29. Troadec JD, Marien M, Darios F, Hartmann A, Ruberg M, Colpaert F, Michel PP. Noradrenaline provides long-term protection to dopaminergic neurons by reducing oxidative stress. J Neurochem 2001; 79:200–210.
30. Werner P, Di Rocco A, Prikhojan A, Rempel N, Bottiglieri T, Bressman S, Yahr M. COMT-dependent protection of dopaminergic neurons by methionine, dimethinine and S-adenosylmethionine (SAM) against L-dopa toxicity in vitro. Brain Res 2001; 893:278–281.
31. Marin C, Jimenez A, Bonastre M, Vila M, Agid Y, Hirsch EC, Tolosa E. LY293558, an AMPA glutamate receptor antagonist, prevents and reverses levodopa-induced motor alterations in parkinsonian rats. Synapse 2001; 42:40–47.
32. Storch A, Blessing H, Bareiss M. Catechol-O-methyltransferase inhibition attenuates levodopa toxicity in mesencephalic dopamine neurons. Mol Pharmacol 2000; 57:589–594.
33. Takashima H, Tsujihata M, Kishikawa M, Freed WJ. Bromocriptine protects dopaminergic neurons from levodopa-induced toxicity by stimulating D(2‖ receptors. Exp Neurol 1999; 159:98–104.
34. Zou L, Jankovic J, Rowe DB, Xie W, Appel SJ, Le W. Neuroprotection by pramipexole against dopamine- and levodopa-induced toxicity. Life Sci 1999; 64:1275–1285.
35. Carvey PM, Pieri S, Ling ZD. Attenuation of levodopa-induced toxicity in mesencephalic cultures by pramipexole. J Neural Transm 1997; 104:209–228.
36. Cheng N, Maeda T, Kume T, Kaneko S, Kochiyama H, Akaike A, Goshima Y, Misu Y. Differential neurotoxicity induced by L-DOPA and dopamine in cultured striatal neurons. Brain Res 1996; 743:278–283.
37. Serra PA, Esposito G, Enrico P, Mura MA, Migheli R, Delogu MR, Miele M, Desole MS, Grella G, Miele E. Manganese increases L-DOPA auto-oxidation in the striatum of the freely moving rat: potential implications to L-DOPA long-term therapy of Parkinson's disease. Br J Pharmacol 2000; 130:937–945.
38. Olanow CW, Youdim MHB. Iron and neurodegeneration: prospects for neuroprotection. Olanow CW, Jenner P, Youdim MBH, eds. Neurodegeneration and Neuroprotection in Parkinson's Disease. London: Academic Press, 1996:55–67.
39. Velez-Pardo C, Del Rio MJ, Verschueren H, Ebinger G, Vaugquelin G. Dopamine and iron induce apoptosis in PC12 cells. Pharmacol Toxicol 1997; 80:76–84.
40. Mena MA, Casarejos MJ, Carazo A, Paino CL, Garcia de Yebenes J. Glia conditioned medium protects fetal rat midbrain neurons in culture from L-dopa toxicity. Neuroreport 1996; 7:441–445.
41. Mena MA, Casarejos MJ, Carazo A, Paino CL, Garcia de Yebenes J. Glia protects fetal midbrain dopamine neurons in culture from L-DOPA toxicity through multiple mechanisms. J Neural Transm 1997; 104:317–328.
42. Mena MA, Davila V, Sulzer D. Neurotrophic effect of L-DOPA in postnatal midbrain dopamine neuron/cortical astrocyte cultures. J Neurochem 1997; 69:1398–1408.
43. Desagher S, Glowinski J, Premont J. Astrocytes protect neurons from hydrogen peroxide toxicity. J Neurosci 1996; 16:2553–2562.
44. Engele J, Bohn MC. The neurotrophic effects of fibroblast growth factors on dopaminergic neurons in vitro are mediated by mesencephalic glia. J Neurosci 1991; 11:3070–3078. Erratum in: J Neurosci 1992; 2:685.
45. Hoffer BJ, Hoffman A, Bowenkamp K, Huettl P, Hudson J, Martin D, Lin LF, Gerhardt GA. Glial cell line-derived neurotrophic factor reverses toxin-induced injury to midbrain dopaminergic neurons in vivo. Neurosci Lett 1994; 182:107–111.

46. Takeshima T, Shimoda K, Sauve Y, Commissiong JW. Astrocyte dependent and independent phases of the development and survival of rat embryonic day 14 mesencephalic neurons in culture. Neurosci 1994; 60:809–823.
47. Takeshima T, Johnston JM, Commissiong JW. Oligodendrocyte-type-2 astrocyte (O2A) progenitors increase the survival of rat mesencephalic, dopaminergic neurons from death induced by serum deprivation. Neurosci Lett 1994; 166:178–182.
48. Han SK, Mytilineou C, Cohen G. L-DOPA up-regulates glutathione and protects mesencephalic cultures against oxidative stress. J Neurochem 1996; 66:501–510.
49. Koshimura K, Tanaka J, Murakami Y, Kato Y. Effects of dopamine and L-DOPA on survival of PC12 cells. J Neurosci Res 2000; 62:112–119.
50. Migheli R, Godani C, Sciola L, Delogu MR, Serra PA, Zangani D, De Natale G, Miele E, Desole MS. Enhancing effect of manganese on L-DOPA-induced apoptosis in PC12 cells: role of oxidative stress. J Neurochem 1999; 73:1155–1163.
51. Hefti F, Melamed E, Bhawan J, Wurtman RJ. Long-term administration of levodopa does not damage dopaminergic neurons in the mouse. Neurology 1981; 31:1194–1195.
52. Perry TL, Yong VW, Ito M, Foulks JG, Wall RA, Godin DV, Clavier RM. Nigrostriatal dopaminergic neurons remain undamaged in rats given high doses of L-dopa and carbidopa chronically. J Neurochem 1984; 43:990–993.
53. Reches A, Fahn S. Chronic dopa feeding of mice. Neurology 1982; 32:684–685.
54. Fornai F, Battaglia G, Gesi M, Giorgi FS, Orzi F, Nicoletti F, Ruggieri S. Time-course and dose-response study on the effects of chronic L-DOPA administration on striatal dopamine levels and dopamine transporter following MPTP toxicity. Brain Res 2000; 887:110–117.
55. Blunt SB, Jenner P, Marsden CD. Suppressive effect of L-dopa on dopamine cells remaining in the ventral tegmental area of rats previously exposed to the neurotoxin 6-hydroxydopamine. Mov Disord 1993; 8:129–133.
56. Naudin B, Bonnett JJ, Costentin J. Acute L-dopa pretreatment potentiates 6-hydroxydopamine-induced toxic effects on nigro-striatal dopamine neurons in mice. Brain Res 1995; 701:151–157.
57. Spencer JP, Jenner A, Aruoma OI, Evans PJ, Kaur H, Dexter DT, Jenner P, Lees AJ, Marsden DC, Halliwell B. Intense oxidative stress damage promoted by L-dopa and its metabolites: implications for neurodegenerative disease. FEBS Lett 1994; 353:246–250.
58. Dziewczapolski G, Murer G, Agid Y, Gershanik O, Raisman-Vozari R. Absence of neurotoxicity of chronic L-dopa treatment in 6-hydroxydopamine lesioned rats. Neuroreport 1997; 8:975–979.
59. Murer MG, Dziewczapolski G, Menalled LB, Garcia MC, Agid Y, Gershanik O, Raisman-Vozari R. Chronic levodopa is not toxic for remaining dopamine neurons, but instead promotes their recovery, in rats with moderate nigrostriatal lesions. Ann Neurol 1998; 43:561–575.
60. Datla KP, Blunt SB, Dexter DT. Chronic L-DOPA administration is not toxic to the remaining dopaminergic nigrostriatal neurons, but instead may promote their functional recovery, in rats with partial 6-OHDA or FeCL(3) nigrostriatal lesions. Mov Disord 2001; 16: 424–434.
61. Camp DM, Loeffler DA, LeWit PA. L-DOPA does not enhance hydroxyl radical formation in the nigrostriatal dopamine system of rats with a unilateral 6-hydroxydopamine lesion. J Neurochem 2000; 74:1229–1240.
62. Cleren C, Vilpoux, C, Dourmap N, Bonnett JJ, Costentin J. Acute interactions between L-dopa and the neurotoxic effects of 1-methyl-4-phenylpyridinium or 6-hydroxydopamine in mice. Brain Res 1999; 830:314–319.
63. Clement MV, Long LH, Ramalingam J, Halliwell B. The cytotoxicity of dopamine may be an artifact of cell culture. J Neurochem 2002; 81:414–421.
64. Rajput AH, Fenton ME, Birdi S, Macaulay R. Is levodopa toxic to human substantia nigra? Mov Disord 1997; 12:634–638.
65. Quinn N, Parkes D, Jonata I, Marsden CD. Preservation of the substantia nigra and locus coeruleus in a patient receiving levodopa (2kg) plus decarboxylase inhibitor over a four-year period. Mov Disord 1986; 1:65–68.
66. Hoehn MMM. Parkinsonism treated with levodopa: progression and mortality. J Neural Transm 1983; 19(suppl):253–264.
67. Diamond SG, Markham CH, Hoehn MM, McDowell FH, Muenter MD. Multicenter study of Parkinson's mortality with early versus later dopa treatment. Ann Neurol 1987; 22:8–12.
68. Martilla RJ, Kuopio AM, Rinne UK. Survival in Parkinson's disease: early levodopa treatment enhances life expectancy. New Trends Clin Neuropharm 1994; 8:120–121.
69. Gwinn Hardy K, Evidente VGH, Waters C, Muenter MD, Hardy J. L-Dopa slows progression of familial Parkinson's disease. Lancet 1999; 353:1850–1851.

70. Rajput AH, Uitti RJ, Ho M, Offord K, Rajput A, Barsan P. Current survival profile in parkinsonism. New Trends Clin Neuropharm 1994; 8:121–122.
71. Uitti RJ, Ahlskog JE, Maraganore DM, Muenter MD, Atkinson EJ, Cha RH, O'Brien PC. Levodopa therapy and survival in idiopathic Parkinson's disease: Olmsted county project. Neurology 1993; 43:1918–1926.
72. Yahr MD, Wolf A, Antunes JL, Miyoshi K, Duffy P. Autopsy findings in parkinsonism following treatment with levodopa. Neurology 1972; 22(suppl):56–71.
73. Le WD, Rowe DB, Jankovic J, Xie W, Appel SH. Effects of cerebrospinal fluid from patients with Parkinson disease on dopaminergic cells. Arch Neurol 1999; 56:194–200.
74. Kordower JH, Freeman TB, Snow BJ, Vingerhoets FJ, Mufson EJ, Sanberg PR, Hauser RA, Smith DA, Nauert GM, Perl DP, et al. Neuropathological evidence of graft survival and striatal reinnervation after the transplantation of fetal mesencephalic tissue in a patient with Parkinson's disease. N Engl J Med 1995; 332:1118–1124.
75. Whone AL, Remy P, Davis, MR, Sabolek M, Nahmias C, Stoessl AJ, Walts RL, Brooks DJ. The REAL PET study. Slow progression of early Parkinson's disease treated with ropinirole compared with levodopa. Neurology 2002; 58(suppl 3):A82–A83.
76. Marek K, Seibyl J, Shoulson I, Holloway R, Kieburtz K, McDermott M, Kamp C, Shinaman A, Fahn S, Lang A, Weiner W, Welsh M. Dopamine transporter brain imaging to assess the effects of pramipexole vs. levodopa on Parkinson disease progression. JAMA 2002; 287:1653–1661.
77. Przuntek H, Welzel D, Blumner E, Danielczyk W, Letzel H, Kaiser HJ, Kraus PH, Riederer P, Schwarzmann D, Wolf H, et al. Bromocriptine lessens the incidence of mortality in L-dopa-treated parkinsonian patients: Prado study discontinued. Eur J Clin Pharmacol 1992; 43:357–363.

6

Levodopa Therapy

Alejandro A. Rabinstein

University of Miami School of Medicine, Miami, Florida, U.S.A.

Lisa M. Shulman and William J. Weiner

University of Maryland School of Medicine, Baltimore, Maryland, U.S.A.

I. INTRODUCTION

In the history of therapy for Parkinson's disease (PD), there is no more important event than the discovery of levodopa-replacement therapy. The introduction of this agent in 1967 (1) was nothing short of a revolution in the treatment of PD. Very early in the use of levodopa it became apparent that the drug had remarkable efficacy in treating the major motor symptoms of PD, that it was associated with certain adverse events, and that it was not a cure, nor did it appear to slow progression of PD. It was a powerful and extremely useful symptomatic treatment.

When dopamine agonists were introduced in the early 1970s (2), the accepted clinical practice was to initiate treatment with levodopa and to introduce the agonist when motor fluctuations and dyskinesias began. This was an efficacious strategy, and over time clinical practice evolved to balance levodopa and agonist use. The combined judicious use of both agonists and levodopa has resulted in better management of PD.

This chapter will explore some of the basic mechanisms of levodopa action, its efficacy in PD, and the controversary surrounding its use in early PD.

II. PHARMACOKINETICS OF LEVODOPA

Levodopa (L-3,4-dihydroxyphenylalanine) is a large neutral amino acid synthesized endogenously from L-tyrosine by the catalytic action of the enzyme tyrosine hydroxylase. Endogenous and exogenous levodopa are converted to dopamine by the activity of L-aromatic amino acid decarboxylase (L-AAAD, also known as dopa decarboxylase). Tyrosine hydroxylase is the rate-limiting enzyme highly specific to catecholaminergic neurons specialized in the synthesis of dopamine and only found in the brain, sympathetic ganglia and nerves, and adrenal medulla. In contrast, L-AAAD is not rate limiting (i.e., its activity is not regulated by changes in the intensity of dopaminergic transmission) (3) and shows a rather ubiquitous distribution, being present in a variety of neurons as well as kidney, liver, intestinal, and cerebral endothelial cells (4). Therefore, a considerable proportion of exogenous levodopa is decarboxylated to dopamine in peripheral sites. Levodopa may also be metabolized to 3-*O*-methyldopa (3-OMD) by the enzyme catechol-*O*-methyltransferase (COMT) present in liver and red blood cells. In fact, even in the presence of a peripheral decarboxylase inhibitor, only 10% of exogenously administered levodopa may reach the brain (5).

Dopamine is inactivated by the enzymes monoamine oxidase (MAO) and COMT. MAO is a mitochondrial enzyme that exists in two forms, MAO-A and MAO-B, which differ in substrate preference, inhibitor specificity, tissue and cell distribution, and immunological properties (6). MAO-A is predominantly expressed in catecholaminergic nerurons, whereas MAO-B is mostly found in serotoninergic neurons (7). In the brain, COMT is mostly localized in glial cells. Oxidation of dopamine forms dihydroxyphenylacetic acid, and its *O*-methylation produces 3-methoxytyramine. The common end product of dopamine catabolism is homovanillic acid (HVA), which is excreted in the urine.

Levodopa is mostly absorbed in the proximal part of the small intestine by an active saturable carrier system for large neutral amino acids. The rate of gastric emptying determines the rate of levodopa intestinal absorption. Gastric emptying is delayed by food (especially fatty food) (8) and becomes more erratic with age (9). Therefore, levodopa is ideally administered 30–60 minutes before meals to maximize absorption. Since levodopa must compete with other large neutral amino acids for its absorption, rescheduling or restriction of protein intake may be useful in some patients with advanced PD (10). Levodopa absorption may also be reduced or delayed by increased gastric acidity and by certain drugs, such as other dopaminergic agents, antimuscarinics, tricyclic anti depressants, and ferrous sulfate (11). In contrast, diets rich in insoluble fiber (12) could enhance levodopa absorption. Metoclopramide can also increase levodopa absorption (13), but its use cannot be widely recommended in patients with PD due to its antidopaminergic properties.

In clinical practice, levodopa is almost invariably administered in combination with a peripheral decarboxylase inhibitor (carbidopa or benserazide). At usual doses, these decarboxylase inhibitors do not cross the blood-brain barrier, thus reducing the peripheral metabolism of levodopa. This results in a nearly twofold increase in plasma levodopa elimination half-life (14) and a 75% reduction in total dose required (15).

After intestinal absorption and first passage through the liver via portal circulation, levodopa reaches the systemic circulation. Levodopa clearance then follows biphasic kinetics. During the short distribution phase (30 min), levodopa enters various tissue reservoirs, most notably the skeletal muscle, and crosses the blood-brain barrier using a saturable bidirectional transport system specific for neutral amino acids (16). As in the intestinal mucosa, high protein load may negatively influence levodopa transport across the blood-brain barrier (17). In patients with advanced PD, ventricular cerebral spinal fluid (CSF) concentrations are 12% of plasma levels and peak levodopa concentrations occur 1–2 hours after peak plasma levels. Plasma and CSF pharmacokinetic parameters are highly correlated, but clinical improvement and worsening, as well as the onset of dyskinesias, are more closely related to the changes of levodopa and dopamine in the CSF (18).

III. MECHANISM OF ACTION OF LEVODOPA

The classic hypothesis regarding the central mechanism of action of levodopa assumes that after crossing the blood-brain barrier, the drug enters presynaptic nerve terminals of hyperactive surviving nigrostriatal dopaminergic neurons. In these terminals, levodopa is decarboxylated by residual L-AAAD and stored as dopamine to be released into the synaptic cleft (19). However, accruing evidence indicates that central effects of levodopa are considerably more complex than previously thought. In fact, despite extensive research efforts, the central handling and mechanism of action of levodopa remain the source of controversy and uncertainty.

The exact sites of exogenous levodopa decarboxylation remain to be fully elucidated. L-AAAD activity has been shown in striatal serotoninergic terminals (20,21), capillary endothelium (22), glial cells (23), various nonmonoaminergic intrastriatal neurons such as small aspiny interneurons (24) and medium-sized spiny projection neurons (25), and extra-striatal neurons in different locations (26). However, the results of studies assessing the conversion of levodopa to dopamine in these sites have often yielded conflicting results (23,24,27). Some investigators have even suggested that levodopa itself could produce a response without previous conversion into dopamine by directly acting on dopamine D2 receptors (28,29), but the prevailing view is that conversion to dopamine is indeed necessary for the principal levodopa actions to occur (21).

The precise mode of presynaptic storage and release of levodopa also remains unclear. Animal experiments have shown that reserpine-induced dysfunction of synaptic vesicles in dopaminergic neurons has little impact on striatal dopamine levels after levodopa administration (30). Also, electrochemical studies in animal models showed that direct electrical neuronal stimulation to manipulate the firing rate of dopaminergic neurons had no significant effect on the levels of striatal dopamine after exogenous levodopa administration (31). These results defy the traditional model of phasic release of levodopa from stores in synaptic vesicles. Instead, it has been suggested that dopamine could form extravesicular cytosolic pools in the nerve terminals of nigrostriatal dopaminergic neurons (30). After reaching a certain intraneuronal concentration threshold, dopamine might then leak into the synaptic cleft and produce tonic receptor stimulation. However, repeated levodopa administration increases the spontaneous firing rate of dopaminergic cells in dopamine-depleted rats (31), suggesting that phasic dopamine release occurs in response to exogenous levodopa.

Postsynaptically, matters are not much clearer. Sensitivity to levodopa effects is greater in dopamine-denervated striatum compared with intact striatum (21,32). In addition to this denervation hypersensitivity of dopamine receptors, reuptake of dopamine is reduced in denervated striatum (21). Thus, as denervation progresses, more dopamine would become available in the synaptic cleft to act on increasingly hypersensitive postsynaptic receptors. The relative importance of different dopamine receptors has been the subject of much investigation. D1 agonists, mixed D1/D2 agonists, and D2 antagonists, but not D2 agonists increase striatal C-fos expression (33), a cell marker of dopamine-induced postsynaptic responses. It is possible that levodopa acts mainly by activating D1 receptors, with D2 receptors playing a facilitatory role.

A positron emission tomography (PET) study using 18-fluorodeoxyglucose to quantify regional metabolic abnormalities in patients with PD demonstrated that exogenous levodopa reduces the abnormal expression of metabolic activity commonly observed with PD (thalamic and lentiform hypermetabolism coupled with cortical hypometabolism) (34). This suggests that the response to levodopa therapy in PD could result from the modulation of cortico-striato-pallido-thalamocortical pathways. Event-related functional magnetic resonance imaging (MRI) has also been successfully used to study the effects of levodopa treatment on PD (35).

IV. LEVODOPA FOR THE TREATMENT OF PD: PRACTICAL CONSIDERATIONS

Levodopa is the single most effective drug for the treatment of the motor symptoms of PD and benefits virtually all patients with a pathologically confirmed diagnosis (36). It improves quality of life and reduces morbidity and mortality in patients with PD (37–39). However, levodopa does not arrest the underlying neurodegenerative process, and over time therapy begins to fail. Motor symptoms become more refractory, and nonmotor symptoms (e.g., dementia, psychiatric disturbances, dysautonomia) often develop. In addition, increasing duration and severity of the disease and prolonged use of levodopa are associated with the appearance of motor complications, most notably dyskinesias and motor fluctuations.

Levodopa is routinely administered orally in combination with a peripheral decarboxylase inhibitor. Carbidopa is the peripheral decarboxylase inhibitor used in the United States, whereas benserazide is used in other parts of the world. Carbidopa/ levodopa is available in dosages of 10/100, 25/100, and 25/250. There is also a controlled-release formulation offered in doses of 25/100 and 50/200. Benserazide/levodopa is available in doses of 25/100 and 50/200, with a controlled-release form available in doses of 50/200. Controlled-release formulations are less well absorbed than immediate-release formulations, and doses 20–30% higher may be needed to achieve an equivalent clinical effect. Supplemental carbidopa may be prescribed in dosages of up to 300 mg/day to patients receiving effective doses of levodopa-carbidopa who continue to have nausea and vomiting due to insufficient inhibition of peripheral decarboxylation. Domperidone, a peripheral dopamine antagonist, may also be very effective in controlling these side effects, but it is not available in the United States. Liquid preparations of levodopa may be useful in the management of patients who have extreme problems with motor fluctuations or have developed swallowing difficulties.

When initiating therapy with levodopa, it is advisable to start with low doses and titrate the dosage gradually to minimize the risk of acute side effects. The general principle should be to use the lowest dose that provides a satisfactory clinical response. Restriction of levodopa to delay the onset of motor complications cannot be advocated in the presence of parkinsonian symptoms resulting in functional impairment (40). When patients fail to respond to high doses of levodopa (800–1000 mg/d), the diagnosis of PD should be reassessed (36). Studies suggest that sustained response to levodopa is dependent on the timing and amount of the single doses of the drug (40,41). Thus, time intervals between doses must be individually adjusted for maximally lasting efficacy.

Unfortunately, benefit from levodopa declines and adverse effects increase over time (42). Long-term levodopa therapy is associated with the occurrence of various motor complications (Table 1). Dyskinesias and motor fluctuations may be observed in nearly 40% of patients after 4–6 years of levodopa treatment (43). Fluctuating nonmotor symptoms may also emerge in the later stages of the disease (44), including neuropsychiatric disturbances that may be exacerbated by levodopa. Also, late features of PD, such as freezing, postural and gait instability, and autonomic dysfunction, tend to be nonresponsive to levodopa therapy (45).

Temporary levodopa withdrawal (drug holiday) has been suggested as a potentially useful strategy to restore the efficacy of the drug in patients with advanced PD, possibly by favoring an upregulation of dopamine receptors (46–49). However, these drug holidays place patients at high risk for serious complications such as aspiration pneumonia, deep

Table 1 Motor Complications of Levodopa Therapy

Motor fluctuations
Wearing-off phenomenon (at the end of each dose)
On-off phenomenon (unpredictable timing)
Dose failures
Freezing episodes
Dyskinesias
Peak dose dyskinesia
Dyskinesia-improvement-dyskinesia syndrome (diphasic dyskinesias)
Dystonia

venous thrombosis, pressure sores, and even malnutrition. Abrupt cessation of levodopa may also result in manifestations similar to those seen in patients with neuroleptic malignant syndrome (50). At best, this intervention may improve the efficacy of levodopa for just a few months, and it is rarely used in clinical practice (51).

V. LEVODOPA SIDE EFFECTS AND LATE COMPLICATIONS

Adverse events related to levodopa are common. The most frequent clinically relevant side effects observed during the early phases of levodopa treatment are nausea and vomiting, postural hypotension, and somnolence. Nausea can be ameliorated by taking the medication with food, but this recommendation may lead to decreased absorption of the drug. Nausea and postural hypotension are related to excessive peripheral dopamine activity. Thus, increasing the dose of the peripheral decarboxylase inhibitor (carbidopa or benserazide) can be helpful. Other early side effects are much less common, and sometimes idiosyncratic. They include skin rash, darkening of the urine, diaphoresis, positive Coombs' test, and hemolytic anemia. Nonfatal cardiac arrhythmias have been reported in patients taking levodopa, but the incidence of arrhythmias in these patients is comparable to that observed in age-matched control subjects.

Psychiatric side effects may become problematic as the disease progresses. Although the appearance of psychiatric symptoms often follows an increase in levodopa dose or the addition of a dopaminergic or anticholinergic agent, occasionally these symptoms appear without an obvious precipitant. Vivid dreams and nightmares are commonly the first manifestations. Visual illusions and hallucinations, sometimes with retention of insight, often follow. Delusions and rarely auditory hallucinations are found in more severe cases. Depression frequently affects patients with PD, but levodopa does not appear to have any consistent effect on depression (52,53). However, levodopa can occasionally precipitate manic states in PD, as well as non-PD, patients (54). Dementia is a late but serious problem in 20–40% of patients with PD. While psychotic symptoms and organic confusional states induced by dopaminergic drugs may clear rapidly after withdrawal of the implicated medications, the cognitive dysfunction of patients with established dementia will not respond to this intervention. Psychiatric symptoms may fluctuate in late stages of the disease, adding even more complexity to their management.

For practical purposes, the motor complications of levodopa may be divided into two subgroups: motor fluctuations and dyskinesias. Motor fluctuations may be defined as alternating periods of good motor function ("on periods" during which the patient is responding to the drug) and periods of impaired motor function ("off" periods with suboptimal or lack of response to the medication). Early in the course of the disease, patients respond to a single dose of levodopa for several hours despite the short plasma half-life of the drug (55), and may even tolerate missing doses with little or no symptoms. These benefits are related to the "long-duration response" (LDR) of chronically administered levodopa. Early on, LDR is measured in days and it may last several weeks. The LDR alone could represent up to one third of the therapeutic activity of levodopa (56), but the LDR is difficult to distinguish from the short-duration response (SDR) (i.e., the motor response occurring immediately following a single dose of levodopa and lasting only a few hours) in clinical practice. The LDR is inversely related to disease severity and duration (7,57); the decline in the LDR over time reflects the incremental inadequacy of central dopamine handling in advanced PD and may play a pivotal role in the development of motor complications.

With advancing PD, the motor benefits after a single dose of levodopa become progressively shorter, finally approaching the plasma half-life of the drug that remains unchanged throughout the course of the disease (56). Also, the levodopa concentration required to achieve the maximal therapeutic response increases with time as the disease worsens (58). The clinical correlate of these pharmacodynamic changes is known as "wearing off," a deterioration of the motor status toward the end of the interval between doses. At this stage, patients may also begin to experience more rapid and unpredictable fluctuations of motor function between doses, a complication known as the "on-off" phenomenon.

First described by Cotzias et al. over 30 years ago (1), levodopa-induced dyskinesias are involuntary, choreiform, or athetoid movements that occur in response to administration of the medication. These movements may involve virtually any part of the body. Dystonia is a less frequent form of levodopa-induced dyskinesia and must be differentiated from the dystonia observed during "off" periods due to insufficient medication. Dyskinesias are commonly observed in combination with motor fluctuations and may also exhibit a fluctuating course. These fluctuating dyskinesias may follow the pattern described as diphasic dyskinesias or dyskinesia-improvement-dyskinesia (D-I-D) (59).

Dyskinesias usually respond to the reduction or elimination of levodopa, but often these changes result in disabling worsening of the parkinsonian symptoms. As PD progresses, finding a levodopa schedule able to provide adequate motor benefit while avoiding dyskinesias eventually becomes an impossible task. At that point a compromise should be discussed with the patient, now forced to accept either some dyskinesias during "on" periods or some parkinsonian symptoms during "off" periods. The comparative effects of dyskinesias and of PD symptoms on the patient's quality of life should guide the therapeutic plan.

Patients treated in the prelevodopa era experienced dyskinesias much earlier after onset of levodopa treatment than patients included in later series who received levodopa from the time of first diagnosis of the disease (60). This discrepancy may be explained by differences in disease duration and severity. Indeed, the severity of PD at the time of levodopa initiation is inversely correlated with the interval to development of dyskinesias (61). In the present era, patients treated with levodopa for 4–6 years have approximately a 40% likelihood of experiencing motor complications (motor fluctuations or dyskinesias) (60). This proportion continues to increase with time; in a recent clinico-pathological study, the overall prevalence of motor complications in a series of patients with a mean duration of illness of nearly 16 years was 71% (42). It is possible that every patient with PD treated with levodopa is destined to develop motor complications at some point.

The pathophysiology of levodopa-induced motor complications is unclear. Different investigators have postulated that their occurrence might be related to pulsatile stimulation of dopamine receptors (62,63), alterations in dopamine receptor signaling (64,65), downstream changes in protein and genes (66), and abnormalities in nondopamine transmitter systems (such as glutaminergic and opioid) (67,68). All these events combine to produce alterations in the firing patterns that signal between the basal ganglia and the cortex (69,70). The current theory is that in patients with PD, abnormal pulsatile stimulation of striatal dopamine receptors replaces the normally predominant tonic firing of dopaminergic neurons due to the loss of striatal dopaminergic terminals that results in reduced dopamine storage capacity. Pulsatile stimulation also occurs with the intermittent administration of exogenous levodopa. As the disease advances, the brain becomes more dependent on the levels of administered levodopa and hence more susceptible to pulsatile stimulation. These concepts suggest that continuous delivery of levodopa could be a helpful strategy to minimize the long-term risk of motor complications (71).

VI. CONTROVERSIES SURROUNDING LEVODOPA USE

A. Should Dopamine Agonists Be Used Instead of Levodopa for Treating Early PD?

Recent prospective, randomized, double-blind, long-term trials have been designed to compare dopamine agonists versus levodopa for treating early PD. Initial treatment with ropinirole versus levodopa was compared in a 5-year prospective, randomized, double-blind trial in patients with early symptomatic PD (72). A total of 268 patients were enrolled; 179 were randomly assigned to initial treatment with ropinirole and 89 to levodopa. The rates of patients completing the 5-year follow-up were similar in both groups (47% in the ropinirole group and 51% in the levodopa group). However, more patients in the levodopa group completed the study without additional open label levodopa supplementation (required by 64% of the patients initially treated with ropinirole vs. 34% of those started on levodopa). There was a significant reduction in cumulative incidence of dyskinesia in the ropinirole group, regardless of levodopa supplementation. Overall, dyskinesia developed in 36 of the 177 patients in the ropinirole group (20%) and in 40 of the 88 in the levodopa group (45%) as assessed by item 32 of the Unified Parkinson's Disease Rating Scale (UPDRS). Before the addition of supplementary levodopa, only 5% of patients in the ropinirole group had developed dyskinesias versus 36% in the levodopa group. The hazard ratio for remaining free of dyskinesias in the ropinirole group as compared with the levodopa group was 2.82 [95% confidence interval (CI) 1.78–4.44; $p < 0.001$]. Disabling dyskinesias developed in 8% of patients on ropinirole and 23% of patients on levodopa (hazard ratio 3.02; $p = 0.0020$). However, despite this favorable result in terms of incidence of dyskinesias, patients who received initial treatment with ropinirole had slightly worse scores for activities of daily living (Part II of the UPDRS) at the end of the study than patients in the levodopa group. Among patients who completed the study, those initially started on levodopa had significantly greater improvement in motor function as assessed by Part III of the UPDRS (mean difference between treatments 4.48 points; $p = 0.008$) and less freezing while walking. Wearing-off effects were slightly less prominent in the ropinirole group. There was no significant difference in the incidence of neuropsychiatric adverse events between the two groups (24% incidence in the ropinirole group vs. 17% in the levodopa group), but the incidence of hallucinations was higher in patients who had been started on ropinirole (17% vs. 6% of patients on levodopa). There were no reports of sleep attacks in either group. Rates of early withdrawal were similar in both groups.

Another double-blind clinical trial conducted by the Parkinson Study Group, the CALM-PD study, compared the use of pramipexole versus levodopa in early PD (73). Three hundred and one early symptomatic PD patients were randomized in a double-blind fashion to receive either pramipexole plus placebo or placebo and levodopa. Initial results were reported for patients prospectively followed for 23.5 months. After week 11, investigators were allowed to introduce open-label supplementary levodopa to treat residual disability. The primary endpoint was the occurrence of any of three dopaminergic motor complications: wearing off, on-off effects, and dyskinesias. Twenty-eight percent of patients assigned to initial pramipexole therapy reached the primary endpoint as compared with 51% of patients in the levodopa group (hazard ratio 0.44, 95% CI 0.30–0.66; $p < 0.0001$), with the largest difference occurring in the subset of patients with dyskinesias. Forty-eight percent of patients in the pramipexole group required supplemental levodopa as opposed to 36% in the levodopa group ($p = 0.03$). The mean improvement in total UPDRS scores from baseline to the end of the follow-up was significantly greater ($p = 0.0002$) in the patients initially treated with levodopa (mean difference between scores 4.8).

A study comparing cabergoline with levodopa also found that the frequency of motor complications was reduced in patients initially started on the dopamine agonist (74). Motor complications occurred in 34% of the levodopa group and 22% of patients receiving cabergoline over the 3–5 years of follow-up ($p < 0.02$). Similar to the experience with other dopamine agonists, improvement in motor disability was superior with levodopa.

These clinical trials indicate that in patients with PD who require initiation of dopaminergic treatment, either levodopa or a dopamine agonist may be used. If improving motor disability is considered the first priority, levodopa is a better choice. Conversely, a dopamine agonist should be the preferred agent when the focus is on delaying the incidence of motor complications (75).

Novel functional neuroimaging techniques now offer new opportunities to assess the effect of levodopa and dopamine agonists on PD progression. A study by the Parkinson Study Group was designed to evaluate the rates of in vivo dopamine neuron degeneration after initial treatment with levodopa or pramipexole in early PD in a subset of the CALM-PD population (76). Single photon emission computed tomography (SPECT) was used to measure the uptake of 2β-carboxymethoxy-3β(4-iodophenyl) tropane—a dopamine transporter and a biomarker for striatal dopaminergic terminals—labeled with iodine 123 ([^{123}I] β-CIT). Patients were imaged serially, and the primary outcome measure was the percentage change from baseline in striatal [^{123}I] β-CIT uptake after 46 months. Patients treated initially with pramipexole had a reduced loss of striatal uptake of the radionucleide compared with the patients in the levodopa group. At the end of the follow-up, the degree of reduction in [^{123}I] β-CIT uptake correlated with the change in UPDRS score, an important finding since this correlation between imaging and clinical outcomes had been disputed in prior studies (77,78). The authors favored the hypothesis that pramipexole may have a protective effect on the process of degeneration of dopamine neurons. A relative reduction in the loss of ^{18}F-dopa uptake after 2 years of treatment with ropinirole compared with a group of patients treated with levodopa has also been reported (79). Nevertheless, the interpretation of these imaging studies has been criticized (80–84), and the claim that dopamine agonists may grant neuroprotective advantages seems premature (85). Further studies are needed before firm conclusions can be reached.

B.   When Initiating Levodopa Therapy, Is the Sustained-Release Formulation Any Better?

Controlled-release levodopa has been shown to produce consistent rises in plasma levodopa levels that last 3–4 hours longer than those achieved with standard levodopa formulations (86). This property has made controlled-release levodopa a useful alternative in the management of advanced patients with PD who experience motor fluctuations (87). In addition, experimental evidence suggesting that pulsatile stimulation of striatal dopamine receptors may play a role in the induction of levodopa-related motor complications has spurred interest in the use of controlled-release formulations for early treatment of PD.

Only one study compared sustained-release and immediate-release levodopa preparations using a prospective, randomized, double-blind design (88). In this multicenter study, patients had a relatively low incidence of dyskinesias over 5 years of follow-up (20.6% of patients receiving immediate-release levodopa vs. 21.6% of patients in the controlled-release group). The only difference noted between the treatment groups was a greater improvement in activities of daily living scores in the controlled-release group (mean change of -0.8 compared with $+0.2$ in patients receiving the standard formulation; $p = 0.031$). The results of this study failed to produce sufficient evidence to recommend controlled-release levodopa over immediate-release levodopa when initiating dopaminergic treatment. Since its design required that both formulations be initiated with twice-daily dosing, this study did not adequately address the role of pulsatile stimulation of striatal dopamine receptors in the pathogenesis of dyskinesias and motor fluctuations.

VII.   CONCLUSIONS

Levodopa remains the most effective treatment for PD. More than 30 years of widespread use of this agent has produced no evidence of levodopa-induced toxic effects in patients with PD. Levodopa has improved the quality of life in PD patients, from those with early disease to those with very advanced disease.

REFERENCES

1. Cotzias GC, Van Woert MH, Schiffer LM. Aromatic amino acids and modification of parkinsonism. N Eng J Med 1967; 276:374–379.
2. Calne DB, Teychenne PF, Claveria LE, Eastman R, Greenacre JK, Petrie A. Bromocriptine in parkinsonism. Br Med J 1974; 4:442–444.
3. Lovenberg W, Victor SJ. Regulation of tryptophan tyrosine hydroxylase. Life Sci 1974; 14:2337–2353.
4. Rahman MK, Nagatsu T, Kato T. Aromatic L-amino acid decarboxylase activity in central and peripheral tissues and serum of rats with L-DOPA and L-5-hydroxytryptophan as substrates. Biochem Pharmacol 1981; 30:645–649.
5. Kaakkola S. Clinical pharmacology, therapeutic use and potential of COMT inhibitors in Parkinson's disease. Drugs 2000Jun; 59(6):1233–1250.
6. Abell, CW. Monoamine oxidase A and B from human liver and brain. Methods Enzymol 1987; 142:638–650.
7. Deleu D, Northway MG, Hanssens Y. Clinical pharmacokinetic and pharmacodynamic properties of drugs used in the treatment of Parkinson's disease. Clin Pharmacokinet 2002; 41(4):261–309.
8. Baruzzi A, Contin M, Riva R, Procaccianti G, Albani F, Tonello C, Zoni E, Martinelli P. Influence of meal ingestion time on pharmacokinetics of orally administered levodopa in parkinsonian patients. Clin Neuropharmacol 1987; 10:527–537.
9. Contin M, Riva R, Martinelli P, Albani F, Baruzzi A. Effect of age on the pharmacokinetics of oral levodopa in patients with Parkinson's disease. Eur J Clin Pharmacol 1991; 41:463–466.
10. Karstaedt PJ, Pincus JH. Protein redistribution diet remains effective in patients with fluctuating parkinsonism. Arch Neurol 1992; 49:149–151.
11. Pfiefer RF. Antiparkinsonian agents. Drug interactions of clinical significance. Drug Safety 1996; 14:343–354.

12. Astarloa R, Mena MA, Sanchez V, de la Vega L, de Yebenes JG. Clinical and pharmacokinetic effects of a diet rich in insoluble fiber on Parkinson disease. Clin Neuropharmacol 1992; 15:375–380.
13. Mearrick PT, Wade DN, Birkett DJ, Morris J. Metoclopramide, gastric emptying and L-dopa absorption. Austr NZ J Med 1974; 4:144–148.
14. Gancher ST, Nutt JG, Woodward WR. Peripheral pharmacokinetics of levodopa in untreated, stable, and fluctuating parkinsonian patients. Neurology 1987; 37:940–944.
15. Cedarbaum JM. Clinical pharmacokinetics of anti-parkinsonian drugs. Clin Pharmakinetics 1987; 13:141–178.
16. Pardridge WM, Oldendorf WH. Transport of metabolic substrates through the blood-brain barrier. J Neurochem 1977; 28:5–12.
17. Nutt JG, Woodward WR, Carter JH, Trotman TL. Influence of fluctuations of plasma large neutral amino acids with normal diets on the clinical response to levodopa. J Neurol Neurosurg Psychiatry 1989; 52:481–487.
18. Olanow CW, Gauger LL, Cedarbaum JM. Temporal relationships between plasma and cerebrospinal fluid pharmacokinetics of levodopa and clinical effect in Parkinson's disease. Ann Neurol 1991; 29:556–559.
19. Hornykiewicz O. The mechanisms of action of L-dopa in Parkinson's disease. Life Sci 1974; 15: 1249–1259.
20. Arai R, Karasawa N, Geffard M, Nagatsu T, Nagatsu I. Immunohistochemical evidence that central serotonin neurons produce dopamine from exogenous L-DOPA in the rat, with reference to the involvement of aromatic L-amino acid decarboxylase. Brain Res 1994; 667:295–299.
21. Lopez A, Munoz A, Guerra MJ, Labandeira-Garcia JL. Mechanisms of the effects of exogenous levodopa on the dopamine-denervated striatum. Neuroscience 2001; 103:639–651.
22. Melamed E, Hefti F, Wurtman RJ. Decarboxylation of exogenous L-DOPA in rat striatum afer lesions of the dopaminergic nigrostriatal neurons: the role of striatal capillaries. Brain Res 1980; 198:244–248.
23. Tsai MJ, Lee EH. Characterization of L-DOPA transport in cultured rat and mouse astrocytes. J Neurosci Res 1996; 43:490–495.
24. Mura A, Jackson D, Manley MS, Young SJ, Groves PM. Aromatic L-amino acid decarboxylase immunoreactive cells in the rat striatum: a possible site for the conversion of exogenous L-DOPA to dopamine. Brain Res 1995; 704:51–60.
25. Tashiro Y, Kaneko T, Sugimoto T, Nagatsu I, Kikuchi H, Mizuno N. Striatal neurons with aromatic L-amino acid decarboxylase-like immunoreactivity in the rat. Neurosci Lett 1989; 100:29–34.
26. Schneider JS, Sun ZQ, Roeltgen DP. Effects of dihydrexidine, a full dopamine D-1 receptor agonist, on delayed response performance in chronic low dose MPTP-treated monkeys. Brain Research 1994; 663:140–144.
27. Melamed E, Hefti F, Liebman J, Schlosberg AJ, Wurtman RJ. Serotonergic nerones are not involved in action of L-dopa in Parkinson's disease. Nature 1980; 283:772–774.
28. Nakamura S, Yue JL, Goshima Y, Miyamae T, Ueda H, Misu Y. Non-effective dose of exogenously applied L-dopa itself stereoselectively potentiates postsynaptic D2 receptor-mediated locomotor activities of conscious rats. Neurosci Lett 1994; 170:22–26.
29. Fisher A, Biggs CS, Eradiri O, Starr MS. Dual effects of L-3,4-dihydroxyphenylalanine on aromatic L-amino acid decarboylase, dopamine release and motor stimulation in the reserpine-treated rat: evidence that behaviour is dopamine independent. Neuroscience 2000; 95:97–111.
30. Melamed E, Globus M, Uzzan A, Rosenthal J. Is dopamine formed from exogenous L-dopa stored within vesicles in striatal dopaminergic nerve terminals: implications for L-dopa's mechanism of action in Parkinson's disease. Neurology 1995; 35(suppl 1):118.
31. Hefti F, Melamed E. Dopamine release in rat striatum after administration of L-dopa as studied with in vivo electrochemistry. Brain Res 1981; 225:333–346.
32. Abercrombie ED, Bonatz AE, Zigmond MJ. Effects of L-dopa on extracellular dopamine in striatum of normal and 6-hydroxydopamine-treated rats. Brain Res 1990; 525:36–44.
33. Robertson GS, Fibiger HC. Neuroleptics increase c-fos expression in the forebrain: contrasting effects of haloperidol and clozapine. Neuroscience 1992; 46:315–328.
34. Feigin A, Fukuda M, Dhawan V, Przedborski S, Jackson-Lewis V, Mentis MJ, Moeller JR, Eidelberg D. Metabolic correlates of levodopa response in Parkinson's disease. Neurology 2001; 57:2083–2088.
35. Haslinger B, Erhard P, Kampfe N, Boecker H, Rummeny E, Schwaiger M, Conrad B, Ceballos-Bauman AO. Event-related functional magnetic resonance imaging in Parkinson's disease before and after levodopa. Brain 2001; 124:558–570.
36. Hughes Aj, Ben-Shlomo Y, Daniel SE, Lees AJ. What features improve the accuracy of clinical diagnosis in Parkinson's disease: a clinic pathologic study. Neurology 1992; 42:1142–1146.

37. Yahr MD. Levodopa. Ann Intern Med 1975; 83:675–682.
38. Diamond SG, Markham CH, Hoehn MM, McDowell FH, Muenter MD. Multi-center study of Parkinson mortality with early versus later dopa treatment. Ann Neurol 1987; 22:8–12.
39. Scigliano G, Musicco M, Soliveri P, Piccolo I, Girotti F, Giovannini P, Caraceni T. Mortality associated with early and late levodopa therapy initiation in Parkinson's disease. Neurology 1990; 40:265–269.
40. Quattrone A, Zappia M, Aguglia U, Branca D, Colao R, Montesanti R, Nicoletti G, Palmieri A, Parlato G, Rizzo M. The subacute levodopa test for evaluating long-duration response in Parkinson's disease. Ann Neurol 1995; 38:389–395.
41. Zappia M, Oliveri RL, Bosco D, Nicoletti G, Branca D, Caracciolo M, Napoli ID, Gambardella A, Quattrone A. The long-duration response to L-dopa in the treatment of early PD. Neurology 2000; 54:1910–1915.
42. Rajput AH, Fenton ME, Birdi S, Macaulay R, George D, Rozdilsky B, Ang LC, Senthilselvan A, Hornykiewicz O. Clinical-pathological study of levodopa complications. Mov Disord 2002; 17:289–296.
43. Ahlskog JE, Muenter MD. Frequency of levodopa-related dyskinesias and motor fluctuations as estimated from the cumulative literature. Mov Disord 2001; 16:448–458.
44. Riley DE, Lang AE. The spectrum of levodopa-related fluctuations in Parkinson's disease. Neurology 1993; 43:1459–1464.
45. Klawans HL. Individual manifestations of Parkinson's disease after ten or more years of levodopa. Mov Disord 1986; 1:187–192.
46. Direnfeld LK, Feldman RG, Alexander MP, Kelly-Hayes M. Is L-DOPA drug holiday useful? Neurology 1980; 30:785–788.
47. Weiner WJ, Koller WC, Perlik SJ, Nausieda P, Klawans HL. Drug holiday and management of Parkinson disease. Neurology 1980; 30:1257–1261.
48. Corona T, Rivera C, Otero E, Stopp L. A longitudinal study of the effects of an L-dopa drug holiday on the course of Parkinson's disease. Clin Neuropharmacol 1995; 18:325–332.
49. Nutt JG, Carter JH, Woodward WR. Effect of brief levodopa holidays on the short-duration response to levodopa: evidence for tolerance to the antiparkinsonian effects. Neurology 1994; 44:1617–1622.
50. Sechi GP, Tanda F, Mutani R. Fatal hyperpyrexia after withdrawal of levodopa. Neurology 1984; 34:249–251.
51. Koller WC, Weiner WJ, Perlik SJ, Nausieda PA, Goetz CG, Klawans HL. Complications of long term levodopa therapy: Long term efficacy of drug holiday. Neurology 1981; 31:473–476.
52. Marsh GG, Markham CH. Does levodopa alter depression and psychopathology in Parkinsonism patients?. J Neurol Neurosurg Psychiatry 1973; 36:925–935.
53. Shulman LM, Taback R, Bean J, Mellman TA, Weiner, WJ. The comorbidity of the non-motor symptoms of Parkinson's disease. Mov Disord 2001; 16:507–510.
54. Peet M, Peters S. Drug-induced mania. Drug Safety 1995; 12:146–153.
55. Muenter MD, Tyce GM. L-dopa therapy of Parkinson's disease: plasma L-dopa concentration, therapeutic response, and side effects. Mayo Clin Proc 1971; 46:231–239.
56. Nutt JG, Holford NH. The response to levodopa in Parkinson's disease: imposing pharmacological law and order. Ann Neurol 1996; 39:561–573.
57. Zappia M, Bosco D, Plastino M, Nicoletti G, Branca D, Oliveri RL, Aguglia U, Gambardella A, Quattrone A. Pharmacodynamics of the long-duration response to levodopa in PD. Neurology 1999; 53:557–560.
58. Contin M, Riva R, Martinelli P, Albani F, Baruzzi A. Relationship between levodopa concentration, dyskinesias, and motor effect in parkinsonian patients: a 3-year follow-up study. Clin Neuropharmacol 1997; 20:409–418.
59. Muenter MD, Sharpless NS, Tyce GM, Darley FL. Patterns of dystonia ("I-D-I" and "D-I-D-") in response to 1-dopa therapy for Parkinson's disease. Mayo Clin Proc 1977; 52:163–174.
60. Ahlskog JE, Nishino H, Evidente VG, Tulloch JW, Forbes GS, Caviness JN, Gwinn-Hardy KA. Persistent chorea triggered by hyperglycemic crisis in diabetics. Mov Disord 2001; 16:890–898.
61. Kostic VS, Marinkovic J, Svetel M, Stefanova E, Przedborski S. The effect of stage of Parkinson's disease at the onset of levodopa therapy on development of motor complications. Eur J Neurol 2002; 9:9-14.
62. Juncos JL, Engber TM, Raisman R, Susel Z, Thibaut F, Ploska A, Agid Y, Chase Y. Continuous and intermittent levodopa differentially affect basal ganglia function. Ann Neurol 1989; 25:473–478.
63. Da la Fuente-Ferandez R, Lu JQ, Sossi V, Jivan S, Schulzer M, Holden JE, Lee CS, Ruth TJ, Calne DB, Stoessl AJ. Biochemical variations in the synaptic level of dopamine precede motor fluctuations in Parkinson's disease: PET evidence of increased dopamine turnover. Ann Neurol 2001; 49:298–303.

64. Muriel MP, Bernard V, Levey AI, Laribi O, Abrous DN, Agid Y, Bloch B, Hirsch EC. Levodopa induces a cytoplasmic localization of D1 dopamine receptors in striatal neurons in Parkinson's disease. Ann Neurol 1999; 46:103–111.

65. Hwang WJ, Yao WJ, Wey SP, Shen LH, Ting G. Downregulation of striatal dopamine D2 receptors in advanced Parkinson's disease contributes to the development of motor fluctuation. Eur Neurol 2002; 47:113–117.

66. Calon F, Grondin R, Morissette M, Goulet M, Blanchet PJ, Di Paolo T, Bedard PJ. Molecular basis of levodopa-induced dyskinesias. Ann Neurol 2000; 47:S70–78.

67. Dunah AW, Wang Y, Yasuda RP, Kameyama K, Huganir RL, Wolfe BB, Standaert DG. Alterations in subunit expression, composition, and phosphorylation of striatal N-methyl-D-aspartate glutamate receptors in a rat 6-hydroxydopamine model of Parkinson's disease. Mol Pharmacol 2000; 57:342–352.

68. Henry B, Brotchie JM. Potential of opioid antagonists in the treatment of levodopa-induced dyskinesias in Parkinson's disease. Drugs Aging 1996; 9:149–158.

69. Boraud T, Bezard E, Bioulac B, Gross CE. Dopamine agonist-induced dyskinesias are correlated to both firing pattern and frequency alterations of pallidal neurons in the MPTP-treated monkey. Brain 2001; 124:546–557.

70. Bezard E, Brotchie JM, Gross CE. Pathophysiology of levodopa-induced dyskinesia: potential for new therapies. Nature Rev Neurosci 2001; 2:577–588.

71. Nutt JG, Obeso JA, Stocchi F. Continuous dopamine-receptor stimulation in advanced Parkinson's disease. Trends in Neurosci 2000; 23(10 suppl):S109–115.

72. Rascol O, Brooks DJ, et al for the 056 Study Group. A five-year study of the incidence of dyskinesia in patients with early Parkinson's disease who were treated with ropinirole or levodopa. N Engl J Med 2000; 342:1484–1491.

73. Parkinson Study Group. Pramipexole versus levodopa as initial treatment for Parkinson disease—a randomized controlled trial. JAMA 2000; 284:1931–1938.

74. Rinne UK, Bracco F, Couza C, et al. Early treatment of Parkinson's disease with carbegoline delays the onset of motor complications. Drugs 1998; 55(suppl 1):23–30.

75. Miyasaki JM, Martin W, Suchowersky O, Weiner WJ, Lang AE. Practice parameter: initiation of treatment for Parkinson's disease: an evidence-based review. Report of the Quality Standards Subcommittee of the American Academy of Neurology. Neurology 2002; 58:11–17.

76. Parkinson Study Group. Dopamine transporter brain imaging to assess the effects of pramipexole versus levodopa on Parkinson disease progression. JAMA 2002; 287:1653–1661.

77. Marek K, Innis R, Van Dick C, et al. [I^{123}]beta-CIT SPECT imaging assessment of the rate of Parkinson's disease progression. Neurology 2001; 57:2089–2094.

78. Morrish P, Rakshi J, Bailey D, et al. Measuring the rate of progression and estimating the preclinical period of Parkinson's disease with [^{18}F]dopa PET. J Neurol Neurosurg Psychiatry 1998; 64:314–319.

79. Whone A, Remy P, Davis MR, et al. The REAL-PET study: slower progression in early Parkinson's disease treated with ropinirole compared with L-dopa. Neurology 2002; 58(suppl 3):A82-A83.

80. Ahlskog JE, Maraganore DM, Uitti RJ, Uhl GR. Dopamine transporter brain imaging to assess the effects of pramipexole versus levodopa on Parkinson disease progression (letter to the editor). JAMA 2002; 288:311.

81. Albin RL, Nichols TE, Frey KA. Dopamine transporter brain imaging to assess the effects of pramipexole versus levodopa on Parkinson disease progression (letter to the editor). JAMA 2002; 288:311–312.

82. Morrish PK. Dopamine transporter brain imaging to assess the effects of pramipexole versus levodopa on Parkinson disease progression (letter to the editor). JAMA 2002; 288:312.

83. Ahlskog JE. Slowing Parkinson's disease progression: recent dopamine agonist trials. Neurology 2003; 60:381–389.

84. Albin RL, Frey KA. Initial agonist treatment of Parkinson disease: a critique. Neurology 2003; 60:390–394.

85. Wooten GF. Agonists vs levodopa in PD: the thrilla of whitha. Neurology 2003; 60:360–362.

86. Goetz CG, Tanner CM, Shannon KM, et al. Controlled-release levodopa/carbidopa (CR4-Sinemet) in Parkinson's disease patients with and without motor fluctuations. Neurology 1988; 38: 1143–1146.

87. Hutton JT, Morris JL, Bush DF, et al. Multicenter controlled study of Sinemet CR vs Sinemet (25/100) in advanced Parkinson's disease. Neurology 1989; 39(suppl 2):67–72.

88. Koller WC, Hutton JT, Tolosa E, et al. Immediate-release and controlled-release carbidopa/levodopa in PD: a 5-year randomized multicenter study. Carbidopa/Levodopa Study Group. Neurology 1999; 53:1012–1019.

7

Levodopa Infusion

Justo Garcia de Yébenes, Pedro García Ruiz, and Alba Serrano

Facultad de Medicina, Universidad Autónoma de Madrid, Madrid, Spain

I. RATIONALE FOR LEVODOPA INFUSIONS IN PARKINSON'S DISEASE

The clinical response of patients with Parkinson's disease (PD) to treatment with levodopa changes over time from an excellent effect at the initial stages of the disease, the "honeymoon period", to a complicated response after several years of disease progression. While almost all patients present a sustained clinical benefit from levodopa at the beginning of the disease, only 25% continue to show a smooth response after 5 years of treatment (1) (Table 1).

The presence of levodopa-induced fluctuations is related to the disappearance of the long-term response (2), a motor improvement that lasts for several days, and the progressive shortening of the short-term response. The short-duration improvement is thought to be related to the effect of "circulating" levodopa and to the presence of dopamine in the synaptic cleft of dopaminergic neurons. Since the half-life of levodopa is 0.60–1.08 hours (3), the short-term improvement lasts for no more than 1 or 2 hours.

Patients that show a sustained improvement are those who are able to reuptake dopamine from the intersynaptic space, store it in synaptic vesicles, and release it according to the activation of different neurons. Carlsson (4) compared early and advanced patients with PD with the experimental models of dopamine deficiency induced by α-methyltyrosine and reserpine. In patients with advanced disease it is thought to be a lack of feedback inhibition of dopamine release and, therefore, no regulation of the storage of the neurotransmitter (4). For that reason, in patients with on-off syndrome there is a correlation between the clinical status and the levels of levodopa in plasma and the ratio between plasma levodopa and large neutral amino acids (5).

The pharmacokinetics of levodopa is altered in the striatum, which is deprived of dopamine innervation. That alteration has been found in rats (6) and monkeys (7) with dopaminergic lesions and humans with PD (8). The levels of dopamine in the striatum of rats with unilateral nigrostriatal lesions induced by 6-hydroxydopamine (6-OHDA)

Table 1   Clinical Responses in 330 Patients After 5 Years of Levodopa Treatment

Response	Number of patients (%)
Fluctuations	142 (43)
Dyskinesia	67 (19)
Fluctuations and dyskinesia	36 (11)
Toxicity at subtherapeutic doses	14 (4)
Good smooth response	83 (25)
Complete loss of effect	27 (8)

Source: Modified from Ref. 1.

treated with levodopa, increase less in the ipsilateral striatum than in the side contralateral to the lesion (6). The levels of levodopa, dopamine, and its metabolites, 3-methoxytyramine (3MT) and dihydroxyphenyl acetic acid (DOPAC), were reduced in the striatum ipsilateral to the injected hemibrain in monkeys with unilateral dopaminergic lesions (Fig. 1) induced by intracarotid administration of 1-methyl-4-phenyl-1,2,3,6-tetrahydropyridine (MPTP) (7). ^{18}F-fluorodopa uptake and retention of ^{18}F-fluorodopa metabolites in patients with PD are related to disease severity (8–11).

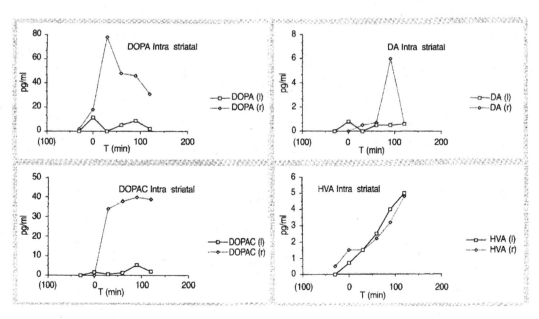

Figure 1   Retention of levodopa (upper left), dopamine (upper right), DOPAC (lower left), and HVA (lower right), as measured by intracerebral dialysis in the corpora striatal of one monkey with a unilateral lesion of the left hemibrain by MPTP, 0.4 mg/kg, injected into the left carotid artery. (l) Left, denervated striatum; (r) right, contralateral, control striatum. The animal was infused with levodopa, 25 mg/kg, and carbidopa, 5 mg/kg, at time 0, and the dialysates were collected for periods of 30 minutes before and 120 minutes after the infusion of levodopa. DOPAC, Dihydroxyphenyl acetic acid; HVA, homovanillic acid; MPTP, 1-methyl-4-phenyl-1,2,3,6-tetrahydropyridine.

If the ability to store dopamine in vesicles is reduced with the progression of the disease, either by reduction of the number of dopamine terminals in the striatum or by inhibition of the feedback-mediated inhibition of release by these terminals at the moments of high activation of the system, the therapeutic effect of levodopa may depend on the maintenance of steady levels of amino acids. Continuous infusion of levodopa or dopamine agonists is a putative alternative, though not easy to perform in the usual clinical setting. These infusions, however, in addition to their technical difficulties, raise important theoretical questions. It is not known whether the activation of a given nigrostriatal dopamine synapse, which in general is produced in a phasic pattern following the depolarization of the nigrostriatal dopaminergic neuron, by a continuous flow of the neurotransmitter or its precursor, produces a persistent activation of the postsynaptic striatal target or if the initial response is followed by tolerance, priming, or reverse tolerance. There is debate about whether the net postsynaptic effect depends on the "number" of receptors occupied by the neurotransmitter or on the "rate" of occupation, aggregation, and internalization of the complex neurotransmitter-receptor. If the dopaminergic neurotransmission in the striatum follows some of these models, it would be difficult to expect a clinically relevant or longstanding response to continuous infusion of levodopa or dopamine agonists. The importance of the "diffuse" effect of a neurotransmitter or receptor agonist that acts upon many striatal dopaminergic synapses in a hormonal fashion and the selective neuronal firing of a few dopaminergic neurons to facilitate the different patterns of human motor behavior is unknown.

II. DUODENAL INFUSIONS

Duodenal infusions of levodopa have the theoretical advantage of bypassing the upper gastrointestinal system, avoiding irregularities of gastric emptying and anatomical abnormalities of the esophagus and stomach, while assuring stable levels of levodopa in plasma. A summary of the conditions that may produce problems for absorption of levodopa is presented in Table 2. Some of these problems, such as giant esophageal diverticula (Fig. 2), may be solved by appropriate surgical techniques, and others, such as slow or irregular gastric emptying, by a fiber-rich diet (12) or prokinetics (13,14).

Several authors have reported their experience with long-term continuous intra-duodenal infusion of levodopa through naso-duodenal or trans-abdominal catheters (15–18). In some of these studies the patients were followed for several years, and the improvement obtained by duodenal infusions was confirmed by opto-electronic devices that reduce the risk of overestimation of placebo effects. The number of patients included in these studies continues to be small. The indication for the treatment was fluctuations

Table 2 Anatomical and Functional Problems That May Interfere with Levodopa Absorption and May Be Solved by Duodenal Infusion

Anatomical problems:	Esophageal stenosis or giant diverticula, hiatal hernia, pyloric stenosis
Functional problems:	Untreatable vomiting, slow or irregular gastric emptying, functional closing of pylorus by dopamine

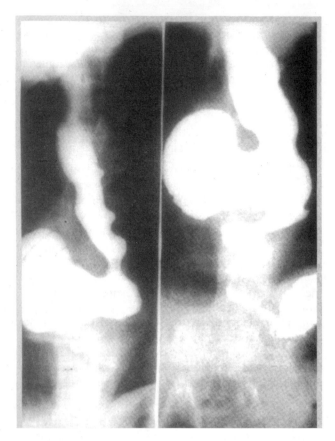

Figure 2 Giant esophageal diverticulus in a 72-year-old patient with unpredictable responses to oral levodopa. At times the patient responded very well to the medication, but at other times he would not improve at all if the medication was retained in the diverticulus or would develop dyskinesias if several doses of medication were discharged downward from the diverticulus to the stomach. After two episodes of aspiration pneumonia, the upper gastrointestinal system was examined with a barium contrast. Surgical correction of the diverticula solved the problem of fluctuations and unpredictable responses to oral levodopa.

resistant to conventional therapy. More precise indications should be defined and confirmed by double-blind studies. Mechanical and physical problems, the main reason for discontinuation of the therapy, remain to be solved.

III. PARENTERAL INFUSIONS

Parenteral infusions of levodopa, dopamine agonists, and other antiparkinsonian drugs have been tried for more than a quarter of a century. The first trial was performed by Shoulson et al. (19) in five patients with PD with predictable wearing off. The intravenous infusion of levodopa with oral administration of carbidopa improved the fluctuations for up to 4 hours, but it produced orthostatic hypotension. Several years later different authors showed that off periods could be improved by intravenous infusion of levodopa for several hours added to their regular oral treatment with levodopa and large aromatic amino acid decarboxylase inhibitors (20–23). The beneficial effect of intravenous levodopa could be blocked by oral administration of large neutral amino acids (23), suggesting that these compounds compete not only with the absorption of levodopa in the gut but also with its transport across the blood-brain barrier. It was also shown that large levels of 3-*O*-methyldopa (3-OMD), a catechol-*ortho*-methyl–transferase–mediated metabolite of levodopa, blocked the cerebral uptake of levodopa in animals (24).

One of the problems of intravenous levodopa infusions is that the drug is very insoluble at neutral pH, barely 1 mg/mL, which makes it necessary for the patient to carry large equipment, which is impractical in a normal environment. For these reasons intravenous infusions of levodopa are very useful as a research tool examining the mechanisms involved in fluctuations and on-off syndromes, but not very practical for most patients in everyday conditions.

Some strategies were used to increase levodopa solubility and, consequently, to reduce the size of the infusion equipment. Esters of levodopa and different alcohols that are soluble and could be hydrolyzed in the patient's body after their administration, releasing the amino acid and the respective alcohol, were considered as interesting pro-drugs. Levodopa methyl ester was widely used and proved effective as an antiakinetic agent (25). Levodopa methyl ester, however, raised concerns of toxicity since each molecule of the ester would eventually be hydrolyzed to one molecule of levodopa and also to one molecule of methanol. Though the amount of methanol produced to administer from 500 mg to 1 g of levodopa daily would probably not be too high, there are concerns about using a compound that inhibits mitochondrial function in a disease where abnormalities of mitochondrial activity have been reported for many years. More recently, an ester of levodopa and ethanol, levodopa ethyl ester, has been prepared. This compound is also soluble, and its risk of toxicity is lower.

The most common side effects of short-term intravenous infusions of levodopa are usually related to the production or aggravation of dyskinesia (22). Another concern is the induction or aggravation of hallucinations. In one study of five patients with PD with visual hallucinations prior to intravenous infusion of levodopa, the patients did not hallucinate during continuous or pulsatile intravenous infusions, for up to 4 hours (26). The patients were much more stimulated than in normal conditions, and this experimental stimulation could have had a suppressor effect on hallucinations.

The difficulty to perform studies examining the clinical effect of levodopa infusion in the normal patient environment and the lack of double-blind studies makes it difficult to assess the clinical value of these techniques. Intravenous infusions of levodopa have been performed in patients with PD investigated by $H_2^{15}O$/positron emission tomography (PET) (27) and ^{18}F-fluorodeoxyglucose/PET (28) in order to study the effect of levodopa on activation of motor responses and its metabolic correlates. The first of these studies revealed that levodopa-induced clinical improvement correlated with activation of the basal ganglia and thalamus and that levodopa-induced impairment of motor accuracy correlated with activation of the cerebellar vermis (27). The second study revealed that levodopa infusion improved the scores of the Unified Parkinson's Disease Rating Scale (UPDRS) and that the clinical improvement correlated with a reduction of ^{18}F-fluorodeoxyglucose uptake in the cortex and the basal ganglia (28), the typical metabolic pattern of PD. Although these results suggest that the infusion of levodopa has clinical value, long-term double-blind placebo-controlled infusion studies are needed (29).

Due to the limitations of solubility of levodopa, other compounds with antiakinetic properties have been considered for parenteral infusion in patients with PD. Lisuride, a water-soluble ergot derivative with D2 dopamine receptor agonist properties, was considered promising for intravenous or subcutaneous infusion (30). Long-term results of lisuride infusion were disappointing. In addition to subcutaneous nodules at the points of injection, most patients developed severe psychiatric side effects, including hallucinations and hypersexuality.

The most successful dopamine agonist used in continuous subcutaneous infusion for long-term treatment of levodopa-related complications in patients with PD is apomorphine (31–34). One study of 19 patients with severe unpredictable refractory motor fluctuations and disabling levodopa-induced dyskinesias revealed that continuous subcutaneous infusion with apomorphine monotherapy for a minimum duration of 2.7 years during the waking hours produced a mean reduction of 65% in the severity of dyskinesia and a mean reduction of 85% in frequency and duration. In addition, after discontinuation of levodopa there was a concomitant reduction in "off" time from 35 to 10% of the waking day (31). Another study included 64 patients treated with a mean daily dose of 93 mg, of apomorphine. Forty-five of the patients converted to monotherapy and were followed for a mean of 4–108 months (33).

The antidyskinetic effect of apomorphine may be related to several factors, including the antidyskinetic effect of D1 agonists and the pattern of continuous infusion of the agonist. Continuous stimulation of dopamine receptors produces less dyskinesia than pulsatile stimulation. This is related to a less profound effect of continuous stimulation of dopamine receptors on the enhancement of synthesis of pro-met-enkephalin in the globus pallidus lateralis (35) than that of pulsatile stimulation. Continuous administration of apomorphine has also been reported to be neuroprotective of dopaminergic neurons in MPTP-treated mice (34), while pulsatile administration of this compound did not have any neuroprotective effect.

In addition to levodopa and dopamine agonists, other compounds have been tested in continuous parenteral infusion for the treatment of fluctuations and dyskinesias in patients with PD (Table 3). Amantadine is an old antiparkinsonian agent with a complex pharmacological profile. Amantadine is now considered a noncompetitive antagonist of the N-methyl-D-aspartate (NMDA) receptor in addition to having other properties, such

Table 3 Parenteral Infusion of Levodopa and Other Compounds for the Treatment of Fluctuations in Parkinson's Disease

Compound	Results
Levodopa and derivatives	Good results on fluctuations in short-term studies performed in clinical research centers; absence of long-term studies in normal clinical setting; problems of solubility of the drug
Apomorphine	Good results on fluctuations and dyskinesia in long-term studies of intravenous and mostly subcutaneous infusion; some patients in monotherapy; preliminary but promising data about neuroprotection
Other dopamine agonists	Little use with the exception of substitutive therapy during levodopa suppression
Amantadine	Preliminary data showed antidyskinetic effect

as being an anticholinergic agent and a promoter of dopamine release. A study was performed in nine PD patients with motor fluctuations and disabling peak dose dyskinesias. These patients received their first morning levodopa dose, followed by a 2-hour intravenous infusion of amantadine (200 mg) or placebo, on two different days. The severity of parkinsonian deficits and dyskinesias was assessed according to the UPDRS motor and the Abnormal Involuntary Movement Scale (AIMS) every 15 minutes during the infusion and for 3 hours thereafter, while patients were taking their usual oral antiparkinsonian therapy (36). Intravenous infusion of amantadine improved levodopa-induced dyskinesias by 50% without any loss of the antiparkinsonian benefit. The authors concluded that their results suggested that agents with a pharmacological profile as inhibitors of excitatory amino acids could be valuable in the treatment of levodopa-induced complications. Given the mixed pharmacological profile of amantadine, the clinical value of this study requires confirmation with other compounds with more selective NMDA modulatory effects and with more prolonged infusions and testing.

IV. INTRACEREBRAL INFUSIONS

The feasibility, safety, and efficacy of intracerebral infusions of levodopa, dopamine, or dopamine agonists in patients with PD are not known. This method of administration offers some possible advantages over parenteral infusions. In terms of the pharmacokinetics, the effects of intracerebral infusions do not depend on the diet since the active compound is directly placed in the brain and does not have to compete with large neutral amino acids for transport across the blood-brain barrier. Furthermore, there is no need to infuse a pro-drug, such as levodopa, that requires decarboxylation to be converted to dopamine, which itself could be infused. Another advantage of intracerebral infusion is that the active compound could be selectively administered to the brain nuclei involved in the motor aspects of the disease, mostly the dorsolateral striatum, without the simultaneous stimulation of the limbic system or cortical areas whose dopaminergic neurotransmission is an important element for the development of psychiatric complications of antiparkinsonian treatments.

Intracerebroventricular (ICV) infusion of dopamine and dopamine agonists counteracts the behavioral and biochemical effects of unilateral lesions of the nigrostriatal dopaminergic neurons with 6-OHDA and akinesia induced by monoamine depletion after chronic treatment with reserpine (37,38). In the case of reserpine-depleted rats, ICV infusion of dopamine was coupled to systemic administration of monoamine oxidase inhibitors. The experiments in rodents lasted up to 4 weeks, and the drug was delivered through a delivery system connected to an osmotic minipump that could be replaced after 1–4 weeks of infusion. In rodents there were no significant side effects of the treatment or the delivery system with the exception of a black deposit of dopamine-derived compounds at the wall of the ventricle (Fig. 3) in some animals. The presence of this deposit led to the investigation of the putative toxicity of dopamine to dopamine neurons in vitro, which led to conflicting results (39,40).

The infusion of dopamine or dopamine agonists in primates can suppress motor fluctuations for up to 17 weeks (37,38). Rhesus and cynomolgus monkeys with MPTP-induced parkinsonism received parenteral treatments with intramuscular injections of bromocriptine, 1–4 mg/kg, pergolide, 0.1–0.5 mg/kg, apomorphine, 0.5–1.0 mg/kg, and (+)-4-propyl-9-hydroxynaphthoxacine (PHNO) 0.09 mg/kg. All agents produced

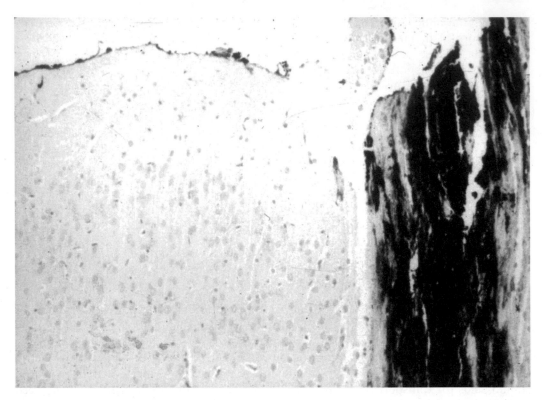

Figure 3 Pigment in the ventricular wall of a rat infused with dopamine in the lateral ventricle.

dose-dependent improvement of akinesia but increased fluctuations and dyskinesia regardless of the pharmacological profile of the compounds (selective for D2, bromocriptine, and PHNO; nonselective for D1 or D2, apomorphine, or pergolide). The intracerebral infusion of dopamine, 25 mg/h, (+) deprenyl, 0.2 mg/h, or PHNO, 30–120 µg/kg/d, greatly improved akinesia without fluctuations or dyskinesia.

There were, however, problems with the experiments in monkeys. In one of two animals infused with dopamine, there was a deposit of black pigment in the ventricle. The programmable electronic pumps used for infusion were too large for the monkeys and produced pressure necrosis of the skin covering them and loss of the pump in two cases. One animal fought ferociously against the implanted delivery system, though it was totally implanted under the skin, and disconnected it in two cases. Another animal, pulling away a specially designed monkey jacket placed around her chest, with a pocket holding a motor activity counting device, produced a traumatic lesion of the carotid artery. Finally, one of the animals had a surgical hemiplegia during the implantation of the ventricular catheter. In summary, the results were promising, but the model was inadequate.

The infusion of dopaminergic compounds into the nervous system of patients with PD requires solving the following experimental issues: site of infusion, device, requirements of the delivery system, drugs to be infused, and solvent. Some of the putative solutions to these problems are presented in Table 4.

Table 4 Experimental Issues for Intracerebral Continuous Administration of Compounds

Component	Issues
Site of infusion	The dorsolateral striatum is more appropriate than the ventricle
Infusion pump	Must be programmable with different rates of infusion according to the patient schedule and individual activities
Kind of delivery system	Should allow diffusion of the active compound to the whole striatum, be easily removable and rechargeable; resistant to drugs and environment
Active compound	Stable at body temperature, soluble at neutral pH, diffusible, and selective for dopamine neurons
Solvent	Nontoxic, stable, and resistant to sterilization

V. CONCLUSIONS

Though the use of infusion of dopaminomimetic compounds has been investigated extensively as a putative method for the treatment of patients with PD and fluctuations induced by oral medication, few of the available treatments have confirmed their value in the general clinical setting. Enteral infusions of levodopa may be useful in some patients with PD with anatomical or functional problems of the gastrointestinal tract, though other medical or surgical approaches may be more useful in most cases.

With respect to the use of parenteral infusions of levodopa, the future of this technique requires the availability of a very soluble levodopa pro-drug that could be infused in a small volume of solvent. Subcutaneous infusions of dopamine agonists are limited to that of apomorphine and can be helpful to some patients after long-term application. Intracerebral infusion of dopaminomimetics in patients with PD is not recommended.

REFERENCES

1. Fahn S. Adverse effects of levodopa. In: Olanow CW, Lieberman AN, eds. The Scientific Basis for the Treatment of Parkinson's Disease. Park Ridge, NJ: Parthenon Publishing Group, 1992:89–112.
2. Nutt JG, Carter JH, van Houten L, Woodward WR. Short- and long-duration responses to levodopa during the first year of levodopa therapy. Ann Neurol 1997; 42:349–355.
3. Nutt JG, Fellman JH. Pharmacokinetics of levodopa. Clin Neuropharmacol 1984; 7:35–49.
4. Carlsson A. Are "on-off" effects during chronic L-DOPA treatment due to faulty feedback control of the nigrostriatal dopamine pathway? J Neural Transm 1983; 19(suppl):153–161.
5. Eriksson T, Magnusson T, Carlsson A, Linde A, Granerus A-K. "On-off" phenomenon in Parkinson's disease: correlation to the concentration of DOPA in plasma. J Neural Transm 1984; 59:229–240.
6. Spencer SE, Wooten GF. Altered pharmacokinetics of L-DOPA metabolism in rat striatum deprived of dopaminergic innervation. Neurology 1984; 34:1105–1108.

7. Garcia de Yebenes J, Rojo A. Tratamiento con L-DOPA de la enfermedad de Parkinson. Continua Neurol 2000; 3(suppl):67–82.
8. Torstenson R, Hartvig P, Langstrom B, Westerberg G, Tedroff J. Differential effects of levodopa on dopaminergic function in early and advanced Parkinson's disease. Ann Neurol 1997; 41:334–340.
9. Marek K, Innis R, van Dyck C, Fussell B, Early M, Eberly S, Oakes D, Seibyl J. [^{123}I]Beta-CIT SPECT imaging assessment of the rate of Parkinson's disease progression. Neurology 2001; 57:2089–2094.
10. Leenders KL, Oertel WH. Parkinson's disease: clinical signs and symptoms, neural mechanisms, positron emission tomography, and therapeutic interventions. Neural Plast 2001; 8:99–110.
11. Khan NL, Brooks DJ, Pavese N, Sweeney MG, Wood NW, Lees AJ, Piccini P. Progression of nigrostriatal dysfunction in a parkin kindred: an [18F]dopa PET and clinical study. Brain 2002; 125:2248–2256.
12. Astarloa R, Mena MA, Sánchez V, de la Vega L, de Yebenes JG. Clinical and pharmacokinetic effects of a diet rich in insoluble fiber on Parkinson's disease. Clin Neuropharmacol 1992; 15:375–380.
13. Diaz Neira W, Sanchez Bernardos V, Mena MA, Garcia de Yebenes J. Efecto del cisapride sobre los niveles plasmaticos de L-DOPA y la respuesta clinica en la enfermedad de Parkinson. Arch Neurobiol 1994; 57:26–30.
14. Neira WD, Sanchez V, Mena MA, de Yebenes JG. The effects of cisapride on plasma L-DOPA levels and clinical response in Parkinson's disease. Mov Disord 1995; 10:66–70.
15. Kurlan R, Rubin AJ, Miller C, Rivera-Calimlim L, Clarke A, Shoulson I. Duodenal delivery of levodopa for on-off fluctuations in parkinsonism: preliminary observations. Ann Neurol 1986; 20:262–265.
16. Syed N, Murphy J, Zimmerman T Jr, Mark MH, Sage JI. Ten years' experience with enteral levodopa infusions for motor fluctuations in Parkinson's disease. Mov Disord 1998; 13:336–338.
17. Nilsson D, Hansson LE, Johansson K, Nystrom C, Paalzow L, Aquilonius SM. Long-term intraduodenal infusion of a water based levodopa-carbidopa dispersion in very advanced Parkinson's disease. Acta Neurol Scand 1998; 97:175–183.
18. Nilsson D, Nyholm D, Aquilonius SM. Duodenal levodopa infusion in Parkinson's disease—long-term experience. Acta Neurol Scand 2001; 104:343–348.
19. Shoulson I, Glaubiger GA, Chase TN. On-off response. Clinical and biochemical correlations during oral and intravenous levodopa administration in parkinsonian patients. Neurology 1975; 25:1144–1148.
20. Quinn N, Parkes JD, Marsden CD. Control of on/off phenomenon by continuous intravenous infusion of levodopa. Neurology 1984; 34:1131–1136.
21. Quinn N, Marsden CD, Parkes JD. Complicated response fluctuations in Parkinson's disease: response to intravenous infusion of L-DOPA. Lancet 1982; 2:412–415.
22. Hardie RJ, Lees AJ, Stern GM. On-off fluctuations in Parkinson's disease. A clinical and neuro-pharmacological study. Brain 1984; 107:487–506.
23. Nutt JG, Woodward WR, Hammerstad JP, Carter JH, Anderson JL. The "on-off" phenomenon in Parkinson's disease. Relation to levodopa absorption and transport. N Engl J Med 1984; 310:483–488.
24. Gervas JJ, Muradas V, Bazan E, Aguado EG, de Yebenes JG. Effects of 3-OM-DOPA on monoamine metabolism in rat brain. Neurology 1983; 33:278–282.
25. Cooper DR, Marrel C, Testa B, Van de Waterbeemd H, Quinn N, Jenner P, Marsden CD. L-DOPA methyl ester—a candidate for chronic systemic delivery of L-DOPA in Parkinson's disease. Clin Neuropharmacol 1984; 7:89–98.
26. Goetz CG, Pappert EJ, Blasucci LM, Stebbins GT, Ling ZD, Nora MV, Carvey PM. Intravenous levodopa in hallucinating Parkinson's disease patients: high-dose challenge does not precipitate hallucinations. Neurology 1998; 50:515–517.
27. Feigin A, Ghilardi MF, Fukuda M, Mentis MJ, Dhawan V, Barnes A, Ghez CP, Eidelberg D. Effects of levodopa infusion on motor activation responses in Parkinson's disease. Neurology 2002; 59:220–226.
28. Feigin A, Fukuda M, Dhawan V, Przedborski S, Jackson-Lewis V, Mentis MJ, Moeller JR, Eidelberg D. Metabolic correlates of levodopa response in Parkinson's disease. Neurology 2001; 57:2083–2088.
29. De la Fuente-Fernandez R, Ruth TJ, Sossi V, Schulzer M, Calne DB, Stoessl AJ. Expectation and dopamine release: mechanism of the placebo effect in Parkinson's disease. Science 2001; 293:1164–1166.
30. Obeso JA, Martinez-Lage JM, Luquin MR, Bolio N. Intravenous lisuride infusion for Parkinson's disease. Ann Neurol 1983; 14:252.

31. Colzi A, Turner K, Lees AJ. Continuous subcutaneous waking day apomorphine in the long-term treatment of levodopa induced interdose dyskinesias in Parkinson's disease. J Neurol Neurosurg Psychiatry 1998; 64:573–576.
32. Stocchi F, Vacca L, De Pandis MF, Barbato L, Valente M, Ruggieri S. Subcutaneous continuous apomorphine infusion in fluctuating patients with Parkinson's disease: long-term results. Neurol Sci 2001; 22:93–94.
33. Manson AJ, Turner K, Lees AJ. Apomorphine monotherapy in the treatment of refractory motor complications of Parkinson's disease: long-term follow-up study of 64 patients. Mov Disord 2002; 17:1235–1241.
34. Battaglia G, Busceti CL, Cuomo L, Giorgi FS, Orzi F, De Blasi A, Nicoletti F, Ruggieri S, Fornai F. Continuous subcutaneous infusion of apomorphine rescues nigro-striatal dopaminergic terminals following MPTP injection in mice. Neuropharmacology 2002; 42:367–373.
35. Zeng BY, Jolkkonen J, Jenner P, Marsden CD. Chronic L-DOPA treatment differentially regulates gene expression of glutamate decarboxylase, preproenkephalin and preprotachykinin in the striatum of 6-hydroxydopamine-lesioned rat. Neuroscience 1995; 66:19–28.
36. Ruzicka E, Streitova H, Jech R, Kanovsky P, Roth J, Rektorova I, Mecir P, Hortova H, Bares M, Hejdukova B, Rektor I. Amantadine infusion in treatment of motor fluctuations and dyskinesias in Parkinson's disease. J Neural Transm. 2000; 107:1297–1306.
37. De Yebenes JG, Fahn S, Jackson-Lewis V, Mena MA. The effect of intracerebroventricular infusion of (+)-4-propyl-9-hydroxynapthoxacine (PHNO) through a totally implanted drug delivery system in rats with dopamine deficiency. Mov Disord 1987; 2:291–299.
38. De Yebenes JG, Fahn S, Jackson-Lewis V, Jorge P, Mena MA, Reiriz J. Continuous intracerebro-ventricular infusion of dopamine and dopamine agonists through a totally implanted drug delivery system in animal models of Parkinson's disease. J Neural Transm 1988; 27(suppl):141–160.
39. Mena MA, Pardo B, Casarejos MJ, Garcia de Yebenes J. Neurotoxicity of L-DOPA on catecholamine-rich neurons. Mov Disord 1992; 7:23–31.
40. Mena MA, Davila V, Bogaluvsky J, Sulzer D. A synergistic neurotrophic response to L-dihydroxy-phenylalanine and nerve growth factor. Mol Pharmacol 1998; 54:678–686.

8

Bromocriptine

Kelly E. Lyons and Rajesh Pahwa

University of Kansas Medical Center, Kansas City, Kansas, U.S.A.

José Martin Rabey

Assaf Harofeh Medical Center and Tel Aviv University, Zerifin, Israel

The occurrence of motor fluctuations and dyskinesia after chronic levodopa therapy led to the investigation of new therapeutic strategies for the treatment of Parkinson's disease (PD) (1). One strategy was the use of dopamine agonists as an adjunct to levodopa with the intention of reducing levodopa-induced motor complications by lowering the dose of levodopa (2). Dopamine agonists act directly on the dopamine receptors, eliminating the need for conversion to dopamine and subsequent difficulties with absorption and transport across the blood-brain barrier. In addition, dopamine agonists have a longer half-life than levodopa, resulting in more continuous postsynaptic dopamine receptor stimulation. In 1974, bromocriptine was the first dopamine agonist approved for the treatment of PD in the United States (3,4). This chapter will focus on the pharmacokinetics, clinical studies, and adverse effects of bromocriptine.

I. PHARMACOKINETICS

Bromocriptine mesylate (Parlodel) is a semi-synthetic ergot alkaloid with strong dopamine agonist activity. It is a D2 receptor agonist and a weak D1 receptor antagonist with 5HT2 antagonistic effects and mild adrenergic effects. Peak plasma bromocriptine levels are typically obtained after 70–100 minutes (5,6). Ninety percent undergoes first-pass hepatic metabolism, and therefore the oral bioavailability is less than 10%. The elimination half-life of bromocriptine is approximately 5–8 hours, and only about 5% is excreted unchanged in the urine.

Bromocriptine is typically initiated at 1.25 mg/d (half of a 2.5 mg tablet) and increased by 1.25 mg/week to 1.25 mg three times per day with meals. It is then increased by 2.5 mg every 2–4 weeks until efficacy is obtained. The usual dose range is 10–40 mg in divided doses three times per day with meals. Safety has not been established for doses over 100 mg/d.

II. CLINICAL STUDIES AND EFFICACY

There have been multiple studies examining the effects of bromocriptine as monotherapy when compared to placebo, other dopamine agonists, and levodopa in early PD (Table 1) and as an adjunct to levodopa in advanced disease (Tables 2, 3). This chapter will focus primarily on the larger, double-blind, randomized studies.

A. Monotherapy

In a double-blind, parallel-group study of 21 de novo PD patients, bromocriptine was found to be superior to placebo in controlling parkinsonian symptoms (7). In two double-blind studies, de novo PD patients were randomized to receive either bromocriptine or levodopa as monotherapy. After approximately 5 months, the bromocriptine and levodopa groups demonstrated equivalent control of parkinsonian symptoms (8,9). Rinne (10) compared 76 PD patients on bromocriptine monotherapy in which supplemental levodopa could be added as needed to 217 patients on levodopa monotherapy. After 5 years he found that the bromocriptine group with additional low-dose levodopa experienced similar efficacy levels as the higher-dose levodopa monotherapy group, but the bromocriptine group had fewer motor complications (10). Several other studies have compared bromocriptine with necessary levodopa supplementation to levodopa monotherapy (11–14). The majority of these studies have demonstrated that levodopa is more efficacious than bromocriptine monotherapy, but with the addition of supplemental levodopa the bromocriptine groups experience similar efficacy with fewer motor fluctuations and dyskinesias compared to levodopa alone. Mizuno et al. (15) reported a double-blind study comparing bromocriptine and pergolide. After 8 weeks of treatment, the two groups experienced similar efficacy. Korczyn et al. (14) compared the efficacy of bromocriptine and ropinirole in de novo PD patients. At 6 months ropinirole was significantly more potent than bromocriptine, with a 35% reduction in Unified Parkinson's Disease Rating Scale (UPDRS) scores compared to 27% with bromocriptine. These results were maintained for up to 3 years. Details of the above-mentioned studies can be found in Table 1.

B. Adjunctive Therapy to Levodopa

Bromocriptine was first introduced in advanced PD patients with levodopa-induced motor complications. In studies in which either bromocriptine or placebo was added to levodopa, bromocriptine was consistently found to be superior to placebo in controlling motor symptoms of PD (17–19). In one study the use of bromocriptine allowed for up to a 74% mean reduction in levodopa dose (17). Since bromocriptine had been more beneficial than placebo when added to levodopa and in some cases was able to reduce levodopa doses, it was suggested that bromocriptine might be beneficial in slowing the development of motor complications if it were added to levodopa prior to the onset of motor fluctuations and dyskinesias (20–22). Several investigators completed studies in which either bromocriptine or placebo was added to levodopa prior to the development of motor complications. The majority of these studies demonstrated no differences in the control of motor symptoms between groups receiving both levodopa and bromocriptine and groups receiving levodopa alone. However, motor complications as well as total levodopa dose were often significantly less in the combination groups when compared to levodopa alone (20–22). Details of the above-mentioned studies are shown in Table 2.

Table 1 Selected Studies of Bromocriptine as Monotherapy in Early Parkinson's Disease

Study (Ref.)	Design	n	Duration	Drugs[a]	Outcome
Staal-Schreinemachers et al. 1986 (7)	Double-blind, placebo-controlled	21	6 months	Bromocriptine up to 15 mg Placebo	Bromocriptine had superior efficacy to placebo
Libman et al. 1986 (8)	Double-blind, levodopa-controlled	49	19.5 weeks	Bromocriptine 24 mg Levodopa 252 mg	Bromocriptine and levodopa had equal efficacy
Riopelle et al. 1987 (9)	Double-blind, levodopa-controlled	77	5.5 months	Bromocriptine 26 mg Levodopa 262 mg	Bromocriptine and levodopa had equal efficacy
Rinne, 1987 (10)	Uncontrolled, nonrandomized, levodopa-controlled	76	5 years	Bromocriptine 13.7 mg + levodopa 592 mg Levodopa 795 mg	Bromocriptine with supplemental levodopa as needed equivalent to higher-dose levodopa monotherapy with fewer motor complications
Herskovitz et al. 1988 (11)	Randomized, open-label	86	31 months	Levodopa 556 mg Bromocriptine 12.6 mg Levodopa 572 mg + bromocriptine 7.5 mg	No differences between treatment groups; 50% of bromocriptine group received supplemental levodopa
PD Research Grp UK, 1993 (12)	Randomized, open-label	782	1 year 3 years	Levodopa 420 mg Levodopa 352 mg + selegiline 10 mg Bromocriptine 36 mg	At 1 year both levodopa groups were more efficacious than bromocriptine; at 3 years 32% on bromocriptine monotherapy and motor complications were less frequent
Hely et al. 1994 (13)	Randomized, open-label	126	5 years	Bromocriptine 32 mg Levodopa $\leq$600 mg	Levodopa had increased efficacy compared to bromocriptine at 1 year; bromocriptine with supplemental levodopa had more efficacy than levodopa alone and fewer motor complications

(Continued)

Table 1 (*continued*)

Study (Ref.)	Design	n	Duration	Drugs[a]	Outcome
Montastruc et al. 1994 (14)	Randomized, open-label	60	5 years	Bromocriptine 52 mg Levodopa 569 mg	Bromocriptine with supplemental levodopa after an average of 2.7 years had equivalent efficacy to levodopa alone
Mizuno et al. 1995 (15)	Double-blind, pergolide-controlled	98	8 weeks	Pergolide 1.43 mg Bromocriptine 15.1 mg	Bromocriptine and pergolide had equivalent efficacy
Korczyn et al. 1999 (16)	Double-blind, ropinirole-controlled	335	3 years	Ropinirole 12 mg Bromocriptine 24 mg	Ropinirole was superior to bromocriptine in activities of daily living scores; motor complications were infrequent in both groups

[a] Average dose used in study.

Table 2 Selected Studies of Bromocriptine as an Adjunct to Levodopa in Parkinson's Disease

Study (Ref.)	Design	n	Duration	Drugs[a]	Outcome
Kartzinel et al. 1996 (17)	Double-blind, placebo-controlled (fluctuators)	20	6 months	Bromocriptine 79 mg + stable levodopa / Stable levodopa + placebo	Mean dose of levodopa reduced 74% in bromocriptine group; bromocriptine improved total disability by 19% compared to placebo
Hoehn and Elton, 1985 (18)	Double-blind, placebo-controlled (fluctuators)	36	10 months	Bromocriptine 20 mg + stable levodopa / Stable levodopa + placebo	Bromocriptine superior to placebo; bromocriptine 37% improvement over baseline; over 70% on bromocriptine had improvement in motor complications
Toyokura et al. 1985 (19)	Randomized placebo control (fluctuators)	222	2 months	Bromocriptine 16.7 mg + stable levodopa / Stable levodopa + placebo	Bromocriptine superior to placebo particularly in akinesia, gait difficulties, and wearing off; 29% of the bromocriptine and 15% of placebo had moderate to marked improvement
Nakanishi et al. 1992 (20)	Randomized, open-label (disease < 5 years)	416	5 years	Bromocriptine 11 mg + levodopa 387 mg / Levodopa alone 407 mg	Symptom ratings were comparable; motor complications were less in the combined group
Przuntek et al. 1996 (21)	Randomized (newly diagnosed)	674	42 months	Levodopa 308 mg + bromocriptine 14 mg / Levodopa alone 439 mg	Control of motor symptoms was comparable; motor complications were less in the combined group: 20 vs. 29%; bromocriptine allowed 31% reduction in levodopa
Gimenez-Rolden et al. 1997 (22)	Double-blind, placebo-controlled (levodopa < 6 months)	50	8 months	Bromocriptine 15 mg + levodopa 465 mg / Levodopa 507 mg + placebo	No reduction in levodopa dose with bromocriptine compared to placebo
Gimenez-Rolden et al. 1997 (22)	Open-label	50	44 months	Bromocriptine 24 mg + levodopa 15 mg / Levodopa 726 mg + placebo	Significant reduction in levodopa dose with bromocriptine compared to placebo

[a] Average dose used in study.

Table 3 Selected Studies of Bromocriptine Compared to Other Antiparkinsonian Medications as Adjuncts to Levodopa in Parkinson's Disease

Study (Ref.)	Design	n	Duration	Drugs[a]	Outcome
LeWitt et al. 1983 (23)	Double-blind, crossover	24	7–10 (each arm)	Bromocriptine 42 mg + levodopa Pergolide 3.3 mg + levodopa	Comparable efficacy between the two drugs
Mizuno et al. 1995 (15)	Double-blind, randomized	192	8 weeks	Bromocriptine 14.6 mg + levodopa Pergolide 1.24 mg + levodopa	Comparable efficacy with a trend toward greatest improvement with pergolide
Pezzoli et al. 1995 (24)	Single-blind, crossover	57	12 weeks (each arm)	Bromocriptine 24.2 mg + levodopa Pergolide 2.3 mg + levodopa	Significant improvement compared to baseline for both drugs but pergolide was superior in most measures
Inzelberg et al. 1996 (25)	Double-blind, randomized	44	9 months	Bromocriptine 22 mg + levodopa Cabergoline 3.18 mg + levodopa	Significant improvement for both drugs compared to baseline, no difference between the two drugs
LeWitt et al. 1982 (26)	Double-blind, crossover	26	7–10 weeks (each arm)	Bromocriptine 56.5 mg + levodopa Lisuride 4.5 mg + levodopa	Comparable efficacy between the two drugs with greater improvement with bromocriptine for akinesia
Laihinen et al. 1992 (27)	Double-blind, crossover	20	8 weeks (each arm)	Bromocriptine 15 mg + levodopa Lisuride 1.3 mg + levodopa	30% improvement for both drugs compared to baseline
Guttman et al. 1997 (28)	Double-blind, placebo-controlled	247	9 months	Bromocriptine 22.6 mg + levodopa Pramipexole 4–5 mg + levodopa Placebo + levodopa	Both drugs had significantly greater improvement than placebo, motor score improved 35% with pramipexole and 24% with bromocriptine
Tolcapone Study Group, 1999 (29)	Open-label, randomized	146	8 weeks	Bromocriptine 224 mg + levodopa Tolcapone 600 mg + levodopa	Both drugs had comparable efficacy in motor scores; levodopa dose was reduced by 16.5% with tolcapone and 4% with bromocriptine

[a] Average dose used in study.

Several studies have compared the efficacy of bromocriptine to other antiparkinsonian medications. Studies have shown that when added to levodopa, bromocriptine and pergolide both provide improvement in motor functioning, but pergolide tends to be slightly more potent than bromocriptine (15,23,24). In a study in which either bromocriptine or cabergoline was added to levodopa, significant motor improvement was seen with both drugs, and there were no differences between the two drugs (25). Two double-blind, crossover studies comparing bromocriptine and lisuride as an adjunct to levodopa found comparable motor benefit with the two drugs (26,27). A double-blind placebo-controlled study compared bromocriptine, pramipexole and placebo in combination with levodopa. Both drugs demonstrated significantly greater improvement in motor functioning when compared to placebo. However, pramipexole improved UPDRS motor scores by 35%, while they were improved by only 24% with bromocriptine (28). In another study, either bromocriptine or tolcapone was added to levodopa therapy. The two drugs demonstrated comparable improvements in motor scores, but levodopa dose was reduced by 16.5% with tolcapone and only 4% with bromocriptine (29). Details of the above-mentioned studies can be found in Table 3.

III. SAFETY AND TOLERABILITY

Bromocriptine is typically safe and well tolerated when used as monotherapy or as adjunctive therapy to levodopa in early and advanced PD patients. Side effects are consistent with those of other dopaminergic drugs and include nausea, vomiting, orthostatic hypotension, leg edema, somnolence, hallucinations, and psychosis. The incidence and severity of these side effects can be reduced by a slow gradual titration schedule. A rare but possibly serious side effect of bromocriptine is pleuropulmonary or peritoneal fibrosis, which is associated with ergot derivatives (30).

IV. CONCLUSION

Bromocriptine was the first dopamine agonist approved for the treatment of PD in the United States. As monotherapy, bromocriptine has been shown to be beneficial in controlling the motor symptoms of PD when compared with placebo. In early disease, bromocriptine taken alone or with low doses of levodopa, when necessary, may reduce the appearance of motor complications when compared to taking levodopa alone. Bromocriptine has also been shown to improve motor functioning and reduce motor complications as an adjunct to levodopa when compared to placebo. Multiple antiparkinsonian medications have been compared to bromocriptine. Cabergoline and lisuride where shown to be comparable to bromocriptine in improving motor functioning in PD. Comparisons of bromocriptine to pergolide, pramipexole, and ropinirole demonstrate that all drugs improve motor functioning in PD, and the degree of improvement may be less with bromocriptine. However, there is currently no clear proof that one dopamine agonist is superior to the others in clinical practice, and if a loss of effect or no effect is seen with one agonist, a switch to a different dopamine agonist may be beneficial. Tolcapone was shown to have comparable effects on motor function compared to bromocriptine, but it allowed for a much greater reduction in levodopa dose. With the development of new and potentially more potent agents for the treatment of PD and the relatively high cost of bromocriptine, it is no longer commonly used for the treatment of PD.

REFERENCES

1. Marsden CD, Parkes JD . "On-off" effects in patients with Parkinson's disease on chronic levodopa therapy. Lancet 1976; 1:292–296.
2. Kartzinel R, Calne DB. Studies with bromocriptine — Part 1. "On-off" phenomena. Neurology 1976; 26:508–510.
3. Calne DB, Teychenne PF, Claveria LE, Eastman R, Greenacre JK, Petrie A. Bromocriptine in parkinsonism. Br Med J 1974; 4:442–444.
4. Calne DB, Teychenne PF, Leigh PN, Bamji AN, Greenacre JK. Treatment of parkinsonism with bromocriptine. Lancet 1974; 2:1355–1356.
5. Friis ML, Gron U, Larsen NE, Pakkenberg H, Hvidberg EF. Pharmacokinetics of bromocriptine during continuous oral treatment of Parkinson's disease. Eur J Clin Pharmacol 1979; 15:275–280.
6. Schran HF, Bhuta SI, Schwarz HJ, Thorner MO. The pharmacokinetics of bromocriptine in man. Adv Biochem Psychopharmacol 1980; 23:125–139.
7. Staal-Schreinemachers AL, Wesseling H, Kamphuis DJ, Burg WVD, Lakke JP. Low-dose bromocriptine therapy in Parkinson's disease: double-blind, placebo-controlled study. Neurology 1986; 36:291–293.
8. Libman I, Gawel MJ, Riopelle RJ, Bouchard S. A comparison of bromocriptine (Parlodel) and levodopa-carbidopa (Sinemet) for treatment of "de novo" Parkinson's disease patients. Can J Neurol Sci 1987; 14:576–580.
9. Riopelle RJ. Bromocriptine and the clinical spectrum of Parkinson's disease. Can J Neurol Sci 1987; 14(suppl 3):455–459.
10. Rinne UK. Early combination of bromocriptine and levodopa in the treatment of Parkinson's disease: a 5-year follow-up. Neurology 1987; 37:826–828.
11. Herskovits E, Yorio A, Leston J. Long-term bromocriptine treatment in de novo parkinsonian patients. Medicina 1988; 48:345–350.
12. Parkinson's Disease Research Group in the United Kingdom. Comparisons of therapeutic effects of levodopa, levodopa and selegiline, and bromocriptine in patients with early, mild Parkinson's disease: three year interim report. BMJ 1993; 307:469–472.
13. Hely MA, Morris JG, Reid WG, O'Sullivan DJ, Williamson PM, Rail D, Broe GA, Margries S. The Sydney Multicentre Study of Parkinson's Disease: a randomised, prospective five year study comparing low dose bromocriptine with low dose levodopa-carbidopa. J Neurol Neurosurg Psychiatry 1994; 57:903–910.
14. Montastruc JL, Rascol O, Senard JM, Rascol A. A randomised controlled study comparing bromocriptine to which levodopa was later added, with levodopa alone in previously untreated patients with Parkinson's disease: a five year follow-up. J Neurol Neurosurg Psychiatry 1994; 57:1034–1038.
15. Mizuno Y, Kondo T, Narabayashi H. Pergolide in the treatment of Parkinson's disease. Neurology 1995; 45(suppl 3):S13–S21.
16. Korczyn AD, Brunt ER, Larsen JP, Nagy Z, Poewe WH, Ruggieri S. A 3-year randomized trial of ropinirole and bromocriptine in early Parkinson's disease. The 053 Study Group. Neurology 1999; 53:364–370.
17. Kartzinel R, Teychenne P, Gillespie MM, Perlow M, Gielen AC, Sadowsky DA, Calne DB. Bromocriptine and levodopa (with or without carbidopa) in parkinsonism. Lancet 1976; 2:272–275.
18. Hoehn MM, Elton RL. Low dosages of bromocriptine added to levodopa in Parkinson's disease. Neurology 1985; 35:199–206.
19. Toyokura Y, Mizuno Y, Kase M, Sobue I, Kuroiwa Y, Narabayashi H, Uono M, Nakanishi T, Kameyama M, Ito H, et al. Effects of bromocriptine on parkinsonism. A nation-wide collaborative double-blind study. Acta Neurol Scand 1985; 72:157–170.
20. Nakanishi T, Iwata M, Goto I, Kanazawa I, Kowa H, Mannen T, Mizuno Y, Nishitani H, Ogawa N, Takahashi A, Tashiro K, Tohgi H, Yanagisawa N. Nation-wide collaborative study on the long-term effects of bromocriptine in the treatment of parkinsonian patients. Final Report. Eur Neurol 1992; 32(suppl 1):9–22.
21. Przuntek H, Welzel D, Gerlach M, Blumner E, Danielczyk W, Kaiser HJ, Kraus PH, Letzel H, Riederer P, Uberla K. Early institution of bromocriptine in Parkinson's disease inhibits the emergence of levodopa-associated motor side effects. Long-term results of the PRADO study. J Neural Transm 1996; 103:699–715.
22. Gimenez-Roldan S, Tolosa E, Burguera JA, Chacon J, Liano H, Forcadell F. Early combination of bromocriptine and levodopa in Parkinson's disease: a prospective randomized study of two parallel

groups over a total follow-up period of 44 months including an initial 8-month double-blind stage. Clin Neuropharmacol 1997; 20:67–76.

23. LeWitt PA, Ward CD, Larsen TA, Raphaelson MI, Newman RP, Foster N, Dambrosia JM, Calne DB. Comparison of pergolide and bromocriptine therapy in parkinsonism. Neurology 1983; 33:1009–1014.

24. Pezzoli G, Martignoni E, Pacchetti C, Angeleri V, Lamberti P, Muratorio A, Bonuccelli U, DeMari M. A cross-over, controlled study comparing pergolide with bromocriptine as an adjunct to levodopa for the treatment of Parkinson's disease. Neurology 1995; 45(suppl 3):S22–S27.

25. Inzelberg R, Nisipeanu P, Rabey JM, Orlov E, Catz T, Kippervasser S, Schechtman E, Korczyn AD. Double-blind comparison of cabergoline and bromocriptine in Parkinson's disease patients with motor fluctuations. Neurology 1996; 47:785–788.

26. LeWitt PA, Gopinathan G, Ward CD, Sanes JN, Dambrosia JM, Durso R, Calne DB. Lisuride versus bromocriptine treatment in Parkinson's disease: a double-blind study. Neurology 1982; 32:69–72.

27. Laihinen A, Rinne UK, Suchy I. Comparison of lisuride and bromocriptine in the treatment of advanced Parkinson's disease. Acta Neurol Scand 1992; 86:593–595.

28. Guttman M, International Pramipexole-Bromocriptine Study Group. Double-blind comparison of pramipexole and bromocriptine treatment with placebo in advanced Parkinson's disease. Neurology 1997; 49:1060–1065.

29. The Tolcapone Study Group. Efficacy and tolerability of tolcapone compared with bromocriptine in levodopa-treated parkinsonian patients. Mov Disord 1999; 14:38–44.

30. Ben-Noun L. Drug-induced respiratory disorders: incidence, prevention and management. Drug Saf 2000; 23:143–164.

9
Pergolide

Maria Bozi and Kailash P. Bhatia

University College London, London, England

I. INTRODUCTION

Dopamine agonists were first introduced for the treatment of Parkinson's disease (PD) as adjunctive therapy to levodopa in an attempt to reduce the levodopa-induced motor complications. The first agents to be tried were ergot derivatives, which have long been known to possess dopamine receptor agonistic activity (1). Bromocriptine was the first oral ergot dopamine agonist licensed and marketed for the treatment of PD in the mid-1970s (2). A decade later, another semisynthetic ergot derivative, pergolide, more potent than bromocriptine and with a longer half-life, was tested in patients with late-stage PD and approved for use in 1989 (3,4).

II. PHARMACOLOGY

A. Mechanism of Action

Pergolide mesylate (8-β-methyl-thiomethyl-6-N-propylegoline) is a synthetic ergoline dopamine agonist that has dose-dependent D2/D1 receptor activity (5). It has high intrinsic activity at D2 receptors, while it exerts its D1 agonistic activity only at high concentrations through stimulation of adenylate cyclase activity. There is experimental data to support that, like other dopamine agonists, pergolide at low doses may act predominantly on presynaptic dopamine autoreceptors, inhibiting dopamine synthesis (6). It has been suggested that the apparent higher sensitivity of dopamine autoreceptors accounts for this paradoxical effect of small compared to large doses of some dopamine agonists (7). Like most ergot derivatives, pergolide also acts on nondopamine receptors such as adrenergic, serotoninergic, and muscarinic receptors.

Pergolide has been shown to induce contralateral turning in 6-hydroxydopamine (6-OHDA)-lesioned rats, which is blocked by D2 or mixed D1/D2 antagonists, indicating that its motor effect results from stimulation of striatal dopamine receptors (8). Pergolide-induced turning is not affected by dopamine depletion caused by pretreatment with reserpine or α-methylparatyrosine (AMPT), suggesting that pergolide exerts its anti-parkinsonian activity independently of dopamine (9).

Pergolide inhibits the secretion of prolactin in humans. It also causes a transient rise in serum concentrations of growth hormone and a decrease in serum concentrations of luteinizing hormone.

B. Pharmacokinetics

Pergolide is rapidly absorbed from the gastrointestinal tract and reaches peak plasma concentrations within 1–3 hours. Its half-life ranges between 15 and 42 hours, being longer than that of most dopamine agonists with the exception of cabergoline (65 h) (10). Pergolide binds highly to plasma proteins, so it may interact with other drugs that affect protein binding such as phenytoin, warfarin, and macrolides.

III. PERGOLIDE IN CLINICAL PRACTICE

Dopamine agonists possess some theoretical advantages over levodopa: (a) they exert their action directly, stimulating the dopamine receptors and thus bypassing the degenerating nigrostriatal neurons, (b) they do not depend on a pool of decarboxylase enzymes for conversion into the active drug, (c) they do not compete with dietary amino acids for active transport across the gut epithelium and blood-brain barrier, and (d) they do not produce toxic metabolites or free radicals (11).

In theory, pergolide should have an advantage over other dopamine agonists due to its unique agonistic activity on both D1 and D2 dopamine receptors. Although the function of D1 receptors in the treatment of patients with PD is not fully understood, there is considerable evidence indicating that additional D1 receptor stimulation may be necessary for the optimization of the antiparkinsonian effect (12–14). In 1-methyl-4-phenyl-1,2,3,6-tetrahydropyridine (MPTP)–treated monkeys the combined administration of CY 208-24 (a selective D1 agonist) with a long-acting preparation of bromocriptine (a D2 receptor agonist and a weak D1 receptor antagonist) ameliorated motor function at doses at which the separate administration of these drugs was ineffective (15). The stimulation of D1 receptors alone also seems to mediate antiparkinsonian activity. In a study conducted in humans, the administration of ABT-431, a selective D1 receptor agonist, to patients with PD resulted in antiparkinsonian efficacy of similar magnitude to levodopa (16). The relative contribution of dopamine D1 and D2 receptor function to the generation of dyskinesias remains a matter of controversy. Dopamine D2 agonists have been shown to induce dyskinesias in experimental models (17). On the contrary, there have been reports of D1 receptor agonists inducing fewer dyskinesias than D2 agonists and even having a beneficial effect on repeated administration (18,19). Therefore, the dual action of pergolide on D1 and D2 receptors could theoretically contribute to its superior antiparkinsonian efficacy and reduced potency to induce dyskinesias compared to other dopamine agonists devoid of D1 agonism.

Pergolide has been used in clinical practice both as monotherapy in de novo PD patients and as adjunctive therapy to levodopa in patients with fluctuating disease. There are relatively few controlled studies evaluating its efficacy as compared to the more recent agonists (20). This is partly due to the lack of well-defined methodology guidelines for clinical trials at the time that pergolide was introduced (21). This chapter will summarize the data available from the most methodologically sound clinical trials on the efficacy, safety, and tolerability of pergolide in the treatment of PD.

IV. EFFICACY OF PERGOLIDE IN CONTROLLING PARKINSONISM

A. Pergolide as Monotherapy in Early Disease

The efficacy of pergolide as monotherapy in the early stages of PD has been assessed in two large double-blind studies: one compared to placebo and one versus levodopa (22,23) (Table 1). Additional data are also provided by a three-arm study conducted in a mixed population of patients with both early and advanced disease. The long-term open-label arm of this study provides the only information available on the long-term efficacy of pergolide.

Barone et al. in 1999 performed a 3-month double-blind placebo-controlled study conducted in 105 patients with PD of less that 3 years duration who were randomized to receive either pergolide or placebo (mean age approximately 62 years) (22). Efficacy assessments included the Unified Parkinson's Disease Rating Scale (UPDRS), the Clinical Global Impression (CGI), and the Schwab and England Activities of Daily Living (ADL) scores. The primary outcome measure was the number of responders defined as having at least a 30% reduction in the UPDRS motor scale. Secondary endpoints were changes from baseline to last visit in the UPDRS total, ADL and motor scores, CGI, and Schwab and England ADL. At a mean daily dose of 2.06 ± 0.76 mg, pergolide proved to be more effective than placebo, as signified by the greater percentage of responders in the pergolide-treated group (57% vs. 17% in the placebo group). All other endpoints showed a significant improvement with pergolide compared to placebo. CGI scores revealed a total of 48% of patients treated with pergolide rated as "very much improved" or "much improved" versus 6% of patients treated with placebo. Six patients in the pergolide group and two in the placebo group withdrew from the study because of adverse events. The adverse events reported were similar to those reported with other dopamine agonists. Only anorexia, nausea, vomiting, and dizziness occurred significantly more often with pergolide than with placebo ($p < 0.05$).

A 1-year interim analysis of a 3-year double-blind randomized study of pergolide versus levodopa in early stage PD using PErgolide L-dopa MOnotherapy–Positron Emission Tomography (PELMO-PET) was presented (23). A total of 294 patients were treated with pergolide or levodopa to assess the long-term efficacy and safety of pergolide when used as monotherapy. A further objective was to determine whether monotherapy with pergolide could delay the onset of motor complications compared with levodopa. After 1 year the mean daily dose for pergolide was 2.5 mg and 466 mg for levodopa. Both treatments produced a significant improvement in UPDRS ADL and motor scores from baseline at the 1-year evaluation. A responder analysis (defined as patients with $> 30\%$ improvement in the UPDRS motor) showed similar results (53% in the pergolide and 54% in the levodopa group). Changes in the CGI severity scale reached statistical significance only in the levodopa group. At the end of 1 year, 79% of pergolide-treated patients and 84% of levodopa-treated patients remained in the study, demonstrating that both drugs have significant antiparkinsonian efficacy that persists for at least 1 year.

Prior to these studies, Mizuno et al. in 1995 conducted an uncontrolled open-label study in 86 patients with PD who had not received levodopa and 314 patients already on levodopa treatment but with unsatisfactory response (24). The mean daily dose of pergolide in this group over the 8-week follow-up period was 0.85 ± 0.57 mg up to a maximum of 5 mg. Among the 86 de novo patients, 82 remained in the study. Of the remaining patients, 7 (8.5%) showed marked improvement, 32 (39%) moderate improvement, 32 (39%) mild improvement, and 11 (13.4%) showed either no improvement or worsening.

Table 1 Pergolide Monotherapy in De Novo PD Patients: Randomized Clinical Trials

Study (Ref.)	Design	Duration (months)	No. of patients	Mean daily drug dose (mg)	Efficacy measures	Results
Barone et al., 1999 (22)	Double-blind, placebo-controlled	3	105	P: 2.06	UPDRS (ADL, motor) Schwab & England, ADL, CGI	Significant improvement of UPDRS (overall score, ADL, motor), CGI and Schwab & England compared to placebo
PELMO-PET (1-year interim), 2000 (23)	Double-blind, levodopa-controlled	12	294	P: 2.51 L: 466	UPDRS (part II–III) Schwab & England, ADL, CGI	Significant improvement of UPDRS (ADL, motor) with both treatments, but greater with levodopa; significant improvement of CGI only with levodopa; similar % of responders in both groups

P = pergolide; L = levodopa; ADL = activities of daily living; CGI = clinical global impression; UPDRS = Unified Parkinson's Disease Rating Scale.

The short-term (8-week) double-blind bromocriptine-controlled arm of this study demonstrated beneficial effects of pergolide and bromocriptine in 345 de novo and levodopa-treated patients (24). In the de novo group, 49 patients were randomized to pergolide and 49 to bromocriptine. The mean maintenance daily doses of pergolide and bromocriptine were 1.43 and 15.1 mg, respectively. Both treatments significantly improved most of the items studied (i.e., tremor, rigidity, akinesia, retropulsion, short-stepped gait, masked face, hygiene, feeding, and dressing) to a similar degree. The occurrence of side effects was also comparable in both treatment groups.

The long-term open-label study conducted by the same investigators provides the only published information on the long-term (>1 year) efficacy of pergolide when used as monotherapy in early stage PD (24). Sixty-two de novo patients who received pergolide as initial antiparkinsonian treatment were followed for 2–4 years. Among them, 28 patients required levodopa supplementation at some point during follow-up. By the end of the first year, 32 of 62 patients dropped out or required levodopa supplementation because of side effects, disease progression, unsatisfactory response to pergolide, or other reasons. Only 18 of 62 patients retained the initial improvement and continued on pergolide monotherapy by the end of the third year. Additional data on the long-term efficacy of pergolide as mono-therapy are expected when the results of the 3-year levodopa-controlled PELMO-PET study are published. According to preliminary unpublished results of this study, 52% of the de novo patients who were assigned to pergolide could remain on monotherapy for the 3-year duration of the study versus 62% of patients in the levodopa group (25).

B. Pergolide as Add-On Therapy to Levodopa

Pergolide was first introduced in the early 1980s as an adjunctive treatment to levodopa in patients with motor complications (3,4). Since then a number of small trials have been performed to evaluate its usefulness in patients with unsatisfactory response to levodopa (26–31). Large randomized trials have compared the efficacy of pergolide as add-on treatment to levodopa with placebo and bromocriptine.

1. Placebo-Controlled Studies

In 1994 Olanow et al. published the results of a multicenter double-blind placebo-controlled study in 376 patients with moderately severe dyskinesia or end-of-dose deterioration (mean age 63 years, mean duration of disease 11 years) (32). Patients randomized to pergolide were receiving a mean daily dose of 2.94 mg at the end of 6-months. Motor function and ADL were assessed during the on state using weighted rating scales. Other assessment criteria were an evaluation of dyskinesias on a 0–4 scale and a quantitative estimate of the number of hours of off-time. Attempts were made to reduce the dosage of levodopa. Approximately 30 subjects dropped out in each group. Pergolide permitted a significant reduction in the mean levodopa dose of 24.7% versus 4.9% in patients randomized to placebo ($p < 0.001$). Pergolide significantly improved the motor and ADL scores as compared to placebo with significant improvement in most of the parameters assessed. Off-time was reduced by 1.8 hours per day compared with 0.2 hours with placebo ($p < 0.001$). At study endpoint, 56% of pergolide and 25% of placebo patients had an improvement in total parkinsonian score of $>25\%$ ($p < 0.001$), while 24% in the pergolide and 5% in the placebo group had an improvement of $>50\%$ ($p < 0.001$). The introduction of the trial medication was followed by the development or worsening of dyskinesias in 62% of the pergolide-treated patients versus 25% of the placebo-treated patients ($p < 0.05$). However, they could be efficiently managed by a reduction in levodopa dosage so that by the end of the study dyskinesias were not significantly different in the two groups (Table 2). Other adverse events included nausea, dyspepsia, hallucinations, insomnia, and drowsiness and occurred more frequently in the pergolide than in the placebo group. Hallucinations were the most troublesome and led to the withdrawal of eight pergolide-treated and three placebo-treated patients. Rare adverse reactions noticed in the pergolide group included erythromelalgia in two patients and pleural effusion and leucopenia in one patient each. Adverse events lead to the withdrawal of 9.5% of pergolide-treated and 4.3% of placebo-treated patients.

2. Bromocriptine-Controlled Studies

The findings of four randomized bromocriptine-controlled studies—two double-blind (24,33), one single-blind (34), and one open-label, crossover study (35) performed in a variety of patients with PD (Table 3)—will be summarized in this section.

Le Witt et al. conducted the first double-blind comparative study of pergolide and bromocriptine in 1983 (33). This was a two-period, crossover study performed in a mixed population of 27 patients with PD (15 with motor fluctuations, 9 stable with good response to levodopa, and 3 de novo patients). The period of treatment ranged from 7 to 10 weeks. The mean optimal daily dose was 3.3 mg for pergolide and 42.7 mg for bromocriptine. Most patients improved with both treatments with no significant difference between the two groups. The adverse event profile was also similar with both agents.

Pezzoli et al. in 1994 carried out a single-blinded crossover comparative study of pergolide versus bromocriptine in 68 patients with PD who showed a declining response to levodopa (34). Both drugs were administered for 12 weeks. The average daily dose of pergolide was 2.3 mg and of bromocriptine 24.2 mg. Addition of pergolide or bromocriptine resulted in a significant improvement in efficacy endpoints [New York University Parkinson's Disease Scale (NYUPDS) and modified CGI scale] compared to baseline. Direct comparison of the two treatments showed pergolide to be more effective than bromocriptine in daily living scores ($p = 0.020$) and motor scores ($p = 0.038$). There was a significant improvement in dyskinesia and dystonia scores with pergolide compared with levodopa alone but no significant differences were shown between the two treatment groups.

The short-term (8-week) double-blind bromocriptine-controlled trial conducted by Mizuno et al. (24) included both de novo and more advanced patients already on levodopa. Ninety-three patients in the add-on group were assigned to pergolide and 99 to bromocriptine. Pergolide (mean daily dose 1.24 mg) and bromocriptine (mean daily dose 14.6 mg) both improved most of the endpoints studied. Although there was a tendency for a greater improvement with pergolide than bromocriptine, the difference did not reach statistical significance.

In 1996 Boas et al. published a 24-week open-label crossover study in 33 levodopa-treated patients with suboptimal control of motor complications (35). The mean daily doses of pergolide and bromocriptine at the end of the study were 3.6 and 21.7 mg, respectively. A significant improvement in UPDRS motor scores over baseline was observed with both treatments ($p < 0.05$). The improvement was reported to be significantly greater with pergolide than with bromocriptine ($p < 0.01$). Levodopa dosage was reduced by 26% with pergolide versus 10% with bromocriptine ($p < 0.01$).

V. PREVENTION OF MOTOR COMPLICATIONS

The putative role of dopamine agonists in preventing or delaying the onset of motor complications related to dopaminergic treatment has become a growing area of interest

Table 2 Pergolide as Add-On to Levodopa in PD Patients with Advanced Disease

Study (Ref.)	Design	Duration (months)	No. of patients	Mean age	Mean disease duration (y)	Mean daily drug dose	Efficacy measures	Results
Olanow et al., 1994 (32)	Double-blind, placebo-controlled	6	376	63	11	2.9 mg	Modified CURS	Significant improvement of CURS (motor and ADL) with pergolide
							Dyskinesias 0–4 scale	No difference in dyskinesias at end of study between the two groups
							Number of hours off	Reduction of hours off by 1.8 h/d with pergolide vs. 0.2 h/d with placebo
							Levodopa dose reduction	Reduction of mean levodopa dose by 24.7% with pergolide vs. 4.9% with placebo

CURS = Columbia University Rating Scale; ADL = activities of daily living.

Table 3 Comparative Trials of Pergolide with Bromocriptine

Study (Ref.)	Design	Duration	No. of patients	Characteristics	Mean daily drug dose	Efficacy measures	Results
Le Witt et al., 1983 (33)	Double-blind, crossover	7–18 weeks	24	3 de novo 9 stable 15 fluctuators	P: 3.3 Br: 42.7	Duvoisin scale Reaction time and movement time	Similar efficacy
Pezzoli et al., 1994 (34)	Single-blind, crossover	12 weeks for each treatment	68	All fluctuators	P: 2.3 Br: 24.2	NYUPDS CGI	Greater improvement in NYUPDS with pergolide
Mizuno et al., 1995 (24)	Double-blind parallel group	8 weeks	345	98 de novo 192 fluctuators	P: 1.4 Br: 15.1 P: 1.2 Br: 14.6	UPDRS CGI	Similar efficacy in de-novo pts; greater improvement in UPDRS in fluctuators with pergolide, but not statistically significant
Boas et al., 1996 (35)	Open-label, crossover	12 weeks for each treatment	33	All fluctuators	P: 3.6 Br: 21.7	UPDRS Levodopa dose reduction	Greater improvement in UPDRS and greater decrease in levodopa dose 26% vs. 10% with pergolide

W = Weeks; NYUPDS = New York University Parkinson's Disease Scale; CGI = Clinical Global Improvement; UPDRS = Unified Parkinson's Disease Rating Scale; P = pergolide; Br = bromocriptine.

and research. It has been postulated that motor complications may develop in response to pulsatile stimulation of striatal dopamine receptors and that long-acting dopaminergic agents may reduce the risk of motor fluctuations and dyskinesias by producing more continuous or tonic stimulation (36). Several trials involving bromocriptine, cabergoline, ropinirole, and pramipexole provide data to support this hypothesis (37–40). Information on the potential of pergolide to delay the onset of motor complications is limited and derives from the long-term open-label study by Mizuno et al. and from partial results of the 3-year PELMO-PET study.

In the study conducted by Mizuno et al., 62 de novo PD patients received pergolide and were followed for 2–4 years (24). The incidence of "wearing off" was 8.8% in patients who could continue on pergolide monotherapy, while it reached 42.9% in those who required levodopa supplementation. Dyskinesias developed in 14.7% of patients who remained on pergolide monotherapy and in 21.5% of patients who received levodopa add-on therapy. It is possible that patients in the latter group had more severe disease.

Partial results are available from the PELMO-PET study. A total of 294 untreated PD patients were randomized to receive either pergolide or carbidopa/levodopa. Dose titration of the study drug was permitted throughout the 3-year follow-up period. The average daily dose of pergolide reached 3.2 mg and that of levodopa 504 mg. Open-label levodopa supplementation was not allowed. More patients in the levodopa group completed the study (62% vs. 52% in the pergolide group). Adverse events and a perceived lack of efficacy accounted for the withdrawals and were more common in the pergolide group. A 1-year interim analysis showed that the time to onset of motor complications was significantly longer with pergolide (41). Preliminary results from the same study showed that at the end of the 3 years, motor complications were more frequent with levodopa compared with pergolide treatment (33% vs. 17%; $p = 0.067$). Similarly, levodopa-treated patients were more likely to develop dyskinesias (approximately 40% vs. 20% of pergolide treated patients; $p = 0.004$) (25).

However, the results that show delay of motor complications when treatment is initiated with a dopamine agonist must be interpreted with caution. In the relevant trials, patients treated with agonists had significantly poorer motor scores. It is possible that treatment intensity was lower in the agonist arms resulting in lower incidence of dyskinesias. Moreover, it is not surprising that individuals in the agonist arms had less "wearing off." Dopamine agonists have longer half-lives than levodopa, so the reduced incidence of motor fluctuations is probably not a result of initial agonist treatment but of their pharmacokinetic properties (42).

VI. CONTROL OF MOTOR COMPLICATIONS

The development of motor fluctuations and dyskinesias related to levodopa therapy necessitated the testing of other agents such as dopamine agonists in an attempt to achieve better motor control. However, there is only one large double-blind placebo-controlled trial evaluating the efficacy of pergolide in the treatment of patients with motor complications (32). In this study by Olanow et al., pergolide significantly reduced "wearing off" without aggravating dyskinesias.

High doses of pergolide have also been proposed to enable a drastic reduction of the levodopa dosage and improve motor complications. While Lang et al. (4) in 1982 failed to demonstrate improvement of dyskinesias with high doses of pergolide (range of dosage

0.4–15 mg/d), subsequent reports favored a beneficial effect. First, Mear et al. reported benefits of pergolide monotherapy in advanced PD patients (43). Following this report, Facca and Sanchez-Ramos treated 13 patients with severe incapacitating dyskinesias with high doses of pergolide trying to establish pergolide monotherapy without diminishing antiparkinsonian efficacy (44). Patients had an average age of 65.9 years and average duration of disease of 12.9 years. In five patients levodopa was withdrawn and replaced by pergolide monotherapy for 6–18 months. Early morning akinesia prevented the complete withdrawal of levodopa in the rest of patients. The average daily dose of levodopa was reduced to 12% of the average dose at baseline. Pergolide was used at a mean dose of 6.5 mg/d, and the highest dose used as monotherapy was 10 mg/d. The severity of dyskinesias assessed using the Abnormal Involuntary Movement Scale (AIMS) was significantly reduced (AIMS scores decreased from 32.5 to 7.15 after pergolide). Moreover, the percentage of the day that patients were dyskinetic decreased dramatically from 70.9 to 13%. At the same time, the percentage of time "off" was reduced from 26 to 16%. After 6 years, three patients remained levodopa-free and the improvement of dyskinesias and motor fluctuations was maintained (45). A large multicenter open-label trial involved 62 PD patients with advanced disease (46). All patients were treated with a minimum daily pergolide dose of 4.5 mg. The mean pergolide dosage that allowed a 50% reduction in the levodopa dose was 8.25 mg/d (range: 4.5–24 mg/d). In 14 patients, levodopa was discontinued. The duration of "off" periods was significantly decreased from an average of 7.3 to 1.7 hours per day. These findings are interesting but need confirmation by large double-blind trials.

VII. SAFETY AND TOLERABILITY

Pergolide is generally well tolerated when used both as monotherapy and adjunctive treatment. The 1-year interim analysis of the PELMO-PET study showed that 79.1% of the pergolide-treated patients and 83.6% of the levodopa-treated patients completed the first year of the study (41). The adverse event rate was significantly higher for pergolide (85.1%) than for levodopa (71.2%; $p = 0.004$), but serious adverse events occurred at a similar frequency in both groups. In the double-blind placebo-controlled study by Barone et al., 6 of a total of 53 patients in the pergolide and 2 of a total of 52 patients in the placebo group withdrew because of adverse events. Dropout rates because of adverse events reported by Olanow et al.(32) were 9.5% with pergolide and 4.3% with placebo.

Side effects commonly associated with the use of pergolide are similar to those reported with other dopamine agonists. These include nausea, vomiting, anorexia, dyspepsia, asthenia, dry mouth, dizziness, insomnia, nervousness, delusions, hallucinations, and somnolence. Gastrointestinal symptoms are the most common. When pergolide is added to levodopa, it can induce or worsen preexisting dyskinesias. The most common adverse events during the two large randomized trials of pergolide in de novo and fluctuating patients are summarized in Table 4. Pergolide, like other ergot compounds, can cause pleuropulmonary, pericardial, and retroperitoneal fibrosis, erythromelalgia (a painful reddish discoloration of the skin particularly in the distal part of the legs), and digital vasospasm. Serosal fibrosis, believed to be an idiosyncratic reaction, usually develops approximately 2 years after the initiation of treatment. The discontinuation of the offensive drug partially reverses the condition (54–56). Ankle edema is seen with ergot as well as nonergot compounds (50).

Table 4 Adverse Events with Pergolide Treatment

Pergolide monotherapy[a] ($n = 53$)		Pergolide adjunct therapy[b] ($n = 189$)	
Event	%	Event	%
Nausea[c]	32.1	Dyskinesia[c]	62
Somnolence	15.1	Nausea[c]	24
Dizziness[c]	13.2	Hallucinations[c]	14
Insomnia	9.4	Drowsiness[c]	10
Vomiting[c]	9.4	Insomnia[c]	8
Anorexia[c]	7.5	Nasal congestion[c]	7
Asthenia	7.5	Dyspepsia[c]	6
Dyspepsia	7.5	Dyspnea[c]	5
Dry mouth	3.8		
Nervousness	3.8		
Rhinitis	3.8		

[a]From Ref. 22.
[b]From Ref. 32.
[c]Adverse events that were significantly different in pergolide and placebo groups.

There have been some concerns in the past that pergolide may have a cardiotoxic effect. Asymptomatic ventricular arrhythmias were detected in parkinsonian patients on pergolide using Holter monitoring (58). Subsequent studies did not confirm an association of pergolide with cardiac side effects (59,60). Recently, three cases of patients with severe, unexplained tricuspid regurgitation were described (61). Additional significant left sided valve regurgitation was noted in two. Echocardiography and histological examination of the surgically explanted valves revealed abnormalities strikingly similar to those associated with carcinoid-, ergot-, and fenfluramine-induced valve disease. Carcinoid valvular disease was excluded. All three patients were taking pergolide and none had received any of the other drugs. Therefore, it was suggested that an association between pergolide and valvular heart disease might exist.

Sedative effects have been attributed to all dopamine agonists. Increased concern has followed recent reports of sudden sleep episodes while driving in patients receiving pramipexole and ropinirole (55). Although this effect of "irresistible sleepiness" was initially thought to be restricted to nonergot agonists, there is evidence that this is likely a class effect common to all dopamine agonists and closely related to daytime somnolence (56,57). Similarly, pergolide is not devoid of sedative effects and several cases of "sleep attacks" have been reported in association with its use (56,58). However, there is some suggestion that sleep episodes may occur less frequently with pergolide than with the nonergot dopamine agonists (59,60). The absence of well-conducted clinical trials does not allow for definitive conclusions.

To reduce the risk of side effects pergolide is initiated at a low dose, which is then titrated gradually. The simultaneous administration of domperidone, a peripheral dopamine receptor antagonist improves gastrointestinal tolerability. The highest recommended dose of pergolide is 5 mg. However, higher doses have been reported with good long-term tolerability. It is thus possible that the ergoline-derived dopamine agonists may not have been deployed to their full therapeutic potential in either clinical trials or clinical practice (61).

VIII. PERGOLIDE AND MORTALITY

Data on mortality associated with the use of pergolide is limited. There is one open-label retrospective uncontrolled analysis of mortality data from clinical trials involving 1330 patients with PD treated with pergolide as an adjunct to levodopa (62). When compared to the general population of the same age, gender, and race distribution, the ratio of observed to expected deaths was 2.3 for the same period of observation. This was consistent with ratios with levodopa and levodopa combination treatments.

IX. NEUROPROTECTIVE PROPERTIES

There has been a growing interest in the putative neuroprotective effects of dopamine agonists. Theoretically, dopamine agonists could provide neuroprotection by producing (a) a levodopa-sparing effect, thus diminishing the potential toxic effects of dopamine metabolism, (b) a reduction in dopamine synthesis via stimulation of presynaptic dopamine autoreceptors, (c) direct antioxidant effects, and (d) restoration of the inhibition to the subthalamic nucleus (STN) with subsequent diminution of STN-mediated excitotoxicity (63,64). The majority of evidence to support the neuroprotective effects of dopamine agonists derives from in vitro and in vivo studies. Two large longitudinal clinical studies evaluated the potential of ropinirole and pramipexole to delay disease progression using fluorodopa positron emission tomography (PET) and β-CIT single photon emission computed tomography (SPECT) scans as markers of neuronal degeneration (65,66).

Data to support the putative neuroprotective properties of pergolide are limited. In vitro studies have shown that pergolide has neuroprotective effects under conditions of elevated oxidative stress in cell cultures (67,68). In an animal study, the administration of pergolide in the diet of rats for 2 years diminished the age-related changes in nigral dopamine neurons and striatal dopamine terminals compared to control animals (69). The 3-year randomized European PELMO-PET study will evaluate, among other efficacy and safety endpoints, the relative effects of pergolide and levodopa monotherapy on disease progression using fluorodopa PET scans. The preliminary results showed a similar degree of decline in striatal fluorodopa uptake in both levodopa- and pergolide-treated patients during the 3-year follow-up period (23).

X. COMPARISON OF PERGOLIDE WITH OTHER ANTIPARKINSONIAN AGENTS

So far there is no convincing evidence to support superiority of a certain dopamine agonist over other agents of the same class. Pergolide has not been proven more efficacious than bromocriptine, although some small, uncontrolled or short-term studies have reported superior symptomatic control with pergolide (24,33,70). A 10:1 dose conversion ratio of bromocriptine to pergolide has been proposed. Few comparative studies of pergolide with the newer nonergot agonists exist. They have concluded that a rapid (overnight) switch from pergolide to pramipexole or ropinirole is safe, but no superiority of the newer agonists over pergolide could be established. Pergolide was converted to pramipexole or ropinirole at dose equivalence ratios of 1:1 and 1:6 respectively (71–73).

Data evaluating the relative efficacy of pergolide to other antiparkinsonian agents such as monoamine oxidase (MAO)-B and catechol-O-methyl transferase (COMT) inhibitors is still very limited. A short-term open-label study compared the efficacy, safety, and tolerability of pergolide to tolcapone in 203 patients with fluctuating response to levodopa (74). Both drugs provided similar improvements in efficacy variables with the exception of improvement in quality of life, which was significantly greater with tolcapone. Tolcapone was better tolerated and had a more favorable adverse event profile than pergolide. Further long-term double-blind randomized trials are needed to evaluate the efficacy of pergolide relative to other dopamine agonists and antiparkinsonian agents.

XI. CONCLUSIONS

Pergolide has been used in clinical practice for over 20 years. Clinical experience and information available from clinical trials have proven pergolide to be a safe and effective drug for the treatment of PD when used both as monotherapy in de novo patients or as an adjunct to levodopa in patients with more advanced disease. More information is awaited on its long-term efficacy, while the neuroprotective properties and possible role in delaying the onset of motor complications of pergolide as well as other dopamine agonists are still unclear and are being tentatively investigated.

REFERENCES

1. Goldstein M, Lieberman A, Lew J, Asano T, Rosenfeld M, Makman M. Interaction of pergolide with central dopaminergic receptors. Neurobiology 1980; 77:3725–3728.
2. Kartzinel R, Teychenne P, Gillespie MM, Perlow M, Gielen AC, Sadowsky DA, Calne DB. Bromocriptine and levodopa (with or without carbidopa) in parkinsonism. Lancet 1976; 2:272–275.
3. Lieberman A, Goldstein M, Leibowitz M, Neophytides A, Kupersmith M, Pact V, Kleinberg D. Treatment of advanced Parkinson disease with pergolide. Neurology 1981; 31:675–682.
4. Lang AE, Quinn N, Brincat S, Marsden CD, Parkes JD. Pergolide in late-stage Parkinson disease. Ann Neurol 1982; 12:243–247.
5. Langtry HD, Clissold SP. Pergolide. A review of its pharmacological properties and therapeutic potential in Parkinson's disease. Drugs 1990; 39:491–506.
6. White FJ, Wang RY. Pharmacological characterization of dopamine autoreceptors in the rat ventral tegmental area: microiontophoretic studies. J Pharmacol Exp Ther 1984; 231:275–280.
7. Skirboll LR, Grace AA, Bunney BS. Dopamine auto- and postsynaptic receptors: electrophysiological evidence for differential sensitivity to dopamine agonists. Science 1979; 206:80–82.
8. Arnt J, Hyttel J. Differential involvement of dopamine D-1 and D-2 receptors in the circling behaviour induced by apomorphine, SK & F 38393, pergolide and LY 171555 in 6-hydroxydopamine-lesioned rats. Psychopharmacology (Berl) 1985; 85:346–352.
9. Duvoisin RC, Heikkila RE, Manzino L. Pergolide-induced circling in rats with 6-hydroxydopamine lesions in the nigrostriatal pathway. Neurology 1982; 32:1387–1391.
10. Rubin A, Lemberger L, Dhahir P. Physiologic disposition of pergolide. Clin Pharmacol Ther 1981; 30:258–265.
11. Montastruc JL, Rascol O, Senard JM. Treatment of Parkinson's disease should begin with a dopamine agonist. Mov Disord 1999; 14:725–730.
12. Ahlskog JE, Muenter MD, Bailey PA, Stevens PM. Dopamine agonist treatment of fluctuating parkinsonism. D-2 (controlled-release MK-458) vs combined D-1 and D-2 (pergolide). Arch Neurol 1992; 49:560–568.
13. Vermeulen RJ, Drukarch B, Sahadat MC, Goosen C, Wolters EC, Stoof JC. The dopamine D1 agonist SKF 81297 and the dopamine D2 agonist LY 171555 act synergistically to stimulate motor behavior of 1-methyl-4-phenyl-1,2,3,6-tetrahydropyridine-lesioned parkinsonian rhesus monkeys. Mov Disord 1994; 9:664–672.
14. Jackson DM, Hashizume M. Bromocriptine induces marked locomotor stimulation in dopamine-depleted mice when D-1 dopamine receptors are stimulated with SKF38393. Psychopharmacology (Berl) 1986; 90:147–149.

15. Goldstein M, Lieberman AN, Takasugi N, Shimizu Y, Kuga S. The antiparkinsonian activity of dopamine agonists and their interaction with central dopamine receptor subtypes. Adv Neurol 1990; 53:101–106.

16. Rascol O, Blin O, Thalamas C, Descombes S, Soubrouillard C, Azulay P, Fabre N, Viallet F, Lafnitzegger K, Wright S, Carter JH, Nutt JG. ABT-431, a D1 receptor agonist prodrug, has efficacy in Parkinson's disease. Ann Neurol 1999; 45:736–741.

17. Blanchet PJ, Gomez-Mancilla B, Di Paolo T, Bedard PJ. Is striatal dopaminergic receptor imbalance responsible for levodopa-induced dyskinesia? Fundam Clin Pharmacol 1995; 9:434–442.

18. Blanchet PJ, Gomez-Mancilla B, Bedard PJ. DOPA-induced "peak dose" dyskinesia: clues implicating D2 receptor-mediated mechanisms using dopaminergic agonists in MPTP monkeys. J Neural Transm Suppl 1995; 45:103–112.

19. Pearce RK, Jackson M, Smith L, Jenner P, Marsden CD. Chronic L-DOPA administration induces dyskinesias in the 1-methyl-4-phenyl 1,2,3,6-tetrahydropyridine-treated common marmoset (Callithrix Jacchus). Mov Disord 1995; 10:731–740.

20. Goetz CG, Koller WC, Powe W, Rascol O, Sampaio C. DA Agonists-ergot derivatives: pergolide. Mov Disord 2002; 17(suppl 4):S79–S82.

21. Begg C, Cho M, Eastwood S, Horton R, Moher D, Olkin I, Pitkin R, Rennie D, Schulz KF, Simel D, Stroup DF. Improving the quality of reporting of randomized controlled trials. The CONSORT statement. JAMA 1996; 276:637–639.

22. Barone P, Bravi D, Bermejo-Pareja F, Marconi R, Kulisevsky J, Malagu S, Weiser R, Rost N. Pergolide monotherapy in the treatment of early PD: a randomized, controlled study. Pergolide Monotherapy Study Group. Neurology 1999; 53:573–579.

23. Lledo A, Hundermer HP, van Laar T, Quail D, Rost N, Nohria V, Wolters EC, Schwarz J, Oertel W. Long-term efficacy of pergolide monotherapy in early-stage Parkinson's disease. One-year interim analysis of a 3-year double-blind randomised study of pergolide versus levodopa [abstr]. Mov Disord 2000; 15(suppl 3):126.

24. Mizuno Y, Kondo T, Narabayashi H. Pergolide in the treatment of Parkinson's disease. Neurology 1995; 45(suppl 3):S13–S21.

25. Hubble JP. Long-term studies of dopamine agonists. Neurology 2002; 58(suppl 1):S42–S50.

26. Sage JI, Duvoisin RC. Pergolide therapy in Parkinson's disease: a double-blind, placebo-controlled study. Clin Neuropharmacol 1985; 8:260–265.

27. Olanow CW, Alberts MJ. Double-blind controlled study of pergolide mesylate in the treatment of Parkinson's disease. Clin Neuropharmacol 1987; 10:178–185.

28. Ahlskog JE, Muenter MD. Treatment of Parkinson's disease with pergolide: a double-blind study. Mayo Clin Proc 1988; 63:969–978.

29. Diamond SG, Markham CH, Treciokas LJ. Double-blind trial of pergolide for Parkinson's disease. Neurology 1985; 35:291–295.

30. Jankovic J. Long-term study of pergolide in Parkinson's disease. Neurology 1985; 35:296–299.

31. Jeanty P, Van den Kerchove M, Lowenthal A, De Bruyne H. Pergolide therapy in Parkinson's disease. J Neurol 1984; 231:148–152.

32. Olanow CW, Fahn S, Muenter M, Klawans H, Hurtig H, Stern M, Shoulson I, Kurlan R, Grimes JD, Jankovic J, et al. A multicenter double-blind placebo-controlled trial of pergolide as an adjunct to Sinemet in Parkinson's disease. Mov Disord 1994; 9:40–47.

33. LeWitt PA, Ward CD, Larsen TA, Raphaelson MI, Newman RP, Foster N, Dambrosia JM, Calne DB. Comparison of pergolide and bromocriptine therapy in parkinsonism. Neurology 1983; 33:1009–1014.

34. Pezzoli G, Martignoni E, Pacchetti C, Angeleri VA, Lamberti P, Muratorio A, Bonuccelli U, De Mari M, Foschi N, Cossutta E, et al. Pergolide compared with bromocriptine in Parkinson's disease: a multicenter, crossover, controlled study. Mov Disord 1994; 9:431–436.

35. Boas J, Worm-Petersen J, Dupont E, Mikkelsen B, Wermuth L. The levodopa dose-sparing capacity of pergolide compared with that of bromocriptine in an open-label, cross-over study. Eur J Neurol 1996; 3:44–49.

36. Olanow CW, Obeso JA. Preventing levodopa-induced dyskinesias. Ann Neurol 2000; 47(4 suppl 1): S167–S178.

37. Parkinson Study Group. Pramipexole vs levodopa as initial treatment for Parkinson's disease. JAMA 2000; 284:1931–1938.

38. Rinne UK, Bracco F, Chouza C, et al. Early treatment of Parkinson's disease with cabergoline delays the onset of motor complications. Results of a double-blind levodopa controlled trial. The PkDS009 Study Group. Drugs 1998; 55 (suppl 1):23–30.

39. Rascol O, Brooks DJ, Korczyn AD, et al. A five-year study of the incidence of dyskinesia in patients with early Parkinson's disease who were treated with ropinirole or levodopa. N Engl J Med 2000; 342:1484–149.

40. Rinne UK. Brief communications: early combination of bromocriptine and levodopa in the treatment of Parkinson's disease: a 5-year follow-up. Neurology 1987; 37:826–828.

41. Hundemer HP, Lledo A, van Laar T, Quail D, Oertel W, Schwarz J, Wolters E. The safety of pergolide monotherapy in early-stage Parkinson's disease. One-year interim analysis of a 3-year double-blind, randomised study of pergolide versus levodopa [abstr]. Mov Disord 2000; 15(suppl 3):115.

42. Albin RL, Frey KA. Initial agonist treatment of Parkinson disease: a critique. Neurology 2003; 60:390–394.

43. Mear JY, Barroche G, de Smet Y, Weber M, Lhermitte F, Agid Y. Pergolide in the treatment of Parkinson's disease. Neurology 1984; 34:983–986.

44. Facca A, Sanchez-Ramos J. High-dose pergolide monotherapy in the treatment of severe levodopa-induced dyskinesias. Mov Disord 1996; 11:327–329.

45. Bonuccelli U, Colzi A, Del Dotto P. Pergolide in the treatment of patients with early and advanced Parkinson's disease. Clin Neuropharmacol 2002; 25:1–10.

46. Trenkwalder C, Winkenlmann J, Hundemer HP, Oehlwein C, Storch A, Polzer U, Schwarz J. High-dose treatment of Parkinson's disease with pergolide [abstr]. Mov Disord 2000; 15:132.

47. Shaunak S, Wilkins A, Pilling JB, Dick DJ. Pericardial, retroperitoneal, and pleural fibrosis induced by pergolide. J Neurol Neurosurg Psychiatry 1999; 66:79–81.

48. Lund BC, Neiman RF, Perry PJ. Treatment of Parkinson's disease with ropinirole after pergolide-induced retroperitoneal fibrosis. Pharmacotherapy 1999; 19:1437–1438.

49. Balachandran KP, Stewart D, Berg GA, Oldroyd KG. Chronic pericardial constriction linked to the antiparkinsonian dopamine agonist pergolide. Postgrad Med J 2002; 78:49–50.

50. Tan EK, Ondo W. Clinical characteristics of pramipexole-induced peripheral edema. Arch Neurol 2000; 57:729–732.

51. Leibowitz M, Lieberman A, Goldstein M, Neophytides A, Kupersmith M, Gopinathan G, Mehl S. Cardiac effects of pergolide. Clin Pharmacol Ther 1981; 30:718–723.

52. Tanner CM, Chhablani R, Goetz CG, Klawans HL. Pergolide mesylate: lack of cardiac toxicity in patients with cardiac disease. Neurology 1985; 35:918–921.

53. Kurlan R, Miller C, Knapp R, Murphy G, Shoulson I. Double-blind assessment of potential pergolide-induced cardiotoxicity. Neurology 1986; 36:993–995.

54. Pritchett AM, Morrison JF, Edwards WD, Schaff HV, Connolly HM, Espinosa RE. Valvular heart disease in patients taking pergolide. Mayo Clin Proc 2002; 77:1280–1286.

55. Frucht S, Rogers JD, Greene PE, Gordon MF, Fahn S. Falling asleep at the wheel: motor vehicle mishaps in persons taking pramipexole and ropinirole. Neurology 1999; 52:1908–1910.

56. Ferreira JJ, Galitzky M, Montastruc JL, Rascol O. Sleep attacks and Parkinson's disease treatment. Lancet 2000; 355:1333–1334.

57. Ondo WG, Dat Vuong K, Khan H, Atassi F, Kwak C, Jankovic J. Daytime sleepiness and other sleep disorders in Parkinson's disease. Neurology 2001; 57:1392–1396.

58. Schapira AH. Sleep attacks (sleep episodes) with pergolide. Lancet 2000; 355:1332–1333.

59. Homann CN, Wenzel K, Suppan K, Ivanic G, Kriechbaum N, Crevenna R, Ott E. Sleep attacks in patients taking dopamine agonists: review. BMJ 2002; 324:1483–1487.

60. Schlesinger I, Ravin PD. Dopamine agonists induce episodes of irresistible daytime sleepiness. Eur Neurol 2003; 49:30–33.

61. Navan P, Bain PG. Long term tolerability of high dose ergoline derived dopamine agonist therapy for the treatment of Parkinson's disease. J Neurol Neurosurg Psychiatry 2002; 73:602–603.

62. Sayler ME, Street JS, Bosomworth JC, Potvin JH, Kotsanos JG. Analysis of mortality in pergolide-treated patients with Parkinson's disease. Neuroepidemiology 1996; 15:26–32.

63. Olanow CW, Jenner P, Brooks D. Dopamine agonists and neuroprotection in Parkinson's disease. Ann Neurol 1998; 44(3 Suppl 1):S167–S174.

64. Le WD, Jankovic J. Are dopamine receptor agonists neuroprotective in Parkinson's disease?. Drugs Aging 18; 2001:389–396.

65. Marek K, Seibyl J, Shoulson I, et al. Dopamine transporter brain imaging to assess the effects of pramipexole vs levodopa on Parkinson's disease: a four-year randomised controlled trial. Neurology 2002; 58:A81–A82.

66. Whone A, Remy P, Davis M et al. The REAL-PET study: slower progression in early Parkinson's disease treated with ropinirole compared to L-dopa. Neurology 2002; 58:A82–A83.

67. Gille G, Rausch WD, Hung ST, Moldzio R, Janetzky B, Hundemer HP, Kolter T, Reichmann H. Pergolide protects dopaminergic neurons in primary culture under stress conditions. J Neural Transm 2002; 109:633–643.

68. Uberti D, Piccioni L, Colzi A, Bravi D, Canonico PL, Memo M. Pergolide protects SH-SY5Y cells against neurodegeneration induced by H(2)O(2). Eur J Pharmacol 2002; 434:17–20.

69. Felten DL, Felten SY, Fuller RW, Romano TD, Smalstig EB, Wong DT, Clemens JA. Chronic dietary pergolide preserves nigrostriatal neuronal integrity in aged-Fischer-344 rats. Neurobiol Aging 1992; 13:339–351.

70. Goetz CG, Tanner CM, Glantz RH, Klawans HL. Chronic agonist therapy for Parkinson's disease: a 5-year study of bromocriptine and pergolide. Neurology 1985; 35:749–751.

71. Hanna PA, Ratkos L, Ondo WG, Jankovic J. Switching from pergolide to pramipexole in patients with Parkinson's disease. J Neural Transm 2001; 108:63–70.

72. Goetz CG, Blasucci L, Stebbins GT. Switching dopamine agonists in advanced Parkinson's disease: is rapid titration preferable to slow? Neurology 1999; 52:1227–1229.

73. Canesi M, Antonini A, Mariani CB, Tesei S, Zecchinelli AL, Barichella M, Pezzoli G. An overnight switch to ropinirole therapy in patients with Parkinson's disease. Short communication. J Neural Transm 1999; 106:925–929.

74. Koller W, Lees A, Doder M, Hely M. Randomized trial of tolcapone versus pergolide as add-on to levodopa therapy in Parkinson's disease patients with motor fluctuations. Mov Disord 2001; 16:858–866.

10
Pramipexole

Fabrizio Stocchi
"Neuromed," Pozzilli (IS), Italy

I. INTRODUCTION

Parkinson's disease (PD) is a neurodegenerative disorder primarily affecting the dopaminergic neurons in the nigrostriatal pathway (1–3). Supplementation of the dopaminergic system with levodopa treatment was a major breakthrough in the treatment of PD (4,5). However, levodopa-induced motor complications and narrowing of the levodopa therapeutic window over time has limited treatment benefits for many patients with PD (6,7). The development of dopamine receptor agonists has provided an important pharmacotherapeutic strategy for the treatment of PD. Pramipexole (Mirapex®), one such agent, is the subject of this chapter.

Pramipexole is a nonergot dopamine receptor agonist with selectivity for the D_2 family of dopamine receptors (8–10). Comprehensive preclinical studies have shown that pramipexole improves motor symptoms in animal models of PD (11–16). A variety of double-blind, placebo-controlled clinical studies have established the effectiveness and safety of pramipexole in early and advanced PD (17–26). As an adjunct to levodopa, pramipexole treatment improves dyskinesias, lengthens on time, and reduces off time (23,25,26).

Preclinical studies suggest that pramipexole may have disease-modifying properties. Extensive studies have demonstrated the ability of pramipexole to provide neuroprotection in diverse in vitro (27–33) and in vivo (34–42) models of neurodegeneration in PD. The results of imaging studies using β-CIT and single photon emission computed tomography (SPECT) are consistent with pramipexole's preclinical neuroprotection data. Although the clinical relevance of pramipexole's neuroprotective properties in preclinical studies has not been established, these experiments suggest that pramipexole may provide neuroprotection through unique mechanisms both dependent and independent of its activation of dopamine receptors (29,43). Further investigations in clinical studies will elucidate the clinical utility of pramipexole for neuroprotection.

II. CHEMISTRY AND PHARMACODYNAMICS

Pramipexole dihydrochloride [(*S*)-2-amino-4,5,6,7-tetrahydro-6-propylamine-benzothiazole dihydrochloride monohydrate] is a synthetic aminobenzothiazole derivative. The addition of the *N*-propylamino group makes pramipexole a potent dopamine receptor agonist. The chemical structure of pramipexole—both *R*(+) and *S*(−) enantiomers—is shown in Figure 1 (44).

   In vitro experiments with cloned human dopamine receptors as well as in vivo experiments have demonstrated that pramipexole has approximately a 7- to 10-fold greater affinity for the D_3 receptor than for the D_2 receptor (8–10). Unlike ergot-type agonists, pramipexole shows very little binding to nondopamine receptors. Pramipexole shows weak binding to the α-adrenergic receptors, but the binding affinity is approximately 200 times lower than to the D_3 receptor. Pramipexole binding to serotonin receptors is negligible (8).

   Extensive preclinical studies have examined the mechanism of action of pramipexole in vitro and in vivo (11–16). These studies have led to the hypothesis that, at low doses, pramipexole acts on D_2/D_3 presynaptic autoreceptors to prevent the release of dopamine, whereas at high doses pramipexole activates postsynaptic D_2/D_3 receptors. Because

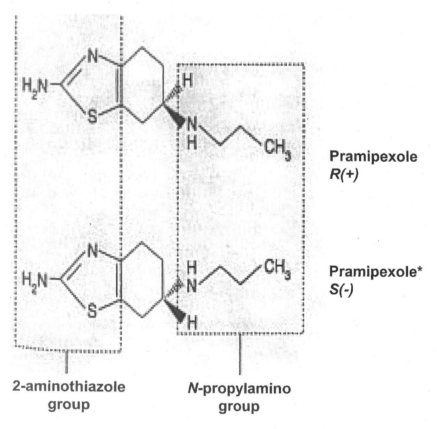

Figure 1 Chemical structure of pramipexole. *denotes commercial compound. (Courtesy of F. N. Johnson, Marius Press, Lancashire, UK.)

presynaptic dopamine receptors are severely depleted due to dopaminergic neuronal degeneration, the primary action of pramipexole in PD appears to be on D_2/D_3 postsynaptic neurons (11).

In experiments in which striatal dopamine was depleted with toxic agents or dopaminergic function was blocked by dopamine receptor antagonists, pramipexole reversed parkinsonian symptoms in both primate (12,15,16) and rodent models (12–14). Haloperidol-induced dyskinesia in monkeys was reversed by pramipexole, and the extent of relief was dose dependent (12). Pramipexole also relieved reserpine-induced rigidity and akinesia in rats (13).

Unilateral degeneration of the substantia nigra with the toxin 6-hydroxydopamine (6-OHDA) causes contralateral circling in rats after levodopa administration. Postsynaptic striatal neurons on the lesioned side are hyperstimulated by levodopa after prolonged dopamine depletion and, thus, become dominant over the normal striatal neurons on the untreated side of the animal. In this model, pramipexole caused rats to move in a circular motion away from the destroyed side (14). Pramipexole-induced circling can be inhibited by the D_2 antagonist haloperidol, presumably through inhibition of the hypersensitive postsynaptic receptors (12). Similar results have been observed in monkeys that have sustained permanent neuronal damage after unilateral 1-methyl-4-phenyl-1,2,3,6-tetrahydropyridine (MPTP) treatment. These animals responded to pramipexole with contralateral circling soon after the damage was sustained and remained sensitive to pramipexole 5–6 years later (12,15,16).

These preclinical results support the utility of pramipexole for the treatment of motor symptoms in PD.

III. PHARMACOKINETICS

Pramipexole is rapidly absorbed after oral administration, with a bioavailability of greater than 90%. It is eliminated primarily through excretion by the kidneys, with 90% of the unmetabolized drug recovered in urine (45). Since there is minimal hepatic metabolism, hepatic insufficiency is unlikely to have a significant effect on the elimination of pramipexole. There is minimal interaction with the cytochrome P450 enzyme system, indicating a reduced chance of drug-drug interaction with commonly prescribed drugs such as antibiotics, antifungals, antidepressants, and antiarrhythmics (45–47).

Pramipexole has linear pharmacokinetics over the clinically relevant range of doses and has an elimination half-life of 8 hours in healthy subjects and of 12 hours in subjects over 65 years of age (47). The longer half-life in subjects over 65 years of age is due to the approximately 30% lower total clearance in these patients, an age-related reduction in glomerular filtration rate resulting in reduced renal clearance (45,48). Clinical trials

Table 1 Pharmacokinetics of Selected Dopamine Agonists

Dopamine agonist	Oral bioavailability	Site of metabolism or excretion	Half-life (h)
Bromocriptine	8	Hepatic metabolism	3–8
Pergolide	20	Hepatic metabolism	15–27
Ropinirole	55	Hepatic metabolism	6
Pramipexole	>90	Renal excretion	8–12

indicate that the increased half-life in elderly patients does not affect the safety or efficacy of pramipexole in these patients. For comparison, the pharmacokinetics of pramipexole and other dopamine agonists are shown in Table 1 (45,49).

IV. CLINICAL EFFICACY

Pramipexole has been shown to be effective for treating early and advanced PD in many short-term and long-term double-blind trials (17–23,25,26,50). As monotherapy in early PD, pramipexole improved activities of daily living (ADL) and motor scores on the Unified Parkinson's Disease Rating Scale (UPDRS) scales II (ADL) and III, (motor) respectively (17–19). In a direct comparison with levodopa, pramipexole significantly delayed motor complications and dyskinesia (25,26). Long-term, open-label studies suggest that some patients may be maintained on pramipexole monotherapy for more than 3 years before supplemental levodopa is required to control motor symptoms (51). In advanced PD, pramipexole was found to be effective for reducing UPDRS ADL and motor scores when used as an adjunct with levodopa and was also found to be levodopa sparing (23). In a population that included patients with early and late PD, pramipexole was shown to improve tremor, a symptom that may not be well controlled by levodopa (24).

A. Efficacy of Pramipexole in Early Parkinson's Disease

1. Placebo-Controlled Trials

The clinical efficacy of pramipexole in early PD was evaluated in double-blind, randomized, placebo-controlled trials that included over 600 patients (Table 2) (17–19). Patients were classified as having early PD as determined by Hoehn and Yahr Stages I to III. Levodopa was not allowed in any of the trials, but stable doses of selegiline and anticholinergics were. The UPDRS was used to evaluate improvements in PD symptoms in all trials.

Shannon and colleagues (19) reported significant improvement in motor function as early as week 3, and by the end of the study UPDRS III motor scores improved by 25% from baseline in the pramipexole group compared with placebo, which worsened 6.9% from baseline ($p < 0.0001$) (Fig. 2). UPDRS II (ADL) scores improved by 22% in the pramipexole group compared with a worsening of 4.8% in the placebo group ($p < 0.0001$) (Fig. 2). The mean daily dose of pramipexole for those that entered the maintenance phase was 3.8 mg. The majority of patients in both treatment groups finished the study (83% and 80% for pramipexole and placebo, respectively). Nausea, constipation, insomnia, and visual hallucinations occurred significantly more often in patients treated with pramipexole compared with placebo.

2. Comparative Study of Pramipexole with Levodopa

The CALM-PD (Comparison of the Agonist Pramipexole Versus Levodopa on Motor Complications of Parkinson's Disease) study is a multicenter, parallel-group, double-blind, randomized trial comparing pramipexole with levodopa as initial therapy for patients with early PD (25,26). The primary endpoint of this study was the time to the onset of any of the three dopaminergic motor complications: wearing-off, on-off effects, or dyskinesias. Both 2-year data (25) and 4-year data (26) have been published, the latter as an abstract.

Table 2 Randomized, Placebo-Controlled Trials for the Treatment of Early and Late Parkinson's Disease

Study (Ref.)	n	Trial length, weeks	Titration phase weeks (target dose)	Levodopa allowed[a]	Disease severity	UPDRS II improvement vs. placebo (p-value)	UPDRS III improvement vs. placebo (p-value)	Total UPDRS (p-value)
Hubble et al., 1995 (17)	56	9	6 (4.5 mg)	−	Early	Improved (<0.005)	Improved ($0.05 < p < .01$)[b]	NA
Parkinson Study Group, 1997 (18)	264	10	6 (dose-ranging)	−	Early	NA	NA	Improved all doses (<0.005)
Shannon et al., 1997 (19)	335	31	7 (4.5 mg)	−	Early	Improved (<0.0001)	Improved (<0.0001)	NA
Molho et al., 1995(20)	24	10	7 (4.5 mg)	+	Late	Improved (<0.05)	Decrease less than placebo[c] (>0.05)	NA
Wermuth, 1998 (21)	69	12	7 (5.0 mg)	+	Late	Improved (<0.002)	Improved (<0.1)	Improved (<0.02)
Guttman, 1997 (50)	246	36	11–12 (4.5 mg, avg.)	+	Late	Improved (<0.0002)	Improved ($=0.0006$)	NA
Pinter et al., 1999 (22)	77	12	7 (5 mg)	+	Late	Improved (<0.01)	Improved (<0.001)	NA
Lieberman, 1997 (23)	360	31	7 (4.5)	+	Late	Improved (<0.0001)	Improved (<0.01)	NA

[a]Levodopa dosage reduction could occur during the study.
[b]Patient numbers in group not sufficient to attain statistical significance.
[c]Patients may have been at maximum motor performance with levodopa before initiation of study.
NA = not available; UPDRS = Unified Parkinson's Disease Rating Scale.

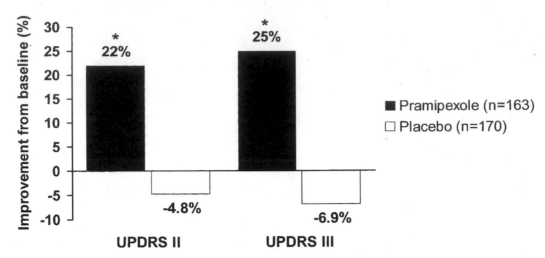

Figure 2 Improvement from baseline in UPDRS scores in early Parkinson's disease. $^*p < 0.0001$. (From Ref. 19.)

Patients with early PD were randomized to initial treatment with pramipexole plus placebo or levodopa plus placebo (25,26). The subjects were escalated to 4.5 mg of pramipexole or 150/600 mg of carbidopa/levodopa during the first 10 weeks. Subjects were permitted to adjust study medication dosages to 1.5, 3.0, or 4.5 mg in the pramipexole arm or to 75/300, 112.5/450, or 150/600 mg in the carbidopa/levodopa arm. Subjects in both groups were permitted to receive supplemental open-label levodopa if necessary during the maintenance period after week 10. After month 24, subjects were allowed to alter the dosage level of the original study medication.

The baseline characteristics for the CALM-PD study are shown in Table 3 (25). The severity of disease for the pramipexole and the levodopa groups was similar based

Table 3 Baseline Characteristics in the CALM-PD Trial

Variable	Levodopa	Pramipexole
Age (y)	61.5 (10.1)	60.9 (10.5)
Men (%)	64	66
Years since PD diagnosis	1.5 (1.4)	1.8 (1.7)
Prior levodopa (%)	26	20
Baseline selegiline (%)	33.1	37.3
Hoehn and Yahr stage:		
1–1.5	33.1	33.3
2–2.5	63.6	60.7
3	3.3	6.0
Total UPDRS	32.5 (12.7)	31.1 (12.8)
MMSE score	29.2 (1.4)	29.3 (1.1)

Data are expressed as mean (SD) unless otherwise specified.
PD = Parkinson's disease; UPDRS = Unified Parkinson's Disease Rating Scale; MMSE = Mini-Mental State Examination.

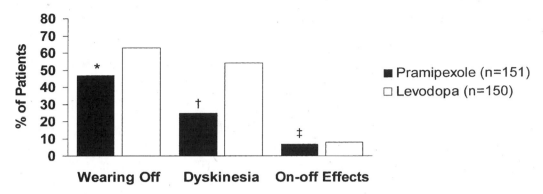

Figure 3 Motor complications over 4 years: pramipexole vs. levodopa. $^*p \le 0.0001$; $^†p = 0.01$. (From Ref. 26.)

on Hoehn and Yahr staging. Previous treatment with levodopa and selegiline at the beginning of the study was similar between groups. Treatment groups were balanced with respect to baseline UPDRS and Mini-Mental State Exam (MMSE) scores, with no statistically significant differences between groups.

Over a 4-year study period, initial monotherapy with pramipexole increased the time before the first occurrence of any one of the three dopaminergic complications (dyskinesias, wearing off, on-off effects) compared with levodopa (Fig. 3) (26). A total of 74% of the patients randomized to levodopa developed any of the three dopaminergic complications compared with 52% of those randomized to pramipexole [hazard ratio (HR): 0.48; 95% CI: 0.35–0.67; $p < 0.0001$]. The risk of wearing off among pramipexole-treated patients was approximately 25% less than the risk for patients treated with levodopa. Wearing off occurred in 47% of patients in the pramipexole group compared with 63% of those in the levodopa group (H: 0.67; 95% CI: 0.49–0.93; $p < 0.02$) (Fig. 3). The risk of dyskinesias for patients receiving pramipexole was reduced by more than 50% compared with patients receiving levodopa; 25% of the pramipexole group experienced dyskinesias compared with 54% of the levodopa group at the end of 4 years (HR: 0.37; 95% CI: 0.25–0.56; $p < 0.0001$) (Fig. 3). In contrast, improvement in total UPDRS scores was greater with levodopa than with pramipexole (3.6 vs. –0.98 units; $p < 0.01$) (26).

Pramipexole was generally well tolerated in patients during the first 2 years of the trial (4-year tolerability results not yet reported) (25). Somnolence, hallucinations, generalized edema, and peripheral edema occurred at a significantly higher rate in the pramipexole group overall, but only edema was significantly higher than levodopa during the maintenance phase.

B. Efficacy of Pramipexole in Advanced Disease

The symptoms of PD are more difficult to control in patients with advanced disease (52). These patients have increased parkinsonism due to dopaminergic degeneration, and many also suffer from motor complications induced by levodopa therapy. The development of motor fluctuations and dyskinesias appears to reflect a progressive narrowing of the therapeutic window for levodopa (6). The threshold level of levodopa exposure required to achieve a therapeutic response progressively increases. At the same time, the threshold

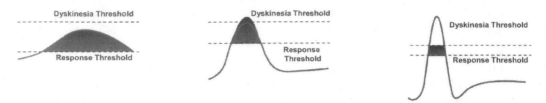

Figure 4 Response to levodopa and progression of Parkinson's disease.

level above which levodopa causes dyskinesia decreases (Fig. 4). In patients with advanced PD, it may therefore become impossible to achieve a levodopa dose with an antiparkinsonian effect without causing dyskinesias. In some patients, surgery or subcutaneous infusion of dopaminergic agents are the only ways of controlling serious dyskinesias in late-stage PD (52–58).

Randomized, double-blind, placebo-controlled trials evaluated pramipexole as adjunctive therapy in advanced PD (Table 2) (20–23,50). Patients who were enrolled in these studies had advanced PD (Hoehn and Yahr stages II to IV) and were experiencing levodopa-induced motor complications. All patients were receiving stable doses of carbidopa/levodopa. Other antiparkinsonian medications were allowed at stable doses in all studies except the trial conducted by Molho and colleagues, where selegiline and sustained-release levodopa were not allowed (20). The dose of pramipexole was escalated generally over 7 weeks to the maximum tolerated dose (4.5 mg). Reduction in the levodopa dose was allowed during some studies at the discretion of the investigator.

In a large trial ($n = 360$) conducted by Lieberman and colleagues (23), patients were followed for a 24-week maintenance period after a 7-week dose escalation period. Significant improvements in UPDRS II and III scores were observed among patients in the pramipexole group versus those in the placebo group (Fig. 5). The percent change from baseline in the UPDRS II ADL scores during off time for pramipexole versus placebo was 24% versus 5%, respectively ($p \leq 0.0001$), and for the UPDRS III motor scores, the change from baseline was 25% versus 12%, respectively ($p = 0.01$). The average daily off time was

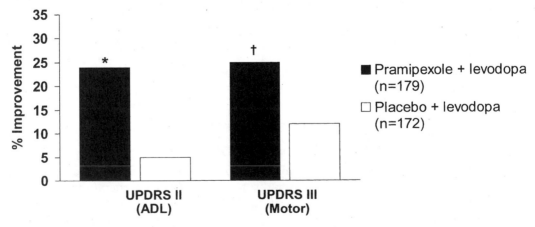

Figure 5 Improvement from baseline in UPDRS scores for pramipexole in combination with levodopa in advanced Parkinson's disease. *$p \leq 0.015$; †$p = 0.001$; ‡$p = 0.34$. (From Ref. 23.)

reduced by 31% in the pramipexole group ($p < 0.0006$), and the duration of on time was extended by approximately 2 hours. In addition, dyskinesias and off time improved with pramipexole compared with placebo as evaluated by the UPDRS IV scores (treatment-induced motor complications). Improvement in UPDRS IV scores was 24% versus 3% for the pramipexole group and the levodopa group, respectively ($p \leq 0.0001$) (23). The improvements in UPDRS scores with pramipexole occurred despite a reduction in the levodopa dose. The mean reduction from baseline of the levodopa dose was 27% in the pramipexole group compared with a 5% reduction in the placebo group at week 31 ($p < 0.0001$) (23). Similar results were found in an open-label trial designed to evaluate levodopa sparing in patients receiving pramipexole as an adjunct to levodopa; 72% of patients had a levodopa dose reduction of at least 20% (59).

C. Pramipexole Efficacy for Tremor in Early and Advanced Parkinson's Disease

A cardinal characteristic of PD is rest tremor, which is found in approximately 70–75% of patients (60). Tremor-predominant PD may become disabling if postural or kinetic components exist (61). In a double-blind, randomized, placebo-controlled trial, 84 patients with early or advanced PD and drug-resistant tremor were given either placebo ($n = 40$) or pramipexole ($n = 44$) as an adjunct to levodopa. The trial had a 7-week dose titration

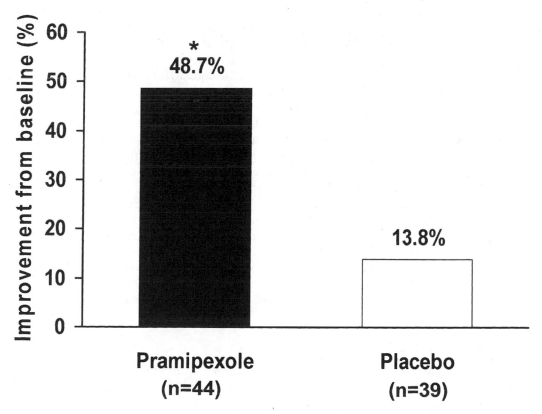

Figure 6 Improvement in tremor in early and advanced Parkinson's disease populations. *$p < 0.0001$. (From Ref. 24.)

phase, followed by a 4-week maintenance period (24). Stable doses of other anti-parkinsonian medications were allowed.

Pramipexole significantly improved tremor compared with placebo (24). The mean absolute difference in the change in tremor score (subscale of UPDRS III) was −4.4 points (95% CI −6.2 to −2.5; $p < 0.0001$), which corresponds to a 34.7% improvement for pramipexole over placebo (Fig. 6). Similar results were found in the trial of Lieberman and colleagues in advanced PD. In this trial there was a 65% improvement in tremor for the pramipexole group compared with 46% for patients receiving levodopa only (23).

V. SAFETY AND TOLERABILITY OF PRAMIPEXOLE

Generally, pramipexole was well tolerated in randomized, placebo-controlled trials of early and late PD (17–23,25,26,50). An approximately equal percentage of patients in the pramipexole groups (0–20%) and the placebo groups (0–40%) discontinued PD studies. In trials of late PD, the reasons for discontinuation were more likely due to adverse events (AEs) in the pramipexole groups and worsening of symptoms in the placebo groups (62). AEs that occurred more frequently with pramipexole than levodopa were somnolence, hallucinations, and gastrointestinal (GI) symptoms. However, in some trials the difference between pramipexole and placebo or levodopa for some AEs was not significant. For instance, in the trial by Lieberman and colleagues in patients with advanced disease, only hallucinations occurred at a greater frequency than placebo (23), and in the trial by the Parkinson Study Group in patients with early disease, hallucinations were significantly worse than with levodopa only in the dose-escalation phase (25).

When treating patients with dopaminergic agents, orthostatic hypotension, somnolence, and GI symptoms can occur (62). Orthostatic hypotension does not appear to be a significant AE for pramipexole, since it did not occur at a greater rate than placebo in clinical trials (62). In controlled trials with pramipexole, somnolence occurred at a greater rate than placebo, primarily in early PD. Furthermore, in the CALM-PD study, somnolence, hallucinations, and GI symptoms occurred more frequently during the escalation phase than during the maintenance phase (25). In general, dopamine agonists tend to cause GI disturbances and constipation. These AEs appear to be more of an issue in early PD, although the reason for this is unclear.

Sudden onset of sleep has been associated with dopaminergic agents in a small percentage of PD patients (63). A recent review has suggested that there are two types of sudden sleep episodes; those with a prodrome of sedation or drowsiness and those without previous warning (64). The latter occurs rarely in PD patients (63). Additional studies are necessary to assess the prevalence of sudden onset of sleep in PD patients taking no medication as well as in the general population. There are currently no guidelines on preventing or treating sudden onset of sleep in PD patients.

VI. PRAMIPEXOLE AND DEPRESSION

Depression occurs in approximately 40% of patients with PD, but in some studies estimates are as high as 70% (65). Depressive symptoms may be related to both the biological features and psychological effects of the disease. Although differences in neuropathology have been noted in depressed versus nondepressed PD patients, the interpretation of these results is not clear (66,67).

There is a theoretical neurophysiological basis for a relationship between the biological effects of PD and depression. It has been proposed that dopaminergic neurons may have an important role in depression, since serotonergic neurons in the limbic forebrain ultimately converge on dopaminergic neurons in the nucleus accumbens, which is involved in the control of mood and emotions (68). This suggests that dopaminergic signaling may be an integral part of serotonergic treatment, and thus may provide a target for the treatment of depression. Dopaminergic dysfunction in the nigrostriatal pathway may affect dopaminergic transmission in other areas of the brain that control mood (69,70). Furthermore, there is ample evidence that dopamine is involved in other psychiatric diseases, including schizophrenia (70).

Evidence that dopaminergic therapy may be valuable for treating depression comes from studies showing that the D_2 agonists piribedil and bromocriptine possess anti-depressive potential (71,72). Agents that raise dopamine levels, such as bupropion and dopaminomimetics (amineptine and minaprine), have rapid-onset antidepressive effects, raising interest in the potential therapeutic value of dopaminergic agents for treating depression (73). Regardless of the etiological relationship between depression and PD, depression in PD is a major factor associated with poor quality of life (74,75).

In a double-blind, randomized, placebo-controlled, parallel-group trial by Corrigan and colleagues, pramipexole was evaluated for the treatment of major depression in patients without PD (76). Patients received either pramipexole 0.375 mg ($n = 36$), 1.0 mg ($n = 35$), 5 mg ($n = 33$), fluoxetine 20 mg ($n = 35$), or placebo ($n = 35$) for 8 weeks. The Hamilton Psychiatric Rating Scale for Depression (HAM-D) was used to assess changes in depressive symptoms. The HAM-D is a 17-item scale that assesses depressed mood, vegetative and cognitive symptoms of depression, and coexisting anxiety symptoms. In this study, all treatment groups had similar HAM-D baseline scores. After 8 weeks, patients in the pramipexole groups overall were significantly improved compared with placebo ($p < 0.05$) (76). In a comparison by dosage group, those in the pramipexole 1.0 mg group showed significant improvement compared with placebo ($p < 0.01$); the pramipexole 5 mg group had the highest improvement compared with placebo, but the number of patients in this group was not large enough for statistical analysis due to patient discontinuations. These results suggest that pramipexole may be as effective as 20 mg of fluoxetine for the treatment of major depression.

The effects of pramipexole on depression in patients with advanced PD were evaluated in a prospective observational study ($n = 657$). Most patients were receiving levodopa at baseline ($n = 610$). Pramipexole was escalated to a maximum dose of 4.5 mg over 4 weeks. Clinical efficacy was evaluated at 63 ± 35 days (mean $\pm$ SD) after baseline assessments. Patients with moderate to severe PD (Hoehn and Yahr stage II or III) were evaluated for changes in depressive symptoms using the Snaith-Hamilton Pleasure Scale (SHAPS-D) (77). This questionnaire consists of 14 items designed to measure the ability to experience pleasure over four domains, including interests/pastimes, social interaction, sensory experience, and food/drink. Although all patients were tested for depressive symptoms using the SHAPS-D scale, only those patients who had persistent or severe depression at baseline ($n = 135$) were included in the SHAPS-D analysis. There was a significant mean ($\pm$SD) improvement of 3.54 ± 3.91 points on the SHAPS-D scale compared with baseline after approximately 9 weeks of therapy with pramipexole ($p < 0.001$). This prospective, observational study suggests that double-blind, placebo-controlled studies should be carried out to further evaluate the utility of pramipexole for treating depression in PD patients (78).

VII. PRECLINICAL EVIDENCE FOR PRAMIPEXOLE NEUROPROTECTION

A. Apoptosis and Parkinson's Disease

Loss of dopaminergic neurons in the substantia nigra pars compacta (SNpc) leads to the cardinal symptoms of motor dysfunction in PD (79). Dopaminergic neurons appear to be at increased risk for degeneration, since dopamine metabolism generates reactive oxygen species (ROS) and free radicals (80). Furthermore, one of the earliest defects in PD is the reduction of the glutathione-dependent detoxification system, which normally eliminates ROS and free radicals generated by the metabolism of dopamine.

There is increasing evidence that apoptosis (programmed cell death) is the primary mechanism whereby dopaminergic neurons degenerate in the SNpc (81–83). Apoptosis is characterized by condensation of chromatin and deoxyribonucleic acid (DNA) fragmentation followed by cell death. Oxidative stress, reduction of mitochondrial membrane potential, and excitotoxicity appear to be major contributory factors that cause apoptotic cell death in the SNpc (81,84,85).

The study of apoptosis in PD (both in vitro and in vivo) utilizes toxins that induce cellular dysfunction and death (Table 4). The induction phase of apoptosis occurs after an intra- or extracellular insult, which triggers nuclear activation of proapoptotic genes, such as p53 and Bax (81). Activation of caspases, which are proteases normally present in the cytoplasm as proenzymes, is a critical step in the induction phase of apoptosis (86). The interaction of the tumor necrosis factor-α (TNF-α) family of receptors (TNFR1, DR3, and Fas-Apo-1) with their respective ligands can lead to the direct activation of the caspase cascade (87). After ligand binding, these "death" receptors form a multimeric complex that can directly activate downstream caspases (88). In toxin-based in vitro models (e.g., MPTP-exposed cells), the release of cytochrome c (caused by the loss of mitochondrial membrane potential) and the opening of the mitochondrial permeability transition pore (PTP) appear to be the major inducing factors of apoptosis (89,90). Once

Table 4 Models for Pramipexole Neuroprotection

Experimental agent	Protect against	Models (Ref.)
Levodopa	Reversible/oxidative stress	Embryonic MES cells (27,28)
		MES 23.5 cells (109)
		Cerebral granular cells (30)
MPTP	Oxidative stress	SH-SY5Y cells (31,32)
		Marmosets (34)
		Mice (35,77)
		Rats (38)
Rotenone	Oxidative stress	SH-SY5Y cells (99)
6-OHDA	Oxidative stress	Rats (39,40)
3-Acetylpyridine	Excess glutamate, toxic NO formation	Rats (42)
Methamphetamine	Dopamine-related oxidative stress	Mice (41)
Ischemic damage	Oxidative stress	Gerbils (110)
TNF-α	Activation of caspase cascade	MES cells (27)

6-OHDA = 6-hydroxydopamine;   MPTP = 1-methyl-4-phenyl-1,2,3,6-tetrahydropyridine;   NO = nitric oxide; TNF-α = tumor necrosis factor-α; MES cells = mesencephalic cells; SH-SY5Y cells = human neuroblastoma cell line.

cytochrome c is released, it is available to bind to another proapoptotic protein, Apaf-1, which triggers the activation of the caspase cascade, leading to the final stage of apoptosis and cell death. Although the models that generate the current hypothesis of apoptotic cell death do not mimic the pathologic conditions in PD, there is evidence that mitochondrial damage and release of cytochrome c may be key components in the pathogenesis of PD (83,91).

Apoptosis is counteracted by a number of antiapoptotic proteins such as Bcl-2 and Bcl-xl. These are transmembrane proteins that inhibit the release of cytochrome c from mitochondria by inhibiting the proapoptotic protein Bax. This membrane protein allows ion flux across the mitochondrial membranes and, thus, a disruption of the mitochondrial membrane potential (92). Inhibitor-of-apoptosis proteins (IAPs) are a family of proteins that inhibit the activation of specific caspases. Trophic factors such as insulin-like growth factor-I (IGF-I) and basic fibroblast growth factor (bFGF) are antiapoptotic, since they appear to protect Bcl-2 and Bcl-xl from inactivation (93).

Excess glutamate causes excitotoxicity through activation of N-methyl-D-aspartate (NMDA) receptors leading to excess intracellular Ca^{2+} and nitric oxide production (94,95). Nitric oxide can cause mitochondrial oxidative stress and induce proapoptotic nuclear enzymes that degrade DNA when overexpressed (95). Recent evidence suggests that excitotoxicity can cause apoptosis through a caspase-independent pathway that involves induction of apoptosis-inducing factor (AIF). Release of this proapoptotic factor from mitochondria is also inhibited by Bcl-2 (96).

B. Pramipexole Neuroprotective Activity In Vitro

Extensive in vitro (27–33) and in vivo studies (34–42) have evaluated the neuroprotective properties of pramipexole. Although studies in cells and animals do not precisely match the conditions seen in PD, these models have been valuable for investigating the neuroprotective properties of dopamine agonists (Table 4).

1. Evidence for Protection by Pramipexole from In Vitro Levodopa Toxicity

Ling and colleagues reported that pramipexole is a potent dopamine agonist for protecting embryonic mesencephalic (MES) cells from cell death caused by levodopa toxicity (27,28). In this in vitro system, pramipexole induced the expression of an autotrophic protein and protected it from oxidation. Although other D_3 agonists (7-OH-DPAT and PD128, 907) appear to be capable of producing a protective factor, they do not protect against levodopa-induced neurotoxicity, nor are they able to prevent the oxidation of this factor (28). Additionally, these experiments raise interest in non–receptor-mediated neuroprotective properties of pramipexole, since other experiments with MES 23.5 cells have shown that the protection from 6-OHDA toxicity in this system is not dependent on dopamine receptor activity (29). The receptor-independent activities of pramipexole were confirmed in primary cultures of cerebellar granule cells. Both enantiomers of pramipexole, R(+) and S(−), protected against levodopa toxicity, suggesting a receptor-independent mechanism of protection (30).

2. In Vitro Protection of Pramipexole Against MPTP/MPP$^+$-Induced Toxicity

The metabolite of MPTP, N-methyl-4-phenyl-pyridinium (MPP$^+$), has been shown to be actively transported into dopamine neurons by the dopamine transporter (97). Long-term, low-dose MPTP/MPP$^+$ causes slow nigral-striatal degeneration, which is quite similar to the degeneration process in PD (98). Using the toxin MPTP, Kitamura and colleagues showed that preincubation of neuroblastoma SH-SY5Y cells with pramipexole, talipexole, or bromocriptine protected these cells from MPP^+-induced apoptosis (31,32). The levels of cellular ROS were lowered, as well as p53 (nuclear activator of apoptosis). Activation of proapoptotic caspase-3 and -9 was inhibited, and induction of the antiapoptotic protein Bcl-2 occurred.

Pramipexole treatment also maintained the mitochondrial membrane potential in MPP^+-treated neuroblastoma SH-SY5Y cells, preventing the opening of the PTP and the release of apoptotic factors (33). Interestingly, pramipexole also was shown to protect against mitochondrial damage and apoptosis caused by the widely used insecticide rotenone (99). Rotenone is thought to have a mechanism of neuronal damage similar to that of MPP^+.

3. Protection Against TNF-α-Induced Toxicity by Pramipexole

In a series of experiments conducted by Carvey and colleagues, it was found that TNF-α specifically induces the loss dopaminergic neurons, using tyrosine hydroxylase (TH) as a marker. Loss of TH-containing dopaminergic neurons occurred without affecting other neurons in the culture (27). When MES cells were incubated with pramipexole and TNF-α, approximately equal numbers of dopaminergic neurons survived as in those incubated with culture medium alone, indicating that pramipexole provides excellent protection from TNF-α toxicity in this system. Olanzapine, a dopamine receptor antagonist, was somewhat protective against dopamine toxicity in this system, but provided no protection against TNF-α. Pramipexole's protection against TNF-α toxicity is particularly encouraging, since there is evidence of increased TNF-α activity in the substantia nigra in PD patients (100).

C. In Vivo Evidence of Pramipexole's Neuroprotective Properties

1. Pramipexole Protects Against MPTP-Induced Neurotoxicity in Monkeys

Jenner and colleagues demonstrated that marmosets treated with MPTP suffered acute loss of greater than 50% of TH-positive neurons in the substantia nigra (34). When these monkeys were pretreated with pramipexole for 5 days before MPTP treatment, significantly fewer neurons were lost compared with those treated with MPTP alone (188 vs. 124 cells, respectively: $p < 0.05$). Animals treated with pramipexole during or after acute MPTP treatment did not differ significantly from animals receiving MPTP treatment alone, suggesting that neuroprotective mechanisms in this acute neuro-degeneration animal model require the presence of pramipexole prior to neuronal insult, possibly through induction of antiapoptotic factors. Evidence of protection from MPTP-induced neurotoxicity has been observed in mice (35–37) and rats (38).

2. Pramipexole Protects Against 6-OHDA – and Methamphetamine-Induced Neurotoxicity

Pramipexole also protects against the neurotoxic agents methamphetamine and 6-OHDA. These agents cause mitochondrial oxidative damage and produce hydroxyl radicals in dopaminergic neurons. In rats, pramipexole protects dopaminergic neurons from neurotoxic free radicals produced by 6-OHDA toxicity (39,40) and provides almost 100% protection of dopaminergic neurons in mice treated with methamphetamine (41).

3. Pramipexole Protects Against Excitotoxicity

3-Acetylpyridine (3-AP) causes the degeneration of the inferior olivary nucleus and fibers that innervate Purkinje cells, causing severe impairment of motor coordination in rats

(101). 3-AP–induced depletion of cyclic guanine nucleotide (cGMP) and adenosine triphosphate (ATP) in the cerebellum interferes with the chemical gradient required to prevent the excess release of glutamate. Excess glutamate causes excitotoxicity through overactivation of the NMDA receptor on dopaminergic neurons (102). Administration of pramipexole or bromocriptine (dosed before and after 3-AP administration) provided neuroprotection against neuronal damage caused by 3-AP (42). Both agents also significantly attenuated the reduction in cGMP and ATP, restored motor coordination, and prevented the loss of inferior olivary nucleus neurons caused by pretreatment with 3-AP. It is unclear what role pramipexole and bromocriptine play in this system, but recent evidence suggests that NMDA-induced neurotoxicity may act, at least partially, through a caspase-independent mechanism (96).

VIII. BRAIN IMAGING FOR EVALUATION OF DOPAMINERGIC FUNCTION IN PATIENTS TREATED WITH PRAMIPEXOLE

SPECT brain imaging is a sensitive technique for evaluating the dopaminergic system and is suitable for use in large clinical trials (103,104). Using radioligands such as $[^{123}I]\beta$-CIT, SPECT can accurately distinguish PD patients from normal controls. This technique utilizes changes in the uptake of $[^{123}I]\beta$-CIT by the dopamine transporter protein (DAT), which normally is responsible for transporting dopamine into neurons and can be used as a measure of dopaminergic function (105). As dopaminergic neuronal function is lost during the progression of PD, the intensity of radioactive labeling with $[^{123}I]\beta$-CIT decreases (104,106).

SPECT images of healthy controls compared with PD patients at Hoehn and Yahr Stage I demonstrate the symmetrical striatal activity of normal subjects compared with the asymmetrical reduction in striatal activity of PD patients (105). In one study, Marek

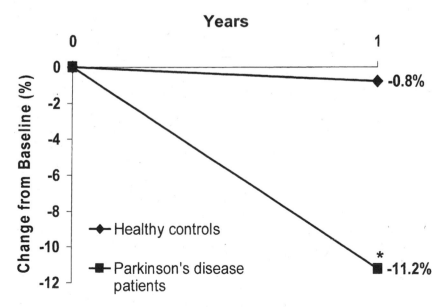

Figure 7 Annual reduction in β-CIT uptake in Parkinson's disease vs. age-matched controls. *$p < 0.0001$. (From Ref. 105.)

and colleagues estimated the mean annual reduction in striatal $[^{123}I]\beta$-CIT uptake at 11.2% for patients with PD compared with 0.8% for age-matched healthy controls (Fig. 7). In this study the rate of decline in $[^{123}I]\beta$-CIT uptake was not dependent on the severity of disease (105).

The CALM-PD β-CIT substudy evaluated the effect of initial treatment with pramipexole or levodopa on the percent change from baseline in striatal β-CIT uptake (107). The study was conducted with SPECT imaging, using the biomarker $[^{123}I]\beta$-CIT. The participants in the study were a subset of patients ($n = 82$) from the CALM-PD study (25). Patients were scanned at baseline and at 22, 34, and 46 months during the study. At baseline there was a similar reduction in striatal $[^{123}I]\beta$-CIT uptake in both treatment groups, consistent with a diagnosis of early PD. SPECT imaging at 10 weeks with a sample of patients from each treatment group showed no significant change in $[^{123}I]\beta$-CIT uptake.

At each time point during the study, there was a statistically significant difference between the two treatment groups. The pramipexole group had a significantly reduced loss of $[^{123}I]\beta$-CIT uptake in the striatum, putamen, and caudate compared with the levodopa group (Fig. 8) (107). Over 46 months, the mean percent decrease in striatal $[^{123}I]\beta$-CIT uptake from baseline was 16.0% in the pramipexole group compared with 25.5% in the levodopa group ($p = 0.01$). The levodopa group had an approximately 40% greater rate of decline than the pramipexole group. Similar preservation of dopaminergic function was also observed with the dopamine agonist ropinirole. In this study, positron emission tomography (PET) analysis, measuring ^{18}F-dopa uptake, was used to evaluate ropinirole versus levodopa (108). Although the clinical relevance of these imaging data is not fully understood, and it is not clear if the results may be influenced by a pharmacological effect of dopaminergic agonists on biomarker measurements, these results are promising and may support a role for pramipexole as a disease-modifying agent.

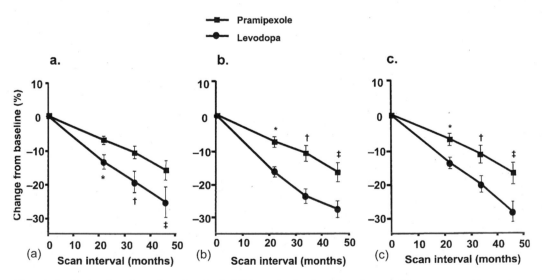

Figure 8 Reduction from baseline in β-CIT uptake in the (a) striatum, (b) putamen, (c) caudate over 4 years: pramipexole vs. levodopa. (a) $^*p = 0.004$; $^{\dagger}p = 0.009$; $^{\ddagger}p = 0.01$; (b) $^*p = 0.005$; $^{\dagger}p = 0.001$; $^{\ddagger}p = 0.03$; (c) $^*p = 0.02$; $^{\dagger}p = 0.04$; $^{\ddagger}p = 0.01$. (From Ref. 107.)

IX. CONCLUSIONS

Pramipexole is a safe and well-tolerated dopamine agonist for the treatment of PD. Clinical trials in early and advanced PD show that pramipexole is effective and may be used as monotherapy for an extended period of time, delaying the need for levodopa therapy and thus avoiding levodopa-induced motor complications. Motor function is improved with pramipexole during the on time, and the duration of off time is reduced. Tremor is also significantly improved with pramipexole therapy as shown in a study that included a patient population with early and advanced PD. Moreover, pramipexole has demonstrated potential for treating patients with depression.

Neuroimaging is rapidly becoming a reliable tool for diagnosing neurodegenerative diseases and monitoring the progression of disease. SPECT neuroimaging demonstrates that pramipexole significantly slows the reduction of β-CIT uptake in the striatum, putamen, and caudate compared with levodopa. Further studies on pramipexole will clarify the clinical significance of the SPECT imaging results and any potential clinical disease-modifying benefits it may possess.

It is presently unclear whether the in vitro and in vivo neuroprotective properties of pramipexole are reflected in the results from the neuroimaging studies. The preservation of dopaminergic function is the ultimate goal of parkinsonian therapy. Although models for demonstrating neuroprotection duplicate many of the conditions found in PD, more research about the exact nature of dopaminergic neurodegeneration in humans is needed before definitive conclusions can be drawn. However, there is accumulating evidence that, as a class, dopamine agonists may provide neuroprotection and that pramipexole has unique neuroprotective properties. Although the biochemical mechanism of pramipexole's neuroprotective effects are not fully elucidated, its ability to provide protection through activities that are dopamine receptor dependent and independent suggest that there may be multiple mechanisms whereby pramipexole may provide neuroprotection.

REFERENCES

1. Schapira AH. Science, medicine, and the future: Parkinson's disease. BMJ 1999; 318(7179):311–314.
2. Siderowf A. Parkinson's disease: clinical features, epidemiology and genetics. Neurol Clin 2001; 19(3):565–578, vi.
3. Lang AE, Lozano AM. Parkinson's disease (second of two parts). N Engl J Med 1998; 339(16):1130–1143.
4. Cotzias GC, Van Woert MH, Schiffer LM. Aromatic amino acids and modification of parkinsonism. N Engl J Med 1967; 276(7):374–379.
5. Tolosa E, Marti MJ, Valldeoriola F, Molinuevo JL. History of levodopa and dopamine agonists in Parkinson's disease treatment. Neurology 1998; 50(6 suppl 6):S2–S10.
6. Obeso JA, Olanow CW, Nutt JG. Levodopa motor complications in Parkinson's disease. TINS 2000; 23(10):S2–S7.
7. Hauser R, Zesiewicz T. Parkinson's Disease. 3rd ed. Coral Springs: FL: Merit Publishing International, Incorporated, 2002.
8. Piercey MF, Hoffmann WE, Smith MW, Hyslop DK. Inhibition of dopamine neuron firing by pramipexole, a dopamine D3 receptor-preferring agonist: comparison to other dopamine receptor agonists. Eur J Pharmacol 1996; 312(1):35–44.
9. Sautel F, Griffon N, Levesque D, Pilon C, Schwartz JC, Sokoloff P. A functional test identifies dopamine agonists selective for D3 versus D2 receptors. NeuroReport 1995; 6(2):329–332.
10. Coldwell MC, Boyfield I, Brown T, Hagan JJ, Middlemiss DN. Comparison of the functional potencies of ropinirole and other dopamine receptor agonists at human D2(long), D3 and D4.4 receptors expressed in Chinese hamster ovary cells. Br J Pharmacol 1999; 127(7):1696–1702.
11. Maj J, Rogoz Z, Skuza G, Kolodziejczyk K. The behavioural effects of pramipexole, a novel dopamine receptor agonist. Eur J Pharmacol 1997; 324(1):31–37.

12. Mierau J, Schingnitz G. Biochemical and pharmacological studies on pramipexole, a potent and selective dopamine D2 receptor agonist. Eur J Pharmacol 1992; 215(2–3):161–170.

13. Lorenc-Koci E, Wolfarth S. Efficacy of pramipexole, a new dopamine receptor agonist, to relieve the parkinsonian-like muscle rigidity in rats. Eur J Pharmacol 1999; 385(1):39–46.

14. Prikhojan A, Brannan T, Yahr MD. Comparative effects of repeated administration of dopamine agonists on circling behavior in rats. J Neural Transm 2000; 107(10):1159–1164.

15. Domino EF, Ni L, Zhang H, Kohno Y, Sasa M. Talipexole or pramipexole combinations with chloro-APB (SKF 82958) in MPTP-induced hemiparkinsonian monkeys. Eur J Pharmacol 1997; 325(2–3):137–144.

16. Domino EF, Ni L, Zhang H, Kohno Y, Sasa M. Effects of pramipexole on contraversive rotation and functional motor impairments in 1-methyl-4-phenyl1,2,3,6-tetrahydropyridine-induced chronic hemiparkinsonian monkeys. J Pharmacol Exp Ther 1998; 287(3):983–987.

17. Hubble JP, Koller WC, Cutler NR, Sramek JJ, Friedman J, Goetz C, Ranhosky A, Korts D, Elvin A. Pramipexole in patients with early Parkinson's disease. Clin Neuropharmacol 1995; 18(4):338–347.

18. The Parkinson Study Group. Safety and efficacy of pramipexole in early Parkinson disease. A randomized dose-ranging study. JAMA 1997; 278(2):125–130.

19. Shannon KM, Bennett JP Jr, Friedman JH. Efficacy of pramipexole, a novel dopamine agonist, as monotherapy in mild to moderate Parkinson's disease. The Pramipexole Study Group. Neurology 1997; 49(3):724–728.

20. Molho ES, Factor SA, Weiner WJ, Sanchez-Ramos JR, Singer C, Shulman L, Brown D, Sheldon C. The use of pramipexole, a novel dopamine (DA) agonist, in advanced Parkinson's disease 2. J Neural Transm Suppl 1995; 45:225–230.

21. Wermuth L. A double-blind, placebo-controlled, randomized, multi-center study of pramipexole in advanced Parkinson's disease. Eur J Neurol 1998; 5(3):235–242.

22. Pinter MM, Pogarell O, Oertel WH. Efficacy, safety, and tolerance of the non-ergoline dopamine agonist pramipexole in the treatment of advanced Parkinson's disease: a double blind, placebo controlled, randomised, multicentre study. J Neurol Neurosurg Psychiatry 1999; 66(4):436–441.

23. Lieberman A, Ranhosky A, Korts D. Clinical evaluation of pramipexole in advanced Parkinson's disease: results of a double-blind, placebo-controlled, parallel-group study. Neurology 1997; 49(1):162–168.

24. Pogarell O, Gasser T, van Hilten JJ, Spieker S, Pollentier S, Meier D, Oertel WH. Pramipexole in patients with Parkinson's disease and marked drug resistant tremor: a randomised, double blind, placebo controlled multicentre study. J Neurol Neurosurg Psychiatry 2002; 72(6):713–720.

25. The Parkinson Study Group. Pramipexole vs levodopa as initial treatment for Parkinson disease: a randomized controlled trial. JAMA 2000; 284(15):1931–1938.

26. Holloway RG. the Parkinson Study Group. Pramipexole versus levodopa as initial treatment for Parkinson disease: a four-year randomized controlled trial. Neurology 2000; 58:A81–A82.

27. Carvey PM, Pieri S, Ling ZD. Attenuation of levodopa-induced toxicity in mesencephalic cultures by pramipexole. J Neural Transm 1997; 104(2–3):209–228.

28. Ling ZD, Robie HC, Tong CW, Carvey PM. Both the antioxidant and D3 agonist actions of pramipexole mediate its neuroprotective actions in mesencephalic cultures. J Pharmacol Exp Ther 1999; 289(1):202–210.

29. Le WD, Jankovic J, Xie W, Appel SH. Antioxidant property of pramipexole independent of dopamine receptor activation in neuroprotection. J Neural Transm 2000; 107(10):1165–1173.

30. VonVoigtlander PF, Fici GJ, Althaus JS. Pharmacological approaches to counter the toxicity of dopa. Amino Acids 1998; 14(1–3):189–196.

31. Kakimura J, Kitamura Y, Takata K, Kohno Y, Nomura Y, Taniguchi T. Release and aggregation of cytochrome c and alpha-synuclein are inhibited by the antiparkinsonian drugs, talipexole and pramipexole. Eur J Pharmacol 2001; 417(1–2):59–67.

32. Kitamura Y, Kosaka T, Kakimura JI, Matsuoka Y, Kohno Y, Nomura Y, Taniguchi T. Protective effects of the antiparkinsonian drugs talipexole and pramipexole against 1-methyl-4-phenylpyridinium-induced apoptotic death in human neuroblastoma SH-SY5Y cells. Mol Pharmacol 1998; 54(6): 1046–1054.

33. King DF, Cooper JM, Schapira AHV. Pramipexole protects against MPP+ toxicity in SHSY5Y cells by maintaining mitochondrial membrane potential. Neurology 2001; 56(8):A377–A378.

34. Jenner P, Iravani MM, Haddon CO, Johnston LC, Jackson MJ, Smith L, Rose S, Schapira A. Pramipexole protects against MPTP-induced nigral dopaminergic cell loss in primates [abstr]. Neurology 2002; 58(7 suppl 3):A494.

35. Zou L, Xu J, Jankovic J, He Y, Appel SH, Le W. Pramipexole inhibits lipid peroxidation and reduces injury in the substantia nigra induced by the dopaminergic neurotoxin 1-methyl-4-phenyl-1,2,3,6-tetrahydropyridine in C57BL/6 mice. Neurosci Lett 2000; 281(2–3):167–170.

36. Kitamura Y, Kohno Y, Nakazawa M, Nomura Y. Inhibitory effects of talipexole and pramipexole on MPTP-induced dopamine reduction in the striatum of C57BL/6N mice. Jpn J Pharmacol 1997; 74(1):51–57.

37. Anderson DW, Neavin T, Smith JA, Schneider JS. Neuroprotective effects of pramipexole in young and aged MPTP-treated mice. Brain Res 2001; 905(1–2):44–53.

38. Cassarino DS, Fall CP, Smith TS, Bennett JP, Jr. Pramipexole reduces reactive oxygen species production in vivo and in vitro and inhibits the mitochondrial permeability transition produced by the parkinsonian neurotoxin methylpyridinium ion. J Neurochem 1998; 71(1):295–301.

39. Ferger B, Teismann P, Mierau J. The dopamine agonist pramipexole scavenges hydroxyl free radicals induced by striatal application of 6-hydroxydopamine in rats: an in vivo microdialysis study. Brain Res 2000; 883(2):216–223.

40. Vu TQ, Ling ZD, Ma SY, Robie HC, Tong CW, Chen EY, Lipton JW, Carvey PM. Pramipexole attenuates the dopaminergic cell loss induced by intraventricular 6-hydroxydopamine. J Neural Transm 2000; 107(2):159–176.

41. Hall ED, Andrus PK, Oostveen JA, Althaus JS, VonVoigtlander PF. Neuroprotective effects of the dopamine D2/D3 agonist pramipexole against postischemic or methamphetamine-induced degeneration of nigrostriatal neurons. Brain Res 1996; 742(1–2):80–88.

42. Sethy VH, Wu H, Oostveen JA, Hall ED. Neuroprotective effects of the dopamine agonists pramipexole and bromocriptine in 3-acetylpyridine-treated rats. Brain Res 1997; 754(1–2):181–186.

43. Abramova NA, Cassarino DS, Khan SM, Painter TW, Bennett JP Jr. Inhibition by R(+) or S(−) pramipexole of caspase activation and cell death induced by methylpyridinium ion or beta amyloid peptide in SH-SY5Y neuroblastoma. J Neurosci Res 2002; 67(4):494–500.

44. Schneider CS, Mierau J. Dopamine autoreceptor agonists: resolution and pharmacological activity of 2,6-diaminotetrahydrobenzothiazole and an aminothiazole analogue of apomorphine. J Med Chem 1987; 30(3):494–498.

45. Wright CE, Sisson TL, Ichhpurani AK, Peters GR. Steady-state pharmacokinetic properties of pramipexole in healthy volunteers. J Clin Pharmacol 1997; 37(6):520–525.

46. Wynalda MA, Wienkers LC. Assessment of potential interactions between dopamine receptor agonists and various human cytochrome P450 enzymes using a simple in vitro inhibition screen. Drug Metab Dispos 1997; 25(10):1211 1214.

47. Full U.S. Prescribing Information for MIRAPEX. www.mirapex.com. 2003. 3–5.

48. Lieberman A, Minagar A, Pinter MM. The efficacy of pramipexole in the treatment of Parkinson's disease. Rev Contemp Pharmacother 2001; 12:59–86.

49. Watts RL. The role of dopamine agonists in early Parkinson's disease. Neurology 1997; 49(1 suppl 1): S34–S48.

50. Guttman M. Double-blind comparison of pramipexole and bromocriptine treatment with placebo in advanced Parkinson's disease International Pramipexole-Bromocriptine Study Group. Neurology 1997; 49(4):1060–1065.

51. Bressman S, Shulman LM, Tanner CM, Rajput AH, Shannon KM, Wright E. Long-term safety and efficacy of pramipexole in early Parkinson's disease. Mov Disord 2000; 15(suppl 3):112–113.

52. Olanow CW, Watts RL, Koller WC. An algorithm (decision tree) for the management of Parkinson's disease (2001): treatment guidelines. Neurology 2001; 56(11 suppl 5):S1–S88.

53. Stocchi F, Ruggieri S, Vacca L, Olanow CW. Prospective randomized trial of lisuride infusion versus oral levodopa in patients with Parkinson's disease. Brain 2002; 125(pt 9):2058–2066.

54. Vaamonde J, Luquin MR, Obeso JA. Subcutaneous lisuride infusion in Parkinson's disease. Response to chronic administration in 34 patients 2. Brain 1991; 114(pt 1B):601–617.

55. Stocchi F, Bramante L, Monge A, Viselli F, Baronti F, Stefano E, Ruggieri S. Apomorphine and lisuride infusion A comparative chronic study 1. Adv Neurol 1993; 60:653–655.

56. Colzi A, Turner K, Lees AJ. Continuous subcutaneous waking day apomorphine in the long term treatment of levodopa induced interdose dyskinesias in Parkinson's disease. J Neurol Neurosurg Psychiatry 1998; 64(5):573–576.

57. Stibe CM, Lees AJ, Kempster PA, Stern GM. Subcutaneous apomorphine in parkinsonian on-off oscillations 1. Lancet 1988; 1(8582):403–406.

58. Pietz K, Hagell P, Odin P. Subcutaneous apomorphine in late stage Parkinson's disease: a long term follow up 1. J Neurol Neurosurg Psychiatry 1998; 65(5):709–716.

59. Pinter MM, Rutgers AW, Hebenstreit E. An open-label, multicentre clinical trial to determine the levodopa dose-sparing capacity of pramipexole in patients with idiopathic Parkinson's disease. J Neural Transm 2000; 107(11):1307–1323.

60. Paulson HL, Stern MB. Movement Disorders: Neurologic Principles and Practice. New York: McGraw-Hill, 1997:183–199.

61. Marjama-Lyons J, Koller W. Tremor-predominant Parkinson's disease. Approaches to treatment 1. Drugs Aging 2000; 16(4):273–278.

62. Biglan KM, Holloway RG. A review of pramipexole and its clinical utility in Parkinson's disease. Expert Opin Pharmacother 2002; 3(2):197–210.

63. Hobson DE, Lang AE, Martin WR, Razmy A, Rivest J, Fleming J. Excessive daytime sleepiness and sudden-onset sleep in Parkinson disease: a survey by the Canadian Movement Disorders Group. JAMA 2002; 287(4):455–463.

64. Homann CN, Wenzel K, Suppan K, Ivanic G, Kriechbaum N, Crevenna R, Ott E. Sleep attacks in patients taking dopamine agonists: review. BMJ 2002; 324(7352):1483–1487.

65. Cummings JL. Depression and Parkinson's disease: a review. Am J Psychiatry 1992; 149(4): 443–454.

66. Becker PM, Corrigan MH, Kasper S, Lin S-C, Montplaisir J, Szegedi A, Willner P. Clinical efficacy of pramipexole in the treatment of conditions other than Parkinson's disease. Rev Contemp Pharmacother 2001; 12:87–104.

67. Cummings JL, Masterman DL. Depression in patients with Parkinson's disease. Int J Geriatr Psychiatry 1999; 14(9):711–718.

68. Willner P. The mesolimbic dopamine system as a target for rapid antidepressant action. Int Clin Psychopharmacol 1997; 12(12 suppl 3):S7–S14.

69. Burn DJ. Beyond the iron mask: towards better recognition and treatment of depression associated with Parkinson's disease. Mov Disord 2002; 17(3):445–454.

70. Okun MS, Watts RL. Depression associated with Parkinson's disease: clinical features and treatment. Neurology 2002; 58(4 suppl 1):S63–S70.

71. Waehrens J, Gerlach J. Bromocriptine and imipramine in endogenous depression. A double-blind controlled trial in out-patients. J Affect Disord 1981; 3(2):193–202.

72. Post RM, Gerner RH, Carman JS, Gillin JC, Jimerson DC, Goodwin FK, Bunney WE, Jr. Effects of a dopamine agonist piribedil in depressed patients: relationship of pretreatment homovanillic acid to antidepressant response 1. Arch Gen Psychiatry 1978; 35(5):609–615.

73. Rampello L, Nicoletti G, Raffaele R. Dopaminergic hypothesis for retarded depression: a symptom profile for predicting therapeutical responses. Acta Psychiatr Scand 1991; 84(6):552–554.

74. Hobson P, Holden A, Meara J. Measuring the impact of Parkinson's disease with the Parkinson's Disease Quality of Life questionnaire. Age Ageing 1999; 28(4):341–346.

75. Factors impacting on quality of life in Parkinson's disease: results from an international survey. Mov Disord 2002; 17(1):60–67.

76. Corrigan MH, Denahan AQ, Wright CE, Ragual RJ, Evans DL. Comparison of pramipexole, fluoxetine, and placebo in patients with major depression. Depress Anxiety 2000; 11(2):58–65.

77. Snaith RP, Hamilton M, Morley S, Humayan A, Hargreaves D, Trigwell P. A scale for the assessment of hedonic tone the Snaith-Hamilton Pleasure Scale. Br J Psychiatry 1995; 167(1):99–103.

78. Reichmann H, Brecht HM, Kraus PH, Lemke MR. [Pramipexole in Parkinson disease. Results of a treatment observation]. Nervenarzt 2002; 73(8):745–750.

79. Lee CS, Schulzer M, Mak EK, Snow BJ, Tsui JK, Calne S, Hammerstad J, Calne DB. Clinical observations on the rate of progression of idiopathic parkinsonism. Brain 1994; 117(Pt 3):501–507.

80. Hirsch EC, Faucheux B, Damier P, Mouatt-Prigent A, Agid Y. Neuronal vulnerability in Parkinson's disease. J Neural Transm Suppl 1997; 50:79–88.

81. Blum D, Torch S, Lambeng N, Nissou M, Benabid AL, Sadoul R, Verna JM. Molecular pathways involved in the neurotoxicity of 6-OHDA, dopamine and MPTP: contribution to the apoptotic theory in Parkinson's disease. Prog Neurobiol 2001; 65(2):135–172.

82. Mochizuki H, Goto K, Mori H, Mizuno Y. Histochemical detection of apoptosis in Parkinson's disease. J Neurol Sci 1996; 137(2):120–123.

83. Schapira AH. Dopamine agonists and neuroprotection in Parkinson's disease. Eur J Neurol 2002; 9(suppl 3):7–14.

84. Merad-Boudia M, Nicole A, Santiard-Baron D, Saille C, Ceballos-Picot I. Mitochondrial impairment as an early event in the process of apoptosis induced by glutathione depletion in neuronal cells: relevance to Parkinson's disease. Biochem Pharmacol 1998; 56(5):645–655.

85. Jacotot E, Costantini P, Laboureau E, Zamzami N, Susin SA, Kroemer G. Mitochondrial membrane permeabilization during the apoptotic process. Ann NY Acad Sci 1999; 887:18–30.

86. Nunez G, Benedict MA, Hu Y, Inohara N. Caspases: the proteases of the apoptotic pathway. Oncogene 1998; 17(25):3237–3245.

87. Yuan J. Transducing signals of life and death. Curr Opin Cell Biol 1997; 9(2):247–251.

88. Hartmann A, Mouatt-Prigent A, Faucheux BA, Agid Y, Hirsch EC. FADD: A link between TNF family receptors and caspases in Parkinson's disease. Neurology 2002; 58(2):308–310.

89. Cassarino DS, Parks JK, Parker WD, Jr, Bennett JP Jr. The parkinsonian neurotoxin MPP+ opens the mitochondrial permeability transition pore and releases cytochrome c in isolated mitochondria via an oxidative mechanism. Biochim Biophys Acta 1999; 1453(1):49–62.

90. Du Y, Dodel RC, Bales KR, Jemmerson R, Hamilton-Byrd E, Paul SM. Involvement of a caspase-3-like cysteine protease in 1-methyl-4-phenylpyridinium-mediated apoptosis of cultured cerebellar granule neurons. J Neurochem 1997; 69(4):1382–1388.

91. Manfredi G, Beal MF. The role of mitochondria in the pathogenesis of neurodegenerative diseases. Brain Pathol 2000; 10(3):462–472.

92. Sadoul R. Bcl-2 family members in the development and degenerative pathologies of the nervous system. Cell Death Differ 1998; 5(10):805–815.

93. Zawada WM, Kirschman DL, Cohen JJ, Heidenreich KA, Freed CR. Growth factors rescue embryonic dopamine neurons from programmed cell death. Exp Neurol 1996; 140(1):60–67.

94. Ayata C, Ayata G, Hara H, Matthews RT, Beal MF, Ferrante RJ, Endres M, Kim A, Christie RH, Waeber C, Huang PL, Hyman BT, Moskowitz MA. Mechanisms of reduced striatal NMDA excitotoxicity in type I nitric oxide synthase knock-out mice. J Neurosci 1997; 17(18):6908–6917.

95. Mandir AS, Poitras MF, Berliner AR, Herring WJ, Guastella DB, Feldman A, Poirier GG, Wang ZQ, Dawson TM, Dawson VL. NMDA but not non-NMDA excitotoxicity is mediated by Poly (ADP-ribose) polymerase. J Neurosci 2000; 20(21):8005–8011.

96. Cregan SP, Fortin A, MacLaurin JG, Callaghan SM, Cecconi F, Yu SW, Dawson TM, Dawson VL, Park DS, Kroemer G, Slack RS. Apoptosis-inducing factor is involved in the regulation of caspase-independent neuronal cell death. J Cell Biol 2002; 158(3):507–517.

97. Javitch JA, D'Amato RJ, Strittmatter SM, Snyder SH. Parkinsonism-inducing neurotoxin, N-methyl-4-phenyl-1,2,3,6-tetrahydropyridine: uptake of the metabolite N-methyl-4-phenylpyridine by dopamine neurons explains selective toxicity. Proc Natl Acad Sci USA 1985; 82(7):2173–2177.

98. Betarbet R, Sherer TB, Greenamyre JT. Animal models of Parkinson's disease. Bioessays 2002; 24(4):308–318.

99. Schapira AHV, Gu M, King DF, Cooper JM, Jenner P. Pramipexole protects against rotenone toxicity: mechanisms and implications [abstr]. Neurology 2002; 58(7 suppl 3):A495.

100. Hunot S, Dugas N, Faucheux B, Hartmann A, Tardieu M, Debre P, Agid Y, Dugas B, Hirsch EC. FcepsilonRII/CD23 is expressed in Parkinson's disease and induces, in vitro, production of nitric oxide and tumor necrosis factor-alpha in glial cells 1. J Neurosci 1999; 19(9):3440–3447.

101. Balaban CD. Central neurotoxic effects of intraperitoneally administered 3-acetylpyridine, harmaline and niacinamide in Sprague-Dawley and Long-Evans rats: a critical review of central 3-acetylpyridine neurotoxicity. Brain Res 1985; 356(1):21–42.

102. Schulz JB, Henshaw DR, Jenkins BG, Ferrante RJ, Kowall NW, Rosen BR, Beal MF. 3-Acetylpyridine produces age-dependent excitotoxic lesions in rat striatum. J Cereb Blood Flow Metab 1994; 14(6): 1024–1029.

103. Dagher A. Functional imaging in Parkinson's disease. Semin Neurol 2001; 21(1):23–32.

104. Marek K, Jennings D, Seibyl J. Single-photon emission tomography and dopamine transporter imaging in Parkinson's disease 1. Adv Neurol 2003; 91:183–191.

105. Marek K, Innis R, van Dyck C, Fussell B, Early M, Eberly S, Oakes D, Seibyl J. [^{123}I] B-CIT SPECT imaging assessment of the rate of Parkinson's disease progression. Neurology 2001; 57:2089–2094.

106. Innis RB, Seibyl JP, Scanley BE, Laruelle M, Abi-Dargham A, Wallace E, Baldwin RM, Zea-Ponce Y, Zoghbi S, Wang S. Single photon emission computed tomographic imaging demonstrates loss of striatal dopamine transporters in Parkinson disease. Proc Natl Acad Sci USA 1993; 90(24): 11965–11969.

107. Parkinson Study Group. Dopamine transporter brain imaging to assess the effects of pramipexole vs levodopa on Parkinson disease progression. JAMA 2002; 287(13):1653–1661.

108. Whone AL, Remy P, Davis MR, Sabolek M, Nahmias C, Stoessl AJ, Watts RL, Brooks DJ. The REAL-PET study: slower progression in early Parkinson's disease treated with ropinirole compared with l-dopa [abstr]. Neurology 2002; 58(7 suppl 3):A82–A83

11
Ropinirole

Olivier Rascol

Clinical Investigation Centre and INSERM U455, Toulouse, France

Fabienne Ory

Toulouse University Hospital, Toulouse, France

Ropinirole is a second-generation orally active D_2 dopamine agonist that is active both peripherally and centrally (1). It was developed for the treatment of Parkinson's disease (PD) and is approved for this indication in many countries (2). Ropinirole is also being evaluated for the treatment of restless legs syndrome (3).

In theory, this compound has several attractive properties:

- Ropinirole's structure is unique from those of ergoline derivatives. This difference may result in fewer toxic effects, like pulmonary or retroperitoneal fibrosis, as compared with older dopamine agonists.

- Ropinirole is a selective drug for the D_2-like dopamine receptors, showing predominance for the D_3 subtype, with little or no affinity for binding at D_1, α_2, β, 5-HT1, 5HT2, benzodiazepine, and GABA receptors (1,4). This might result in fewer side effects.

- Ropinirole produces alterations in motor behavior indicative of antiparkinsonian activity in animal models of PD, including contralateral rotation in 6-hydroxy-dopamine (6-OHDA)–lesioned rats. It improves motor activity and induces less dyskinesia than levodopa in the 1-methyl-4 phenyl-1,2,3,6-tetrahydropyridine (MPTP) model of parkinsonism in the monkey (5–7). This might result in a lower risk of drug-induced abnormal movements in PD patients as compared with levodopa therapy. Moreover, it has been recently shown in the rat that, unlike levodopa ropinirole does not induce an internalization of D_1 receptors, a mechanism that could be related to some reduction in treatment efficacy and the genesis of motor complications (8).

- Ropinirole exhibits protective effects in various experimental models of neuronal cell death (9). This might result in putative neuroprotective properties with a positive impact on the progression of PD.

I. CLINICAL PHARMACODYNAMICS OF ROPINIROLE
    IN HEALTHY VOLUNTEERS

Clinical pharmacology studies have shown ropinirole to lower serum prolactin levels, an expected effect of a D_2 dopamine agonist. This effect of ropinirole is seen at single oral doses of 0.08–2.5 mg (10). Low single doses of ropinirole (0.08 mg) in healthy volunteers do not induce significant changes in supine resting heart rate or blood pressure. Higher doses (0.25 mg) frequently result in symptomatic postural hypotension with a blunting of the increase in noradrenaline which normally occurs upon standing (11,12). It is possible that tolerance to the hypotensive effects of the compound develops in humans based on the models of the rat and monkey (13). Domperidone can reduce such hypotensive effects (12). As expected with any dopamine agonist, gastrointestinal effects, particularly nausea, are seen at doses greater than 1 mg (10). Digestive dopaminergic symptoms are also likely to be prevented by the peripheral dopamine antagonist domperidone and may resolve with chronic treatment. A progressive up-titration is recommended, as with any other dopaminergic drug, in order to reduce these potential side effects when initiating treatment with ropinirole. Placebo-controlled studies conducted in healthy volunteers have demonstrated that ropinirole has sedative effects (14). This has also been reported with other dopaminergic agents, including other agonists and levodopa (15).

II. PHARMACOKINETICS

For a complete review of the pharmacokinetics of ropinirole see Ref. 16. Because of frequent nausea and postural effects above 0.8 mg, the pharmacokinetics of ropinirole have been evaluated over a limited single oral dose range in healthy volunteers. Pretreatment with domperidone 20 mg one hour before administration of ropinirole does not alter ropinirole pharmacokinetics (12). Consequently, the oral pharmacokinetics above 1 mg have been characterized under domperidone cover. Pharmacokinetics after single oral administration of ropinirole in parkinsonian patients are within the range of values reported in healthy individuals.

After oral administration, ropinirole is rapidly absorbed, with median time to maximum plasma concentration (T_{max}) observed approximately 1.4 hours after dosing. Bioavailability of ropinirole is approximately 46%. Both peak plasma concentration (C_{max}) and area under the curve (AUC) increase with corresponding dose increase, over the evaluable range of single doses. The overall mean apparent elimination half-life is 3.5 hours (17). The average terminal phase elimination half-life ($T_{1/2}$) of ropinirole in parkinsonian patients is 6 hours. This is longer than that of levodopa. It is recommended to administer ropinirole three times per day. As expected for a drug administered approximately every half-life, there is on average a two fold higher steady-state plasma concentration of ropinirole after repeat oral dosing. Ropinirole shows linear steady-state pharmacokinetics when administrated as an adjunct to levodopa (18).

Co-administration of food does not markedly affect the availability of steady-state ropinirole; C_{max} was decreased by 25% on average and T_{max} was delayed by 2.6 hours in 12 PD patients treated with 6 mg of ropinirole per day (19). Plasma protein binding of the drug is low (10–39%) and is independent of concentration over the therapeutic range. Drug interactions related to plasma protein binding are thus unlikely.

The metabolism of ropinirole is extensive and does not appear to be dependent on the route of administration. Based on in vitro enzymology data, the cytochrome P450 1A2

(CYP 1A2) enzyme is mainly responsible for the oxidative metabolism of ropinirole. None of the known metabolites are expected to be pharmacologically relevant over the proposed dose range. Elimination of ropinirole is believed to be mostly due to hepatic rather than renal clearance mechanisms. In the absence of specific data, ropinirole should be used with caution in subjects with severe renal or hepatic impairment.

The potential exists for drug interactions when ropinirole is coadministered with either a substrate or inhibitor of the CYP 1A2 enzyme. Ropinirole has little potential to inhibit cytochrome P450 at therapeutic doses, but it is possible that co-substrates (e.g., theophylline) or inhibitors (e.g., ciprofloxacin) of CYP 1A2 may influence the steady-state oral clearance of ropinirole. However, coadministration of oral theophylline at therapeutic doses under steady-state conditions did not induce significant changes in the rate or extent of availability of ropinirole (20). No dose adjustment is necessary for digoxin co-administration with ropinirole (21), but ropinirole may elevate the anticoagulant effects of warfarin (22). Ropinirole has no significant effect on the steady-state pharmacokinetics of the combination of levodopa 100 mg/carbidopa 10 mg twice daily and vice versa (23).

III. EFFICACY

The evidence to support the efficacy of interventions for the treatment of PD, including dopamine agonists such as ropinirole, has been extensively reported in an evidence-based review conducted as an initiative of the Movement Disorder Society (24,25).

A. Effect of Ropinirole on Disease Progression

A large 2-year levodopa-controlled trial, the REAL-PET study (26), was conducted prospectively in 186 de novo PD patients and used functional neuroimaging [positron emission tomography (PET)] as the primary endpoint. After 2 years of follow-up, the percentage decrease from baseline in putaminal ^{18}F-DOPA Ki was significantly less pronounced in the ropinirole arm (−14%) than in the levodopa arm (−23%) ($p < 0.01$). Such a result can be considered as an indirect indication of ropinirole's putative neuro-protective properties. However, this type of trial design does not allow a definite conclusion as to the impact of the drug on disease progression for two main reasons. First, there is no placebo arm in the trial, and therefore the difference between ropinirole-treated and levodopa-treated patients could also be due to an unknown levodopa effect. Second, neuroimaging outcomes are only surrogate markers, and such markers require further validation before any assumption can be drawn regarding clinical relevancy.

B. Symptomatic Efficacy of Ropinirole as Monotherapy in Patients with Early PD

There are several randomized double-blind studies to assess ropinirole efficacy as monotherapy: two placebo-controlled parallel trials (27,28), two levodopa-controlled studies, one with a 6-month planned interim analysis (29) and a 5-year final report (30) and another with a 2-year follow-up (26), and one bromocriptine-controlled study with a 6-month planned interim analysis (31) and a 3-year final report (32).

Adler and colleagues (27) conducted a randomized double-blind placebo-controlled parallel-group 6-month study including 241 patients with early PD. Ropinirole (16 mg/d) was significantly superior to placebo on Unified Parkinson's Disease Rating Scale (UPDRS) motor scores (−24% on ropinirole vs. +3% on placebo at endpoint; $p < 0.001$). The subjects who completed this study were included in a 6-month double-blind extension study (33) that showed that the superiority of ropinirole was maintained over placebo during this period. Forty-four percent of the patients completed the 1-year study without the need of levodopa.

Brooks and colleagues (28) also conducted a randomized parallel placebo-controlled 3-month study including 63 de novo PD patients. At endpoint, UPDRS motor scores improved by 43% in the ropinirole group and by 21% in the placebo group ($p = 0.018$).

Rascol and colleagues (29) published a 6-month planned interim analysis of a 5-year randomized levodopa-controlled study conducted in 268 patients with early PD. At 6 months the mean daily dose of ropinirole was 10 mg/d, while that of levodopa was 460 mg/d. Levodopa was slightly (but significantly) more efficacious than ropinirole after 6 months. UPDRS motor scores improved by -32% on ropinirole and by -44% on levodopa ($p < 0.05$). At final evaluation (5-year follow-up), the mean dose of ropinirole was 16.5 mg/d (plus 427 mg/d of complementary levodopa in 66% of the patients) and 753 mg/d of levodopa (including open-label supplement in 36% of the patients). There was no significant difference between the two groups in the mean changes from baseline in UPDRS activities of daily living (ADL) scores among the patients who completed the study [1.6 (worsening) with ropinirole vs. 0.0 with levodopa, NS]. However, there was a slight but significant difference in favor of levodopa for the UPDRS motor scores (0.8 with ropinirole vs. 4.8 with levodopa, 4.48; 95% CI 1.25–7.72; $p < 0.01$). The clinical relevance of this difference is not known. After 5 years, a third of the patients randomized to ropinirole were receiving ropinirole monotherapy without the need for levodopa supplementation.

Whone and colleagues (26) also measured UPDRS motor scores in the REAL-PET study, comparing early ropinirole treatment to early levodopa monotherapy in 186 patients with early PD. After 2 years of follow-up, only 14% of the ropinirole-treated patients required open-label levodopa supplementation, as compared to 8% of the patients randomized to the levodopa arm. However, there was a six-point difference in UPDRS motor scores (maximum = 104) in favor of levodopa (95%, CI 3.54–9.14; $p < 0.001$). The clinical relevance of this difference remains to be defined, especially because a more global assessment of efficacy (percentage of responders on a clinical global impression score) did not show any significant difference between the two treatment arms in this study.

Korczyn and colleagues (31) also published a planned interim analysis after 6 months of a 3-year study that enrolled 335 patients with early PD in a double-blind bromocriptine-controlled parallel-group design. At 6 months at a mean dose of 8.3 mg/d, ropinirole was slightly, but significantly, more efficacious on parkinsonian disability than bromocriptine (16.8 mg/d) (UPDRS percentage reduction: ropinirole = -35% vs. bromocriptine = -27%; $p < 0.05$). At the final 3-year analysis (32), comparable differences were observed in the patients who completed the trial (ropinirole 12 mg/d, bromocriptine 24 mg/d), in UPDRS ADL (ropinirole = 5.83 vs. bromocriptine = 7.28; $p < 0.01$), and UPDRS motor percentage changes (ropinirole = -31% vs. bromocriptine = -22%; NS). Although statistically significant, the difference between groups was small (treatment difference 1.46 points for ADL). After 3 years of treatment, about one third of the patients still treated in the trial received either agonist as monotherapy, without the need of levodopa supplementation.

A retrospective analysis of three of these large randomized trials (27,32,30) suggests that ropinirole monotherapy is effective in treating resting tremor in early PD (34).

In summary, studying ropinirole's efficacy as monotherapy in early PD demonstrates that the compound is significantly superior to placebo. Compared to levodopa, ropinirole (supplemented with low doses of levodopa when needed) was less effective, while it was slightly superior to bromocriptine as measured with the UPDRS. In the absence of a definition of a minimal clinically relevant difference in the UPDRS score, it is not known if such differences have a practical impact in the everyday management of patients with PD. On long-term follow-up (3–5 years), levodopa supplementation was necessary to keep control of parkinsonian symptoms in a majority of patients, but ropinirole mono-therapy could be maintained without levodopa supplementation in 20–30% of the patients.

C. Efficacy of Ropinirole as an Adjunct Treatment to Levodopa

Several open pilot studies have suggested that ropinirole is useful in treating PD patients who are already treated with levodopa (35,36). Three randomized double-blind placebo-controlled studies have been published.

Rascol and colleagues (37) conducted a 3-month randomized placebo-controlled parallel study in 46 levodopa-treated PD patients with motor fluctuations. Ropinirole was administered twice a day. Drug efficacy was assessed using percentage of awake time spent off and patient diaries. At a dose of 3.3 mg/d, ropinirole decreased time spent off by 44% (from 47% at baseline to 27% at endpoint), while placebo had a smaller effect of 24% (from 44% at baseline to 34% at endpoint). This difference did not reach statistical significance in the intention-to-treat analysis ($p = 0.085$) but only in the efficacy-evaluable population ($p = 0.039$), probably because of an insufficient power of the trial due to the small number of patients.

Lieberman and colleagues (38) performed a randomized, parallel, double-blind, placebo-controlled 6-month study in 149 levodopa-treated PD patients with motor fluctuations. The primary endpoint of this trial was complex: the number of patients who achieved a 20% or greater decrease in levodopa dose *and* a 20% or greater reduction in the percentage of time spent off between baseline and final visit using patient diaries. Overall, 35% of ropinirole-treated patients and 13% of the placebo-treated ones met the primary endpoint definition ($p < 0.002$). Patients randomized to ropinirole achieved a greater reduction in total levodopa daily dose (242 mg (−31%); vs. 51 mg (−6%) with placebo; $p < 0.001$).

Brunt and colleagues (39) conducted a 6-month randomized double-blind, bromocriptine-controlled trial in a heterogeneous population of 555 levodopa-treated PD patients. Patient response was assessed using a complex combination of several outcomes measuring levodopa daily dose reduction, UPDRS motor score reduction, reduction in time spent off, and/or clinical global impression. Overall, no clinically relevant differences were observed between the two treatment arms.

To summarize, ropinirole, as an adjunct to levodopa in patients with advanced PD and motor fluctuations, allows a reduction of off time of 2 hours on average when levodopa dose remains constant. The adjunction of ropinirole to levodopa also allows reducing the levodopa daily dose on average by 20%, and when the two above criteria are combined, ropinirole remains superior to placebo in generating significant improvement in patients with motor fluctuations. There is no evidence that ropinirole is more or less effective than another dopamine agonist, like bromocriptine, as an adjunct treatment to levodopa.

Open-label uncontrolled trials suggest that patients already treated with other dopamine agonists like pergolide or pramipexole can be switched overnight to ropinirole safely (40,41). Nevertheless, empirical clinical experience shows that switching from one agonist to another is not so easy in a number of patients. Dose-equivalence ratios have been empirically proposed (1 mg pergolide = 6 mg ropinirole; 2 mg bromocriptine = 1 mg ropinirole). It has also been reported in an open-label design that high-dose therapy with ropinirole (up to 36 mg/d) in PD patients with motor complications improves motor function and reduces the duration of dyskinesia, but randomized controlled trials are necessary to confirm such pilot findings (42).

IV. PREVENTION OF MOTOR COMPLICATIONS

Rascol and colleagues (30) followed 268 de novo PD patients for 5 years in a randomized, double-blind, parallel, levodopa-controlled design. The primary outcome was the occurrence of dyskinesia (item 32 of the UPDRS IV). The analysis of time to dyskinesia showed a significant difference in favor of ropinirole (hazard ratio for remaining free of dyskinesia 2.82; 95% CI 1.78–4.44; $p < 0.001$). At 5 years the cumulative incidence of dyskinesia was 20% with ropinirole and 45% with levodopa. Disabling dyskinesias were also less frequent in the ropinirole group versus levodopa (hazard ratio for remaining free of dyskinesia 3.02; 95% CI 1.52–6.02; $p = 0.002$). At 5 years before levodopa supplementation, dyskinesias were extremely uncommon in the ropinirole group (5%) versus 36% in levodopa-treated patients. Wearing-off was less frequent on ropinirole than levodopa, but the difference was less striking than for dyskinesia. No effect was observed on freezing when walking. A post hoc analysis was also conducted in this trial to determine whether the dyskinesia-sparing benefit achieved with ropinirole therapy was lost when levodopa was added. This analysis showed that the risk of developing dyskinesia on ropinirole early monotherapy was extremely low. Once levodopa was added to ropinirole, there was no clear evidence of a "catch-up" or persisting preventing effect of ropinirole, and the risk of developing dyskinesia rose in parallel to the level observed for levodopa therapy, but delayed by a median of 3 years (43).

In a 3-year, double-blind, bromocriptine-controlled, parallel-group trial, Korczyn and colleagues (32) also looked for time to dyskinesia as a secondary endpoint. Dyskinesia developed in a minority of patients of both arms after 3 years of follow-up, regardless of levodopa supplementation: 7.7% of patients in the ropinirole group and 7.2% in the bromocriptine-treated group. There was no significant difference between the two groups ($p = 0.84$).

Whone and colleagues (26) also measured the occurrence of dyskinesia as a secondary endpoint in the large 2-year levodopa-controlled neuroimaging REAL-PET study conducted in 186 de novo levodopa-naïve patients with PD. After 2 years of follow-up, only 3% of the patients in the ropinirole arm developed dyskinesia, while 27% did in the levodopa arm ($p < 0.0001$).

In summary, treating a patient with early PD with initial ropinirole monotherapy, supplemented with levodopa as a second-line treatment to control parkinsonism, reduces the risk of dyskinesia after 5 years of follow-up. This is achieved at the cost of a significant—although slight—amount of control of parkinsonism, as measured by the UPDRS, and the clinical relevance of this difference remains a matter of controversy.

V. CLINICAL SAFETY

Overall, the safety profile of ropinirole appears similar to that of other dopamine agonists (44). Ropinirole can induce all classical dopaminergic adverse events including nausea, vomiting, hypotension, and psychosis. Such adverse events appeared to have the same incidence and severity in de novo PD patients treated with ropinirole and bromocriptine (32). In spite of a greater selectivity for dopamine receptors and a lack of effect on serotonergic receptors, ropinirole did not induce less psychosis than bromocriptine (32). In a large 5-year levodopa-controlled trial (30), gastrointestinal, cardiovascular, and neuropsychiatric adverse drug reactions were reported to occur with the same frequency in both treatment groups. However, analyzing individual psychiatric adverse reactions shows that hallucinations, for example, were more frequent with ropinirole than levodopa. Leg edema was also commonly reported in patients on ropinirole.

In levodopa-treated dyskinetic PD patients, ropinirole, like other dopamine agonists, increases such abnormal movements, and one can try to manage this problem by partially decreasing the levodopa daily dose. Conversely, when ropinirole is used as a first-line treatment to which levodopa is added later as a complementary treatment, the risk of occurrence of dyskinesia for up to 5 years is three times lower than when levodopa is initiated as monotherapy (26,30,31).

Concerns have been raised regarding episodes of sudden irresistible sleep attacks, and several case reports have been published in patients on ropinirole or pramipexole (45,46). However, similar episodes have also been reported with most other agonists such as pergolide and bromocriptine (47–49), and even with levodopa monotherapy (50) and entacapone (51). Somnolence as an adverse drug reaction was more frequently reported with ropinirole than with placebo in randomized clinical trials (27). The fact that these sleep episodes are truly new adverse drug reactions related to the new nonergot structure of ropinirole or its preferential impact on D_3 receptors remains debated (52). Epidemiological studies have confirmed that inappropriate daytime somnolence is a common problem in patients with PD, that both disease and drugs should be seen as contributing risk factors, and that there is no greater risk for any given agonist (53).

Long-term postmarketing surveillance is still lacking to assess if the use of a nonergot compound, like ropinirole, causes less pulmonary fibrosis than ergot derivatives, although a few case reports suggest that this might be the case (54). Other infrequent side effects, like penile erection, have been reported with ropinirole, as with other dopamine agonists and levodopa (55).

VI. CONCLUSION

Ropinirole is a new nonergoline selective D_2 dopamine agonist. It has antiparkinsonian efficacy both in the early management of the disease, as monotherapy, and later as an adjunct therapy to levodopa. This is documented in several randomized, controlled trials conducted in several hundreds of patients followed up to 5 years. Dopaminergic adverse events (nausea, orthostatic hypotension, psychosis) are in the range of what is expected with a dopamine agonist. As an early treatment, ropinirole can delay the need for levodopa, and this strategy reduces the incidence of long-term motor side effects such as dyskinesia. Currently, only the symptomatic antiparkinsonian effects of ropinirole have been definitively demonstrated. There is a growing interest in the potential neuroprotective properties of dopamine agonists such as ropinirole. However, it is still too early to conclude as to the impact of such medications on disease progression, even if pilot neuroimaging data are compatible with this hypothesis.

It is recommended to initiate ropinirole at a low dose (0.25 mg three times daily) and to titrate over a 4-week period to a dose of 1 mg three times daily. If parkinsonian symptoms are not sufficiently controlled, the dose of ropinirole should be increased progressively until an adequate therapeutic response is established. The minimal efficacious daily dose is usually 6 mg/d. After 6 months of ropinirole monotherapy, the mean daily dose used in clinical trials ranged from 8 to 16 mg/d. After 5 years, the mean dose of ropinirole was 16.5 mg/d. Doses above 24 mg/d have not been investigated in clinical trials, and 24 mg/d is the maximum recommended dose.

REFERENCES

1. Eden RJ, Costall B, Domeney AM, Genard PA, Harvey CA, Kelly ME, Naylor RJ, Owen DAA, Wright A. Preclinical pharmacology of ropinirole (SK&F 101468-A) a novel dopamine D_2 agonist. Pharmacol Bioche Behav 1991; 38:147–154.
2. Matheson AJ, Spencer CM. Ropinirole: a review of its use in the management of Parkinson's disease. Drugs 2000; 60:115–137.
3. Weimerskirch PR, Ernst ME. Newer dopamine agonists in the treatment of restless legs syndrome. Ann Pharmacother 2001; 35:627–630.
4. Tulloch IF. Pharmacological profile of ropinirole, a non ergoline dopamine agonist. Neurology 1997; 49(suppl 1):S58–S62.
5. Pearce RK, Banerji T, Jenner P, Marsden CD. De novo administration of ropinirole and bromocriptine induces less dyskinesia than L-DOPA in the MPTP-treated marmoset. Mov Disord 1998; 13:234–241.
6. Fukuzaki K, Kamenosono T, Kitazumi K, Nagata R. Effects of ropinirole on motor behaviour in MPTP-treated common marmosets. Pharmacol Biochem Behav 2000; 67:121–129.
7. Maratos EC, Jackson MJ, Pearce RKB, Jenner P. Antiparkinsonian activity and dyskinesia risk of ropinirole and L-DOPA combination therapy in drug naïve MPTP-lesioned common marmosets. Mov Disord 2001; 16:631–641.
8. Muriel MP, Orieux G, Hirsch EC. Levodopa but not ropinirople induces an internalisation of D1 dopamine receptors in parkinsonian rats. Mov Disord 2002; 17:1174–1179.
9. Iida M, Miyazaki I, Tanaka K, Kabuto H, Iwata-Ichikawa E, Ogawa N. Dopamine D2 receptor mediated antioxidant and neuroprotective effects of ropinirole, a dopamine agonist. Brain Res 1999; 838:51–59.
10. Acton G, Broom C. A dose rising study of the safety and effects on serum prolactin of SK&FF 101468, a novel dopamine D_2-receptor agonist. Br J Clin Pharmacol 1989; 28:435–441.
11. Acton G, Broom C, Howland K, Manchee K. Effects of the dopaminergic D_2 receptor agonist ropinirole on posturally-induced changes in plasma catecholamines and haemodynamics. Br J Clin Pharmacol 1990; 29:619.
12. De Mey C, Enterling D, Meineke I, Yeulet S. Interactions between domperidone and ropinirole, a novel dopamine D_2-receptor agonist. Br J Clin Pharmacol 1991; 32:483–488.
13. Parker SG, Raval P, Yeulet, Eden RJ. Tolerance to peripheral, but not central, effects of ropinirole, a selective dopamine D_2-like receptor agonist. Eur J Pharmacol 1994; 265:17–26.
14. Ferreira JJ, Galitzky M, Thalamas C, Tiberge M, Montastruc JL, Sampaio C, Rascol O. Effect of ropinirole on sleep onset: a randomised, placebo-controlled study in healthy volunteers. Neurology 2002; 58:460–462.
15. Andreu N, Chalé JJ, Senard JM, Thalamas C, Montastruc JL, Rascol O. L-Dopa-induced sedation : a double-blind cross-over controlled study versus triazolam and placebo in healthy volunteers. Clin Neuropharmacol 1999; 22:15–23.
16. Kaye CM, Nicholls B. Clinical Pharmacokinetics of ropinirole. Clin Phamacokinetics 2000; 39: 243–254.
17. Boothman BR, Spokes EG. Pharmacokinetic data for ropinirole. Lancet 1990; 336:814.
18. Hubble J, Koller WC, Atchison P, Taylor AC, Citeone DR, Zussman BD, Friedman CJ, Hawker N. Linear pharmacokinetic behaviour of rpinirole during multiple dosing in patients with Parkinson's disease. J Clin Pharmacol 2000; 40:641–646.
19. Thalamas C, Rayet S, Brefel C, Eagle S, Lopez-Gil A, Fitzpatrick K, Beerahee A, Montastruc JL, Rascol O. Effect of food on the pharmacokinetics of ropinirole in patients with Parkinson's disease. Mov Disord 1996; 11(suppl 1):138.
20. Thalamas C, Taylor A, Brefel-Courbon C, Eagle S, Fitzpatrick K, Rascol O. Lack of pharmacokinetic interaction between ropinirole and thephylline in patients with Parkinson's disease. Eur J Clin Pharmacol 1999; 55:299–303.

21. Taylor A, Beerahee A, Citerone D, Davy M, Fitzpatrick K, Lopez-Gil A, Stocchi F. The effect of steady-state ropinirole on plasma concentrations of digoxin in patients with Parkinson's disease. Br J Clin Pharmacol 1999; 47:219–222.
22. Bair JD, Oppelt TF. Warfarin and ropinirole interaction. Ann Pharmacother 2001; 35:1202–1204.
23. Taylor AC, Beerahee A, Cyronak M, Leigh TJ, Fitzpatrick KL, Lopez-Gil A, Vakil SD, Burns E, Lennox G. Lack of a pharmacokinetic interaction at steady state between ropinirole and L-DOPA in patients with parkinson's disease. Pharmacotherapy 1999; 19:150–156.
24. Goetz CG, Koller WC, Poewe W, Rascol O, Sampaio C. Management of Parkinson's disease: an evidence-based review. Mov Disord 2002; 17(suppl 4):S1–S166.
25. Rascol O, Goetz CG, Koller WC, Poewe W, Sampaio C. Treatment interventions for Parkinson's disease: an evidence based assessment. Lancet 2002; 359:1589–1598.
26. Whone AL, Remy P, Davis MR, Sabolek M, Nahmias C, Stoessl AJ, Watts RL, Brooks DJ. The REAL-PET study: slower progression in early Parkinson's disease treated with ropinirole compared with L-dopa. Neurology 2002; 58(suppl 3):82–83.
27. Adler CH, Sethi KD, Hauser RA, Davis TL, Hammerstad JP, Bertoni J, Taylor RL, Sanchez-Ramos J, O'Brien CF. Ropinirole for the treatment of early Parkinson's disease. The Ropinirole Study Group. Neurology 1997; 49:393–399.
28. Brooks DJ, Abbott RJ, Lees AJ, Martignoni E, Philcox DV, Rascol O, Roos RA, Sagar HJ. A placebo-controlled evaluation of ropinirole, a novel D2 agonists, as sole dopaminergic therapy in Parkinson's disease. Clin Neuropharmacol 1998; 21:101–107.
29. Rascol O, Brooks DJ, Brunt ER, Korczym AD, Poewe WH, Stocchi F. on the behalf of the 056 study group. Ropinirole in the treatment of early Parkinson's disease: a 6-month interim report of a 5-year L-dopa-controlled study. Mov Disord 1998; 13:39–45.
30. Rascol O, Brooks DJ, Korczyn AD, De Deyn PP, Clarke CE, Lang AE. for the 056 Study Group. A five-year study of the incidence of dyskinesia in patients with early Parkinson's disease who were treated with ropinirole or levodopa. N Engl J Med 2000; 342:1484–1491.
31. Korczyn AD, Brook DJ, Brunt ER, Poewe WH, Rascol O, Stocchi F. Ropinirole versus bromocriptine in the treatment of early Parkinson's disease: a 6-month interim report of a 3-year study. Mov Disord 1998; 13:46–51.
32. Korczyn AD, Brook DJ, Brunt ER, Poewe WH, Rascol O, Stocchi F. Ropinirole versus bromocriptine in the treatment of early Parkinson's disease: a 3-year study. Neurology 1999; 53:364–370.
33. Sethi KD, O'Brien CF, Hammerstad JP, Adler CV, Davis TL, Taylor RL, Sanchez-Ramos J, Bertoni JM, Hauser RA for the ropinirole Study Group. Ropinirole for the treatment of early Parkinson's: disease a 12-month experience. Arch Neurol 1998; 55:1211–1216.
34. Schrag A, Keens J, Warner J. on behalf of the Ropinirole Study Group. Ropinirole for the treatment of tremor in early parkinson's disease. Eur J Neurol 2002; 9:253–257.
35. Kapoor R, Pirtosek Z, Frankel JP, Stern GM, Lees AJ, Bottomley JM, Sree Haran N. Treatment of Parkinson's disease with novel dopamine D2 agonist SK&F 101468. Lancet 1989; i:1445–1446.
36. Kleedorfer B, Stern GM, Lees AJ, Bottomley JM, Sree-Haran N. Ropinirole (SK and F 101468) in the treatment of Parkinson's disease. J Neurol Neurosurg Psychiatry 1991; 54:10.
37. Rascol O, Lees AJ, Senard JM, et al. Ropinirole in the treatment of levodopa-induced motor fluctuations in patients with Parkinson's disease. Clin Neuropharmacol 1996; 19:234–245.
38. Lieberman A, Olanow CW, Sethi K, Swanson P, Waters CH, Fahn S, Hurtig H, Yahr M. The ropinirole sudy group. Neurology 1998; 51:1057–1062.
39. Brunt ER, Brooks DJ, Korkzyn AD, Montastruc JL, Stocchi F. on behalf of the 043 Study Group. A six-month multicentre double-blind bromocriptine-controlled study of the safety and efficacy of ropinirole in the treatment of patients with Parkinson's disease not optimally controlled by L-dopa. J Neural Transm 2002; 109:489–502.
40. Canesi M, Antinoni A, Mariani CB, Tesei S, Zecchinelli AL, Barichella M, Pezzoli G. An overnight switch to ropinirole in patients with Parkinson's disease. J Neural Transm 1999; 106:925–929.
41. Gimenez-Roldan S, Esteban EM, Mateo D. Switching from bromocriptine to ropinirole in patients with advanced Parkinson's disease: open label pilot response to three different dose-ratios. Clin Neuropharmacol 2001; 24:346–351.
42. Müngersdorf M, Sommer U, Sommer M, Reichmann H. High-dose therapy with ropinirole in patietns with Parkinson's disease. J Neural Transm 2001; 108:1309–1317.
43. Lang AE, Rascol O, Brooks DJ, Clarke CE, De Deyn PD, Korczyn AD, Abdalla M. The development of dyskinesia in Parkinson's disease patients receiving ropinirole and given supplemental L-dopa. Neurology 2002; 58(suppl 3):82.

44. Schrag AE, Brooks DJ, Brunt E, Fuell D, Korkzyn A, Poewe W, Quinn NP, Rascol O, Stocchi F. The safety of ropinirole, a selective nonergoline dopamine agonist, in patients with Parkinson's disease. Clin Neuropharmacol 1998; 21:169–175.
45. Frucht S, Rogers JD, Greene PE, Gordon MF, Fahn S. Falling asleep at the wheel: motor vehicle mishaps in persons taking pramipexole and ropinirole. Neurology 1999; 52:1908–1910.
46. Ryan M, Slevin JT, Wells A. Non-ergot dopamine agonist-induced sleep attacks. Pharmacotherapy 2000; 20:724–726.
47. Ferreira JJ, Galitzky M, Montastruc JL, Rascol O. Sleep attacks and Parkinson's disease treatment. Lancet 2000; 355:1333–1334.
48. Ferreira JJ, Desboeuf K, Galitzky M, Thalamas C, Brefel-Courbon C, Fabre N, Senard JM, Montastruc JL, Castro-Caldas A, Rascol O. "Sleep-attacks" and Parkinson's disease: results of a questionnaire survey in a movement disorders out patient clinic. Mov Discord 2000; 15(suppl 3):897.
49. Shapira AH. Sleep attack (sleep episodes) with pergolide. Lancet 2000; 355:1332–1333.
50. Ferreira JJ, Thalamas C, Montastruc JL, Castro-Caldas A, Rascol O. Levodopa monotherapy can induce "sleep attacks" in Parkinson's disease patients. J Neurol 2001; 56:1239–1242.
51. Tracik F, Ebersbach G. Sudden daytime sleep onset in Parkinson's disease: polysomnographic recordings. Mov Disord 2001; 16:500–506.
52. Olanow CW, Schapira AH, Roth T. Waking-up to sleep episodes in Parkinson's disease. Mov Disord 2000; 15:212–215.
53. Hobson DE, Lang AE, Martin WR, Razmy A, Rivest J, Fleming J. Excessive daytime sleepiness and sudden-onset sleep in Parkinson disease: a survey by the Canadian Movement Disorders Group. JAMA 2002; 287:455–463.
54. Lund BC, Neiman RF, Perry PJ. Treatment of Parkinson's disease with ropinirole after pergolide-induced retroperitoneal fibrosis. Pharmacotherapy 1999; 19:1437–1438.
55. Fine J, Lang AE. Dose-induced penile erection in response to ropinirole therapy for Parkinson's disease. Mov Discord 1999; 14:701–702.

12
Cabergoline

Oscar S. Gershanik

Centro Neurológico-Hospital Francés and Instituto de Investigaciones Farmacológicas,
Buenos Aires, Argentina

I. INTRODUCTION

Dopamine agonists have become a fundamental tool in the pharmacological management of Parkinson's disease (PD) as they have shown the capacity to significantly reduce motor disability when used as monotherapy for up to 5 years (1–3). Moreover, initial treatment with dopamine agonists in de novo patients has proven effective in delaying the onset of motor complications (1–3). Cabergoline is a relatively selective dopamine D2 agonist having high affinity for both D2 and D3 receptors (4). Cabergoline produces long-lasting contralateral rotational behavior in 6-hydroxydopamine (6-OHDA) lesioned rats and significant amelioration of parkinsonian symptomatology in 1-methyl-4-phenyl-1,2,3,6-tetrahydropyridine (MPTP)–treated cynomologus monkeys without inducing dyskinesias. It has a long-lasting effect, far beyond that produced by other dopamine agonists (4,5). Cabergoline has a prolonged plasma elimination half-life (approximately 65 hours), allowing for once-daily administration (6,7). It has been shown to be effective in improving parkinsonian symptomatology both as monotherapy and in combination with levodopa in several clinical trials (8,9).

II. PHARMACOLOGY

A. Pharmacodynamic Properties

Cabergoline (1-[(6-allylergolin-8b-yl)carbonyl] -1- [(3-(dimethylamino) propyl]-3-ethyl-urca) is a relatively selective, ergot-derived, dopamine D2 agonist with prolonged steady binding to the receptor in vivo and in vitro for at least 72 hours (Fig. 1) (10). Dopamine receptor binding studies using selective radioligands in rat brain preparations showed that cabergoline has a similar binding profile to pergolide, with high affinity for D2 and D3 receptors and very low affinity for the D1 receptor. Most important is cabergoline's negligible affinity for nondopaminergic receptors such as adrenergic and serotonergic

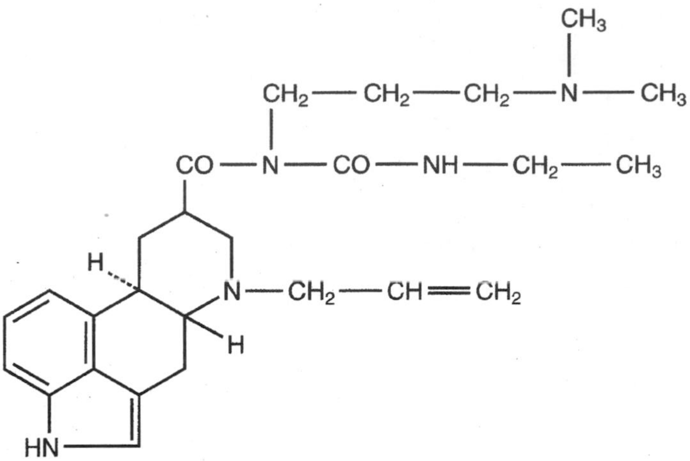

Figure 1 Chemical structure of cabergoline.

receptors (Table 1) (4). An index of its potency and long duration of action as a selective
D2 agonist is reflected by its prolacting-suppressing effect, which is superior to that of bromocriptine (11). A single 0.6 mg dose of cabergoline reduces serum prolactin to levels
obtained with 2.5 mg of bromocriptine, with the effect lasting up to 14 days.

Monkey studies using radiolabeled raclopride and measuring D2 receptor occupancy
by means of positron emission tomography (PET) showed the ability of cabergoline to
cross the blood-brain barrier and have a sustained binding to the receptor lasting
more than 3 days after a single 1-hour intravenous infusion at a dose of 1 mg/kg (10).
Occupancy was determined to range from 59 to 37% from 4 to 68 hours postadministration.

Behavioral studies in animal models of parkinsonism such as the rotational 6-OHDA
lesioned rat and the MPTP-treated monkey provided evidence of its antiparkinsonian
activity (4). Cabergoline, given subcutaneously at doses of 0.5 or 1 mg/kg, was shown
to induce sustained contralateral rotational behavior in the rat, which at 6 hours

Table 1 Dopamine Agonists: Affinity for Different Receptor Types

Drug	Class	Dopamine receptor activity		Other receptor activity	
		D1(D1,D5)	D2(D2,D3,D4)	5HT1/2	α1/2
Bromocriptine	Ergot	Antagonist	Moderate-marked agonist	Agonist	Agonist
Pergolide	Ergot	Agonist	Marked agonist	Agonist	Agonist
Lisuride	Ergot	Variable	Marked agonist	Agonist	None
Cabergoline	Ergot	Very weak agonist	Marked agonist	None	None
Ropinirole	NonErgot	None	Marked agonist (D3 > D2)	None	None
Pramipexole	NonErgot	None	Marked agonist (D3 > D2)	None	Moderate agonist
Apomorphine	NonErgot	Weak agonist	Marked agonist	None	None

postadministration was of a greater magnitude than that of apomorphine, quinpirole, pergolide, or bromocriptine. Animals receiving cabergoline showed persistent rotational activity at 24 hours, when all the other agonists had ceased to be effective. In the cynomologous monkey, cabergoline at doses of 0.1 mg/kg subcutaneously or 2 mg/kg orally was able to significantly reduce parkinsonian symptoms (induced by MPTP) without concomitant dyskinesias (12). Clinical benefit persisted 48–72 hours after the administration of cabergoline. In a similar study aimed at evaluating the effects of chronic administration of cabergoline, the drug was injected daily subcutaneously at doses of 0.2 mg/kg for 22 consecutive days (13). The beneficial effects of the drug became evident 60 minutes after the first injection and were sustained throughout the observation period. Locomotor activity reached its peak on the third day, after which it gradually decreased. Reduction of akinesia scores was not associated with the appearance of abnormal involuntary movements in any of the animals studied. Cabergoline with levodopa in the same animal model was more effective and had a prolonged effect compared to each drug administered alone (14). Moreover, cabergoline abolished levodopa-induced hyperactivity and reduced dyskinesias in these monkeys. In a study addressing the issue of levodopa-induced dyskinesias and the effects of dopamine agonists upon them, MPTP-treated monkeys with a long-standing and stable parkinsonian syndrome with levodopa-induced dyskinesias were treated for 6 weeks with cabergoline (0.125–0.185 mg/kg) (15). After 4 weeks of treatment, dyskinesias were significantly reduced and the antiparkinson effect of cabergoline was maintained. When the animals were again exposed to levodopa 4 days after cabergoline withdrawal, there was a significant reduction in the amount of dyskinesias observed in comparison to that observed before the cabergoline treatment.

A sensitized response to repeated exposure to dopaminergic drugs, particularly short-acting ones, is considered an index of the ability of a given drug to produce motor complications (fluctuations and dyskinesias) in patients under long-term antiparkinson therapy. Rats with a unilateral 6-OHDA nigrostriatal lesion show increased contralateral rotational behavior after repeated administration of dopamine agonists (16). Cabergoline (long-acting dopamine agonist) has been shown to reduce the sensitized response to an apomorphine (short-acting dopamine agonist) challenge in rats previously exposed to levodopa and subsequently treated for 7 days with saline, apomorphine, or cabergoline (17).

B. Pharmacokinetic Properties

Cabergoline has a pharmacokinetic profile characterized by a very long elimination half-life (Table 2). After oral administration, cabergoline achieves peak plasma concentration (C_{max}) in 1–2 hours in both healthy volunteers and PD patients, with an extensive tissue distribution, including the brain (18,19). Elimination half-life has been determined to be 65–110 hours, clearly separating cabergoline from the rest of the dopamine agonists in this regard. Pharmacokinetic parameters remain linear within the 2–7 mg/day dose range (20). The drug is extensively metabolized through hydrolysis, and excretion is mainly achieved through the bile and feces (7). Most important is the fact that cabergoline does not affect the pharmacokinetics of levodopa and is not itself affected by food intake, age, or impaired renal or hepatic function (7,20,21).

C. Other Properties

Dopamine agonists have been shown to have neuroprotective properties in in vitro studies that have been attributed to antioxidant or trophic mechanisms and determined to be

Table 2 Pharmacokinetics of Dopamine Agonists

Drug	Elimination half-life, $t_{1/2}$ (h)
Apomorphine	0.5–1.0
Bromocriptine	3–7
Cabergoline	63–110
Lisuride	1.3–2.5
Pergolide	27
Pramipexole	8–12
Ropinirole	6

mediated both by dopaminergic receptor and nonreceptor effects. Lipid peroxidation was reduced in the brain of nonlesioned rats treated with cabergoline for variable periods of time (22). In a separate study using mice with striatal dopaminergic lesions induced by intracerebroventricularly administered 6-OHDA, the antioxidant and neuroprotective properties of cabergoline were explored (23). The reduced striatal dopamine turnover induced by the injection of 6-OHDA was completely normalized by pretreatment with cabergoline. Moreover, cabergoline was a free radical scavenger in vitro and significantly reduced lipid peroxidation in vitro and in vivo. Furthermore, daily administration of cabergoline to mice significantly increased striatal glutathione (GSH) levels by activation of ribonucleic acid (RNA) expressions of GSH-related enzymes. In addition, repeated administration of cabergoline attenuated both 6-OHDA–induced nigrostriatal dopaminergic dysfunction and dopamine neuronal cell death according to this study.

III. CLINICAL STUDIES

Its pharmacological profile, prolonged steady ligation to D2 receptors, long-lasting elimination half-life, sustained behavioral effects in animal models of parkinsonism, and long-acting effects in suppressing prolactin suggested that cabergoline might be efficacious in the treatment of motor fluctuations and loss of efficacy in PD patients by providing continuous stimulation of dopaminergic receptors with once-daily oral dosing (20).

A. Early Studies

Jori et al. were the first to demonstrate the antiparkinsonian efficacy of cabergoline in an open exploratory study evaluating efficacy, tolerability, and dose response (24). They reported that 29% of PD patients receiving cabergoline had a decrease of $> 25\%$ of the baseline Columbia University Rating Scale (CURS) score after single doses of 1–2 mg. Clinical benefit became apparent within 24 hours and lasted 24 hours. Based on these findings, a study was done to evaluate a once-daily dosing regime. This was again an open, uncontrolled study including 22 patients (14 male, 8 female; mean age 65.6 years). Of these, 13 were newly diagnosed patients, 6 were on levodopa, and 3 had stopped levodopa for different reasons; most of the cases were in Hoehn-Yahr stages II and III with a mean duration of the disease of 3 years. All patients were escalated from 0.75 mg to 1 mg/day; 14 had further increments to 1.25 mg/day, 9 to 1.5 mg/day, and only 4 reached the 2 mg/day dose. Treatment was discontinued in two patients (symptomatic orthostatic hypotension in one case and nocturnal delusions and confusion in another). In 4 additional cases there were reports of adverse events (nausea, hypotension, transient confusion, ankle edema). Twenty-one of the cases were able to complete 2 weeks of treatment, 18 completed 4 weeks, and 11 proceeded to the long-term follow-up phase. Nineteen out of the 22 cases showed an improvement of >25% with reductions in the mean CURS score from 35.9 at baseline to 27.9 after the second week of treatment (1 mg/day) and 26 after 4 weeks (mean daily dose 1.25 mg). At 6 months the majority of patients in the long-term follow-up phase maintained decreases in the CURS score ranging from 35 to 39%. This study demonstrated the feasibility of a once-daily dose regime of a dopamine agonist.

Lera et al. (19) evaluated the long-term efficacy of cabergoline in PD patients with motor fluctuations and dyskinesias on chronic levodopa therapy using the single daily dose regime. In this open study including 36 patients with a mean follow-up period of 14.2 months, the maximum dose reached was much higher than previously used (mean dose 11.3 mg) in an attempt to ascertain not only the efficacy of high doses but also their safety and tolerability. The results obtained were quite encouraging, with significant improvement in the Unified Parkinson's Disease Rating Scale (UPDRS) motor scores both in the off and the on periods (54.8 vs. 25.5 and 20.7 vs. 11.7 respectively), marked reductions in the number of "off" hours (6.8 vs. 1.2 hours), and a significant reduction in the daily levodopa requirement (1,012 vs. 625.9 mg/day). The adverse event profile was similar to that with levodopa and other dopamine agonists. However, the effects were not positive for all patients, and the authors further subdivided the patient population into three groups according to the degree of clinical response observed. Ten of the patients showed a "dramatic" response with an almost complete disappearance of off periods, without enhanced dyskinesia, and reduction of levodopa dosage of 60%. These patients were followed for an extended period of 28.3 months with persistent benefit. In the group of "moderate" responders, 23 patients had a reduction in the severity and duration of off periods, but they also had an increase in the severity of dyskinesias. Three patients were considered to be therapeutic failures as severe off periods reappeared and dyskinesias were worsened. This study was important in determining the wide dose range of cabergoline, allowing for prolonged high-dose administration in combination with levodopa in patients experiencing long-term complications.

In three additional uncontrolled studies (25–27) with similar designs, cabergoline was administered to PD patients on long-term levodopa therapy at a much lower dose (maximum 2.5 mg/day during the titration phase, in two studies further increments up to 5 mg/day were allowed during the treatment phase) for up to 13 weeks. Randomization and dose escalation were performed in a blinded fashion. Results of these trials confirmed the efficacy of cabergoline in improving motor disability and fluctuations in advanced PD patients when used in combination with levodopa (Table 3).

The efficacy and safety of cabergoline was subsequently studied in several phase II and III studies involving a total of approximately 4000 patients in Europe, the Americas, and Japan, yielding comparative results (9).

B. Controlled Studies in Patients Experiencing Motor Fluctuations During Long-Term Levodopa Therapy

There have been five pivotal studies addressing the efficacy of cabergoline in patients with advanced PD (Table 4) (28–32). Of these five studies two were placebo controlled, and three were double-blind comparisons with bromocriptine. In all five studies the baseline and demographic characteristics were similar and matched for age (61–63 years), gender

Table 3 Efficacy of Cabergoline in Improving Motor Disability and Response Fluctuations in Advanced PD Patients When Used in Combination with Levodopa[a]

Trial	No. of patients	Dosage escalation (mg/day)	Duration	Results
Hutton et al., 1993(25)	25	1.0 ($n=19$)	5 weeks escalation	UPDRS ADL (13.3 vs. 9.3)
		1.5 ($n=14$)	8 weeks treatment	UPDRS Motor (14.7 vs. 8.2)
		2.0 ($n=9$)		Mean off-time
		2.5 ($n=4$)		reduction 50%
Lieberman et al., 1993(26)	61	0.5 ($n=12$)	5 weeks escalation	UPDRS ADL
		1.0 ($n=12$)	8 weeks treatment	(16.9 vs. 11.0)
		1.5 ($n=12$)		
				UPDRS Motor (14.8 vs. 11.3)
				Mean off-time reduction 31%
		2.0 ($n=12$)		
		2.5 ($n=12$)		
Ahlskog et al., 1994 (27)	41	0.5–2.5 ($n=8$ or 9 for each dose)	5 weeks escalation 8 weeks treatment	UPDRS ADL (15.7 vs. 9.8) Mean off-time reduction 42%

PD = Parkinson's disease; UPDRS = Unified Parkinson's Disease Rating Scale; ADL = activities of daily living.
[a]Summary of early open-label studies.

distribution, and disease duration (9–14 years). All patients received levodopa in doses ranging from 650 to 1000 mg/day.

In the study by Steiger et al. (28) the effect of cabergoline supplementation on the number of hours spent off was the primary efficacy variable, whereas in Hutton et al.'s study (29) the change in daily levodopa dosage was the primary endpoint. In the three comparative studies with bromocriptine, the rating of clinical improvement in motor disability according to the Clinical Global Impression (CGI) scale was used as a measure of efficacy (30–32). Nonetheless, in all studies patients were evaluated at each visit using the UPDRS, which provided an objective measure of the effects of cabergoline on motor disability.

In the placebo-controlled studies cabergoline was found to be significantly superior to placebo in improving motor fluctuations and reducing the percentage of off time (Table 4) (28,29). Both on and off period motor function were improved, as were activities of daily living. Only in the larger study by Hutton et al. (29) was there a significant reduction in levodopa dosage in cabergoline-treated patients. The overall incidence of adverse events in patients treated with cabergoline was similar to that of placebo (74 vs. 68%), but a few adverse events were more frequently observed in cabergoline patients (hypotension, gastric disturbances, hallucinations, peripheral edema). There was a higher number of

Table 4 Comparison of the Efficacy of Cabergoline (CBG) Versus Placebo (P) or Bromocriptine (BRC) in Patients with Advanced Parkinson's Disease Under Chronic Levodopa Therapy

Trial	No. of patients	Treatment	Reduction in time off (%)	Reduction in levodopa dosage (%)
Placebo-controlled studies				
Steiger et al., 1996 (28)	19	CBG titration (< 22 weeks) 0.5–10 mg	45	45
	18	P	18	38
Hutton et al., 1996 (29)	123	CBG titration (< 10 weeks) 0.5–5 mg	39	18
	65	P	15	3
Comparisons with bromocriptine				
Destee et al., 1996 (30)	191	CBG titration (< 15 weeks) 0.5–6 mg	63	8
	193	BRC titration (< 15 weeks) 5–40 mg	55	3
Schneider et al., 1996 (31)	181	CBG titration (< 13 weeks) 0.5–6 mg	51	8
	185	BRC titration (< 13 weeks) 5–40 mg	45	1
Inzelberg et al., 1996 (32)	22	CBG titration (not mentioned) 0.5–6 mg	50	10
	22	BRC titration (not mentioned) 5 – 40mg 9 months at stable dose	19	9

withdrawals due to intolerable adverse events in the cabergoline- than in the placebo-treated patients—15 and 7%, respectively (28,29).

Comparison studies with bromocriptine did not show significant differences in terms of response rates or effects on levodopa dosage, but there was a non-significant trend in favor of cabergoline with regard to the percentage reduction in off time (Table 4) (30–32). Although adverse event occurrence was similar in both the cabergoline and the bromocriptine groups, there was a higher rate of withdrawal due to intolerable side effects with bromocriptine.

C. Controlled Study in Early Parkinson's Disease

The only controlled study in early PD patients was a multicenter, randomized double-blind 5-year trial performed to assess whether initial therapy with cabergoline alone or in combination with levodopa prevented or delayed the occurrence of long-term motor complications in patients with newly diagnosed PD, as compared with initial levodopa treatment (3,8,33). Additional goals were the evaluation of the clinical effectiveness and tolerability of cabergoline relative to levodopa and the long-term efficacy of cabergoline monotherapy. Four hundred and nineteen patients with newly diagnosed idiopathic PD in Hoehn and Yahr Stages I–III with functional disability warranting

Table 5 Patient Disposition at End of Study Comparing Efficacy of Cabergoline Versus Levodopa in De Novo Patients

Variable	Cabergoline ($n = 211$)	Levodopa ($n = 209$)
Treatment duration (median, days)	1293	1312
Patients not requiring extra levodopa	73 (35.1%)	106 (52.0%)
Cumulative levodopa exposure (mg)	303.8	637.4
Patients reaching the endpoint	47 (22.6%)	70 (34.3%)

pharmacological intervention were enrolled. No patients had been previously treated with levodopa dopamine agonists, or selegiline. Amantadine or anticholinergic treatment had to be withdrawn prior to study entry. This was a multicenter (31 centers in Europe and Latin America), randomized, double-blind, parallel-group, controlled trial in which the patients were randomly assigned to either cabergoline ($n = 211$) or levodopa ($n = 208$). The dose titration was done over ≤ 24 weeks, from an initial dose of cabergoline of 0.25 mg/day and of levodopa of 100 mg/day up to either the optimal dose (i.e., well-tolerated dose that did not produce further clinical improvement over the previous one) or maximum doses of 4 and 600 mg/day, respectively. The goal was to maintain the optimal or maximum tolerated dose until the onset of motor complications or up to 5 years. The primary endpoint was the occurrence of motor complications (fluctuations or dyskinesias) at two consecutive visits. Open-label levodopa was added to both treatment arms when improvement in motor disability decreased below 30% compared to baseline. No other antiparkinsonian treatment was allowed. Preliminary results published at one year showed that up to 62% of the patients randomized to cabergoline could be maintained on monotherapy with persisting clinical improvement compared to baseline (8). The final results of this study are summarized in Table 5 (3,33). The median doses of cabergoline and levodopa used in the trial were 3 and 500 mg/day, respectively. In the cabergoline group, 65% of the patients required additional levodopa compared to 48% of those in the levodopa group. An analysis of the primary efficacy variable showed that 22% of the patients treated with cabergoline ($n = 47$; 4 on cabergoline monotherapy and 43 receiving additional levodopa) reached the endpoint (development of motor complications confirmed at two consecutive 3-month visits) compared to 34% of the patients in the levodopa group ($n = 70$; 17 on a stable levodopa dose and 53 requiring additional levodopa). A Kaplan and Meier estimate of the cumulative risk of developing motor complications showed that it was significantly higher in the levodopa versus cabergoline group (log rank test; $p = 0.0175$). The relative risk of motor complications was consistently higher in the levodopa than in the cabergoline group, and it increased over time (Fig. 2). Applying a Cox model to the analysis of the data showed that the cabergoline group had a greater than 50% lower risk of developing a motor complication than the levodopa group. Furthermore, addition of levodopa more than doubled the risk of motor complications in both treatment groups. The more severe the motor disability at baseline, the higher the risk of motor complications; on the contrary, risk varied inversely with the patient's age at entry. Motor function measured by the UPDRS was one of the secondary variables. Motor disability improved with either treatment for up to 1 year, after which improvement decreased with disease progression. At all evaluation points during the study, mean UPDRS motor scores were slightly but significantly more improved in the levodopa group than in the cabergoline group. After 4 years, patients in the levodopa group maintained an

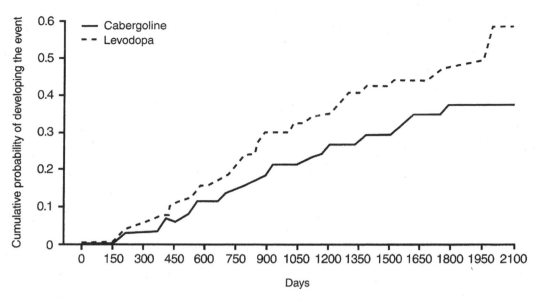

Figure 2 Probability of developing motor complications in patients with early Parkinson's disease treated with cabergoline (alone or with additional levodopa) or levodopa. (Adapted from Ref. 33.)

average 30% improvement in motor disability compared to baseline, while the mean improvement in the cabergoline group was 22% (Fig. 3). More than 35% of the patients in the cabergoline group remained on monotherapy after 5 years.

In summary, both treatments improved motor disability, decreasing UPDRS activities of daily living and motor scores, but development of motor complications was significantly less frequent in patients treated with cabergoline than in levodopa recipients (22% vs. 34%) (3,33). Moreover, the risk of developing motor complications during treatment with cabergoline was more than 50% lower than with levodopa. In patients with early PD, cabergoline was shown to be effective either as monotherapy or combined with levodopa; furthermore, starting treatment with cabergoline significantly delayed the development of motor complications. The results of this study are in agreement with what has been published for other dopamine agonists (e.g., ropinirole, pramipexole), confirming that using a dopamine agonist as the first line of treatment in early PD is beneficial in reducing the risk of motor complications even after the introduction of levodopa (1,2). These studies have also shown that it is possible to maintain some patients on dopamine agonist monotherapy for periods of up to 5 years.

D. Cabergoline for Control of Nocturnal Disabilities in Parkinson's Disease

The long duration of action of cabergoline, allowing for once-daily administration, has been considered to be a unique feature that would make this drug suitable for the management of nocturnal disabilities (bradykinesia, nocturnal pain and discomfort, restlessness). In a comparative study (34) of cabergoline and pergolide, approximately equipotent doses were given once daily at 6 p.m. in an attempt to reduce excessive daytime sleepiness (EDS) as a consequence of reduced nighttime sleep secondary to nocturnal

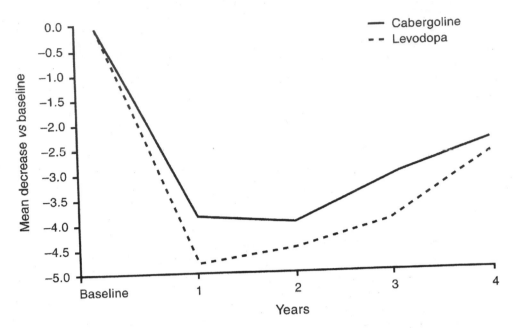

Figure 3 UPDRS motor scores in patients treated with cabergoline or levodopa. (Adapted from Ref. 33.)

motor disabilities. Patients were evaluated by means of the Epworth Sleepiness Scale (ESS) administered before treatment and in the morning following drug administration. Both drugs were shown to reduce ESS scores, with cabergoline being the most effective of the two, although these differences did not reach statistical significance. The same paradigm was used to evaluate the effects of these two drugs on nocturnal dystonic pain. Cabergoline was also shown to be more effective than pergolide in reducing nighttime dystonic pain. The benefit for both symptoms was maintained for up to 6 months. In another study (35) cabergoline was compared to controlled-release levodopa given at night time in an attempt to improve nocturnal akinesia and off period painful dystonia. Cabergoline was significantly superior ($p < 0.05$) to controlled-release levodopa in reducing the number of hours spent off at night as well as nocturnal pain. Based on the few studies available, cabergoline appears to be a valid alternative for the treatment of nocturnal disabilities in PD (for review see Ref. 36).

E. Cabergoline in Combination with Short-Acting Dopamine Agonists

Cabergoline was proposed as the ideal drug to be used in combination with drugs such as pramipexole or ropinirole (short-acting, t.i.d dose regime) due to its different pharmacokinetic properties (long duration of action, once-daily administration). Stocchi and coworkers reported a study using this novel approach (37). The study was conducted as a 3-month prospective open-label pilot trial. Twenty-seven patients with idiopathic PD were included, of which 21 were receiving either pramipexole or ropinirole in combination with levodopa, and 6 were treated with either dopamine agonist. All patients received the dopamine agonist in doses high enough (3.7 mg/d for pramipexole; 17.3 mg/d for ropinirole) to be considered as the maximum effective dose but had not obtained a satisfactory control of symptoms. Clinical assessments were performed by a blind evaluator at regular intervals throughout the study (at baseline, every 2 weeks during the cabergoline titration phase, and every 4 weeks once the optimal dose was achieved). UPDRS motor scores in both the on and the off states, and the Abnormal Involuntary Movements Scale (AIMS) was administered to patients receiving levodopa. Patients receiving a dopamine agonist only were assessed for their best motor state. Levodopa-treated patients also kept a home diary, recording the number of hours spent off to evaluate the effects of the addition of cabergoline on motor fluctuations. Patients on levodopa were kept on a stable dose of the drug (mean daily dose 471.4 ± 239.0 mg/d) during the study period. Cabergoline was started at 0.5 mg given once daily and titrated upwards until maximum benefit was obtained. The mean daily dose of cabergoline used for the levodopa group was 4.04 ± 1.62 mg, while the nonlevodopa group received $3.8 + 0.7$ mg/d. All patients showed further improvement with the addition of cabergoline. In the levodopa group there was significant improvement both for the off period motor state and motor fluctuations with more than 50% reduction of the number of hours spent off. The nonlevodopa group also showed significant improvement in the motor state with a reduction of the motor score of the UPDRS of approximately 38%. All patients tolerated adjunctive cabergoline well, and there were no withdrawals due to adverse effects. Six of the 27 patients reported mild and transient side effects (nausea, ankle edema, hypotension).

IV. DOSAGE AND MODE OF ADMINISTRATION

According to published studies, cabergoline possesses a wide therapeutic range, showing clinically measurable effects in doses as low as 0.5 mg/d and up to 16 mg/d (9,25–27). The usual therapeutic range is 2.5 6 mg/d (1,2,8,38). The usual starting dose is 0.5 mg/d in single-dose administration, in the morning; upward dose titration (0.5 mg increments) can be accomplished at weekly intervals until clinical benefit is observed or limiting side-effects appear (25). Cabergoline has been shown to be effective both as monotherapy in de novo PD patients and as an add-on therapy in patients taking levodopa with or without motor complications (8,28,29). In those cases in whom nocturnal disabilities warrant the addition of cabergoline, the drug may be administered in a single evening dose (34–36).

V. SAFETY

The adverse-event profile of cabergoline is consistent with that of other dopaminergic agonists, including gastrointestinal (nausea, vomiting), cardiovascular (dizziness, orthostatic hypotension), and neuropsychiatric (delusions, hallucinosis) effects (39). In comparative studies of cabergoline with other ergot derivatives (bromocriptine, pergolide) (30–32,40) no significant differences were found in their safety profiles, although there was a trend in favor of cabergoline showing less adverse events.

   In patients with preexisting dyskinesias, cabergoline is likely to aggravate them, as has been observed with other dopamine agonists (27). There is evidence that when cabergoline is used as an initial therapy it may delay the onset and reduce the long-term risk of the occurrence of motor complications, especially dyskinesia (3,33). Moreover, this benefit is carried over even after levodopa supplementation becomes necessary.

Ankle edema and pericardial or pleural fibrosis as observed with other ergot compounds have been occasionally reported with cabergoline (33,41,42).

The effect of cabergoline on sleep (EDS and sleep "attacks") has not been specifically addressed in any of the published clinical trials, and sleep problems were reported without further details. A single case has been reported of a patient receiving cabergoline and levodopa in whom sleep "attacks" developed after the addition of entacapone (43). Moreover, in a retrospective study analyzing the prevalence of EDS and sleep "attacks" in patients receiving either cabergoline, pramipexole, or levodopa, not a single case of sleep "attacks" was detected (44).

REFERENCES

1. Rascol O, Brooks DJ, Korczyn AD, De Deyn PP, Clarke CE, Lang AE. A five-year study of the incidence of dyskinesia in patients with early Parkinson's disease who were treated with ropinirole or levodopa. 056 Study Group. N Engl J Med 2000; 342(20):1484–1491.
2. Parkinson Study Group. Pramipexole vs levodopa as initial treatment for Parkinson disease: a randomized controlled trial. JAMA 2000; 284(15):1931–1938.
3. Rinne UK. A 5 year double blind study with cabergoline versus levodopa in the treatment of early Parkinson's disease (abstr). Parkinsonism Related Disord 1999; 5(suppl):S84.
4. Carfagna N, Caccia C, Buonamici M, et al. Biochemical and pharmacological studies on cabergoline, a new putative antiparkinsonian drug (abstr). Soc Neurosci Abs 1991; 17:1075.
5. Arai N, Isaji M, Miyata H, Fukuyama J, Mizuta E, Kuno S. Differential effects of three dopamine receptor agonists in MPTP-treated monkeys. J Neural Transm [Park Dis Dement Sect] 1995; 10(9991):55–62.
6. Lera G, Vaamonde J, Muruzabal J, Obeso JA. Cabergoline: a long-acting dopamine agonist in Parkinson's disease. Ann Neurol 1990; 28(4):593–594.
7. Battaglia R, Strolin Benedetti M, Mantegani S, Castelli MG, Cocchiara G, Dostert P. Disposition and urinary metabolic pattern of cabergoline, a potent dopaminergic agonist in rat, monkey and man. Xenobiotica 1993; 23:1377–1389.
8. Rinne UK, Bracco F, Chouza C, Dupont E, Gershanik O, Marti Masso JF, Montastruc JL, Marsden CD, Dubini A, Orlando N, Grimaldi R. Cabergoline in the treatment of early Parkinson's disease: results of the first year of treatment in a double-blind comparison of cabergoline and levodopa. Neurology 1997; 48(2):363–368.
9. Marsden CD. Clinical experience with cabergoline in patients with advanced Parkinson's disease treated with levodopa. Drugs 1998; 55(suppl 1):17–22.
10. Bergstrom M, Hartvig P, Nava C, et al. Effects of cabergoline on striatal dopamine receptor binding and dopamine synthesis. In vivo study in monkey with positron emission tomography (abstr). Proceeding of the European Neuroscience Association 1995:192.
11. Ferrari C, Barbieri C, Caldara R, Mucci M, Codecasa F, Paracchi A, Romano C, Boghen M, Dubini A. Long-lasting prolactin-lowering effect of cabergoline, a new dopamine agonist, in hyperprolactinemic patients. J Clin Endocrinol Metab 1986; 63(4):941–945.
12. McArthur RA, Brughera M, Cervini MA. The effect of the D2 agonist cabergoline on MPTP-induced parkinsonism in monkeys. In: Beninger RJ, Palomo T, Arcer T Dopamine Disease States. Madrid: CYM Press, 1996:67–81.
13. Nomoto M, Kita S, Iwata S-I, Kaseda S, Fukuda T. Effects of acute or prolonged administration of cabergoline on parkinsonism induced by MPTP in common marmosets. Pharmacol Biochem Behav 1998; 59(3):717–721.
14. Arai N, Isagy M, Kojima M, Mizuta E, Kuno S. Combined effects of cabergoline and l-dopa on parkinsonism in MPTP-treated cynomologus monkeys. J Neural Transm 1996; 103:1307–1316.
15. Tahar AH, Gregoire L, Bangassoro E, Bedard PJ. Sustained cabergoline treatment reverses levodopa-induced dyskinesias in parkinsonian monkeys. Clin Neuropharmacol 2000; 23(4):195–202.
16. Henry B, Crossman AR, Brotchie JM. Characterization of enhanced behavioral responses to L-Dopa following repeated administration in the 6-hydroxydopamine-lesioned rat model of Parkinson's disease. Exp Neurol 1998; 151:334–342.
17. Kashihara K, Manabe Y, Murakami T, Abe K. Effects of short- and long-acting dopamine agonists on sensitized dopaminergic neurotransmission in rats with unilateral 6-OHDA lesions. Life Sci 2002; 70:1095–1100.

18. Persiani S, Pianezzola E, Broutin F, Fonte G, Strolin Benedetti M. Radioimmunoassay for the synthetic ergoline derivative cabergoline in biological fluids. J Immunoassay 1992; 13:457–476.
19. Lera G, Vaamonde J, Rodriguez M, Obeso JA. Cabergoline in Parkinson's disease: long-term follow-up. Neurology 1993; 43(12):2587–2590.
20. Fariello RG. Pharmacodynamic and pharmacokinetic features of cabergoline: rationale for use in Parkinson's disease. Drugs 1998; 55(suppl 1):10–16.
21. Del Dotto P, Colzi A, Pardini C, Lucetti C, Dubini A, Grimaldi R, Bonuccelli U. Cabergoline improves motor disability without modifying L-DOPA plasma levels in fluctuating Parkinson's disease patients. J Neural Transm 1995; 45(suppl):259–265.
22. Nicoletta Finotti, Laura Castagna, Antonio Moretti, Fulvio Marzatico. Reduction of lipid peroxidation in different rat brain areas after cabergoline treatment. Pharmacol Res 2000; 42(4):287–291.
23. Yoshioka M, Tanaka K, Miyazaki I, Fujita N, Higashi Y, Asanuma M, Ogawa N. The dopamine agonist cabergoline provides neuroprotection by activation of the glutathione system and scavenging free radicals. Neurosci Res 2002; 43:259–267.
24. Jori MC, Franceschi M, Giusti MC, Canal N, Piolti R, Frattola L, Bassi S, Calloni E, Mamoli A, Camerlingo M. Clinical experience with cabergoline, a new ergoline derivative, in the treatment of Parkinson's disease. Adv Neurol 1990; 53:539–43.
25. Hutton JT, Morris JL, Brewer MA. Controlled study of the antiparkinsonian activity and tolerability of cabergoline. Neurology 1993; 43(3):613–616.
26. Lieberman A, Imke S, Muenter M, Wheeler K, Ahlskog JE, Matsumoto JY, Maraganore DM, Wright KF, Schoenfelder J. Multicenter study of cabergoline, a long-acting dopamine receptor agonist, in Parkinson's disease patients with fluctuating responses to levodopa/carbidopa. Neurology 1993; 43(10):1981–1984.
27. Ahlskog JE, Muenter MD, Maraganore DM, Matsumoto JY, Lieberman A, Wright KF, Wheeler K. Fluctuating Parkinson's Disease. Treatment with the long-acting dopamine agonist cabergoline. Arch Neurol 1994; 51:1236–1241.
28. Steiger MJ, El Debas T, Anderson T, Findley LJ, Marsden CD. Double-blind study of the activity and tolerability of cabergoline versus placebo in parkinsonians with motor fluctuations. J Neurol 1996; 243(1):68–72.
29. Hutton JT, Koller WC, Ahlskog JE, Pahwa R, Hurtig III, Stern MB, Hiner BC, Lieberman A, Pfeiffer RF, Rodnitzky RL, Waters CH, Muenter MD, Adler CH, Morris JL. Multicenter, placebo-controlled trial of cabergoline taken once daily in the treatment of Parkinson's disease. Neurology 1996; 46(4):1062–1065.
30. Destee A, Schneider E, Gershanik O, Dom R, Tichy J, Korczyn AD, Caraceni T, Lakke JPWF, Szczudlik A, Lees A, Chouza C, Kostic V, and the CBG Study Group. Efficacy and tolerability of cabergoline compared to bromocriptine in patients suffering from levodopa associated motor complications (not on treatment with DA-agents)(abstr). Mov Disord 1996; 22(suppl 1): S226–S269.
31. Schneider E, Gershanik O, Dom R, Tichy J, Korczyn AD, Caraceni T, Lakke JPWF, Szczudlik A, Lees A, Chouza C, Kostic V, and the CBG Study Group. Efficacy and tolerability of cabergoline compared to bromocriptine in patients suffering from levodopa associated motor complications (on treatment with DA-agents) (abstr). Mov Disord 1996; 11(suppl 1): S227–S269.
32. Inzelberg R, Nisipeanu P, Rabey J M, Orlov E, Catz T, Kippervasser S, Schechtman E, Korczyn AD. Double-blind comparison of cabergoline and bromocriptine in Parkinson's disease patients with motor fluctuations. Neurology 1996; 47:785–788.
33. Rinne UK, Bracco F, Chouza C, Dupont E, Gershanik O, Marti Masso JF, Montastruc JL, Marsden CD. Early Treatment of Parkinson's disease with cabergoline delays the onset of motor complications. Results of a double-blind levodopa controlled trial. Drugs 1998; 55(suppl 1):23–30.
34. Chaudhuri RK, Gathani T, Agapito C, et al. Comparative study of the effect of pergolide and cabergoline on nocturnal disabilities in Parkinson's disease: a single blind study (abstr). Parkinsonism Relat Disord. 1999; 5(suppl):S70.
35. Chaudhuri KR, et al. The use of cabergoline in nocturnal parkinsonian disabilities causing sleep disruption: a parallel study with controlled-release levodopa. Eur J Neurol. 1999; 6(suppl 5):S11–S15.
36. Chaudiri KR. Twenty-four-hour symptom control in Parkinson's disease, with emphasis on management of nocturnal disabilities. Eur Neurol. 2001; 46(suppl 1):1–2.
37. Stocchi F, Berardelli A, Vacca L, Thomas A, De Pandis MF, Modugno N, Valente M, Ruggieri S. Combination of two different dopamine agonists in the management of Parkinson's disease. Neurol Sci 2002; 23:S115–S116.
38. Navan P, Bain PG. Long term tolerability of high dose ergoline derived dopamine agonist therapy for the treatment of Parkinson's disease. J Neurol Neurosurg Psychiatry 2002; 73(5):602–603.

39. DA agonists—ergot derivatives: cabergoline: management of Parkinson's disease. Mov Disord 2002; 17 (suppl 4):S68–S71.

40. Ulm G, Schüler P. on behalf of the MODAC Study Group. Cabergolin versus Pergolid. Eine videoverblindete, randomisierte, multizentrische Crossover-studie. Akt Neurologie 1999; 25:360–365.

41. Geminiani G, Fetoni V, Genitrini S, Giovannini P, Tamma F, Caraceni T. Cabergoline in Parkinson's disease complicated by motor fluctuations. Mov Disord 1996; 11(5):495–500.

42. Ling LH, Ahlskog JE, Munger TM, Limper AH, Oh JK. Constrictive pericarditis and pleuropulmonary disease linked to ergot dopamine agonist therapy (cabergoline) for Parkinson's disease. Mayo Clin Proc 1999; 74:371–375.

43. Tracik F, Ebersbach G. Sudden daytime sleep onset in Parkinson's disease: polysomnographic recordings. Mov Disord 2001; 16(3):500–506.

44. Pal S, Bhattacharya KF, Agapito C, Chaudhuri KR. A study of excessive daytime sleepiness and its clinical significance in three groups of Parkinson's disease patients taking pramipexole, cabergoline and levodopa mono and combination therapy. J Neural Transm 2001; 108(1):71–77.

13
Apomorphine and Rotigotine

Stephen Gancher*

Oregon Health Sciences University, Portland, Oregon, U.S.A.

Stephan Behrens

Schwarz Biosciences, Monheim, Germany

I. INTRODUCTION

The development of levodopa-induced dyskinesias and fluctuations continues to be a major challenge in the long-term management of Parkinson's disease (PD). These adverse motor effects are rare with initial therapy but develop in most patients over years of treatment. In many patients, fluctuations between immobility, intolerable "on" chorea, and painful "off" dystonia become as disabling as tremor and bradykinesia.

To a large extent these problems reflect undesirable pharmacological properties of levodopa; it is rapidly cleared from plasma, is absorbed erratically, and is transported into the brain by a carrier system that can be saturated by dietary amino acids. Treatments to enhance the absorption of levodopa and delay its clearance include controlled-release formulations of levodopa, Catehol-O-methyltransferase (COMT) inhibitors and low-protein diets, but these are inadequate in many patients.

Many of these problems can be treated by the addition of a dopamine agonist. These drugs lessen the severity of off periods, improve off dystonia, and allow the total daily dose of levodopa to be lowered, which may reduce dyskinesias. Also, by reducing the use of levodopa, there may be a reduction in metabolic stress from the formation of free radicals. In support of this idea, recent studies using functional brain imaging demonstrated a slower loss of basal ganglia signal in patients initiating treatment with dopamine agonists in comparison to levodopa (1,2).

However, there are a number of limitations in the use of the currently available dopamine agonists. First, they are prone to cause side effects. These are similar to those

---

**Current affiliation*: Northwest Permanente, Portland, Oregon, U.S.A.

produced by levodopa but may be more frequent. Some side effects, such as nausea and hypotension, are self-limited and can be effectively managed in most patients by starting the drug at low doses and increasing slowly. Other side effects, such as sedation and confusion, are less manageable and may limit the maximally tolerated dose of drug. A second problem is that dopamine agonists are not as effective as levodopa over time. Although dopamine agonists can be used alone in patients with mild PD, almost all patients eventually require the addition of levodopa.

In this chapter two novel dopamine agonists, apomorphine and rotigotine, are discussed. Each drug has unique properties; apomorphine is a short-acting, potent drug that can reverse periods of parkinsonism (off periods), and rotigotine is administered by a long-acting, transdermal formulation.

II. APOMORPHINE

Apomorphine is different in its actions and uses than other dopamine agonists. Apomorphine has a very rapid onset of effect and is rapidly cleared. These properties allow apomorphine to be best used as a "rescue" treatment in patients with severe motor fluctuations.

A. History

Apomorphine is a very old drug. It was discovered in 1869 that morphine, when heated, yielded a compound that induced motor hyperactivity and stereotyped motor behaviors in animals. It was also recognized to have potent sedating and emetic properties, and it was tried clinically in the late 1800s in a variety of neurological and psychiatric disorders. Because it is quick acting after subcutaneous or intramuscular injection and is a potent emetic, it was widely used in emergency rooms and was used as an aversive treatment for alcoholism (3). Apomorphine was also recognized to have effects on reducing decerebrate rigidity in animals (3) and was first tried in patients with PD in the early 1950s by Schwab et al. (4).

Apomorphine was further studied by Cotzias (5,6) and others beginning in the early 1970s. When administered by subcutaneous injection, it was found to produce severe nausea. Oral administration was better tolerated, but required large doses. After azotemia developed in many of the patients studied (7), the clinical use of apomorphine in PD was largely abandoned.

Domperidone, a dopaminergic antagonist that has minimal central nervous system (CNS) effect can reduce or eliminate many of the side effects of apomorphine (8), and this discovery has allowed much of the current research and use of apomorphine to be performed.

B. Chemistry and Pharmacology

1. Physical Properties

Apomorphine is a rearrangement product of morphine, which is formed by exposing morphine to a strong acid under pressure. It is a polycyclic hydrocarbon which retains a dopamine-like structure as part of the molecule. It is unstable in aqueous solution, auto-oxidizing to form a turquoise-colored reaction product, but is stable when prepared with antioxidants or when stored in powdered form.

2. Pharmacokinetics

Absorption

Apomorphine is quickly and virtually completely absorbed following subcutaneous injection, with peak plasma levels achieved within 5–10 minutes in most patients. The volume of distribution and peak levels are similar to levels achieved after intravenous administration. Apomorphine is rapidly cleared from plasma; its elimination half-life is approximately 30 minutes following subcutaneous injection. There is no apparent storage of apomorphine in subcutaneous tissues; its clearance following a subcutaneous infusion is similar to intravenous infusion (9). Effective doses for PD treatment are in the 1–4 mg (25–50 μg/kg) range. Apomorphine can be absorbed by other routes, including sublingual, intranasal, and rectal administration, and efforts are being made to deliver apomorphine transdermally. Of these formulations, the sublingual route has been most extensively studied. Following sublingual administration of 2–4 mg tablets, apomorphine is absorbed, but more slowly than following subcutaneous adminstration; peak levels are attained in 40–60 minutes, and the drug is cleared with an apparent elimination half-life of 3 hours. Peak levels and area under the curves are smaller than in comparison to subcutaneous administration, mostly likely reflecting the drugs rapid metabolism. Using an older formulation of apomorphine tablets, intended for dissolution into saline and subcutaneous injection, sublingual apomorphine was found to be approximately 10–22% bioavailable in comparison to subcutaneous administration (10).

Distribution and Metabolism

Apomorphine is rapidly and extensively distributed through tissues; its volume of distribution is up to two times body weight (11). It is highly protein bound, but is also lipophilic and rapidly diffuses into brain and cerebrospinal fluid (CSF) compartments following subcutaneous or intravenous administration. Apomorphine is rapidly cleared from plasma by a first-pass hepatic metabolism, mostly by glucuronidation and sulfation; these metabolites are excreted in the bile (12). In addition, apomorphine is very prone to oxidation and may auto-oxidize in vivo (11). There is also a minor pathway involving o-methylation; peak plasma concentrations of apomorphine were found to be slightly higher following administration of the COMT inhibitor tolcapone (13). Higher blood levels are achieved in patients with renal and hepatic disease (14). Because of this rapid and near-complete metabolism, oral administration of apomorphine is not useful. Very low plasma levels are achieved, with less than 5% bioavailability, due to first-pass hepatic metabolism (15).

3. Pharmacological Actions and Uses in Parkinson's Disease

Following subcutaneous injection, apomorphine produces an improvement in motor signs that is qualitatively similar to levodopa. Like levodopa and other dopamine agonists, it produces a number of other effects, including hypotension, nausea, diaphoresis, and sedation. At high doses (10 mg or more) apomorphine is an effective emetic. At very low doses apomorphine can induce penile erections.

Diagnostic Testing

In patients with PD, apomorphine has been used to predict the response to levodopa, with a sensitivity and specificity similar but not superior to a levodopa challenge (16). A positive response has been found to predict benefit to subthalamic nucleus stimulation (16). Because of its quick action, apomorphine challenges have been used during deep brain surgeries in studies of neurophysiological activity (18).

Subcutaneous Administration

Apomorphine is used in the long-term treatment of PD in patients with motor fluctuations. It can be administered by subcutaneous bolus injections as well as by an infusion pump. An extensive, evidence-based review of the use of apomorphine has been recently reported (19).

Subcutaneous Bolus Injections

When used as a bolus injection, patients typically self-administer apomorphine 4–6 times per day during off periods. The injections are typically administered subcutaneously through clothing, in the abdominal wall or upper thigh, and reduce symptoms in approximately 15 minutes. Typically, a 2–3 mg subcutaneous bolus injection improves symptoms for 60–90 minutes, with higher doses producing a longer duration of action.

It is effective for over 90% of off periods (20) and, when used repeatedly, reduces the duration of off periods by 50% or more (21,22). In addition to improving typical symptoms of parkinsonism, such as bradykinesia and tremor, bolus injections of apomorphine can be used to improve other symptoms, including intractable pain (23). Used in this way, apomorphine is generally more effective than oral dopamine agonists or COMT inhibitors.

Subcutaneous Infusion

Apomorphine can also be administered by subcutaneous infusion, using an external infusion pump. Used in this fashion, apomorphine reduces both the frequency as well as the severity of off periods, may allow the doses of other medications to be lowered, and has been found to also significantly lessen the severity and duration of levodopa-induced dyskinesias (19,24). Apomorpine infusions are usually administered during the day. The constant infusion of apomorphine does result in a degree of tolerance (25); this effect is not seen when apomorphine is infused during waking hours.

Other Routes of Intermittent Administration

Owing to its high lipid solubility, apomorphine may also be administered by intranasal, sublingual, and rectal routes, all of which have the advantage of painless, easy administration.

Intranasal Administration

Apomorphine is rapidly absorbed following intranasal administration and is quick acting. A small placebo-controlled trial found it to be effective when used in a manner similar to subcutaneous bolus administration (26). Intranasally administered apomorphine is also used in long-term treatment of patients, but nasal stuffiness, vestibulitis, and crusting are common problems with its administration (27). It is mainly used as a short-term treatment in place of other routes.

Sublingual Administration

Apomorphine can also be absorbed sublingually. When used in patients with PD, the latency to effect is longer than following subcutaneous injection, and doses of up to 10 times the subcutaneous route are needed (28). Although some of the delay in effect is due to time needed for dissolution of the sublingual tablets, even sublingual administration of a concentrated solution of apomorphine still results in delays of nearly 30 minutes in some patients (29). Similar to the intranasal route, irritation of the oral mucosa has been noted in some patients, but there have been several small series reporting sustained benefit over months (30–32).

4. Side Effects

Apomorphine is prone to cause a variety of acute and chronic side effects. These are similar to the effects shared with oral dopamine agonists but are more pronounced. The most common side effect following administration of apomorphine is nausea. This adverse effect is very common following initial doses of apomorphine, particularly in patients naive to other dopamine agonists, but lessens with repeated doses. Vomiting is unusual with doses used in PD. Orthostatic hypotension, sweating, bradycardia, pallor, yawning, and other dysautonomic side effects also are common with apomorphine, occurring in approximately one third of patients. The nausea and many of the other acute side effects are likely to be due to stimulation of the chemoreceptor trigger zone and other dopamine receptors that lie outside the blood-brain barrier and are greatly attenuated by domperidone. Pretreatment with domperidone for 2–4 days at 60–80 mg per day prior to initiating treatment with apomorphine reduces the incidence of nausea and allows higher doses of apomorphine to be administered. Most patients are able to discontinue domperidone after several days or weeks of apomorphine treatment. However, some patients continue to struggle with nausea or other side effects despite use of domperidone. The reason is unclear, but this may be due to stimulation of basal ganglia endogenous opioid receptors by apomorphine, as naloxone partially blocks the motor effects of apomorphine (33). Other acute side effects are rare but may include syncope and hypotension.

Long-term systemic side effects of apomorphine are also uncommon. Although severe azotemia occurred in patients treated with oral apomorphine, no effects on liver or renal function tests have been noted in any of the acute or chronic studies utilizing apomorphine by parenteral routes. Rarely patients have developed a Coombs-positive hemolytic anemia and increases in pancreatic enzymes during chronic apomorphine treatment (34,35), but other abnormalities in blood counts have not been noted.

In addition to systemic side effects, local side effects commonly occur following administration of apomorphine. It is irritating to the subcutaneous tissues. Subcutaneous nodules are almost universally noted following infusions or injections of apomorphine, and rare subcutaneous necrosis may occur. These nodules may interfere with drug absorption, but they are manageable by rotation of infusion or injection sites or by temporarily substituting nasal apomorphine. Some of these local problems may be due to the low pH of available apomorphine formulations, and efforts are being made to improve the tolerability of apomorphine in the subcutaneous tissues.

III. ROTIGOTINE

Rotigotine is a nonergolinic dopamine agonist developed as a new continuous transdermal delivery system. The rotigotine development is based on long-term experience with other transdermal delivery systems addressing recent needs raised by such a pharmacological treatment and the compound itself.

A. Pharmacology

Rotigotine is a derivative of the 2-aminotetralins (Fig. 1) and a nonergolinic dopamine receptor agonist. It is highly lipophilic and readily diffuses across the blood-brain barrier. Rotigotine binds to dopamine receptors with the highest affinity to D3 and D2 receptors and demonstrates biological activities, similar to typical dopamine D2 agonists, in both in vivo and in vitro studies.

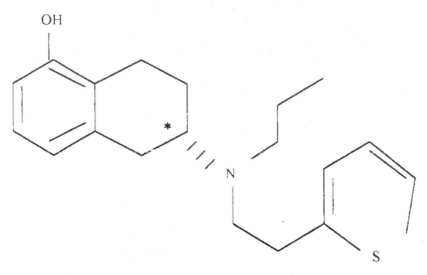

Figure 1 Chemical structure of rotigotine. The chiral carbon is designated by an asterisk.

Biochemical assays include inhibition of the acetylcholine release in rabbit brain slices by electrical stimulation inhibition of the dopamine synthesis in rats induced by gamma butyryl lactone, inhibition of striatal dopamine release in rats, and inhibition of prolactin release in rats and monkeys after rotigotine administration.

Behavioral effects typical of dopamine agonists include induction of motor hyperactivity and stereotypies in rats and monkeys without brain lesions, as well as rotational behavior in rats and monkeys with 6-hydroxydopamine lesions.

The rotigotine patch is intended to be replaced every 24 hours. The patch was designed to deliver a certain ideally constant amount of the dopamine agonist through the skin for a period of at least 24 hours. Compared to tablets or capsules, the advantage of this transdermal delivery system is related to the continuous release of the compound through the skin as long as the patch is in place. This should result in more stable plasma levels of this dopamine agonist. This is of importance, because intermittent administration of levodopa or dopamine agonists with a pulsatile stimulation of the dopamine receptor may contribute to motor complications (36,37). On the other hand, continuous dopaminergic

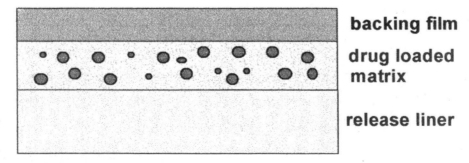

Figure 2 Schematic structure of rotigotine: cross-sectional view of the patch.

receptor stimulation in the CNS not only results in fewer side effects caused by peak and trough plasma levels, but leads to fewer motor fluctuations in late-stage PD patients.

The patch contains three major components: flexible tan-colored backing film, a self-adhesive drug-loaded matrix, and a release liner (Fig. 2). A steady-state plasma concentration is achieved after approximately 12 hours. With multiple applications of rotigotine every 24 hours, stable plasma levels are maintained. The substance has a half-life of approximately 4–5 hours. The plasma protein binding is approximately 90%. Rotigotine is metabolized, and phase 1 metabolites and conjugates are mainly eliminated by renal and biliary routes.

B. Clinical Experience

In a large double-blind, parallel-group, placebo-controlled study of rotigotine mono-therapy, patients with early PD (Hoehn and Yahr stage 3 or less) were treated with rotigotine patches at varying daily doses over a 3-month period. Two hundred and fifty-four patients treated with rotigotine showed an improvement of motor symptoms compared to 62 placebo-treated patients. In this 3-month study with rotigotine mono-therapy, dosages of rotigotine at 9.0, 13.5, and 18.0 mg/d (corresponding to patch sizes of 20, 30, and 40 cm^2) demonstrated a statistically significant improvement in PD symptoms as measured by the Unified Parkinson's Disease Rating Scale (UPDRS), with the two highest doses demonstrating the greatest efficacy. The average improvement in UPDRS part II and III comparing rotigotine treatment vs. placebo reached 31% in the 9.0 mg group and 49% and 51% in the groups treated with 13.5 and 18.0 mg (38).

In another study, over 300 patients with advanced PD were treated with rotigotine at 9.0, 18.0, and 27 mg/d in addition to levodopa in a double-blind, placebo-controlled trial of transdermal rotigotine over a 3-month period. Inclusion criteria included a minimum dose of 300 mg/d of levodopa and motor fluctuations with at least 2.5 off hours per day. The effect of rotigotine was measured by self-reported diaries. Results showed a decrease in off time without an increase of disabling dyskinesia in the on motor stage. The 77 patients with severe motor fluctuations showed a reduction in off time of 2.4 hours per day when treated with a daily dose of 27 mg (60 cm^2) rotigotine. However, the group of 81 placebo-treated PD patients were found to exhibit a reduction in average off time of 1.8 hours per day (39).

An open-label trial conducted in advanced PD patients showed that with rotigotine add-on therapy the mean daily levodopa dose could be reduced by one third without worsening of the clinical symptoms. In the same trial placebo-treated patients could reduce their daily levodopa dose by only 7% (40).

C. Adverse Effects

Rotigotine-treated patients in early PD reported that the most frequent adverse events were nausea and vomiting, dizziness, headache, drowsiness, sleepiness, and fatigue. Besides the typical dopaminergic adverse event profile, skin reactions at the patch application site occurred slightly more frequent in the rotigotine-treated group compared to placebo. In summary, all adverse events mentioned have been also reported under placebo but with a lower incidence. Eight percent of the rotigotine-treated patients and 5% of the placebo-treated patients discontinued the study due to the adverse events.

Patients with motor fluctuations reported as most common adverse events nausea and vomiting, dizziness, headache, as well as skin reactions at the patch application site.

The skin reactions occurred more frequently in the higher rotigotine dosage group than in the lower one. Seven percent of rotigotine-treated patients discontinued the study medication due to the most common adverse events of nausea and vomiting and patch application site reactions. Three percent of placebo-treated patients discontinued the study medication due to these adverse events.

In general, skin reactions were transient; the severity was slight and moderate. These application site reactions on the skin recovered completely after removing the patch. A systematic daily change of the patch application site was not possible due to the study protocol. This was changed in follow-up studies.

In summary, based on the available study results, it can be concluded that rotigotine is well tolerated in early and advanced PD patients. As well, rotigotine administration leads to improvement of motor symptoms in PD.

REFERENCES

1. Marek K, Seibyl J, Shoulson I, Holloway R, Kieburtz K, McDermott M, Kamp C, Shinaman A, Fahn S, Lang A, Weiner W, Welsh M. Dopamine transporter brain imaging to assess the effects of pramipexole vs levodopa on Parkinson disease progression. JAMA 2002; 287:1653–1661.
2. Whone AL, Watts RL, Stoessl AJ, et al. Slower progression of Parkinson's disease with ropinirole versus levodopa: the REAL-PET study. Ann Neurol 2003; 54:93–101.
3. Neumeyer JL, Lai S, Baldessarini RJ. Historical highlihgts of the chemistry, pharmacology, and early clinical uses of apomorphine. In: Gesa GL, Corsini GU, eds. Apomorphine and Other Dopaminomimetics. Vol. 1: Basic Pharmacology. New York: Raven Press, 1981: 1–17.
4. Schwab RS, Amador LV, Lettvin JY. Apomorphine in Parkinsons disease. Trans Am Neurol Accoc 1951; 76:251–253.
5. Duby SE, Cotzias GC, Papavasilious PS, Lawrence WH. Injected apomorphine and orally administered levodopa in parkinsonism. Neurology 1972; 27:474–480.
6. Cotzias GC, Papavasilious PS, Fehling C, Kaufman B, Mena I. Similarities between neurological effects of L-DOPA and of apomorphine. N Engl J Med 1970; 282:31–33.
7. Cotzias GC, Papavasilious PS, Tolosa ES, Mendez J, Bell-Midura M. Treatment of Parkinson's disease with aporphines. N Engl J Med 1976; 294:567–572.
8. Corsini GU, Gessa GL, Del Zompo M, Mangoni A. Therapeutic efficacy of apomorphine combined with an extra-cerebral inhibitor of dopamine receptors in Parkinson's disease. Lancet 1979; 1:954–956.
9. Gancher ST, Woodward WR, Boucher B, Nutt JG. Peripheral pharmacokinetics of apomorphine in humans. Ann Neurol 1989; 26:232–238.
10. Gancher ST, Nutt JG, Woodward WR. Absorption of apomorphine by various routes in parkinsonism. Mov Disord 1991; 6:212–216.
11. Neef C, van Laar T. Pharmacokinetic-pharmacodynamic relationships of apomorphine in patients with Parkinson's disease. Clin Pharmacokinet 1999; 37:257–271.
12. Premkumar ND, Velagaleti PR, Ramanathan R, Ronsen B, Kukulka MJ, Bopp BA. Disposition and metabolism of apomorphine following subcutaneous administration in a bile duct-cannulated beagle dog (abstr). wwww.abclabs.com/dd/idd_posters/adme/tapapodog.pdf.
13. Ondo WG, Hunter C, Vuong KD, Jankovic J. The pharmacokinetic and clinical effects of tolcapone on a single dose of sublingual apomorphine in Parkinson's disease. Parkinsonism Relat Disord. 2000; 6:237–240.
14. Clinical monograph, Uprima® (apomorphine HCl tablets) sublingual. Presentation to the Urology Subcommittee of the Advisory Committee for Reproductive Health Drugs, April 10, 2000. TAP HOLDINGS INC. Data on file in the Food and Drug Administration.
15. Baldesswarini RJ, Arana GW, Kula NS, Campbell A, Harding M. Preclinical studies of the pharmacology of aporphines. In: Gessa GL, Corsini GU, eds. Apomorphine and the Other Dopaminomimetics. Vol. 1: Basic Pharmacology. New York: Raven Press, 1981: 219–228.
16. Clarke CE, Davies P. Systematic review of acute levodopa and apomorphine challenge tests in the diagnosis of idiopathic Parkinson's disease. J Neurol Neurosurg Psychiatry 2000; 69:590–594.
17. Pinter MM, Alesch F, Murg M, Helscher RJ, Binder H. Apomorphine test: a predictor for motor responsiveness to deep brain stimulation of the subthalamic nucleus. J Neurol 1999; 246:907–913.

18. Lozano AM, Lang AE, Levy R, Hutchison W, Dostrovsky J. Neuronal recordings in Parkinson's disease patients with dyskinesias induced by apomorphine. Ann Neurol 2000; 47(4 suppl 1):141–146.
19. Goetz CG, Koller WC, et al. Dopamine agonists: non-ergot derivatives: apomorphine. Mov Disord 2002; 17(suppl 4):S83–S89.
20. Dewey RB, Hutton JT, Le Witt PA, et al. A randomized, double-blind, placebo-controlled trial of subcutaneously injected apomorphine for parkinsonian off-state events. Arch Neurol 2001; 58:1385–1392.
21. Hughes AJ, Bishop S, Kleedorfer B, Turjanski N, Fernandez W, Lees AJ, Stern GM. Subcutaneous apomorphine in Parkinson's disease: response to chronic administration for up to five years. Mov Disord 1993; 8:165–170.
22. Poewe W, Wenning GK. Apomorphine: an underutilized therapy for Parkinson's disease. Mov Disord 2000; 15:789–794.
23. Factor SA, Brown DL, Molho ES. Subcutaneous apomorphine injections as a treatment for intractable pain in Parkinson's disease. Mov Disord 2000; 15:167–169.
24. Colzi A, Turner K, Lees AJ. Continuous subcutaneous waking day apomorphine in the long term treatment of levodopa induced interdose dyskinesias in Parkinson's disease. J Neurol Neurosurg Psychiatry 1998; 64:573–576.
25. Gancher ST, Nutt JG, Woodward WR. Time course of tolerance to apomorphine in parkinsonism. Clin Pharmacol Ther 1992; 52:504–510.
26. Dewey RB, Maraganore DM, Ahlskog JE, et al. A double-blind, placebo-controlled study of intranasal apomorphine spray as a rescue agent for off-states in Parkinson's disease. Mov Disord 1998; 13:782–778.
27. Esteban Munoz J, Marti MJ, Marin C, Tolosa E. Long-term treatment with intermittent intranasal or subcutaneous apormorphine in patients with levodopa-related motor fluctuations. Clin Neuropharmacol 1997; 20:245–252.
28. Ondo W, Hunter C, Almaguer M, Gancher S, Jankovic J. Efficacy and tolerability of a novel sublingual apomorphine preparation in patients with fluctuating Parkinson's disease. Clin Neuropharmaol 1999; 22:1–4.
29. Panegyres PK, Graham SJ, Williams BK, Higgins BM, Morris JGL. Sublingual apomorphine solution in Parkinson's disease. Med J Aust 1991; 155:371–374.
30. Montastruc JL, Rascol O, Senard JM, Gualano V, Bagheri H, Houin G, Lees A, Rascol A. Sublingual apomorphine in Parkinson's disease: a clinical and pharmacokinetic study. Clin Neuropharmacol 1991; 14:432–437.
31. Hughes AJ, Webster R, Bovington M, Lees AJ, Stern GM. Sublingual apomorphine in the treatment of Parkinson's disease complicated by motor fluctuations. Clin Neuropharmacol 1991; 14:556–561.
32. Deffond D, Durif F, Tournilhac M. Apomorphine in treatment of Parkinson's disease: comparison between subcutaneous and sublingual routes. J Neurol Neurosurg Psychiatry 1993; 56:101–103.
33. Klintenberg R, Svenningsson P, Gunne L, Andren PE. Naloxone reduces levodopa-induced dyskinesias and apomorphine-induced rotations in primate models of parkinsonism. J Neural Transm 2002; 109:1295–1307.
34. Pinter MM, Helscher RJ, Mundsperger N, Binder H. Transient increase of pancreatic enzymes evoked by apomorphine in Parkinson's disease. J Neural Transm 1998; 105:1237–1244.
35. Poewe W, Kleedorfer B, Wagner M, Bosch S, Schelosky L. Continuous subcutaneous apomorphine infusions for fluctuating Parkinson's disease. Long-term follow-up in 18 patients.
36. Chase TN. The significance of continuous dopaminergic stimulation in the treatment of Parkinson's disease. Drugs 1998; 55(suppl 1):1–9.
37. Verhagen Metman L, Konitsiotis S, Chase TN. Pathophysiology of motor response complications in Parkinson's disease: hypotheses on the why, where and what. Mov Disord 1999; 14:4–8.
38. Fahn S. for the Parkinson Study Group. Rotigotine Transdermal System (SPM 962) is safe and effective as monotherapy in early Parkinson's disease (abstr). Parkinsonism Rel Disord 2001; 7:S55.
39. Quinn N. for the SP 511 Investigators. Rotigotine Transdermal Delivery System (TDS)(SPM 962)— a multi-center, double-blind, randomized, placebo-controlled trial to assess the safety and efficacy of Rotigotine TDS in patients with advanced Parkinson's disease (abstr). Parkinsonism Rel Disord 2001; 7:S66.
40. Verhagen Metman L, Gillespie M, Farmer C, Bibbiani F, Konitsiotis S, Morris M, Shill H, Bara-Jimenez W, Mouradin MM, Chase TN. Continous transdermal dopaminergic stimulation in advanced Parkinson's disease. Clin Neuropharmacol 2001; 24:163–169.

14
Tolcapone

Paul J. Tuite and Brian A. Weisenberg

University of Minnesota, Minneapolis, Minnesota, U.S.A.

I. INTRODUCTION

A. Overview

Tolcapone (3,4-dihydroxy-4'-methyl-5-nitrobenzophenone) is a reversible inhibitor of catechol-O-methyltransferase (COMT), an enzyme responsible for the central and peripheral metabolism of levodopa (1,2). By inhibiting COMT, tolcapone improves the pharmacokinetics of levodopa in patients with fluctuating Parkinson's disease (PD), thereby providing clinical benefits such as decreased motor fluctuations, increased on-time, decreased off-time, and a reduction of the total levodopa dose (3–8).

B. Levodopa Therapy and Motor Fluctuations

After 10 years of levodopa treatment, approximately 70–80% of patients develop motor fluctuations and dyskinesias (9). Motor fluctuations are characterized by fluctuations in mobility where patients have "on" periods, in which they are responsive to medications, and "off" periods, where they are unresponsive or insufficiently responsive to medication. These fluctuations may occur at predictable or unpredicatable times after a dose, or there can be rapid cycling from on to off. As the disease progresses, the response to a single dose of levodopa shortens and eventually approximates the plasma half-life of the drug (60–90 minutes) (10). These changes probably relate to the loss of dopaminergic neurons in the substantia nigra and a decreased ability to store, synthesize, and release dopamine—i.e., the dopamine storage hypothesis (11). Thus, there is limited ability to buffer the oscillating plasma and brain concentrations of levodopa resulting in motor fluctuations. Fluctuations are reduced when levodopa is administered continuously by the intravenous route (12). Based on this and other research, it has been proposed that tonic as opposed to phasic stimulation of dopamine receptors may provide a better clinical benefit and lessened risk of motor complications (10). Researchers have attempted to minimize plasma levodopa fluctuations to address these concerns (13). This has been done by administering levodopa in a controlled-release formulation to provide more stable plasma levels of levodopa and by inhibiting peripheral levodopa metabolism with COMT inhibitors.

C. Rationale for COMT Inhibition

Levodopa is converted to dopamine in the periphery by aromatic amino acid decarboxylase (AADC) and into 3-O-methyldopa (3-OMD) by COMT (Fig. 1) (14). As a result, only 5–10% of orally administered levodopa crosses the blood-brain barrier (15). Carbidopa or benserazide are used to inhibit the activity of AADC in the gut wall, increasing the amount of levodopa that crosses the blood-brain barrier by a factor of 2 and decreasing the amount of levodopa required to produce a clinical benefit by 70–80% (14,16). The inhibition of AADC, however, shifts the metabolism of levodopa to COMT. COMT is a widely distributed enzyme found in the gut wall, liver, kidneys, muscles, erythrocytes, and brain.

Metabolism of levodopa by COMT results in the production of 3-OMD, a nonreactive metabolite with a half-life of approximately 15 hours. 3-OMD competes with levodopa for transport across the blood-brain barrier via the large neutral amino acid (LNAA) transporter, and at high concentrations has been shown to reduce the efficacy of levodopa in animal models and PD patients. This competitive inhibition by 3-OMD

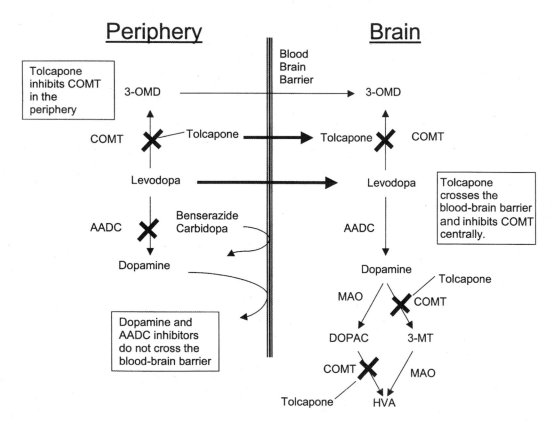

Figure 1 Central and peripheral metabolism of levodopa and the role of tolcapone and AADC inhibitors. AADC = aromatic amino acid decarboxylase; 3-OMD = 3-O-methyldopa; COMT = catechol-O-methyltransferase; MAO = monoamine oxidase; DOPAC = 3,4-dihydroxyphenylacetic acid; HVA = homovanillic acid; 3-MT = 3-methoxytyramine. (Adapted from Ref. 15.)

has not been shown to be clinically significant (17). Thus, by inhibiting COMT and AADC—both avenues for the peripheral metabolism of levodopa—bioavailability of levodopa is increased in the brain (15).

Once levodopa has crossed the blood-brain barrier it can be metabolized centrally by COMT to 3-OMD or by AADC to dopamine (15). However, the central conversion of levodopa into dopamine by AADC is crucial for its clinical benefit. This occurs because inhibitors of AADC such as carbidopa and benserazide do not cross the blood-brain barrier. Subsequently, dopamine is metabolized into 3,4-dihydroxyphenylacetic acid (DOPAC) by monoamine oxidase (MAO) or to 3-methoxytyramine by COMT. DOPAC and 3-MT are then converted to homovanillic acid (HVA) by COMT and MAO. Central inhibition of COMT by tolcapone increases the amount of levodopa converted into dopamine and decreases dopamine metabolism (2,16,18).

II. CLINICAL INFORMATION

A. Pharmacokinetics

Early pharmacokinetic studies investigated tolcapone in single- and multiple-dose administrations with and without concomitant administration of levodopa (Tables 1–3) (19–21). Tolcapone was investigated in 72 healthy young men in a double-blind

Table 1 Pharmacokinetics of Tolcapone[a]

Parameter	Tolcapone single dose		Tolcapone TID regimen[b]	
	100 mg	200 mg	100 mg	200 mg
C_{max} (µg/mL)				
TOL	4.6 ± 2.0	6.3 ± 2.9		
TOL + LDOPA/BEN	4.5 ± 0.8	7.5 ± 1.8	5.1 ± 1.0	7.4 ± 3.3
TOL + LDOPA/CAR	3.8 ± 1.9	8.0 ± 1.5		
t_{max} (h)				
TOL	1.7 ± 1.3	1.8 ± 1.3		
TOL + LDOPA/BEN	0.7 ± 0.3	1.9 ± 1.8	1.2 ± 0.4	1.2 ± 0.5
TOL + LDOPA/CAR	2.6 ± 1.4	2.9 ± 1.3		
AUC (h • µg/mL)				
TOL	12.2 ± 2.3[c]	18.5 ± 5.2		
TOL + LDOPA/BEN	10.2 ± 1.3	24.0 ± 9.8	13.1 ± 1.8	23.9 ± 7.9
TOL + LDOPA/CAR	10.7 ± 3.5	19.6 ± 3.0		
$t_{1/2}$ (h)				
TOL	2.0 ± 0.7[c]	2.1 ± 0.6		
TOL + LDOPA/BEN	1.9 ± 0.3	2.0 ± 0.3	2.8 ± 1.0	2.9 ± 0.5
TOL + LDOPA/CAR	1.7 ± 0.5	1.9 ± 0.45		

C_{max} = maximum plasma concentration; t_{max} = time to maximum plasma concentration; AUC = area under the curve; $t_{1/2}$ = half-life. TOL = Tolcapone; TOL + LDOPA/BEN = Tolcapone Tolcapone co-administered with levodopa/benserazide 100/25 mg; TOL + LDOPA/CAR = Tolcapone co-administered with levodopa/carbidopa 100/25 mg.
[a]Means ± standard deviation; $n = 6$.
[b]After 7 days of treatment.
[c]$n = 5$.
Source: Refs. 19,20,24,25.

Table 2 Pharmacokinetics of Levodopa Co-Administered with Tolcapone[a]

Parameter	Tolcapone single dose		Tolcapone tid dose[b]	
	100 mg	200 mg	100 mg	200 mg
C_{max} (μg/mL)	1.6 ± 0.6	1.3 ± 0.3	1.4 ± 0.9	1.2 ± 0.5
t_{max} (h)	0.9 ± 0.6	0.8 ± 0.5	1.0 ± 0.0	1.0 ± 0.0
AUC (h • μg/mL)	3.3 ± 0.6	3.3 ± 0.6	4.5 ± 2.0	4.1 ± 1.3
$t_{1/2}$ (h)	2.0 ± 0.2	2.3 ± 0.4	2.2 ± 0.5	2.1 ± 0.3

Source: Refs. 24,25.
C_{max} = maximum plasma concentration; t_{max} = time to maximum plasma concentration; AUC = area under the curve; $t_{1/2}$ = half-life.
[a]Levodopa administered as levodopa/benserazide 100/25 mg; means ± standard deviation, $n = 6$.
[b]After 7 days of treatment; $n = 8$.

randomized, placebo-controlled, parallel-group study using single oral tolcapone doses (5, 10, 25, 50, 100, 200, 400, or 800 mg) (20). Another study of 44 healthy young men examined the effects of a placebo or single dose of tolcapone at varying amounts (10, 25, 50, 100, 200, 400, or 800 mg), co-administered with a single dose of levodopa/benserazide (100/25 mg) (19). These two single-dose studies showed that tolcapone is absorbed at all doses (5–800 mg), and the time to reach the maximum plasma concentration, t_{max}, is approximately 2 hours whether or not it is administered with levodopa/benserazide (19,20). The time necessary to decrease the plasma concentration of tolcapone by half (elimination $t_{1/2}$) averaged 2–3 hours.

A study of 62 healthy men and women aged 55–80 years assessed the pharmacokinetics of tolcapone (100, 200, 400, or 800 mg) or placebo given three times a day (21). Each subject received a single unblinded dose of levodopa/benserazide one hour after the first tolcapone or placebo dose of the day. There was no significant difference between the single and multiple dosing regimens for the 100 or 200 mg tolcapone groups as measured by C_{max}, t_{max}, $t_{1/2}$, or the area under the curve (AUC). The pharmacokinetics of tolcapone were linear for these two concentrations. The 400 and 800 mg groups showed no difference between the single and multiple doses as measured by C_{max}, t_{max}, or $t_{1/2}$. However, the average AUC for the multiple tolcapone doses was greater for both the 400 and 800 mg groups. It was suggested that this accumulation occurred due to lower tolcapone metabolism at higher doses. It should be noted, however, that the highest plasma concentration of

Table 3 Tolcapone Pharmacological Data

Bioavailability	Approximately 60%[a]
Volume of distribution	9 L[a]
Total protein binding	> 99.9%[a]
Total clearance	7 L/h[a]
Excretion	Renal 60%, Feces 40%[b]
Metabolism	99% in liver; undergoes glucouronidation, methylation by COMT, and oxidation by cytochrome P450[b]

[a]From Ref. 42.
[b]From Ref. 43.

tolcapone (43.1 μg/mL) observed after a week of 800 mg three times per day (tid) regimen was substantially below the concentration associated with toxicity in animal studies (100 μg/mL).

These single- and multiple-dose tolcapone studies also yielded information on the pharmacokinetics of 3-O-methyltolcapone (3-OMT), a COMT-derived metabolite of tolcapone (19,20). Specifically, there was a dose-dependent increase in t_{max}, but no dose-dependent increase in C_{max}. The elimination $t_{1/2}$ of 3-OMT was 30–40 hours and was not dose-dependent (21). In addition, the concentration of 3-OMT was 35-fold lower than those levels resulting in toxicity in animals.

B. Pharmacodynamics

1. Single-Dose Tolcapone

In addition to studying the pharmacokinetics of tolcapone, the studies mentioned above investigated COMT inhibition by tolcapone and resultant impact on the pharmacokinetics of levodopa and its metabolite 3-OMD (Table 2). The single-dose tolcapone studies showed dose-dependent COMT inhibition in erythrocytes (19–21). The tolcapone concentration to inhibit 50% of erythrocyte COMT activity (EC_{50}) was approximately 1 μg/mL. The time until onset of maximal COMT inhibition (t_{Emax}) was less than 2 hours. The inhibition of COMT activity was reversible, and time to recovery of baseline levels of COMT activity was dose-dependent.

2. Single-Dose Tolcapone with Levodopa + Benserazide

The administration of levodopa/benserazide 100/25 mg had no effect on COMT inhibition by tolcapone at 10–800 mg (19). Time to COMT inhibition remained 1–2 hours. The EC_{50} remained 1 μg/mL, and time to recovery to baseline for 100 and 200 mg was 15–21 hours. Tolcapone doses $\geq$100 mg yielded COMT inhibition greater than 80%.

3. Multiple-Dose Tolcapone

In comparing single- and multiple-dose studies of tolcapone, there was no difference in the EC_{50} values and the degree of COMT inhibition between the two studies, and COMT inhibition remained unchanged with multiple doses (21). The authors concluded that multiple dosing does not lead to pharmacodynamic tolerance.

4. Effect of Single-Dose Tolcapone on Pharmacokinetics of Levodopa

With regard to the effect of tolcapone on levodopa and 3-OMD, single oral tolcapone doses with levodopa/benserazide increased levodopa $t_{1/2}$ and AUC and reduced the mean C_{max} and AUC for 3-OMD, implying inhibition of COMT activity (19). It has also been shown that changing tolcapone doses does not affect the duration and magnitude of COMT inhibition (22,23). In these studies, levodopa t_{max} did not change when administered with tolcapone doses up to 200 mg (24). At tolcapone concentrations >200 mg, the t_{max} for levodopa increased, possibly due to competition for absorption with tolcapone (19). The AUC of levodopa was also increased by tolcapone doses up to 200 mg. The 200 mg dose of tolcapone produced the maximum effect, a twofold increase in levodopa AUC (24,25). This study also found that tolcapone caused levodopa's elimination $t_{1/2}$ to increase without changing its C_{max}. Despite the number of studies that suggest that C_{max} of levodopa is unaffected by co-administration of tolcapone, a recent study reported that C_{max} of levodopa does increase with co-administration of tolcapone and proposed that this may provide an explanation for increased dyskinesias early in the course of tolcapone treatment (26).

5. Effect of Multiple-Dose Tolcapone on Pharmacokinetics of Levodopa

Tolcapone 100–800 mg tid produced the same effect on levodopa and 3-OMD pharmaco-kinetics as seen in the single-dose study (21). More recently, Jorga et al. investigated the pharmacokinetics of levodopa with multiple tolcapone doses in patients with PD (27). Four hundred and twelve patients with fluctuating and nonfluctuating motor symptoms received either placebo or tolcapone in addition to a levodopa decarboxylase inhibitor in three multicenter, parallel, double-blind, placebo-controlled, dose-finding studies. It was shown that the fraction of levodopa metabolized to 3-OMD was reduced by co-administration of tolcapone in a dose-dependent fashion for both fluctuators and non-fluctuators. This led to a decreased clearance of levodopa by 15–25% in fluctuators and 20–30% in nonfluctuators. As a result, the levodopa dosage was reduced during the study, with a resultant total daily levodopa exposure increase of 11% for the 50 mg tid tolcapone dose and 16% for the 200 and 400 mg tid doses. The fluctuations of plasma levodopa ($C_{max} - C_{min}$) were reduced in a dose-dependent fashion. This raises the possibility that the clinical benefit of tolcapone may lie in its ability to reduce plasma fluctuations rather than increase patient exposure to levodopa. This may have some significance related to the research question of possible dose-related toxicity from levodopa either in affecting the rate of disease progression or development of motor complications. Nonetheless, evidence to support the theories of levodopa toxicity remains sparse (28).

C. Clinical Studies with Tolcapone

1. Studies in Patients with Fluctuating Parkinson's Disease

Several pivotal studies have been performed that assessed the use of tolcapone in patients with PD who were experiencing motor fluctuations (Table 4).

In a 6-week, multicenter, double-blind, placebo-controlled study of 151 fluctuating PD subjects, Kurth et al. measured the percent off-time during two 10-hour observational evaluations (at day −1 and day 42) as the primary measure of efficacy (4). Patients in all treatment groups showed a significant reduction in off time after 6 weeks (placebo: −0.4% ± 2.7%; 50 mg tid: −16.6% ± 2.7%; 200 mg tid: −16.1% ± 2.8%; 400 mg tid: −18.1% ± 3.0%). The Unified Parkinson's Disease Rating Scale (UPDRS) motor subscale was also used as a primary measure of efficacy and the AUC was significantly different for all treatment groups (placebo: −11.4 ± 8.6; 50 mg tid: −44.8 ± 8.9; 200 mg tid: −37 ± 8.9; 400 mg tid: −49.1 ± 10.1). As a secondary measure of efficacy the authors quantified on-time with and without dyskinesia during the 10-hour evaluation and found significant increases for all treatment groups compared to placebo (placebo: −1.2 ± 2.8%; 50 mg tid: 16.9 ± 2.9%; 200 mg tid: 16.3 ± 2.6%; 400 mg tid: 16.0 ± 3.2%). Increases in on-time and decreases in off-time were also seen from patient diary evaluations: (a) off-time: placebo: −5%; 50 mg tid: −24%; 200 mg tid: −19%; 400 mg tid: −43%; (b) on-time: placebo: +6%; 50 mg tid: +12%; 200 mg tid: +4%; 400 mg tid: +25%. Levodopa dosage was reduced in all tolcapone-treated groups (placebo: 3.2%; 50 mg tid: 15.4%; 200 mg tid: 26.3%; 400 mg tid: 23.1%), and a significant improvement was observed in an investiga-tor's global assessment (IGA) of change. Other efficacy measures assessed for changes in the UPDRS subscales I (mentation), II (activities of daily living), and III (motor), but there was no significant improvement. Entry criteria for this study included at least three daily doses of immediate-release carbidopa/levodopa, predictable on-times with the first carbidopa/levodopa dosage of the day, and at least two wearing-off episodes lasting a total of more than 2 hours.

Table 4 Long-Term Placebo-Controlled Trials of Tolcapone in Fluctuating and Nonfluctuating Patients

Duration	Dose (mg)	n	Change in on-time (h)[a,b,c]	Change in off-time (h)[a,b,c]	Change in total daily levodopa dose (mg)[a,b]	Change in levodopa intake[a,b]
Fluctuating						
6 weeks	Placebo	28	+0.4	−0.4	−31.2 (29.4)	N/A
	50	25	+0.9	−1.7*	−139 (31)	
	200	26	+0.3	−1.3*	−200 (31)	
	400	26	+1.8	−3.2*	−175 (34)	
6 weeks	Placebo	42	−0.4	−0.1	2.4 (18.0)	N/A
	50	37	+1.6*	−0.9	−56.0 (19.8)	
	200	38	+2.1**	−1.8*	−79.1 (19.9)**	
	400	37	+1.4*	−1.2	−13.3 (20.2)	
3 months	Placebo	66	N/A	−1.4	+15.5 (22.5)	−0.1 (0.1)
	100	69		−2.3	−166.3 (22.3)**	−0.6 (0.1)**
	200	67		−3.2**	−207.1 (22.6)**	−0.7 (0.1)**
6 weeks	Placebo	72	+0.3 (0.3)	−0.3 (0.3)	−0.5 (20.1)	0.0 (0.1)
	100	69	+2.1 (0.3)***	−2.0 (0.3)***	−185.5 (20.6)***	−0.5 (0.1)**
	200	74	+2.3 (0.3)***	−2.5 (0.3)***	−251.5 (19.9)***	−1.2 (0.1)***
3 months	Placebo	58	−0.1 (0.5)	−0.7 (0.4)	−28.9 (26.2)	N/A
	100	60	+1.7 (0.4)	−2.0 (0.3)	−108.9 (23.4)*	
	200	59	+1.7 (0.4)	−1.6 (0.3)	−122.2 (23.9)**	
Nonfluctuating						
6 weeks	Placebo	33	N/A	N/A	−113.9 (22.5)	−1.1 (0.2)
	200	32			−182.0 (23.4)	−1.3 (0.2)
	400	32			−180.6 (23.8)	−1.5 (0.2)
6 months	Placebo	102	N/A	N/A	46.6 (9.6)	N/A
	100	98			−20.8 (9.7)**	
	200	98			−32.3 (9.6)**	

[a]Data given as means with standard error of the mean (SEM) in parentheses where available.
[b]Values calculated by subtracting from baseline.
[c]Changes in on and off time are given as percentage of waking day. In order to provide data in terms of hours in the table, percentages were multiplied by 16 hours.
*$p < 0.05$; **$p < 0.01$; ***$p < 0.001$.

The treatment was well tolerated, with primarily dopaminergic adverse events (dyskinesia and nausea) occurring more in the tolcapone-treated groups than with placebo and being minimized or eliminated by reducing the dosage of carbidopa/levodopa. Other adverse events that occurred more often in the tolcapone-treated groups included postural hypotension, dizziness, and urine discoloration. There was no difference in efficacy between those with and those without adverse events. Furthermore, no remarkable changes in vital signs or laboratory tests were seen. Five patients were withdrawn due to adverse events. Increasing abdominal pain with the 400 mg dose was reported as serious in one instance. This adverse event diminished after discontinuing the trial medication, but returned after initiating higher doses of levodopa. It was suggested that this adverse event was the result of tolcapone potentiating the levodopa, not an effect of the tolcapone itself.

A different 6-week placebo-controlled study, performed by Myllylä and colleagues, measured the effect of tolcapone (50, 200, or 400 mg tid) in 154 PD patients using patient diaries (3). Changes in on- and off-time, the primary measures of efficacy, were significantly improved. The percentage of on-time for the waking day was increased for all doses of tolcapone, with the 200 mg tid dose showing the greatest increase (placebo: −2.1%; 50 mg tid: +10.3%; 200 mg tid: +13.0%; 400 mg tid: +8.9%). Off-time decreased for all doses as well, but only the 200 mg tid dose provided a statistically significant change (placebo: −0.7%; 50 mg tid: −5.9%; 200 mg tid: −11.1%; 400 mg tid: −7.2%). Secondary measures of efficacy included UPDRS subscale scores, IGA scores, and changes in levodopa dose. The IGA scores showed improvement in all treatment groups with the 200 mg tid dose providing the greatest improvement. The UPDRS scores showed no statistically significant improvement, although the activity of daily living (ADL) and motor function scores showed the most improvement in the 200 and 400 mg tid doses. Levodopa was reduced in all tolcapone-treated groups, but only the 200 mg tid dose provided a significant reduction (placebo: 2.4 mg; 50 mg tid: −56.0; 200 mg tid: −79.1; 400 mg tid: −13.3 mg). Overall, 100 out of 154 subjects experienced an adverse event, but only 7 (4 in the 200 mg tid group and one each in the other groups) experienced a serious adverse event. Of these, 2 in the 200 mg tid group reported hallucinations and confusion resulting in hospitilization. Ten patients withdrew from the study (placebo: 3; 50 mg tid: 2; 200 mg tid: 1; 400 mg tid: 3). The most frequent adverse events were levodopa-related, and only dyskinesia, nausea, and muscle cramps occurred more in tolcapone-treated patients than in placebo. No changes in vital signs, laboratory values, or electrocardiogram (ECG) abnormalities could be attributed to tolcapone. Patients in tolcapone-treated groups had fewer incidences of vital sign abnormalities.

A double-blind, placebo-controlled, multicenter study measured the efficacy of tolcapone (100 or 200 mg tid) using patient diaries in 202 fluctuating PD patients (5). Using off-time as a primary measure of efficacy, Rajput and colleagues demonstrated 48% (3.25 hours) less off-time after 3 months in patients taking 200 mg of tolcapone three times a day. The 100 mg tid tolcapone regimen reduced off-time by 32% (2.3 hours), but this was not statistically significant. Results of secondary efficacy measures included a reduction of total daily levodopa dosage for both tolcapone treatment groups (100 mg tid: −21%; 200 mg tid: −23.9%; and placebo increased 1.5%), significant improvements in wearing off, lessening of the severity of PD symptoms, and improvement in overall efficacy for both tolcapone treatment regimens as measured by IGA scores. UPDRS subscales I, II, III, and the total score were not significantly improved. Twenty-eight percent of the patients continued study participation for an additional 9 months, and those who experienced a reduction in off-time at 3 months maintained this benefit at 12 months. Subjects were allowed to increase their levodopa dose in this continuation study to maintain benefit. Within the group of continuing patients, 80% of 100 mg tid patients and 88% of the 200 mg tid patients showed improvement in IGA scores at 12 months compared to 30% of placebo-treated patients. Entry criteria for this study included patients who were taking carbidopa/levodopa at least four times a day (or three times a day if two of the three were a controlled-release formula), had been treated with levodopa for at least a year, and had a clinical response to levodopa.

Nearly all of the patients in the study experienced at least one adverse event, but most were mild or moderate and were side effects commonly associated with levodopa treatment. Overall, 18% of patients (37) withdrew from the study due to adverse events. Dyskinesia developed or worsened in 18% of placebo, 51% of 100 mg tid, and 64% of

200 mg tid-treated groups, but was never a reason for withdrawal from the study. Diarrhea was the most frequent nondopaminergic adverse event and the most common reason given for withdrawal, followed by hallucinations, muscle cramps, confusion, and nausea. Few clinically significant differences in vital signs, ECG, or laboratory tests were observed between treatment groups. Five tolcapone-treated patients (3 in 100 mg tid, 2 in 200 mg tid groups) showed elevated aspartate (AST) and alanine aminotransferase (ALT) concentrations; one in the 200 mg tid group showed levels three to five times normal and withdrew as a result. Results of this patient's liver tests following withdrawal from the study were not reported.

Another study evaluated 215 fluctuating PD subjects and confirmed the efficacy and tolerability of tolcapone at 100 or 200 mg tid using changes in off-time from baseline as a primary measure of efficacy (7). Analysis of patient diaries after 6 weeks of treatment showed that tolcapone-treated groups experienced a significant reduction in off-time (placebo: -0.3 h; 100 mg tid: -2 h; 200 mg tid: -2.5 h) and increased on-time (placebo: $+0.3$ h; 100 mg tid: $+2.1$ h; 200 mg tid: $+2.3$ h). With regard to secondary measures, IGA scores showed significant improvement in "wearing-off" phenomenon, symptom severity, and overall efficacy in more tolcapone-treated patients than placebo (placebo: 19%; 100 mg tid: 50%; 200 mg tid: 57%), and the total daily levodopa dosage was reduced more in tolcapone-treated patients (placebo: 19%; 100 mg tid: 23%; 200 mg tid: 29%). There were no significant changes in the total or subscale scores of the UPDRS. Entry criteria in this study included patients who had been treated with and responded to carbidopa/levodopa for at least one year, showed predictable wearing off that could not be eliminated by altering the antiparkinsonian medication regimen, and had been taking at least four daily doses of carbidopa/levodopa (or three doses if two of the three were a controlled-release formula) with a minimum of 20 mg of carbidopa per dose of levodopa or total daily carbidopa dose of 70 mg.

Adverse events were experienced in 74, 86, and 97% of the placebo, 100 mg tid, and 200 mg tid groups, respectively, but only 14% were considered severe. Thirteen patients withdrew, 11 due to adverse events. The most frequent adverse events were dopaminergic: dyskinesia, nausea, dystonia, anorexia, confusion, hallucinations, and excessive dreaming. They occurred more frequently in the 200 mg tid dose group, and could be reversed with decreased levodopa. Dyskinesia occurred more often in tolcapone-treated groups than with placebo but was never a reason for withdrawal from the study. The most frequent nondopaminergic adverse events were dizziness, increased sweating, and dry mouth. There were no significant changes in vital signs, ECG, or laboratory tests.

A similar study performed in Europe assessed tolcapone 100 or 200 mg tid in combination with levodopa/benserazide in 177 fluctuating PD patients for 3 months (8). Using self-reported off-time from patient diaries as the primary measure of efficacy, tolcapone-treated groups had less off-time (placebo: -11.1%; 100 mg tid: -31.5%; 200 mg tid: -26.2%), but only the 100 mg tid group achieved statistical significance. On-time, however, was significantly increased in both tolcapone-treated groups (placebo: -1.3%; 100 mg tid: $+21.3\%$, 200 mg tid: $+20.6\%$). Results of secondary measures of efficacy included a significantly decreased mean total daily levodopa dose (placebo: -4.3%; 100 mg tid: -16.3%; 200 mg tid: -18%), improved IGA scores (placebo: 37% of patients; 100 mg tid: 70%, 200 mg tid: 78%), a reduction in UPDRS motor scores for the 200 mg tid tolcapone–treated group, and an improved quality of life as measured by the Sickness Impact Profile (SIP) in both treatment groups.

Some patients continued participation in the study for an additional 6 months beyond the primary 3-month endpoint. For the 100 mg tid group, only the decrease in off-time was maintained, whereas in the 200 mg tid group the increase in on-time and the reduction of levodopa dose were maintained in addition to decreased off-time. The entry criteria for this study included patients who had predictable end-of-dose fluctuations in response to levodopa therapy, had been treated with levodopa for one year with clear improvement, and were on a stable regimen of levodopa/benserazide and any other antiparkinsonian drugs for at least 4 weeks. In this study, both dosages of tolcapone were well tolerated. Twenty-seven patients withdrew due to adverse events. Diarrhea was the only adverse event that led to early withdrawal from the study more often than placebo. The most common levodopa-related adverse event was dyskinesia, followed by hallucinations and orthostatic hypotension. No differences in vital signs or ECG results were observed among the study groups. Abnormal AST and ALT levels were observed in three patients, but only one withdrew from the study.

2. Studies in Patients with Nonfluctuating Parkinson's Disease

Other studies have investigated the use of tolcapone in PD patients without fluctuations. Waters and colleagues conducted a 6-month, double-blind, placebo-controlled study of tolcapone (100 or 200 mg tid) in 298 patients with PD who were receiving levodopa but were not experiencing motor fluctuations (29). This study used UPDRS ADLs as the primary measure of efficacy and was able to show significant improvement in both tolcapone-treated groups. There was also improvement in UPDRS mentation, motor, and total scores for both treatment groups. Fewer patients had fluctuations in the tolcapone-treated groups than those in the placebo group, and patients in the tolcapone-treated groups decreased their total daily levodopa intake (placebo: +12.8%; 100 mg tid: −6%; 200 mg tid: −9%). Patients in both treatment groups also showed improvement in the SIP but only the improvement in the physical subscale was significant. Reductions observed at 6 months in levodopa dosage, and improvements in the UPDRS scores and SIP were maintained through month 12 in patients who completed a continuation study. Selection criteria for this study included patients who were taking carbidopa/levodopa, were stable for at least 4 weeks, had shown improvement with treatment, and had a UPDRS ADL score of 3 or more.

A total of 49 patients withdrew from the study due to adverse events. The only adverse event that led to withdrawal more in the tolcapone-treated group than the placebo group was diarrhea. Common dopaminergic side effects were seen and included nausea, dyskinesia, anorexia, sleep disorders, and vomiting. No significant abnormalities in vital signs or ECGs were observed with tolcapone treatment. Elevated liver enzymes were observed in three (3%) and five (5%) of the 100 and 200 mg tid tolcapone-treated groups, respectively. Four of these patients were withdrawn from the study, and the other four returned to normal while on treatment. All cases of elevated liver enzymes developed within 1–6 months of beginning treatment.

A different study conducted by Dupont et al. investigated the use of tolcapone in stable PD patients whose wearing-off phenomena was controlled by an increase in levodopa dosing frequency (30). In this double-blind, placebo-controlled study, 97 patients were given tolcapone (200 mg tid, 400 mg tid, or placebo) for 6 weeks, at which time the change in levodopa dose from baseline was used as a primary efficacy measure. The observed reduction in total daily levodopa dose was greater with both tolcapone groups than placebo but was not statistically significant (placebo: −19%; 200 mg tid: −27%;

400 mg tid: -25%). Secondary measures of efficacy were IGA of severity of PD symptoms and UPDRS subscale and total scores. After 6 weeks, UPDRS scores were improved most in the 200 mg tid tolcapone group, but only the improvement in ADL scores reached statistical significance. The changes in UPDRS scores were not improved compared to placebo for the 400 mg tid group. The results indicate that the reduction in levodopa dosage in the tolcapone-treated groups did not come at the expense of the other measures of efficacy. Patients receiving tolcapone were then crossed over for an additional 3 weeks to receive the other dosage of tolcapone. Entry criteria included patients who had moderately advanced PD. Selegiline and apomorphine were not allowed during the study, but other antiparkinsonian medications were permitted if the dosage regimen had been stable for 2 months prior to the study.

The most frequently reported dopaminergic adverse events were nausea and dyskinesia. Nausea occurred more frequently in tolcapone-treated groups than with placebo and was occasionally accompanied by vomiting. These episodes occurred more at the beginning of the study and were resolved without treatment. Dyskinesia occurred most in the 200 mg tid tolcapone group. UPDRS scores showed no change in incidence of intensity of painful dyskinesias or early morning dystonias. The duration of dyskinesias did increase slightly in tolcapone-treated groups, but this was not considered statistically significant. Diarrhea was the most frequent adverse event. Four patients withdrew from the study due to adverse events related to treatment. Two patients withdrew due to diarrhea; one withdrew due to hallucinations; and one withdrew due to headache, excessive dreaming, and vomiting. These events resolved without sequelae after the study medication was withdrawn.

III. SAFETY

A. Overview

Clinical trials showed that tolcapone is relatively well tolerated (see previous section). Most adverse events were dopaminergic and were rarely a reason for early withdrawal from treatment. Nondopaminergic adverse events were the most common reason for withdrawal from the studies, but even these were relatively uncommon. Despite the tolerability of tolcapone, there were cases of liver dysfunction that prompted the U.S. Food and Drug Administration (FDA) to recommend monitoring of liver function at the time of approval of tolcapone.

B. Hepatic Failure

Following the previously mentioned work where elevated liver transaminases led to withdrawal from studies (5,8,29), Assal and colleagues reported a fatal case of fulminant hepatic failure attributable to tolcapone in June 1998 (31). Three more cases of liver failure—two of which were fatal—were observed by October 1998 after tolcapone was used by approximately 60,000 patients worldwide (a total of 40,000 patient-years) (32–34). On November 12, 1998, the European Agency for the Evaluation of Medicinal Products (EMEA) recommended the suspension of the marketing authorization for tolcapone (35). In the United States, the FDA advised that a revised label with a boxed warning be issued for the drug (32–34). The revised label includes the following text:

1. Tolcapone should not be used by patients until they have discussed the risks with their physician and the patient has provided written informed consent.

2. Tolcapone should only be used in patients with PD who are experiencing symptom fluctuations and are not responding satisfactorily to, or are not appropriate candidates for other adjunctive therapy.

3. Tolcapone therapy should be withdrawn if patients do not show substantial benefit within 3 weeks of initiation.

4. Tolcapone should not be used in patients who exhibit clinical evidence of liver disease or who have had two serum glutamic-pyruvic transaminase (SGPT/ALT) or glutamic-oxaloacetic transaminase (SGOT/AST) values greater than the upper limits of normal. Patients with severe dyskinesia or dystonia should be treated with caution due to a possible association of tolcapone with rhabdomyolysis.

5. For patients starting treatment with tolcapone serum SGPT/ALT and SGOT/AST values should be determined at baseline and monitored every 2 weeks for the first year, every 4 weeks for the next 6 months, and every 8 weeks thereafter. If the dose is increased to 200 mg tid, liver enzyme monitoring should take place before increasing the dose and then be reinitiated at the frequency above.

6. Patients who develop liver dysfunction while on tolcapone and are withdrawn from the drug may be at increased risk for liver injury if tolcapone is reintroduced. These patients should not ordinarily be considered for retreatment with tolcapone.

7. Tolcapone therapy should be discontinued if SGPT/ALT or SGOT/AST level(s) exceed the upper limits of normal, or if clinical signs and symptoms suggest the onset of hepatic failure (persistent nausea, fatigue, lethargy, anorexia, jaundice, dark urine, pruritis, and right upper quadrant tenderness).

In response to these events, Roche Laboratories Inc. assembled a panel of neurologists and hepatologists to review the cases and make recommendations (34). It was the opinion of the panel that the new FDA labeling requirements were exceptionally restrictive and would cause many patients to unnecessarily stop using the drug. In making their argument, the panel noted that in all cases liver dysfunction developed within the first 6 months of tolcapone treatment, and no other cases developed after that time. Furthermore, the recommended guidelines for monitoring liver function were not followed; in three patients no liver monitoring was performed at all. In two cases, the patients continued receiving tolcapone even after clinical symptoms of liver dysfunction developed. The panel noted that no cases of hepatic dysfunction have been reported when the recommended monitoring schedule was followed. Based on these observations, the panel reached a consensus on the following assertions:

1. Tolcapone is an effective adjunctive treatment to levodopa in patients with fluctuating PD and can be used safely in patients who benefit from the drug and are free of liver dysfunction.

2. It is probably not necessary to restrict the drug to patients who have not responded to other therapies because the risk of developing liver injury is virtually negligible with the new monitoring schedule.

3. If it can be confirmed that liver dysfunction and enzyme abnormalities only occur during the first 6 months of treatment, it may be possible to reduce the frequency of monitoring liver function after 6 months.

4. The requirement that tolcapone be withdrawn if liver enzyme levels are elevated above the upper limit of normal is a stricter standard than has been imposed

on drugs with a known risk of hepatotoxic effects, and may therefore be unnecessarily restrictive. A limit of two to three times the upper limit of normal should be used as a criterion for discontinuing tolcapone.

No literature has been published as of yet addressing these assertions.

C. Neuroleptic Malignant-Like Syndrome

Neuroleptic malignant-like syndrome (NMLS) is a side effect associated with neuroleptic agents and withdrawal of antiparkinsonian medications (36). Currently no defined diagnostic criteria exist, but symptoms seen include hyperthermia, akinesia, altered consciousness, rigidity, autonomic dysfunction, tachypnea, and elevated serum creatinine phosphokinase levels (37,38). The clinical course of NMLS is often marked by the onset of rigidity and autonomic changes, followed within hours by fever and altered levels of consciousness. Aspiration pneumonia often occurs; tachyarrhythmias and hypertension—secondary to autonomic instability—increase the risk of myocardial infarction. Furthermore, rhabdomyolysis from the severe rigidity can lead to acute renal failure (37,38). It is hypothesized that central dopaminergic impairment is responsible for NMLS (39).

There have been two reports of NMLS in patients with PD who were receiving tolcapone. In one instance NMLS occurred concomitantly with acute hepatitis and administration of clozapine (40). While hepatocellular injury and NMLS following tolcapone withdrawal are known side effects, no other reports have been published that describe the occurrence of NMLS concurrent with tolcapone treatment and acute liver injury. The authors of the report conclude that tolcapone withdrawal was responsible for the onset of NMLS because symptoms subsided within 12 hours of withdrawal of medications, and clozapine, which was administered to alleviate hallucinations, was reintroduced with levodopa/benserazide (but without tolcapone) at a lower dose without recurrence of NMLS symptoms. The second report postulates that abrupt withdrawal of tolcapone was responsible for NMLS (41). As in the previous case, the patient developed rigidity, hyperpyrexia, and deterioration of consciousness after withdrawal of tolcapone. Hence, it is suggested that tolcapone be tapered gradually and that dosages of carbidopa/levodopa be adjusted to prevent this adverse effect.

IV. SUMMARY

Tolcapone prolongs the action of levodopa through COMT inhibition, resulting in increased on-time and decreased off-time in PD patients with motor fluctuations. Because of its potential to cause liver injury, patients on tolcapone must be monitored for hepatocellular damage, and those patients who do not show clinical improvement within 3 weeks should be withdrawn from the drug. Although the marketing of tolcapone has been suspended in Canada and the European Union because of reports of hepatic failure, it remains an option for treatment in the United States for patients who have persistent fluctuations despite the use of other antiparkinsonian medications.

REFERENCES

1. Mannisto PT, Kaakkola S. Catechol-O-methyltransferase (COMT): biochemistry, molecular biology, pharmacology, and clinical efficacy of the new selective COMT inhibitors. Pharmacol Rev 1999; 51(4):593–628.

2. Ceravolo R, Piccini P, Bailey DL, Jorga KM, Bryson H, Brooks DJ. 18F-Dopa PET evidence that tolcapone acts as a central COMT inhibitor in Parkinson's disease. Synapse 2002; 43(3):201–207.
3. Myllylä VV, Jackson M, Larsen JP, Baas H. Efficacy and safety of tolcapone in levodopa-treated Parkinson's disease patients with "wearing-off" phenomenon: a multicenter, double-blind, randomized, placebo-controlled trial. Eur J Neurol 1997; 4:333–341.
4. Kurth MC, Adler CH, Hilaire MS, Singer C, Waters C, LeWitt P, Chernik DA, Dorflinger EE, Yoo K. Tolcapone improves motor function and reduces levodopa requirement in patients with Parkinson's disease experiencing motor fluctuations: a multicenter, double-blind, randomized, placebo-controlled trial. Tolcapone Fluctuator Study Group I. Neurology 1997; 48(1):81–87.
5. Rajput AH, Martin W, Saint-Hilaire MH, Dorflinger E, Pedder S. Tolcapone improves motor function in parkinsonian patients with the "wearing-off" phenomenon: a double-blind, placebo-controlled, multicenter trial. Neurology 1997; 49(4):1066–1071.
6. Roberts JW, Cora-Locatelli G, Bravi D, Amantea MA, Mouradian MM, Chase TN. Catechol-O-methyltransferase inhibitor tolcapone prolongs carbidopa/levodopa action in parkinsonian patients. Neurology 1993; 43(12):2685–2688.
7. Adler CH, Singer C, O'Brien C, Hauser RA, Lew MF, Marek KL, Dorflinger E, Pedder S, Deptula D, Yoo K. Randomized, placebo-controlled study of tolcapone in patients with fluctuating Parkinson disease treated with levodopa-carbidopa. Tolcapone Fluctuator Study Group III. Arch Neurol 1998; 55(8):1089–1095.
8. Baas H, Beiske AG, Ghika J, Jackson M, Oertel WH, Poewe W, Ransmayr G. Catechol-O-methyltransferase inhibition with tolcapone reduces the "wearing off" phenomenon and levodopa requirements in fluctuating parkinsonian patients. Neurology 1998; 50(suppl 5): S46–S53.
9. Grandas F, Galiano ML, Tabernero C. Risk factors for levodopa-induced dyskinesias in Parkinson's disease. J Neurol 1999; 246:1127–1133.
10. Obeso JA, Rodriguez-Oroz MC, Chana P, Lera G, Rodriguez M, Olanow CW. The evolution and origin of motor complications in Parkinson's disease. Neurology 2000; 55(suppl 4):S13–S20.
11. Mouridian MM, Juncos JL, Fabbrini G, Chase TN. Motor fluctuations on Parkinson's disease: pathogenetic and therapeutic studies. Ann Neurol 1987; 22:475–479.
12. Chase TN, Baronti F, Fabbrini G, Heuser IJ, Juncos JL, Mouradian MM. Rationale for continuous dopamimetic therapy of Parkinson's disease. Neurology 1989; 39(suppl 2):7–10.
13. Chase TN, Oh JD. Striatal mechanisms and pathogenesis of parkinsonian signs and motor complications. Ann Neurol 2000; 46(suppl 1):S122–S129.
14. Goetz CG. Influence of COMT inhibition on levodopa pharmacology and therapy. Neurology 1998; 50(suppl 5):S26–S30.
15. Kurth M, Adler C. COMT inhibition: A new treatment strategy for Parkinson's disease. Neurology 1998; 50(suppl 5):S3–S14.
16. Rivest J, Barclay CL, Suchowersky O. COMT inhibitors in Parkinson's disease. Can J Neurol Sci 1999; 26(suppl 2):S34–S38.
17. Nutt JG. Effect of COMT inhibition on the pharmacokinetics and pharmacodynamics of levodopa in parkinsonian patients. Neurology 2000; 55(suppl 4):S33–S41.
18. Hanson MR, Galvez-Jimenez N. Catechol-O-methyltransferase inhibitors in the management of Parkinson's disease. Semin Neurol 2001; 21(1):15–22.
19. Dingemanse J, Jorga K, Zürcher G, Schmitt M, Sedek G, Da Prada M, Van Brummelen P. Pharmacokinetic and pharmacodynamic interaction between the COMT inhibitor tolcapone and single dose levodopa. Br J Clin Pharmacol 1995; 40:253–262.
20. Dingemanse J, Jorga KM, Schmitt M, Gieschke R, Fotteler B, Zürcher G, Da Prada M, Van Brummelen P. Integrated pharmacokinetics and pharmacodynamics of the novel catechol-O-methyltransferase inhibitor tolcapone during first administration to humans. Clin Pharmacol Ther 1995; 57:508–517.
21. Dingemanse J, Jorga K, Zürcher G, Fotteler B, Sedek G, Nielsen T, van Brummelen P. Multiple-dose clinical pharmacology of the catechol-O-methyltransferase inhibitor tolcapone in elderly subjects. Eur J Clin Pharmacol 1996; 50:47–55.
22. Jorga KM, Sedek G, Fotteler B, Zurcher G, Nielsen T, Aitken JW. Optimizing levodopa pharmacokinetics with multiple tolcapone doses in the elderly. Clin Pharmacol Ther 1997; 62(3):300–310.
23. Jorga K, Fotteler B, Sedek G, Nielsen T, Aitken J. The effect of tolcapone on levodopa pharmacokinetics is independent of carbidopa/levodopa formulation. J Neurol 1998; 245(4):223–230.
24. Jorga KM. Pharmacokinetics, pharmacodynamics, and tolerability of tolcapone: a review of early studies in volunteers. Neurology 1998; 50(suppl 5):S31–S38.

25. Sedek G, Jorga K, Schmitt M, Burns RS, Leese P. Effect of tolcapone on plasma levodopa concentrations after coadministration with carbidopa/levodopa to healthy volunteers. Clin Neuropharmacol 1997; 20(6):531–541.

26. Muller T, Woitalla D, Schulz D, Peters S, Kuhn W, Przuntek H. Tolcapone increases maximum concentration of levodopa. J Neural Transm 2000; 107(1):113–119.

27. Jorga K, Banken L, Fotteler B, Snell P, Steimer JL. Population pharmacokinetics of levodopa in patients with Parkinson's disease treated with tolcapone. Clin Pharmacol Ther 2000; 67(6):610–620.

28. Rajput AH. The protective role of levodopa in the human substantia nigra. Adv Neurol 2001; 86:327–336.

29. Waters CH, Kurth M, Bailey P, Shulman LM, LeWitt P, Dorflinger E, Deptula D, Pedder S. Tolcapone in stable Parkinson's disease: efficacy and safety of long-term treatment. The Tolcapone Stable Study Group. Neurology 1997; 49(3):665–671.

30. Dupont E, Burgunder JM, Findley LJ, Olsson JE, Dorflinger E. Tolcapone added to levodopa in stable parkinsonian patients: a double-blind placebo-controlled study. Tolcapone in Parkinson's Disease Study Group II (TIPS II). Mov Disord 1997; 12(6):928–934.

31. Assal F, Spahr L, Hadengue A, Rubbia-Brandt L, Burkhard PR, Rubbici-Brandt L. Tolcapone and fulminant hepatitis [letter] [published erratum appears in Lancet 1998 Oct 31;352(9138):1478]. Lancet 1998; 352(9132):958.

32. Tasmar (tolcapone) tablets [product information]. Nutley, NJ: Roche Laboratories Inc., 1998.

33. FDA Talk Paper: New Warnings for Parkinson's Drug Tasmar. 1998, Food and Drug Administration: Rockville, MD.

34. Olanow CW. Tolcapone and hepatotoxic effects. Tasmar Advisory Panel. Arch Neurol 2000; 57(2):263–267.

35. Colosimo C. The rise and fall of tolcapone. J Neurol 1999; 246(10):880–882.

36. Friedman JH, Feinberg SS, Feldman RG. A neuroleptic malignantlike syndrome due to levodopa therapy withdrawal. JAMA 1985; 254(19):2792–2795.

37. Granner MA, Wooten GF. Neuroleptic malignant syndrome or parkinsonism hyperpyrexia syndrome. Semin Neurol 1997; 11(3):228–235.

38. Caroff S. Neuroleptic malignant syndrome. J Clin Psychiatry 1980; 41:79–83.

39. Di Rosa AE, Morgante L, Coraci MA, Crissafulli A, Cacciola G, Di Stefano G, Meduri M, Di Perri R. Functional hyperthermia due to central dopaminergic impairment. Funct Neurol 1988; 3(2): 211–215.

40. Blum MW, Siegel AM, Meier R, Hess K. Neuroleptic malignant-like syndrome and acute hepatitis during tolcapone and clozapine medication. Eur Neurol 2001; 46(3):158–160.

41. Iwuagwu CU, Riley D, Bonoma RA. Neuroleptic malignant-like syndrome in an elderly patient caused by abrupt withdrawal of tolcapone, a-catechol-o-methyl transferase inhibitor. Am J Med 2000; 108(6):517–518.

42. Jorga KM, Fotteler B, Heizmann P, Zurcher G. Pharmacokinetics and pharmacodynamics after oral and intravenous administration of tolcapone, a novel adjunct to Parkinson's disease therapy. Eur J Clin Pharmacol 1998; 54(5):443–447.

43. Jorga K, Fotteler B, Heizmann P. Metabolism and excretion of tolcapone, a novel inhibitor of catechol-O-methyltransferase. Br J Clin Pharmacol 1999; 48:513–520.

15
Entacapone

Kathryn A. Chung and John G. Nutt

Oregon Health and Science University, Portland, Oregon, U.S.A.

I. INTRODUCTION

O-methylation, catalyzed by the enzyme catechol-*O*-methyl transferase (COMT), converts levodopa to a clinically inactive metabolite. One class of antiparkinsonian medications has been developed to inhibit this enzymatic pathway in an attempt to augment the effect of levodopa on Parkinson's disease (PD) symptoms. Subsequent clinical investigation of COMT inhibition in PD patients has led to further refinement of how to utilize these medications. This chapter will focus on entacapone, the most widely used inhibitor of COMT. The biochemistry, pharmacology, toxicology, and clinical controversies surrounding entacapone will be reviewed.

II. COMT BIOCHEMISTRY AND DISTRIBUTION

COMT is a ubiquitous enzyme found in plants and animals. Its function is to eliminate biologically active or toxic catechol compounds. Substrates include levodopa, dopamine, adrenaline, and noradrenaline. Other substrates include ascorbic acid and flavenoids. In humans, COMT is distributed widely, but is concentrated in liver, kidney, and intestinal mucosa (1–4). It is also present in the central nervous system (CNS), in both neurons and glia (5). The enzyme is intracellular in location and present in both a soluble (cytoplasmic) form and a membrane-bound form (1). The latter is found largely in postsynaptic neurons, whereas soluble COMT is located in glia (6). The membrane-bound form, which is functionally the most important form at catecholamine neurotransmitter concentrations that are physiologically relevant, appears to be oriented largely toward the cytoplasmic domain (5,7). Thus, COMT will act on levodopa, dopamine, and other substrates when they are intracellular.

In humans, a single gene, located at q11.2 on chromosome 22, encodes both the membrane-bound and soluble forms of COMT (8). Studies of COMT enzyme activity in red blood cells show a trimodal distribution of activity (9). This is consistent with two codominant alleles of the gene, producing enzymes with low or high methylating activity. The low activity form results from a G-to-A substitution at codons 108 of the soluble and 158 of the membrane-bound form of the COMT gene, with a resulting switch of methionine for valine (10). Studies have suggested that high COMT activity may be more common in Asians than Caucasians (11,12), and that those with high COMT activity may respond to levodopa in a less favorable fashion (11). Recent clinical studies have not confirmed this latter observation. In a study of 73 Korean patients with PD and 29 with multiple system atrophy (MSA), the motor response to levodopa was not influenced by the COMT genotype in either group (13). Other studies have shown that COMT genotype does not affect the levodopa response to the COMT inhibitors tolcapone or entacapone (14,15).

With respect to PD, the pertinent actions of COMT are the methylation of levodopa to 3-O-methyldopa (3-OMD) and of dopamine to 3-methoxytyrosine (3-MT) (Fig. 1). Catecholamines and levodopa are methylated on the hydroxyl group of the 3 carbon of the aromatic ring (1). The reaction is a direct nucleophilic attack by one of the phenolic hydroxyls on the methyl group of S-adenylmethionine. It is an essentially irreversible reaction. O-methylated levodopa is not a substrate for dopamine synthesis. O-methylation of dopamine is a means of terminating its action in the CNS.

Inhibition of O-methylation may be important in PD via several mechanisms. First, inhibition of peripheral COMT could increase absorption of levodopa by reducing its metabolism in gut and liver (reduction of first pass effect), although this mechanism was eventually shown to be of little consequence (16). More importantly, COMT inhibition reduces levodopa metabolism. Second, inhibition of brain COMT could also prolong the action of dopamine by decreasing its intracellular metabolism and enhance dopamine synthesis by reducing central levodopa O-methylation. Third, inhibition of central COMT may preserve methyl donors such as S-adenosyl methionine.

Entacapone is a competitive inhibitor of COMT. Entacapone appears to tightly bind to the substrate binding site of COMT, yet is not a substrate for the methylation reaction.

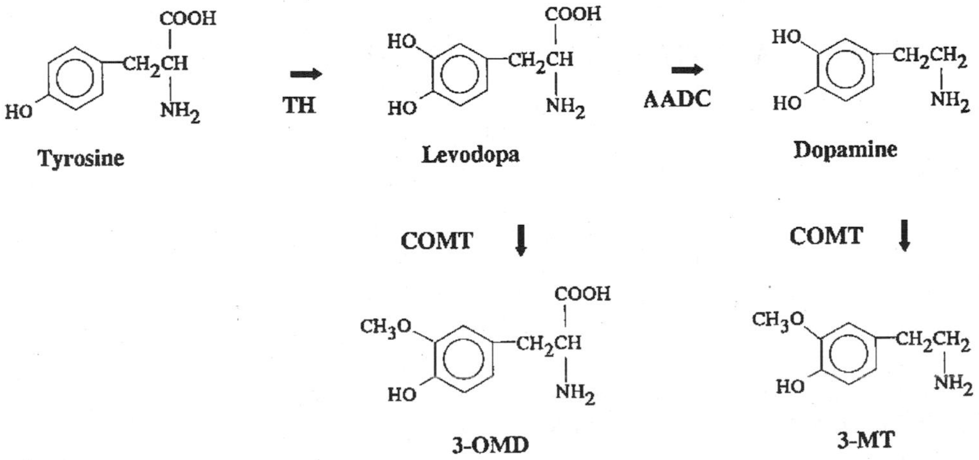

Figure 1 Metabolic pathways for levodopa and dopamine. TH, tyrosine hydroxylase; AADC, aromatic amino acid decarboxylase; COMT, catechol-O-methyltransferase; 3-OMD, 3-O-methyldopa; 3-MT, 3-methoxytyramine. (From Ref. 15a.)

The binding is, however, reversible, and inhibition is reversed as drug levels drop and the drug dissociates from COMT.

III. PHARMACOKINETICS

Entacapone is rapidly and well absorbed after oral administration, with a time to peak plasma concentration (T_{max}) of 0.4 to 0.9 hours (17). Food does not significantly interfere with drug absorption. Bioavailability is estimated at 36% (18). With drug dosage increases peak plasma concentration (C_{max}) and area under the curve (AUC) of entacapone increase linearly (17). Plasma protein binding is 98% in vitro. While the drug is administered in its E-isomer form, in circulation it is converted to the Z-isomer (18,19). Entacapone poorly penetrates the blood-brain barrier (BBB) and thus is considered only a peripheral COMT inhibitor at doses used in humans. This is in contrast to tolcapone, which penetrates the BBB and inhibits peripheral and central COMT (20–22).

Entacapone is eliminated mostly through liver glucuronidization. A small fraction (0.1–0.2%) is found unchanged in urine. In animal studies, approximately 80–90% of the dose is excreted in stool, the remainder in urine (18). The half-life of entacapone is 1–2.2 hours and plasma clearance is 48 L/h (18). The drug does not accumulate with repeated administration (17,19,24).

IV. PHARMACODYNAMICS

Estimates of peripheral inhibition of COMT are obtained with measurements of red blood cell (RBC) COMT activity. Because of the short plasma half-life and reversible inhibition of COMT, entacapone's duration of action is short. For example, a 200 mg dose of enta-capone will inhibit RBC COMT by 60% at peak concentrations (1 hour after administration) and by 10% 4 hours after administration (17,24). Thus, the duration of effect of entacapone is similar to that of regular release cabridopa/levodopa. For these reasons, entacapone is administered with each dose of levodopa.

The effect of different doses of entacapone on inhibition of RBC COMT activity was examined by Heikkinen et al in 21 patients with PD. A 100 mg/dose inhibited COMT activity in RBC by 25%; 200 mg/dose reduced the activity by 33% and a 400 mg/dose reduced it by 32%. The AUC of levodopa increased by 17%, 27% and 37% respectively. The proportion of off time decreased by 11% at 100 mg/dose, by 18% at 200 mg and by 20% at 400 mg, though these results were nonsignificant in the small number of patients studied.

V. LEVODOPA THERAPY AND COMT INHIBITION

If aromatic amino acid decarboxylase (AAAD) is not inhibited by carbidopa or benser-azide, about 70% of levodopa is decarboxylated to form dopamine in the periphery, 10% is methylated to 3-OMD, and much of the remainder may be utilized for melatonin synthesis, leaving only about 1% to penetrate the brain and be converted to dopamine (25,26). When carbidopa or benserazide is concomitantly administered, 3-O-methylation becomes the predominant means of metabolizing levodopa in the periphery meaning loss of potential precursor for striatal dopamine synthesis (27). The result is a substantial rise in the plasma concentration of 3-OMD, which may compete with levodopa for transport by the large neutral amino acid transporter at the BBB (28,29). However, the concentrations of 3-OMD observed in patients is generally a small portion of the total large neutral amino acid pool competing with levodopa for transport at the BBB. Therefore, reduction of 3-OMD is unlikely to be clinically important to the mechanism of action of COMT inhibitors.(28,30) In conclusion, the important action of COMT inhibition (along with AAAD inhibitors) is making more levodopa available to cross into the CNS for decarboxylation to dopamine.

COMT inhibition by entacapone does not change the T_{max} or the C_{max} of levodopa. The observation that T_{max} and C_{max} are unchanged suggests that first-pass metabolism is not altered by entacapone (16,31–34). Levodopa elimination from the plasma is slowed, and thus the AUC is increased by 40–100% (16,31–36). As expected, the O-methylated metabolites 3-OMD and homovanillic acid (HVA) are reduced and dihydrophenylacetic acid (DOPAC) is increased (31,34,35).

A. Single vs Multiple Dose Kinetics

Entacapone will prolong the effect of a single dose of levodopa by 20–70%, without increasing levodopa's C_{max} (16,31–36) (Fig. 2). With repeated dosing of levodopa every 2–4 hours, higher mean plasma concentrations of levodopa may occur (Fig. 3). Due to COMT inhibition, plasma levodopa concentrations are higher at the end of each dose cycle, and the rise in levodopa with the following dose will consequently be higher. In other words, interdose trough levels of levodopa rise as the day wears on; the interdose peaks rise as well but to a lesser extent (16). No further prolongation of levodopa's action occurs compared with acute single dosing. Initial clinical trials indicated that entacapone therapy for 1–8 weeks increased the time the patients were on, and in one study, allowed for a 27% reduction in levodopa dose (16,34,35).

B. Clinical Considerations

The Safety and Efficacy of Entacapone Study Assessing Wearing-off (SEESAW) demonstrated that entacapone led to improved proportion of on time (approximately 1 h/d) as well as a modest improvement in motor scores, despite an average total daily levodopa

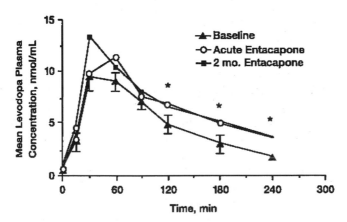

Figure 2 Entacapone prolongs elimination of orally administered levodopa. $^{*}p < 0.05$ compared with baseline. (From Ref. 16.)

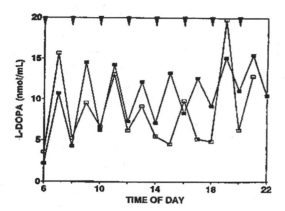

Figure 3 Effect of entacapone on hourly plasma levodopa concentrations. Note that when levodopa is given with (closed boxes) and without (open boxes) entacapone at 2-hour intervals (arrowheads), corresponding plasma levels are more predictable, with less fluctuation between troughs and peaks. (From Ref. 36a.)

dose reduction of about 12% or ~100 mg/day (37). In the Nordic Multicenter Entacapone COMT (NOMECOMT) study, the primary outcome variable was on time over an 18-hour period, and, similar to the SEESAW study, entacapone use resulted in improvement of on time. The average increase of 1.2 hours daily was similar to the 1 hour increase in the SEESAW study, as was the dose reduction in levodopa (average 102 mg) and motor score improvements (38).

The choice of whether to add entacapone or a dopamine agonist to a medication regimen in a fluctuating patient is relevant. A meta-analysis examined the effects of add-on therapy using three different dopamine agonists (pergolide, pramipexole, and ropinirole) or two COMT inhibitors (tolcapone, entacapone) in 1756 patients with PD. Levodopa reduction was significant in all groups, but was most significant for entacapone and pramipexole. Reduction in off time was greatest with pergolide, pramipexole, and entacapone, while side effects were least with ropinirole, pramipexole, and entacapone. There thus appear to be comparable advantages to either class of medication as add-on therapy but a somewhat different spectrum of adverse events (39).

There is controversy about when COMT inhibitors should be added in the course of the disease. Proponents of early use suggest that symptomatic benefit from levodopa is larger, even in those patients without motor fluctuations, though studies that demonstrated this benefit utilized tolcapone (40). Early entacapone use has been hypothesized to lessen the risk of developing motor complications. The mechanism of motor response fluctuations is incompletely understood, but duration of treatment, disease progression, and severity appear to be important contributors. Intermittent pulsatile stimulation of dopamine receptors has been hypothesized to induce levodopa-related motor complications (41). COMT inhibition theoretically might reduce the pulsatility of receptor exposure to levodopa. Of note, controlled-release preparations of levodopa, which theoretically should provide more tonic stimulation of dopamine receptors, have not proven to reduce the incidence of dyskinesias (42,43). Entacapone, which has a very short half-life, may permit less peak and trough fluctuation in levodopa levels, but does not eliminate them.

The use of COMT inhibitors to lessen the risk of motor complications is, an unproven strategy.

Using COMT inhibitors with controlled-release levodopa preparations has not been well studied. The short plasma half-life of entacapone may be a disadvantage with the controlled-release preparation because of its T_{max} of ~2 hours. Theoretically, tolcapone would be a more rational choice given its much longer half-life and thus more sustained COMT inhibition (44). Indeed, one study using 200 mg of entacapone and sustained-release levodopa demonstrated an increase in the AUC of 20% (45) compared to a 45% increase with immediate-release levodopa (16). However, in a study using clinical measures, no difference in entacapone efficacy was distinguishable between subjects receiving immediate release levodopa and those receiving controlled-release levodopa preparations on measures of on time, or Unified Parkinson's Disease Rating Scale (UPDRS) scores (46). Similarly, a study of effects of entacapone on single doses of standard or controlled-release preparations showed comparable prolongation of on time with both preparations (47).

Results of entacapone in stable or nonfluctuating patients have not been published. However, a few studies of tolcapone in stable patients have demonstrated levodopa dose reduction, improvement in activities of daily living (ADL) scores and improvement in motor scores (40,48).

Entacapone has not been studied in levodopa-untreated patients. Because entacapone's actions are peripheral, there is little rationale to do so. A study of tolcapone in untreated PD subjects demonstrated no therapeutic benefit and led to nausea as a common side effect (49). This suggests that tolcapone's central effects on dopamine metabolism are not clinically significant. It also indicates that gastrointestinal (GI) side effects of COMT inhibitors may be a direct effect and not an enhancement of levodopa's GI effects.

With the need for frequent dosing, the cost of entacapone use is not inconsequential. A recent analysis by Palmer et al. in patients who experience off time suggested that entacapone therapy costs $9,327 per quality-adjusted life-year, but with an additional 7.6 months with 25% or less off time per day compared to levodopa treatment alone (50).

Entacapone is now available as a triple combination therapy with carbidopa and levodopa in a tablet form called Stalevo™. The forms of Stalevo™ available are Stalevo™ 50 (carbidopa 12.5 mg, levodopa 50 mg, and entacapone 200 mg), Stalevo™ 100 (carbidopa 25 mg, levodopa 100 mg, entacapone 200 mg), and Stalevo™ 150 (carbidopa 37.5 mg, levodopa 150 mg, entacapone 200 mg).

VI. ADVERSE EFFECTS

Dopaminergic-mediated adverse effects including increased dyskinesia, hallucinations, and orthostasis have been reported with the addition of entacapone to levodopa. These adverse effects can often be attenuated with reductions in levodopa dosage. Since COMT is important in terminating catecholamine effects, theoretically, entacapone could enhance the effects of norepinephrine or epinephrine with consequent risk of cardiac arrthymia or hypertensive effects. While animal studies have shown that such adverse effects are possible with concomitant administration of catecholamines and COMT inhibitors (51), this interaction could not be demonstrated in humans (52,53). A letter describing severe hypertension following ephedrine administration in a patient receiving entacapone has been published, although the report fails to mention, the interval between the last entacapone dose and when ephedrine was administered (54). Less serious side effects reported include constipation, abdominal pain, mouth dryness, and urine discoloration. Diarrhea can be severe and preclude using the drug in a some patients. Liver toxicity has not been reported in clinical trials with entacapone; no significant elevations in alanine aminotransferase (ALT) were noted. This observation suggests that liver toxicity is not a class effect and liver enzyme monitoring is not required with entacapone (55). There has been one controversial report of liver toxicity with entacapone in two patients that resolved with withdrawal of the drug (56).

REFERENCES

1. Guldberg HC, Marsden CD. Catechol-O-methyl transferase: pharmacological aspects and physiological role. Pharmacol Rev 1975:135–206.
2. Nissinen E, Tuominen R, Perhoniemi V, Kaakkola S. Catechol-O methyltransferase activity in human and rat small intestine. Life Sci 1988; 42(25):2609–2614.
3. Schultz E. Catechol-O-methyltransferase and aromatic L-amino acid decarboxylase activities in human gastrointestinal tissues. Life Sci 1991; 49(10):721–725.
4. Sharpless NS, Tyce GM, Owen CA, Jr. Effect of chronic administration of L-dopa on catechol-O-methyltransferase in rat tissues. Life Sci 1973; 12(3):97–106.
5. Mannisto PT, Ulmanen I, Lundstrom K, Taskinen J, Tenhunen J, Tilgmann C et al. Characteristics of catechol-O-methyl-transferase (COMT) and properties of selective COMT inhibitors. Prog Drug Res 1992; 39:291–350.
6. Kaplan GP, Hartman BK, Creveling CR. Immunohistochemical demonstration of catechol-O-methyltransferase in mammalian brain. Brain Res 1979; 167(2):241–250.
7. Roth JA. Membrane-bound catechol-O-methyltransferase: a reevaluation of its role in the O-methylation of the catecholamine neurotransmitters. Rev Physiol Biochem Pharmacol 1992; 120:1–29.
8. Winqvist R, Lundstrom K, Salminen M, Laatikainen M, Ulmanen I. The human catechol-O-methyltransferase (COMT) gene maps to band q11.2 of chromosome 22 and shows a frequent RFLP with BglI. Cytogenet Cell Genet 1992; 59(4):253–257.
9. Weinshilboum RM. Human biochemical genetics of plasma dopamine-beta-hydroxylase and erythrocyte catechol-O-methyltransferase. Hum Genet Suppl 1978; (1):101–112.
10. Lachman HM, Papolos DF, Saito T, Yu YM, Szumlanski CL, Weinshilboum RM. Human catechol-O-methyltransferase pharmacogenetics: description of a functional polymorphism and its potential application to neuropsychiatric disorders. Pharmacogenetics 1996; 6(3):243–250.
11. Rivera-Calimlim L, Reilly DK. Difference in erythrocyte catechol-O-methyltransferase activity between Orientals and Caucasians: difference in levodopa tolerance. Clin Pharmacol Ther 1984; 35(6):804–809.
12. Palmatier MA, Kang AM, Kidd KK. Global variation in the frequencies of functionally different catechol-O-methyltransferase alleles. Biol Psychiatry 1999; 46(4):557–567.
13. Lee MS, Lyoo CH, Ulmanen I, Syvanen AC, Rinne JO. Genotypes of catechol-O-methyltransferase and response to levodopa treatment in patients with Parkinson's disease. Neurosci Lett 2001; 298(2):131–134.
14. Lee MS, Kim HS, Cho EK, Lim JH, Rinne JO. COMT genotype and effectiveness of entacapone in patients with fluctuating Parkinson's disease. Neurology 2002; 58(4):564–567.
15. Chong DJ, Suchowersky O, Szumlanski C, Weinshilboum RM, Brant R, Campbell NR. The relationship between COMT genotype and the clinical effectiveness of tolcapone, a COMT inhibitor, in patients with Parkinson's disease. Clin Neuropharmacol 2000; 23(3):143–148.
15a. Woodward WR, Nutt JG. Catechol-O-methyltransferase inhibitors in the treatment of parkinsonism. In: Koller WC, Paulson G, eds. Therapy of Parkinson's Disease, 2nd ed. New York: Marcel Dekker, 1995:287–297.
16. Nutt JG, Woodward WR, Beckner RM, Stone CK, Berggren K, Carter JH, et al. Effect of peripheral catechol-O-methyltransferase inhibition on the pharmacokinetics and pharmacodynamics of levodopa in parkinsonian patients. Neurology 1994; 44(5):913–919.
17. Keranen T, Gordin A, Karlsson M, Korpela K, Pentikainen PJ, Rita H, et al. Inhibition of soluble catechol-O-methyltransferase and single-dose pharmacokinetics after oral and intravenous administration of entacapone. Eur J Clin Pharmacol 1994; 46(2):151–157.

18. Goetz CG, Koller WC, Poewe W, Rascol O, Sampaio C. Management of Parkinson's disease: an evidence-based review. Move Disord 2002; 17(suppl 4):S45–S51.
19. Package Insert: Comtan (entacapone). 1999. East Hanover, NJ: Orion/Novartis Pharmaceuticals.
20. Mannisto PT, Tuomainen P, Tuominen RK. Different in vivo properties of three new inhibitors of catechol-O-methyltransferase in the rat. Br J Pharmacol 1992; 105(3):569–574.
21. Nissinen E, Linden IB, Schultz E, Pohto P. Biochemical and pharmacological properties of a peripherally acting catechol-O-methyltransferase inhibitor entacapone. Naunyn Schmiedebergs Arch Pharmacol 1992; 346(3):262–266.
22. Mannisto PT, Tuomainen P, Tuominen RK. Different in vivo properties of three new inhibitors of catechol-O-methyltransferase in the rat. Br J Pharmacol 1992; 105(3):569–574.
23. Heikkinen H, Saraheimo M, Antila S, Ottoila P, Pentikainen PJ. Pharmacokinetics of entacapone, a peripherally acting catechol-O-methyltransferase inhibitor, in man A study using a stable isotope techique. Eur J Clin Pharmacol 2001; 56(11):821–826.
24. Rouru J, Gordin A, Huupponen R, Huhtala S, Savontaus E, Korpela K, et al. Pharmacokinetics of oral entacapone after frequent multiple dosing and effects on levodopa disposition. Eur J Clin Pharmacol 1999; 55(6):461–467.
25. Heikkinen H, Nutt JG, LeWitt PA, Koller WC, Gordin A. The effects of different repeated doses of entacapone on the pharmacokinetics of L-dopa and on the clinical response to L-dopa in Parkinson's disease. Clin Neuropharmacol 2001; 24(3):150–157.
26. Nutt JG, Fellman JH. Pharmacokinetics of levodopa. Clin Neuropharmacol 1984; 7(1):35–49.
27. Da Prada M, Keller HH, Pieri L, Kettler R, Haefely WE. The pharmacology of Parkinson's disease: basic aspects and recent advances. Experientia 1984; 40(11):1165–1172.
28. Nutt JG, Woodward WR, Gancher ST, Merrick D. 3-O-Methyldopa and the response to levodopa in Parkinson's disease. Ann Neurol 1987; 21(6):584–588.
29. Muenter MD, Dinapoli RP, Sharpless NS, Tyce GM. 3-O-Methyldopa, L-dopa, and trihexyphenidyl in the treatment of Parkinson's disease. Mayo Clin Proc 1973; 48(3):173–183.
30. Guttman M, Leger G, Cedarbaum JM, Reches A, Woodward W, Evans A, et al. 3-O-Methyldopa administration does not alter fluorodopa transport into the brain. Ann Neurol 1992; 31(6):638–643.
31. Myllyla VV, Sotaniemi KA, Illi A, Suominen K, Keranen T. Effect of entacapone, a COMT inhibitor, on the pharmacokinetics of levodopa and on cardiovascular responses in patients with Parkinson's disease. Eur J Clin Pharmacol 1993; 45(5):419–423.
32. Limousin P, Pollak P, Gervason-Tournier CL, Hommel M, Perret JE. Ro 40–7592, a COMT inhibitor, plus levodopa in Parkinson's disease. Lancet 1993; 341(8860):1605.
33. Keranen T, Gordin A, Harjola VP, Karlsson M, Korpela K, Pentikainen PJ, et al. The effect of catechol-O-methyl transferase inhibition by entacapone on the pharmacokinetics and metabolism of levodopa in healthy volunteers. Clin Neuropharmacol 1993; 16(2):145–156.
34. Kaakkola S, Teravainen H, Ahtila S, Rita H, Gordin A. Effect of entacapone, a COMT inhibitor, on clinical disability and levodopa metabolism in parkinsonian patients. Neurology 1994; 44(1):77–80.
35. Ruottinen HM, Rinne UK. Effect of one month's treatment with peripherally acting catechol-O-methyltransferase inhibitor, entacapone, on pharmacokinetics and motor response to levodopa in advanced parkinsonian patients. Clin Neuropharmacol 1996; 19(3):222–233.
36. Merello M, Lees AJ, Webster R, Bovingdon M, Gordin A. Effect of entacapone, a peripherally acting catechol-O-methyltransferase inhibitor, on the motor response to acute treatment with levodopa in patients with Parkinson's disease. J Neurol Neurosurg Psychiatry 1994; 57(2):186–189
36a. Nutt JG. Effects of catechol-O-methyltransferase (COMT) inhibition on the pharmacokinetics of L-DOPA. Adv Neurol 1996; 69:493–496.
37. Entacapone improves motor fluctuations in levodopa-treated Parkinson's disease patients. Parkinson Study Group. Ann Neurol 1997; 42(5):747–755.
38. Rinne UK, Larsen JP, Siden A, Worm-Petersen J. Entacapone enhances the response to levodopa in parkinsonian patients with motor fluctuations. Nomecomt Study Group. Neurology 1998; 51(5):1309–1314.
39. Inzelberg R, Carasso RL, Schechtman E, Nisipeanu P. A comparison of dopamine agonists and catechol-O-methyltransferase inhibitors in Parkinson's disease. Clin Neuropharmacol 2000; 23(5):262–266.
40. Waters CH, Kurth M, Bailey P, Shulman LM, LeWitt P, Dorflinger E, et al. Tolcapone in stable Parkinson's disease: efficacy and safety of long-term treatment. Tolcapone Stable Study Group. Neurology 1998; 50(5 suppl 5):S39–S45.
41. Obeso JA, Rodriguez-Oroz MC, Rodriguez M, DeLong MR, Olanow CW. Pathophysiology of levodopa-induced dyskinesias in Parkinson's disease: problems with the current model. Ann Neurol 2000; 47(4 suppl 1):S22–S32.

42. Koller WC, Hutton JT, Tolosa E, Capilldeo R. Immediate-release and controlled-release carbidopa/levodopa in PD: a 5-year randomized multicenter study Carbidopa/Levodopa Study Group. Neurology 1999; 53(5):1012–1019.

43. Dupont E, Andersen A, Boas J, Boisen E, Borgmann R, Helgetveit AC, et al. Sustained-release Madopar HBS compared with standard Madopar in the long-term treatment of de novo parkinsonian patients. Acta Neurol Scand 1996; 93(1):14–20.

44. Jorga KM, Fotteler B, Heizmann P, Zurcher G. Pharmacokinetics and pharmacodynamics after oral and intravenous administration of tolcapone, a novel adjunct to Parkinson's disease therapy. Eur J Clin Pharmacol 1998; 54(5):443–447.

45. Ahtila S, Kaakkola S, Gordin A, Korpela K, Heinavaara S, Karlsson M, et al. Effect of entacapone, a COMT inhibitor, on the pharmacokinetics and metabolism of levodopa after administration of controlled-release levodopa-carbidopa in volunteers. Clin Neuropharmacol 1995; 18(1):46–57.

46. Poewe WH, Deuschl G, Gordin A, Kultalahti ER, Leinonen M. Efficacy and safety of entacapone in Parkinson's disease patients with suboptimal levodopa response: a 6-month randomized placebo-controlled double-blind study in Germany and Austria (Celomen study). Acta Neurol Scand 2002; 105(4):245–255.

47. Piccini P, Brooks DJ, Korpela K, Pavese N, Karlsson M, Gordin A. The catechol-O-methyltransferase (COMT) inhibitor entacapone enhances the pharmacokinetic and clinical response to Sinemet CR in Parkinson's disease. J Neurol Neurosurg Psychiatry 2000; 68(5):589–594.

48. Dupont E, Burgunder JM, Findley LJ, Olsson JE, Dorflinger E. Tolcapone added to levodopa in stable parkinsonian patients: a double-blind placebo-controlled study. Tolcapone in Parkinson's Disease Study Group II (TIPS II). Mov Disord 1997; 12(6):928–934.

49. Hauser RA, Molho E, Shale H, Pedder S, Dorflinger EE. A pilot evaluation of the tolerability, safety, and efficacy of tolcapone alone and in combination with oral selegiline in untreated Parkinson's disease patients. Tolcapone De Novo Study Group. Mov Disord 1998; 13(4):643–647.

50. Palmer CS, Nuijten MJ, Schmier JK, Subedi P, Snyder EH. Cost effectiveness of treatment of Parkinson's disease with entacapone in the United States. Pharmacoeconomics 2002; 20(9):617–628.

51. Tornwall M, Mannisto PT. Acute toxicity of three new selective COMT inhibitors in mice with special emphasis on interactions with drugs increasing catecholaminergic neurotransmission. Pharmacol Toxicol 1991; 69(1):64–70.

52. Lyytinen J, Sovijarvi A, Kaakkola S, Gordin A, Teravainen H. The effect of catechol-O-methyltransferase inhibition with entacapone on cardiovascular autonomic responses in L-dopa-treated patients with Parkinson's disease. Clin Neuropharmacol 2001; 24(1):50–57.

53. Illi A, Sundberg S, Koulu M, Scheinin M, Heinavaara S, Gordin A. COMT inhibition by high-dose entacapone does not affect hemodynamics but changes catecholamine metabolism in healthy volunteers at rest and during exercise. Int J Clin Pharmacol Ther 1994; 32(11):582–588.

54. Renfrew C, Dickson R, Schwab C. Severe hypertension following ephedrine administration in a patient receiving entacapone. Anesthesiology 2000; 93(6):1562.

55. Myllyla VV, Kultalahti ER, Haapaniemi H, Leinonen M. Twelve-month safety of entacapone in patients with Parkinson's disease. Eur J Neurol 2001; 8(1):53–60.

56. Fisher A, Croft-Baker J, Davis M, Purcell P, McLean AJ. Entacapone-induced hepatotoxicity and hepatic dysfunction. Mov Disord 2002; 17(6):1362–1365.

16
Anticholinergics

Robert L. Rodnitzky and Winthrop S. Risk II

University of Iowa Hospitals and Clinics, Iowa City, Iowa, U.S.A.

Anticholinergic drugs were the first class of medications found to be an effective treatment for Parkinson's disease (PD). Ordenstein, a student of Charcot, is recognized as having first demonstrated the efficacy of an anticholinergic agent in PD—in this case a naturally occurring belladonna alkaloid (1,2). The pharmacology of these agents was not well understood until 1947, when acetylcholine was identified as a neurotransmitter in the brain (3). Nonetheless, anticholinergic medications, including the later identified synthetic compounds, remained the mainstay of therapy for PD until the introduction of levodopa in the 1960s. Despite the rapidly expanding repertoire of available medical and surgical approaches for the treatment of PD, anticholinergic drugs still have a place in the management of this condition.

I. PHARMACOLOGY

Support of the concept that anticholinergic agents might benefit PD came from the early observation that infusion of an anticholinergic agent into the globus pallidus improved tremor (4). The clinical benefit of orally administered anticholinergic agents in PD has been demonstrated in humans (5) and animals (6). The precise mechanism of action of these agents is unclear. It is generally believed that in PD there is an antagonism between the effect of dopamine and acetylcholine in the basal ganglia. The striatum contains cholinergic interneurons that mediate dense innervation of other cellular elements in this structure (7–9), especially medium spiny neurons (10). A variety of mechanisms have been identified by which cholinergic and dopaminergic systems interact. Activation of D_1 dopamine receptors enhances acetylcholine release, while stimulation of D_2 receptors has the opposite effect (11). Conversely, acetylcholine antagonists have been found to mimic the effect of D_2 stimulation on striatal enkephalin and substance P in experimental animals (12). Acetylcholine receptor blocking agents have been demonstrated to inhibit decarboxylation of levodopa (13).

213

There are two classes of anticholinergic receptors: muscarinic and nicotinic. The anticholinergic agents used in PD block muscarinic receptors, four subtypes of which (M1–M4) have been characterized pharmacologically (14,15). Studies in animals have suggested that blockade of M4, a postsynaptic receptor found on striatal output neurons, might be most effective for blocking tremor (16). Localization studies of the other muscarinic receptor types suggest very specific physiological roles for each (17). The M1 receptor is found predominantly on medium spiny projection neurons, whereas M2 receptors are present in cholinergic neurons. M1 receptors are denser in the striatal matrix in juvenile primates, but are more prevalent in striasomes in the adult. In both instances, M1 receptors are found on synapse-forming spines. It has been suggested that M1- and M2-mediated cholinergic functions in the striatum are highly segregated, with M1 modulating extrinsic extrastriatal glutaminergic and monoaminergic input onto medium spiny gabaergic cells and M2 receptors involved in the autoregulation of acetylcholine release from cholinergic interneurons (17).

A fifth muscarinic receptor subtype (M5) has not been characterized pharmacologically and has no selective high-affinity ligands, although its existence has been determined by the presence of specific M5 messenger ribonucleic acid (mRNA) (18). The potential importance of this receptor in the dopamine/acetylcholine balance in the brain is illustrated by the fact that only M5 mRNA, but not mRNA of any other receptor type, is located near dopamine neurons and D_2 receptors in the substantia nigra and the ventral tegmental area. When dopamine neurons are experimentally destroyed, M5 mRNA is lost, suggesting that this receptor subtype is the principal muscarinic receptor made by dopamine neurons.

Relatively little is known about the pharmacokinetics of anticholinergic drugs (19). Virtually all of the anticholinergic drugs are administered as a hydrochloride salt, except benztropine, which is a mesylate salt. The absorption of most of these agents is relatively rapid. The time for peak plasma concentration (T_{max}) for biperiden, procyclidine, trihexyphenidyl, and diphenhydramine is between 1 and 2.3 hours. Benztropine, however, is absorbed much more slowly ($T_{max} = 7\,h$). The plasma half-lives of trihexyphenidyl (33 h) and biperiden (18–24 h) are relatively long, while those of procyclidine (12 h) and diphenhydramine (4–13 h) are intermediate in length. The plasma level of orally administered biperiden was found to be higher in older animals than in young ones (20), and similar results were found in some studies of diphenhydramine in humans (21,22).

II. EVIDENCE FOR CLINICAL EFFICACY

The benefit of anticholinergic drugs in PD has been studied in several clinical trials. Poorly validated methodologies for assessing clinical changes in PD and variable experimental designs have made interpretation of many of these early studies difficult. Notwithstanding these limitations, an overview of clinical trials involving anticholinergic drugs reveals that most demonstrated a benefit in one or more parkinsonian symptoms. Doshay and colleagues demonstrated the benefit of trihexyphenidyl (23), benztropine (24), and ethopropazine (24) in both tremor and rigidity. In each of these studies a significant number of patients evaluated suffered from postencephalitic parkinsonism rather than idiopathic PD. In later studies, anticholinergic drugs were also evaluated as adjunctive agents in patients receiving levodopa. Bassi et al. (21,25) in an uncontrolled trial, studied the effect of orphenadrine both as monotherapy and as adjunctive therapy in patients receiving levodopa. Improvement was noted in overall disease severity and in disability level in both groups, but was greatest in those in whom the drug was added to levodopa.

Some studies have suggested that anticholinergic drugs may be more useful for treating tremor than akinesia or rigidity. Koller (26) evaluated the relative efficacy of trihexyphenidyl, amantadine, and a low dosage of levodopa for relieving the tremor of PD. Based on accelerometric measurements, tremor amplitude was reduced to a similar degree by both trihexyphenidyl and levodopa (59% vs. 55%) but was improved by less than 25% by amantadine. Schrag et al. (21,27) compared the effects of a single intravenous dose of the anticholinergic drug biperiden with that of a subcutaneous challenge dose of the dopamine agonist apomorphine in 17 patients with PD. In all but one patient, tremor, as assessed by spectral analysis of accelerometric data, responded to both therapies. Rest tremor amplitude was reduced by 98% after apomorphine compared to a 67% reduction after biperiden. Postural tremor amplitude was similarly reduced by the agonist (60%) and biperiden (65%), but neither agent affected tremor frequency. While efficacy for tremor was noted with both agents, the Unified Parkinson's Disease Rating Scale (UPDRS) scores for rigidity and akinesia were only significantly improved by apomorphine. Unlike Koller (28), the authors did not find evidence of a dopamine-unresponsive tremor or a resting tremor with selective anticholinergic responsiveness. A more recent study utilized clinical and electromyographic evaluations to compare the efficacy of the same agent, biperiden, with levodopa as a therapy for tremor. Both agents were more effective for rest tremor than postural tremor, and in both instances the effect of levodopa was superior to that of the anticholinergic agent (29).

III. CLINICAL USE IN PARKINSON'S DISEASE

Although anticholinergic drugs continue to be a valid component of the modern pharmacological armamentarium for PD, the development of more potent therapies for the disease has relegated these preparations to a more limited number of indications.

These drugs are occasionally useful as initial therapy for PD patients whose PD symptoms are minimally disabling. Used in this manner, the mild clinical benefit from anticholinergic drugs may forestall the need for dopaminergic agents, especially levodopa. This is potentially important since there is still controversy as to whether the early use of levodopa may accelerate the underlying illness (30) or hasten onset of dyskinesias and motor fluctuations (31). An added benefit for those whose early symptoms are minimal enough to be adequately treated by anticholinergic drugs is that these agents are considerably less costly than any of the levodopa preparations or dopamine agonists.

It is commonly believed that anticholinergics are somewhat more efficacious for treating tremor than akinesia or rigidity (32). Accordingly, anticholinergics may be an especially good choice in the early mild patient whose predominant symptom is tremor. Similarly, these agents can be considered useful adjuncts to levodopa or dopamine agonist therapy in patients with relatively refractory tremor. This approach is most appropriate in patients below the age of 60 and in those who are not cognitively impaired or suffering from drug-induced hallucinations.

Another use of anticholinergic drugs is in the treatment of dystonia appearing in PD, either as a primary manifestation of the illness or as a drug-induced dystonia (33,34). The benefit is often dose dependent, similar to the effect of these agents in other dystonic disorders. Although dystonia associated with PD may be improved by anticholinergic drugs, it must be kept in mind that these agents can induce or worsen other nondystonic, drug-induced dyskinesias, especially those involving the oro-buccal musculature (35,36).

IV. SPECIFIC ANTICHOLINERGIC PREPARATIONS

A. Orphenadrine

Orphenadrine citrate is a diphenhydramine analogue that is marketed as Norflex® in the United States and most European nations. It is most commonly used as a muscle relaxant, although because of its anticholinergic properties, the hydrochloride salt, marketed as Disipal® in Canada and other nations, is indicated as an antiparkinson agent. This drug may also have some antiglutaminergic properties (37). Orphenadrine is available in 50 mg tablets and 100 mg controlled-release tablets. The usual starting dose is 100 mg of the controlled-release form twice daily or one standard 50 mg tablet three times daily.

B. Procyclidine

Procyclidine hydrochloride, one of several piperidine compounds available to treat PD, is marketed in most nations, including the United States, as Kemadrin®. It is available as a 5 mg scored tablet and in some locations as a 2.5 mg tablet. The usual starting dose is 2.5 mg three times daily.

C. Biperiden

Biperiden hydrochloride is marketed as Akineton® in the United States and many other nations. It is a piperidine compound, available as a 2 mg tablet. The customary starting dosage is 1–2 mg three times daily.

D. Trihexyphenidyl

Trihexyphenidyl hydrochloride is marketed in most nations as Artane®. It is a piperidine compound that is structurally related to biperiden and procyclidine, but trihexyphenidyl is a much more commonly used anticholinergic drug (38). Trihexyphenidyl is available in 2 mg tablets and 5 mg extended-release tablets. The usual starting dose is 1–2 mg three times daily.

E. Benztropine

Benztropine mesylate is a synthetic anticholinergic compound sharing some structural features with both atropine and diphenhydramine. This agent, introduced in 1954, has demonstrated efficacy for PD (39,40) and is the most commonly used anticholinergic for the treatment of drug-induced parkinsonism (41). Benztropine is marketed as Cogentin® in most nations and is available in 0.5, 1, and 2 mg tablets. The usual starting dosage for the treatment of PD is 0.5 mg twice daily. It is also available in parenteral form for intravenous or intramuscular administration.

F. Ethopropazine

Ethopropazine hydrochloride is structurally a phenothiazine, although its pharmacological action is that of an anticholinergic agent, which is the basis of its antiparkinsonian effect. This drug is marketed in Canada as Parsitan®, but it is no longer marketed in the United States. Each tablet contains 50 mg of ethopropazine. A typical starting dosage is 25 mg two or three times daily.

V. ADVERSE EFFECTS

Considering the potential adverse effects of the anticholinergic drugs used in PD is an extremely important factor in determining whether to use these agents in specific patients. The adverse effects of this class of drugs range from symptoms that are mild to those that are seriously disabling. Complicating the situation further is the fact that side effects are not confined to the central nervous system. To a greater extent than almost any other class of antiparkinsonian drugs, anticholinergic agents can result in a wide variety of serious peripheral adverse effects due to the widespread anatomical location of muscarinic acetylcholine receptors found in the parasympathetic nervous system. A further confounding factor is the fact that many patients being treated with anticholinergic PD drugs are concurrently receiving other medications with prominent anticholinergic properties, thereby further increasing the likelihood of unwanted peripheral parasympatholytic and central anticholinergic effects. As an illustration of the widespread use of drugs with anticholinergic activity, one study found that almost 60% of general nursing home residents had received such medications during the past year and even 23% of healthy seniors living at home were found to have had similar pharmacological exposure (42).

VI. PERIPHERAL ADVERSE EFFECTS

The most frequent peripheral side effect of anticholinergic drugs is dryness of the mouth. In many patients, especially those receiving a low dosage of the offending drug, this side effect is a minor inconvenience, and may even improve with time. For others, dryness of the mouth is a welcome occurrence since it can counteract drooling to some extent. However, in some patients, particularly those receiving moderate or high dosages of anticholinergic drugs, dry mouth can be extremely distressing and lead to functional impairment in such activities as chewing and swallowing.

Urinary bladder dysfunction is another anticholinergic side effect, especially in those already experiencing urinary hesitancy. Men with bladder neck obstruction secondary to prostatic hypertrophy are especially prone to this side effect and may occasionally experience urinary retention. In patients with this preexisting symptom, anticholinergic drugs should be avoided if at all possible.

Blurring of vision, like dryness of the mouth, is common and not disabling in most patients receiving low dosages of the anticholinergic PD drugs. This adverse effect is the result of interference with the muscarinic control of ocular accommodation. Drug-induced inhibition of accommodation may result in particular difficulty with near vision, a symptom that can be further complicated by the frequent occurrence of convergence insufficiency in PD patients (43). With larger anticholinergic dosages, visual blurring can become severe enough to contribute to accidents or falls. Another potential ocular complication of anticholinergic therapy is induction or worsening of closed angle glaucoma secondary to the mydriatic effect of these drugs. In some patients not known to be at risk for glaucoma, acute symptoms or pain related to the developing glaucoma may be absent, allowing the condition to progress unnoticed over time. In severe cases, unchecked development of glaucoma related to anticholinergic PD therapy has been reported to lead to permanent blindness (44).

Constipation, a common accompaniment of PD, can be worsened by anticholinergic medications, sometimes contributing to fecal impaction. On rare occasion, this inhibitory effect on gastrointestinal motility has been reported to result in the syndrome of pseudo-obstruction of the colon (45) or megacolon (46). Anticholinergic-induced ileus may be reversed with the use of cholinesterase inhibitors such as neostigmine (47).

Two other peripheral side effects of anticholinergic drugs in PD are extremely rare but potentially serious. Anticholinergic agents can result in an increased heart rate, possibly exacerbating angina or congestive heart failure in susceptible patients. In this regard, orphenadrine has been reported to result in ventricular tachycardia even at low dosages (48). This particular side effect is not solely related to the anticholinergic effect of orphenadrine, but rather may be in part the result of the drug's activity as a sodium channel blocking agent (49).

Acute anticholinergic toxicity is another uncommon, but potentially fatal complication of this class of drugs. This syndrome is most likely to occur in patients receiving other anticholinergic drugs in addition to their antiparkinsonian anticholinergic agents, or in those taking inappropriately high dosages of a prescribed antiparkinsonian drug. The full syndrome consists of hyperthermia, mydriasis, tachycardia, absent bowel sounds, dried mucous membranes, flushed skin, and disorientation (50). The combination of acute disorientation and hyperthermia in such patients can lead to confusion with neuroleptic malignant syndrome (NMS) (51), a condition seen in PD patients who are receiving dopamine blocking antipsychotic agents or who have recently undergone withdrawal of a dopaminergic agent. In PD patients diagnosed with NMS, anticholinergic drugs should be tapered and withdrawn since they can significantly delay recovery from hyperthermia (52).

VII. CENTRAL SIDE EFFECTS

The potential central adverse effects of anticholinergic drugs are largely behavioral and range from a mild but noticeable decrement in cognition to serious and alarming confusion. Cholinergic neurotransmission has long been viewed as playing a major role in memory (53). As such, cholinergic hypofunction has also been demonstrated to play a role in the pathogenesis of the dementia of PD (54,55), although other pathologies such as concurrent Alzheimer's disease (56), cortical Lewy body pathology (56,57), and loss of mesolimbic and mesocortical dopaminergic projections (56–58) have been found to be contributory as well. A loss of cholinergic function, presumably secondary, at least in part, to degeneration in the basal nucleus of Meynert (56,57,59), may be responsible for the subcortico-frontal syndrome that is characteristic of PD dementia (60).

Investigations using functional neuroimaging have demonstrated the detrimental effects of anticholinergic agents on cortical function in PD. Positron emission tomography (PET), performed in PD patients with cognitive impairment resulting from anticholinergic therapy, showed bilateral diffuse decrease of glucose metabolism in the cortex, basal ganglia, thalamus, hippocampus, and cerebellum, all of which improved after cessation of therapy (61). Even in nondemented PD patients, PET studies have revealed a decrease in cerebral blood flow and oxygen metabolic rate in all cortical areas after institution of trihexyphenidyl therapy (62).

Given the putative role of impaired cholinergic transmission in PD dementia, it is not surprising that PD patients are often intolerant of anticholinergic treatment. The potential for anticholinergic drugs to result in behavioral side effects in PD has been demonstrated both by longitudinal evaluation of patients receiving these agents as well as by short-term experimental administration of the drugs. In one study, experimental administration of trihexyphenidyl to nondemented PD patients at low dosages for only one month resulted in a demonstrable decline in recent, but not immediate memory (63). The memory-impairing potential of these drugs, especially new memory acquisition, has also been demonstrated even when administered at standard dosages to normal volunteers (64,65). In another investigation, the experimental administration of a subthreshold dose of scopolamine to healthy subjects had no effect, but more importantly resulted in significantly reduced memory performance in nondemented PD patients (66). The susceptibility of nondemented PD patients to anticholinergic agents is not surprising in view of evidence that such patients, at a relatively early stage of their illness, have abnormalities of cholinergic systems despite their apparently normal cognitive state (67). It is noteworthy, and of clinical importance, that in some of these investigations, elderly subjects became more severely impaired by anticholinergic drugs than did young adults (64,65).

These studies are consistent with the common clinical experience that anticholinergic therapy can further exacerbate the behavioral symptoms of PD patients who are already exhibiting signs of dementia. Such patients are at special risk for developing hallucinations when exposed to this class of drugs. In addition, even cognitively intact PD patients, especially the elderly, are at risk for developing anticholinergic-induced confusion or signs of dementia (68). These concerns are the basis of the generally accepted admonition that anticholinergic medications be used with extreme caution, if at all, in patients over the age of 60, irrespective of their cognitive state (69).

VIII. SUMMARY

Until the 1970s, anticholinergic medications were a mainstay in the treatment of PD. For all but the mildest symptoms of PD, this class of drugs has been supplanted by dopaminergic agents. Anticholinergic drugs may be somewhat more effective for tremor than rigidity or akinesia, but sufficiently rigorous clinical investigations have not yet been carried out to confirm this notion. A number of antiparkinsonian anticholinergic drugs are available, but there is little evidence to suggest the relative superiority of any one agent. While anticholinergic drugs have a role in the treatment of very mild PD, and possibly as antitremor agents in more advanced forms of the illness, clinicians must be aware of the potential central and peripheral side effects of these medications in all PD patients. Special caution should be exercised in using these drugs in the elderly or those with dementia, since these patients are particularly susceptible to the behavioral adverse effects associated with anticholinergic treatment.

REFERENCES

1. Comella CL, Tanner CM. Anticholinergic drugs in the treatment of Parkinson's disease. Koller WC, Paulson G, eds. Therapy of Parkinson's Disease. New York: Marcel Dekker, 1995:109–122.
2. Ordenstein L. Sur la Paralysie et la Sclerose in Plaque Generalise. Paris: Martinet1867.
3. Feldburg W. Present views on the mode of action of acetylcholine in the central nervous system. Physiol Rev 1945; 25:596–642.

4.   Nashold BS. Cholinergic stimulation of the globus pallidus in man. Proc Soc Exp Biol Med 1959; 101:68–69.
5.   Duvoisin RC. Cholinergic-anticholinergic antagonism in parkinsonism. Arch Neurol 1967; 17(2): 124–136.
6.   Mayorga AJ, Cousins MS, Trevitt JT, Conlan A, Gianutsos G, Salamone JD. Characterization of the muscarinic receptor subtype mediating pilocarpine-induced tremulous jaw movements in rats. Eur J Pharmacol 1999; 364(1):7–11.
7.   Woolf NJ. Cholinergic systems in mammalian brain and spinal cord. Prog Neurobiol 1991; 37(6):475–524.
8.   Bergson C, Mrzljak L, Smiley JF, Pappy M, Levenson R, Goldman-Rakic PS. Regional, cellular, and subcellular variations in the distribution of D1 and D5 dopamine receptors in primate brain. J Neurosci 1995; 15(12):7821–7836.
9.   Oh JD, Woolf NJ, Roghani A, Edwards RH, Butcher LL. Cholinergic neurons in the rat central nervous system demonstrated by in situ hybridization of choline acetyltransferase mRNA. Neuroscience 1992; 47(4):807–822.
10. Smith AD, Bolam JP. The neural network of the basal ganglia as revealed by the study of synaptic connections of identified neurones. Trends Neurosci 1990; 13(7):259–265.
11. DiChiara G, Morelli, Consolo S. Modulatory functions of neurotransmitters in the striatum: ACh/dopamine/NMDA interactions. Trends Neurosci 1994; 17(6):228–233.
12. Nisenbaum L. Dopaminergic and muscarinic regulation of striatal enkephalin at substance P messenger RNAs following striatal dopamine denervation: effects of systemic and central administration of quinpirole and scopolamine. Neuroscience 1994; 63(2):435–449.
13. Izurieta-Sanchez P, Sarre S, Ebinger G, Michotte Y. Effect of trihexyphenidyl, a non-selective antimuscarinic drug, on decarboxylation of L-dopa in hemi-Parkinson rats. Eur J Pharmacol 1998; 353(1):33–42.
14. Hersch SM, Levey AI. Diverse pre- and post-synaptic expression of m1-m4 muscarinic receptor proteins in neurons and afferents in the rat neostriatum. Life Sciences 1995; 56(11–12):931–938.
15. Reever CM, Ferrari-DiLeo G, Flynn DD. The M5 (m5) receptor subtype: fact or fiction? Life Sci 1997; 60(13–14):1105–1112.
16. Mayorga AJ, Cousins MS, Trevitt JT, Conlan A, Gianutsos G, Salamone JD. Characterization of the muscarinic receptor subtype mediating pilocarpine-induced tremulous jaw movements in rats. Eur J Pharmacol 1999; 364(1):7–11.
17. Alcantara AA, Mrzljak L, Jakab RL, Levey AI, Hersch SM, Goldman-Rakic PS. Muscarinic m1 and m2 receptor proteins in local circuit and projection neurons of the primate striatum: anatomical evidence for cholinergic modulation of glutamatergic prefronto-striatal pathways. J Comp Neurol 2001; 434(4):445–460.
18. Yeomans J, Forster G, Blaha C. M5 muscarinic receptors are needed for slow activation of dopamine neurons and for rewarding brain stimulation. Life Sci 2001; 68(22–23):2449–2456.
19. Brocks DR. Anticholinergic drugs used in Parkinson's disease: an overlooked class of drugs from a pharmacokinetic perspective. J Pharmacy Pharmaceut Sci 1999; 2(2):39–46.
20. Yokogawa K, Nakashima E, Ichimura F. Effect of fat tissue volume on the distribution kinetics of biperiden as a function of age in rats. Drug Metab Dispos 1990; 18(2):258–263.
21. Labedzki L, Scavone JM, Ochs HR, Greenblatt DJ. Reduced systemic absorption of intrabronchial lidocaine by high-frequency nebulization. J Clin Pharmacol 1990; 30(9):795–797.
22. Simons KJ, Watson WT, Martin TJ, Chen XY, Simons FE. Diphenhydramine: pharmacokinetics and pharmacodynamics in elderly adults, young adults, and children. J Clin Pharmacol 1990; 30(7):665–671.
23. Doshay LJ, Constable K. Artane therapy for parkinsonism: preliminary study of results of 117 cases. JAMA 1949; 140:1317–1322.
24. Doshay LJ. Five-year study of benztropine (Cogentin) methanesulfate. JAMA 1956; 162: 1031–1034.
25. Bassi S, Albizzati MG, Calloni E, Sbacchi M, Frattola L. Treatment of Parkinson's disease with orphenadrine alone and in combination with L-dopa. Br J Clin Pract 1986; 40(7):273–275.
26. Koller WC. Pharmacologic treatment of parkinsonian tremor. Arch Neurol 1986; 43(2):126–127.
27. Schrag A, Schelosky L, Scholz U, Poewe W. Reduction of Parkinsonian signs in patients with Parkinson's disease by dopaminergic versus anticholinergic single-dose challenges. Mov Disord 1999; 14(2):252–255.
28. Koller WC. Dose-response relationship of propranolol in the treatment of essential tremor. Arch Neurol 1986; 43(1):42–43.
29. Milanov I. A cross-over clinical and electromyographic assessment of treatment for parkinsonian tremor. Parkinson Relat Disord 2001; 8(1):67–73.

30. Fahn S. Is levodopa toxic? Neurology 1996; 47(6 suppl 3):S184–S195.
31. Rascol O, Brooks DJ, Korczyn AD, De Deyn PP, Clarke CE, Lang AE. A five-year study of the incidence of dyskinesia in patients with early Parkinson's disease who were treated with ropinirole or levodopa. 056 Study Group. N Engl J Med 2000; 342(20):1484–1491.
32. Olanow CW, Watts RL, Koller WC. An algorithm (decision tree) for the management of Parkinson's disease (2001): treatment guidelines. Neurology 2001; 56(11 suppl 5):S1–S88.
33. Poewe WH, Lees AJ. The pharmacology of foot dystonia in parkinsonism. Clin Neuropharmacol 1987; 10(1):47–56.
34. Giron LT, Jr., Koller WC. Methods of managing levodopa-induced dyskinesias. Drug Safety 1996; 14(6):365–374.
35. Hauser RA, Olanow CW. Orobuccal dyskinesia associated with trihexyphenidyl therapy in a patient with Parkinson's disease. Mov Disord 1993; 8(4):512–514.
36. Linazasoro G. Anticholinergics and dyskinesia. Mov Disord 1994; 9(6):689.
37. Sureda FX, Gabriel C, Pallas M, Adan J, Martinez JM, Escubedo E, et al. In vitro and in vivo protective effect of orphenadrine on glutamate neurotoxicity. Neuropharmacology 1999; 38(5): 671–677.
38. Lamid S, Jenkins RB. Crossover clinical trial of benapryzine and trihexyphenidyl in parkinsonian patients. J Clin Pharmacol 1975; 15(8–9):622–626.
39. Tourtellotte WW, Potvin AR, Syndulko K, Hirsch SB, Gilden ER, Potvin JH, et al. Parkinson's disease: Cogentin with Sinemet, a better response. Prog Neuro-psychopharmacol Biol Psychiatry 1982; 6(1):51–55.
40. Friedman JH, Koller WC, Lannon MC, Busenbark K, Swanson-Hyland E, Smith D. Benztropine versus clozapine for the treatment of tremor in Parkinson's disease. Neurology 1997; 48(4): 1077–1081.
41. Tune LE, McHugh PR, Coyle JT. Management of extrapyramidal side effects induced by neuroleptics. Johns Hopkins Med J 1981; 148(3):149–153.
42. Blazer DG, Federspiel CF, Ray WA, Schaffner W. The risk of anticholinergic toxicity in the elderly: a study of prescribing practices in two populations. J Gerontol 1983; 38(1):31–35.
43. Rodnitzky RL. Visual dysfunction in Parkinson's disease. Clin Neurosci 1998; 5(2):102–106.
44. Friedman Z, Neumann E. Benzhexol-induced blindness in Parkinson's disease. Br Med J 1972; 1(800):605.
45. Howard LM, Markus H. Pseudo-obstruction secondary to anticholinergic drugs in Parkinson's disease. Postgrad Med J 1992; 68(795):70–71.
46. Caplan LH, Naimark A. The transtracheal approach to laryngography. Radiology 1965; 85(3): 439–441.
47. Isbister GK, Oakley P, Whyte IM, Dawson AJ. Treatment of anticholinergic-induced ileus with neostigmine. Ann Emerg Med 2001; 38(6):689–693.
48. Dilaveris P, Pantazis A, Vlasseros J, Gialafos J. Non-sustained ventricular tachycardia due to low-dose orphenadrine. Am J Med 2001; 111(5):418–419.
49. Clark RF. Orphenadrine poisoning and review of physostigmine. J Emerg Med 11(1):97-Feb.
50. Johnson AL, Hollister LE, Berger PA. The anticholinergic intoxication syndrome: diagnosis and treatment. J Clin Psychiatry 1981; 42(8):313–317.
51. Catterson ML, Martin RL. Anticholinergic toxicity masquerading as neuroleptic malignant syndrome: a case report and review. Ann Clin Psychiatry 1994; 6(4):267–269.
52. Susman VL. Clinical management of neuroleptic malignant syndrome. Psychiatric Quarterly 2001; 72(4):325–336.
53. Drachman DA. Memory and cognitive function in man: does the cholinergic system have a specific role? Neurology 2002; 27(8):783–790.
54. Whitehouse PJ, Hedreen JC, White CL, III, Price DL. Basal forebrain neurons in the dementia of Parkinson disease. Ann Neurol 1983; 13(3):243–248.
55. Candy JM, Perry RH, Perry EK, Irving D, Blessed G, Fairbairn AF, et al. Pathological changes in the nucleus of Meynert in Alzheimer's and Parkinson's diseases. J Neurol Sci 1983; 59(2):277–289.
56. Boller F, Mizutani T, Roessmann U, Gambetti P. Parkinson disease, dementia, and Alzheimer disease: clinicopathological correlations. Ann Neurol 1980; 7(4):329–335.
57. Kosaka K. Dementia and neuropathology in Lewy body disease. Adv Neurol 1993; 60:456–463.
58. Rinne JO, Portin R, Ruottinen H, Nurmi E, Bergman J, Haaparanta M, et al. Cognitive impairment and the brain dopaminergic system in Parkinson's disease: [18F]fluorodopa positron emission tomographic study. Arch Neurol 2000; 57(4):470–475.
59. Gaspar P, Gray F. Dementia in idiopathic Parkinson's disease. A neuropathological study of 32 cases. Acta Neuropathol 1984; 64(1):43–52.

60. Bedard MA, Pillon B, Dubois B, Duchesne N, Masson H, Agid Y. Acute and long-term administration of anticholinergics in Parkinson's disease: specific effects on the subcortico-frontal syndrome. Brain Cognition 1999; 40(2):289–313.
61. Nishiyama K, Momose T, Sugishita M, Sakuta M. Positron emission tomography of reversible intellectual impairment induced by long-term anticholinergic therapy. J Neurol Sci 1995; 132(1): 89–92.
62. Takahashi S, Tohgi H, Yonezawa H, Obara S, Yamazaki E. The effect of trihexyphenidyl, an anticholinergic agent, on regional cerebral blood flow and oxygen metabolism in patients with Parkinson's disease. J Neurol Sci 1999; 167(1):56–61.
63. Koller WC. Disturbance of recent memory function in parkinsonian patients on anticholinergic therapy. Cortex 1984; 20(2):307 311.
64. McEvoy JP. A double-blind crossover comparison of antiparkinson drug therapy: amantadine versus anticholinergics in 90 normal volunteers, with an emphasis on differential effects on memory function. J Clin Psychiatry 1987; 48 (suppl):20–23.
65. McEvoy JP, McCue M, Spring B, Mohs RC, Lavori PW, Farr RM. Effects of amantadine and trihexyphenidyl on memory in elderly normal volunteers. Am J Psychiatry 1987; 144(5):573–577.
66. Dubois B, Danze F, Pillon B, Cusimano G, Lhermitte F, Agid Y. Cholinergic-dependent cognitive deficits in Parkinson's disease. Ann Neurol 1987; 22(1):26–30.
67. Ruberg M, Rieger F, Villageois A, Bonnet AM, Agid Y. Acetylcholinesterase and butyrylcholinesterase in frontal cortex and cerebrospinal fluid of demented and non-demented patients with Parkinson's disease. Brain Res 1986; 362(1):83–91.
68. Nishiyama K, Sugishita M, Kurisaki H, Sakuta M. Reversible memory disturbance and intelligence impairment induced by long-term anticholinergic therapy. Intern Med 1998; 37(6):514–518.
69. Olanow CW, Watts RL, Koller WC. An algorithm (decision tree) for the management of Parkinson's disease (2001): treatment guidelines. Neurology 2001; 56(11 suppl 5):S1–S88.

17
Selegiline

Lawrence Elmer

Medical College of Ohio, Toledo, Ohio, U.S.A.

I. INTRODUCTION

Selegiline has been one of the most controversial therapeutic agents available to treat patients with Parkinson's disease (PD). Initially discovered in the 1960s, this drug has been suggested to have potential neuroprotective effects (1), only to be later suspected as a cause of early demise in patients with PD (2). While neither of these extreme viewpoints is widely accepted, selegiline still invokes lively discussion regarding its role as a therapeutic agent for PD. In this chapter, we will review the historical development of selegiline, its mechanism of action, short- and long-term clinical trials, and the current recommendations for its use in the management of PD.

II. HISTORICAL PERSPECTIVE

The history of monoamine oxidase (MAO) inhibitors dates back to the early 1950s to the development of treatments for tuberculosis (1). Iproniazid, a derivative of isoniazid, was found to have psychic energizing effects that were linked to its ability to inhibit MAO (3,4). Investigations of iproniazid as a potential treatment for depression led to widespread acceptance of MAO inhibition as a potentially therapeutic strategy for depressive symptoms, and in the late 1950s a variety of similar compounds were developed.

A side effect of MAO inhibition was soon uncovered by the extensive use of these agents. Patients treated with MAO inhibitors were at risk of developing a hypertensive crisis when there was concomitant consumption of foods, typically cheeses, that contained tyramine (5,6). At this point, research focused on an agent that would inhibit MAO activity without producing the so-called cheese effect.

In the early 1960s, Knoll and colleagues developed a methamphetamine derivative that would inhibit the MAO enzyme system, racemic phenylisopropylmethylpropinylamine HCl, or E-250, which was later renamed deprenyl (7). The levorotatory form of deprenyl, L-deprenyl, demonstrated irreversible inhibition of MAO activity without increasing

223

receptor sensitivity to tyramine (3), suggesting that this compound would be the first MAO inhibitor free of the cheese effect.

In 1968 Johnston synthesized clorgyline, which was chemically similar to deprenyl; however, these two agents had significantly different pharmacological actions (8). Clorgyline was an irreversible inhibitor of a class of MAO activity that preferentially deaminated serotonin and norepinephrine over a synthetic substrate, benzylamine. In contrast, L-deprenyl inhibited a class of MAO activity that preferentially deaminated the synthetic substrates benzylamine and phenylethylamine over the endogenous substrates serotonin and norepinephrine. These differences in substrate specificity, coupled with the observation that deamination of tyramine and dopamine was inhibited by either clorgyline or deprenyl with a biphasic dose-response curve, led to the concept of two separate classes of MAO activity. The MAO-A class of enzymatic activity preferentially deaminates serotonin and norepinephrine, while MAO-B activity preferentially deaminates benzylamine and phenylethylamine. Tyramine and dopamine are substrates for both types of MAO activities (3,9).

The discovery of L-deprenyl was preceded by the pioneering studies of Ehringer and Hornykiewicz (10) implicating dopamine as the primary neurochemical deficiency in postmortem brains of patients afflicted with PD. As dopamine is an endogenous substrate for MAO, investigations shortly followed to determine whether MAO inhibitors could be used to increase dopamine levels and treat symptoms in patients with PD. Unfortunately, the hypertensive crises seen in patients treated with nonspecific MAO inhibitors were also seen in the PD population. In the late 1960s, with the development of L-deprenyl, or selegiline, investigators considered this compound a safer therapeutic agent for the treatment of PD (11) and depression (12) than the nonspecific MAO inhibitors.

III. MECHANISM OF ACTION/PHARMACOLOGY

A. Dopamine Metabolism

The basic pharmacological mechanism of selegiline relates to its ability to inhibit MAO-B activity. In the brain, dopamine is preferentially metabolized by the MAO-B system (13), suggesting that selegiline or similar derivatives may be ideal inhibitors of dopamine degradation in PD. However, some of selegiline's metabolites, including desmethylselegiline and methamphetamine, are pharmacologically active (14). Thus, inhibition of MAO-B is not the sole mode of pharmacological action of selegiline. Selegiline and/or its metabolites also inhibit the reuptake of dopamine and increase the synthesis of dopamine by blocking the presynaptic dopamine autoreceptors that govern the synthesis rate of dopamine (15).

Selegiline is rapidly absorbed from the gastrointestinal tract, reaching peak serum concentrations 1/2 to 2 hours after ingestion. It is a lipophilic molecule, distributed widely throughout the body. Studies with radiolabeled selegiline suggest an apparent volume of distribution of over 300 L, with over 90% of the molecule bound to plasma proteins. In animal studies, selegiline has been shown to distribute more rapidly to the central nervous system than to the periphery. Positron emission tomography (PET) studies have demonstrated that selegiline binds to such areas as the thalamus, striatum, cortex, and brainstem, areas rich in MAO-B content (16,17).

Selegiline is an irreversible inhibitor of MAO-B, and the half-life of its effectiveness is dependent on the time required to synthesize new enzymatic activity. This regeneration of new enzymatic activity usually takes weeks, especially after the majority of the endogenous MAO-B enzyme has been inactivated (14). The inhibition of MAO-B activity in humans following oral administration of selegiline is rapid and complete. MAO-B inhibition in platelets exceeds 90% within hours after oral administration of either 5 or 10 mg of selegiline (18,19). Postmortem examination of PD patients treated with 10 mg selegiline demonstrated almost complete MAO-B inhibition, while residual MAO-A activity was fairly unaffected (20–22). These doses correspond to a brain concentration of 10^{-6} M. Doses significantly higher than this lead to a loss of the MAO-B selectivity and risk of the cheese effect (14).

Five metabolites have been demonstrated in human plasma after the administration of oral selegiline (23,24). The two main metabolites are desmethylselegiline and methamphetamine, which may then be metabolized to amphetamine. Methamphetamine and amphetamine can also be metabolized to pharmacologically inactive parahydroxy derivatives. The role of these metabolites and their potential contribution to the efficacy of selegiline is a matter of extensive discussion.

At low doses, methamphetamine and amphetamine have been known to release dopamine, which may contribute to potential therapeutic benefits in PD patients by increasing striatal dopamine levels. Amphetamines, especially the dextro forms, have also been known to have MAO-A inhibitory properties (25,26). However, in studies examining the concentration of selegiline and its derivatives in cerebrospinal fluid (CSF), the concentration of dextroamphetamines was in the micromolar range, which may be too low to contribute to the efficacy of selegiline (14).

B. Neuroprotective Effects

In addition to its effects on dopamine metabolism, selegiline has a controversial role as a potential neuroprotective agent. This suggestion of neuroprotective effects developed from early observations that selegiline could block the neurotoxic effects of the synthetic narcotic derivative 1-methyl-4-phenyl-1,2,3,6-tetrahydropyridine (MPTP) on nigral neurons (27–29). Intravenous drug users exposed to MPTP developed symptoms of PD which were nearly identical to sporadic forms of PD (30,31). The toxicity of MPTP against nigral neurons is not direct, however, and requires conversion of the parent compound to a toxic derivative 1-methyl-4-phenylpyridinium ion (MPP+), which is mediated by MAO-B activity. MPP+, in turn, is specifically concentrated in dopaminergic neurons and blocks the mitochondrial respiratory chain by inhibiting complex I of the electron transfer chain, contributing to its high specificity for nigral neurons and potent neurotoxicity (32). Selegiline blocks the conversion of MPTP to MPP+ and prevents the resulting nigral neurotoxicity (33).

Subsequent investigations have postulated a multitude of other potential neuroprotective mechanisms associated with selegiline therapy in humans. While outside the scope of this review, the list of possible neurodegenerative mechanisms that selegiline may influence is extensive and includes (a) preventing conversion of environmental pro-toxins (by blocking MAO-B activity) into potential neurotoxic agents, analogous to the MPTP model of nigral neuronal cell death, (b) preventing excessive accumulation and toxicity of oxidative radicals through modification of dopamine metabolism and/or promoting endogenous antioxidant pathways and mechanisms, (c) mimicking endogenous neurotrophic growth factors, leading to repair and regrowth of damaged neurons, and (d) blocking the presumed common pathway of cell death in most neurodegenerative disorders by acting as an antiapoptotic agent and preventing programmed cell death (34,35).

IV. CLINICAL TRIALS—DEPRESSION

Initial studies of selegiline examined its efficacy in treating depression using doses that were relatively MAO-B nonselective (36). In the management of depression, selegiline was found to be useful in patients with depression with or without bipolar features (12). Eleven out of 12 patients had at least 85% inhibition of platelet MAO-B activity after one week of 5 mg/day therapy. After the first week of 5 mg/day, patients were increased to 10 mg/day and then a week later given 15 mg/day. A majority of the patients had greater than 50% reduction in depression despite the absence of a clear correlation with the degree of MAO-B inhibition. One patient developed hypomania and had to be withdrawn from therapy. In this patient population there was a small biphasic effect, with the initial benefit seen within 3 days and further benefit occurring approximately 3 weeks later (37).

V. CLINICAL TRIALS—PARKINSON'S DISEASE

A. Adjunctive Therapy

Levodopa was also introduced in the 1960s as a novel and dramatically effective treatment of PD (38). However, treatment of PD with levodopa resulted in long-term complications including motor fluctuations and dyskinesias. Combination therapy with levodopa and nonselective inhibitors of MAO enhanced the symptomatic improvement seen with levodopa but carried a significant side effect profile, including hypertensive crises (39).

In 1975 Birkmayer and colleagues demonstrated that selegiline potentiated the anti-parkinsonian effects of levodopa therapy when given either parenterally or orally (40,41). In 1977 they reported a clinical trial in 223 PD patients where selegiline was used in combination with levodopa (LD) (42). The addition of selegiline to levodopa resulted in a statistically significant benefit within 60 minutes after the oral dose of selegiline was given, and the benefit was maintained for 1–3 days. These findings were confirmed by subsequent clinical trials (11,43).

In 1983 Birkmayer reviewed his group's experience using selegiline as adjunctive therapy to levodopa in almost 2000 patients over 9 years (44). The primary benefits included improvement of akinesia, decreased frequency and severity of on/off phases, and a reduction in daily motor fluctuations. In addition, patients on selegiline were able to reduce their total daily doses of levodopa and experienced limited side effects from selegiline, most commonly dyskinesias.

Rinne reported 45 PD patients with motor fluctuations following long-term levodopa therapy who were then treated with an open-label trial of selegiline. Over a 1- to 3-month period, 5–10 mg of selegiline daily resulted in a significant improvement in up to 60% of the patients (45).

Similarly, Gerstenbrand and colleagues (46) reported 48 PD patients, all of whom were experiencing decreasing benefits from their therapeutic regimen, which included at least levodopa. Subjects were started on selegiline at a dose of 5–15 mg day to assess therapeutic efficacy. Of 28 patients with an akinetic/rigid form of PD, 13 had a significant response to selegiline. In 14 patients with symptoms of tremor accompanying the akinetic/rigid syndrome, 8 improved significantly with selegiline. A third group of 6 patients with tremor-dominant PD showed no significant improvement in tremor with the addition of selegiline (46).

A large number of double-blind, placebo-controlled trials were published between the years 1977–1989 examining the levodopa-enhancing effects of selegiline (47–61). Over 90% of these studies used 10 mg/day of selegiline. A total of 516 subjects are represented in these 16 trials, 380 (74%) of whom had motor fluctuations. These studies examined either clinical improvement as measured by PD rating scales, reduction of motor fluctuations, reduction in total daily levodopa dosage, or any combination of these three outcome parameters.

When adjunctive selegiline therapy was compared to placebo, in 10/13 studies there was significant improvement in motor fluctuations, in 11/15 studies there was significant improvement in the clinical symptoms of PD, and in 9 studies there was a significant average reduction of 28% in daily levodopa dosage in addition to clinical improvement. The most common side effect was dyskinesia (15,62).

B. Short-Term De Novo Studies

Several large, double-blind, placebo-controlled clinical trials were performed in order to address whether oral selegiline administration could slow the progression of PD in newly diagnosed patients. In most of these studies, the time required until administration of levodopa for control of PD symptoms was considered an indication of delay in the progression of the disease.

The DATATOP (Deprenyl and Tocopherol Antioxidant Therapy of Parkinsonism) study reported interim results in 1989 demonstrating that selegiline delayed the need for levodopa. A total of 800 patients were randomized to receive selegiline (5 mg bid), tocopherol (2000 IU/d, selected for its antioxidant properties), a combination of selegiline and tocopherol, or placebo. The endpoint of this study was the need to initiate levodopa therapy. After an average of 12 months, 97 patients receiving selegiline reached endpoint, while 176 patients not receiving selegiline reached endpoint (63,64).

Similar results were obtained in a smaller study of 54 patients (65). In a double-blind, placebo-controlled study measuring the time until levodopa therapy was required, patients who were randomized to receive placebo averaged 312 days before they required levodopa compared to an average of 549 days in the selegiline group. The difference between the two groups based on Kaplan-Meier survival curves was significant in favor of selegiline. Multiple similar studies corroborated these findings (66–68).

At this point, controversy arose regarding the mechanism of action of selegiline's ability to delay levodopa therapy. Evidence accumulated that selegiline did have mild symptomatic benefits, either directly, or perhaps through its metabolites desmethylselegiline, methamphetamine, or amphetamine. Multiple authors (34, 69–73) argued that the demonstrable symptomatic benefit of selegiline was either sufficient or insufficient to account for the dramatic delay in the need for dopaminergic rescue, thus refuting or supporting the concept of a neuroprotective effect. Long-term analysis of the DATATOP cohort demonstrated differences in the rate of development of motor complications, supporting the use of selegiline and suggesting that long-term selegiline use in PD may alter the clinical course (74,75).

In a double-blind, placebo-controlled trial, 157 de novo PD patients were randomized to receive either selegiline or placebo (76) until levodopa therapy became necessary. At that point, the selegiline or placebo was withdrawn for 8 weeks to evaluate possible symptomatic effects of selegiline. Selegiline was noted to have a wash-in effect at the time of initiation, as there was measurable symptomatic improvement compared to placebo. After the 8-week wash-out period, there was no significant difference in the degree of increased disability seen in the selegiline group compared to placebo. Thus, the benefit attained by patients randomized to receive selegiline did not appear to be solely dependent on a symptomatic effect. In addition, the progression of symptoms from baseline to the end of the wash-out period was significantly slower in the selegiline group when the progression was adjusted by the time to reach the endpoint.

When a semi-annual progression of disability was assessed by different PD rating scales, there were statistically significant differences in favor of the selegiline group. The semi-annual rate of progression of clinical disability decreased by 74–160% as measured by these different scales. The authors attempted to address a major concern of all clinical trials purporting to demonstrate a neuroprotective effect of selegiline—the appropriate length of the wash-out following selegiline therapy, in order to eliminate any residual symptomatic, MAO-B inhibitory effects. In the original DATATOP study, homovanillic acid (HVA, an indirect marker of MAO activity) levels were still decreased at one month following selegiline treatment, but returned to normal after 2 months. By selecting 2 months as the wash-out, the authors argued that they were able to eliminate the symptomatic effects of selegiline, which may have confounded previous trials.

To confound the situation further, a large, multicenter, open-label, prospective trial of selegiline in early PD was published in 1995 (77). In this study, 520 patients were randomized to receive levodopa, selegiline plus levodopa, or bromocriptine, a dopamine receptor agonist. Selegiline dramatically decreased the need for additional doses of levodopa during the study's 4-year follow-up. The mean levodopa dose without selegiline was 635 mg versus 460 mg with selegiline. The mortality rate in the group treated with selegiline after 5 years was significantly higher compared with the group treated with levodopa alone. This study resulted in a new wave of response regarding the use of selegiline in early PD. Previous results were reexamined, mortality rates were calculated, and multiple publications followed, none of which demonstrated any similar data to confirm the findings of this controversial study (78–84).

C. Long-Term Analysis of De Novo Studies

Data from 800 patients with early PD from the DATATOP clinical trial were re-analyzed to evaluate the long-term effects of selegiline (74). Seven percent of the patients had freezing at study entry, and 26% experienced the symptom by the end of follow-up. High baseline risk factors for developing freezing included the onset of PD with a gait disorder, increased rigidity, postural instability, bradykinesia and speech disturbance, and longer disease duration. Selegiline treatment was strongly associated with a decreased risk for developing freezing, while vitamin E had no effect. The authors concluded that selegiline reduced the risk of developing freezing by 53%. This effect only partially faded after selegiline was stopped. This benefit was offset by an increased rate of developing dyskinesias, which occurred in 34% of the selegiline group compared to 19% of the placebo group (75).

In Finland, researchers studied 44 de novo PD patients who were randomized to receive either selegiline or placebo. The patients were examined for 5 years following the point at which all 44 patients required levodopa (85). At the end of 5 years of receiving either selegiline or placebo as well as any additionally required levodopa therapy, patients in the placebo group required an average of 725 mg of levodopa per day compared to 405 mg per day in the selegiline group. No significant differences in mortality were seen between the two groups.

In Germany, 116 de novo patients with PD were randomized in the SELEDO (selegiline plus levodopa) study to receive either selegiline and levodopa or placebo and levodopa and then followed for up to 5 years (86). The dose of levodopa was titrated initially to patient requirements prior to randomization. The average time after randomization until the patients required an additional 50% increase in their dose of levodopa was statistically in favor of the selegiline group—4.9 years versus 2.6 years in the placebo group. The frequency of developing motor fluctuations was not statistically different between the two groups, but showed a trend in favor of the selegiline group. There was no statistically significant difference in mortality between the two groups.

The data from these long-term, prospective, randomized, and blinded trials support the hypothesis that selegiline may modify and possibly slow the progression of PD. The most common adverse effect of selegiline, dyskinesias, appears to be more common among individuals who are already receiving levodopa. Dyskinesia is usually ameliorated through lowering the total daily levodopa dosage. Finally, the possibility that selegiline could potentially contribute to increased mortality rates in PD seems unlikely.

VI. RASAGILINE AND ZYDIS SELEGILINE

Another specific MAO-B inhibitor, n-propargyl-l(R)-aminoindan or rasagiline has recently undergone clinical trials by the Parkinson Study Group in both early and advanced Parkinson's disease. In the TEMPO trial (Rasagiline Mesylate [TVP-1012] in Early Monotherapy for PD Outpatients) 404 early, untreated patients were randomized to receive placebo versus 1 or 2 mg of rasagiline. The change in the total UPDRS score between baseline and 26 weeks of treatment in these subjects was statistically significant in favor of rasagiline at both doses (87). In the PRESTO trial (Parkinson's Rasagiline: Efficacy & Safety in the Treatment of "OFF"), 472 patients with motor fluctuations and at least 2.5 hours of "off" time per day were randomized to receive placebo versus 0.5 or 1.0 mg of rasagiline. The change in the total daily "off" time between baseline and 26 weeks of treatment was significantly reduced in both treatment groups compared to placebo (88).

Zydis selegiline (Zelapar^{TM}) is an orally dissolving table of selegiline. It is available in Europe and is expected to have approval in the United States in 2004. Zydis selegiline was developed as an adjunct to levodopa. The tablet dissolves in saliva on the tongue in seconds and is absorbed into the tissue of the mouth. A daily dose of 1.25 mg of zydis selegiline is equivalent to 10 mg/day of selegiline. Selegiline undergoes first-pass metabolism by the liver to metabolites such as amphetamines and methamphetamines, which can cause adverse effects. The use of the Zydis formulation is hoped to reduce side effects by the avoidance of first-pass hepatic metabolism. In a multicenter, randomized, placebo-controlled study, 163 PD patients with motor fluctuations on stable levodopa received 1.25 mg of Zydis selegiline for 6 weeks followed by 2.5 mg for an additional 6 weeks. A significant reduction in off time and improvements in on and off UPDRS motor scores were observed with the 2.5 mg dose compared to placebo (8).

ACKNOWLEDGMENT

I wish to gratefully acknowledge the assistance of friend and colleague Dr. L. John Greenfield for his editorial comments.

REFERENCES

1. Knoll J. The pharmacology of selegiline ((-)deprenyl). New aspects. Acta Neurol Scand Suppl 1989; 126:83–91.
2. Lees AJ. Comparison of therapeutic effects and mortality data of levodopa and levodopa combined with selegiline in patients with early, mild Parkinson's disease. Parkinson's Disease Research Group of the United Kingdom. BMJ 1995; 311(7020):1602–1607.
3. Knoll J. Deprenyl (selegiline): the history of its development and pharmacological action. Acta Neurol Scand Suppl 1983; 95:57–80.
4. Zeller EA, Barsky J, Fouts JE, Kirchheimer WF, Van Orden IS. Influence of isonicotinic acid hydrazide (INH) and 1-isonicotinic-2-isopropyl hydrazide (IIH) on bacterial and mammalian enzymes. Experientia 1952; 8:349–350.
5. Blackwell B. Hypertensive crisis due to monoamine oxidase inhibitors. Lancet 1963; 11:849–851.
6. Horwitz D, Lovenberg W, Engelmann K, Sjoerdsma A. Monoamine oxidase inhibitors, tyramine and cheese. JAMA 1964; 188:1108–1110.
7. Knoll J, Ecseri Z, Kelemen K, Nievel J, Knoll B. Phenylisopropylmethylpropinylamine (E-250), a new spectrum psychic energizer. Arch Int Pharmacodyn Ther 1965; 155(1):154–164.

8. Johnston JP. Some observations upon a new inhibitor of monoamine oxidase in brain tissue. Biochem Pharmacol 1968; 17(7):1285–1297.
9. Riederer P, Jellinger K, Danielczyk W, Seemann D, Ulm G, Reynolds GP, Birkmayer W, Koppel H. Combination treatment with selective monoamine oxidase inhibitors and dopaminergic agonists in Parkinson's disease: biochemical and clinical observations. Adv Neurol 1983; 37:159–176.
10. Ehringer H, Hornykiewicz. Verteilung von Noradrenalin und Dopamine (3-Hydroxytyramin) im Gehirn des Menschen und ihr Verhalten bei Erkrankungen des extrapyramidalen Systems. Klin Wschr. 1960; 38:1236–1239.
11. Rinne UK. Recent advances in research on parkinsonism. Acta Neurol Scand Suppl. 1978; 67:77–113.
12. Mann J, Gershon S. L-Deprenyl, a selective monoamine oxidase type-B inhibitor in endogenous depression. Life Sci 1980; 26(11):877–882.
13. Glover V, Sandler M, Owen F, Riley GJ. Dopamine is a monoamine oxidase B substrate in man. Nature 1977; 265(5589):80–81.
14. Heinonen EH, Myllyla V, Sotaniemi K, Lamintausta R, Salonen JS, Anttila M, Savijarvi M, Kotila M, Rinne UK. Pharmacokinetics and metabolism of selegiline. Acta Neurol Scand Suppl. 1989; 126:93–99.
15. Heinonen EH, Rinne UK. Selegiline in the treatment of Parkinson's disease. Acta Neurol Scand Suppl. 1989; 126:103–111.
16. Fowler JS, MacGregor RR, Wolf AP, Arnett CD, Dewey SL, Schlyer D, Christman D, Logan J, Smith M, Sachs H, et al. Mapping human brain monoamine oxidase A and B with 11C-labeled suicide inactivators and PET. Science 1987; 235(4787):481–485.
17. Fowler JS, Wolf AP, MacGregor RR, Dewey SL, Logan J, Schlyer DJ, Langstrom B. Mechanistic positron emission tomography studies: demonstration of a deuterium isotope effect in the monoamine oxidase-catalyzed binding of [11C]L-deprenyl in living baboon brain. J Neurochem. 1988; 51(5):1524–1534.
18. Riederer P, Youdim MB, Rausch WD, Birkmayer W, Jellinger K, Seemann D. On the mode of action of L-deprenyl in the human central nervous system. J Neural Transm 1978; 43(3–4):217–226.
19. Riederer P, Youdim MB, Birkmayer W, Jellinger K. Monoamine oxidase activity during (–)-deprenil therapy: human brain post-mortem studies. Adv Biochem Psychopharmacol 1978; 19:377–382.
20. Reiderer P, Reynolds GP. Deprenyl is a selective inhibitor of brain MAO-B in the long-term treatment of Parkinsons's disease. Br J Clin Pharmacol 1980; 9(1):98–99.
21. Riederer P, Youdim MB. Monoamine oxidase activity and monoamine metabolism in brains of parkinsonian patients treated with l-deprenyl. J Neurochem 1986; 46(5):1359–1365.
22. Glover V, Elsworth JD, Sandler M. Dopamine oxidation and its inhibition by (-)-deprenyl in man. J Neural Transm Suppl 1980; 16:163–172.
23. Reynolds GP, Elsworth JD, Blau K, Sandler M, Lees AJ, Stern GM. Deprenyl is metabolized to methamphetamine and amphetamine in man. Br J Clin Pharmacol 1978; 6(6):542–544.
24. Yoshida T, Yamada Y, Yamamoto T, Kuroiwa Y. Metabolism of deprenyl, a selective monoamine oxidase (MAO) B inhibitor in rat: relationship of metabolism to MAO-B inhibitory potency. Xenobiotica 1986; 16(2):129–136.
25. Parkinson D, Callingham BA. Substrate and inhibitor selectivity of human heart monoamine oxidase. Biochem Pharmacol 1979; 28(10):1639–1643.
26. Egashira T, Yamamoto T, Yamanaka Y. Effects of d-methamphetamine on monkey brain monoamine oxidase, in vivo and in vitro. Jpn J Pharmacol 1987; 45(1):79–88.
27. Mytilineou C, Cohen G. Deprenyl protects dopamine neurons from the neurotoxic effect of 1-methyl-4-phenylpyridinium ion. J Neurochem 1985; 45(6):1951–1953.
28. Lewin R. Drug trial for Parkinson's. Science 1987; 236(4807):1420.
29. Fuller RW, Hemrick-Luecke SK, Perry KW. Deprenyl antagonizes acute lethality of1-methyl-4-phenyl-1,2,3,6-tetrahydropyridine in mice. J Pharmacol Exp Ther 1988; 247(2):531–535.
30. Davis GC, Williams AC, Markey SP, Ebert MH, Caine ED, Reichert CM, Kopin IJ. Chronic parkinsonism secondary to intravenous injection of meperidine analogues. Psychiatry Res 1979; 1:249–254.
31. Langston JW, Ballard PA, Tetrud JW, Irwin I. Chronic parkinsonism in humans due to a product of meperidine-analog synthesis. Science 1983; 219:979–980.
32. Chiba K, Trevor A, Castagnoli N Jr. Active uptake of MPP+ a metabolite of MPTP by brain synaptosomes. Biochem Biophys Res Commun 1984; 120:574–578.
33. Heikkila RE, Manzino L, Cabbat FS, Duvoisin RC. Protection against the dopaminergic neurotoxicity of 1-methyl-4-phenyl-1,2,3,6-tetrahydropyridine by monoamine oxidase inhibitors. Nature 1984; 311:467–469.
34. Olanow CW. Deprenyl in the treatment of Parkinson's disease: clinical effects and speculations on mechanism of action. J Neural Transm Suppl. 1996; 48:75–84.
35. Ebadi M, Sharma S, Shavali S, El Refaey H. Neuroprotective actions of selegiline. J Neurosci Res. 2002; 67(3):285–289.

36. Varga E, Tringer L. Clinical trial of a new type promptly acting psychoenergetic agent (phenyl-isopropyl-methylpropinyl-HCl, "E-250"). Acta Med Acad Sci Hung 1967; 23(3):289–295.

37. Mann JJ, Aarons SF, Wilner PJ, Keilp JG, Sweeney JA, Pearlstein T, Frances AJ, Kocsis JH, Brown RP. A controlled study of the antidepressant efficacy and side effects of(-)-deprenyl. A selective monoamine oxidase inhibitor. Arch Gen Psychiatry 1989; 46(1):45–50.

38. Birkmayer W, Hornykiewicz O. Der L 3,4-Dihydroxyphenylalanin (DOPA) Effect bei der Parkinson-akinese. Wien Klin Wochenschr 1961; 73:787–788.

39. Gerstenbrand F, Prosenz P. [On the treatment of Parkinson's syndrome with monoamine oxidase inhibitors alone and in combination with L-dopa]. Praxis 1965; 54(46):1373–1377.

40. Birkmayer W, Danielczyk W, Neumayer E, Riederer P. Dopaminergic supersensitivity in parkinsonism. Adv Neurol 1975; 9:121–129.

41. Birkmayer W, Riederer P, Youdim MB, Linauer W. The potentiation of the anti akinetic effect after L-dopa treatment by an inhibitor of MAO-B, Deprenil. J Neural Transm 1975; 36(3–4):303–326.

42. Birkmayer W, Riederer P, Ambrozi L, Youdim MB. Implications of combined treatment with 'Madopar' and L-deprenil in Parkinson's disease. A long-term study. Lancet 1977; 1(8009):439–443.

43. Csanda E, Antal J, Antony M, Csanaky A. Experiences with L-deprenyl in parkinsonism. J Neural Transm. 1978; 43(3–4):263–269.

44. Birkmayer W. Deprenyl (selegiline) in the treatment of Parkinson's disease. Acta Neurol Scand Suppl. 1983; 95:103–105.

45. Rinne UK. Deprenyl (selegiline) in the treatment of Parkinson's disease. Acta Neurol Scand Suppl. 1983; 95:107–111.

46. Gerstenbrand F, Ransmayr G, Poewe W. Deprenyl (selegiline) in combination treatment of Parkinson's disease. Acta Neurol Scand Suppl. 1983; 95:123–126.

47. Lees AJ, Shaw KM, Kohout LJ, Stern GM, Elsworth JD, Sandler M, Youdim MB. Deprenyl in Parkinson's disease. Lancet 1977; 2(8042):791–795.

48. Stern GM, Lees AJ, Sandler M. Recent observations on the clinical pharmacology of (-) deprenyl. J Neural Transm 1978; 43(3–4):245–251.

49. Schachter M, Marsden CD, Parkes JD, Jenner P, Testa B. Deprenyl in the management of response fluctuations in patients with Parkinson's disease on levodopa. J Neurol Neurosurg Psychiatry 1980; 43(11):1016–1021.

50. Goldstein L. The "on-off" phenomena in Parkinson's disease—treatment and theoretical considerations. Mt Sinai J Med 1980; 47(1):80–84.

51. Eisler T, Teravainen H, Nelson R, Krebs H, Weise V, Lake CR, Ebert MH, Whetzel N, Murphy DL, Kopin IJ, Calne DB. Deprenyl in Parkinson disease. Neurology 1981; 31(1):19–23.

52. Presthus J, Hajba A. Deprenyl (selegiline) combined with levodopa and a decarboxylase inhibitor in the treatment of Parkinson's disease. Acta Neurol Scand Suppl 1983; 95:127–133.

53. Brodersen P, Philbert A, Gulliksen G, Stigard A. The effect of L-deprenyl on on-off phenomena in Parkinson's disease. Acta Neurol Scand 1985; 71(6):494–497.

54. Fischer PA, Baas H. Therapeutic efficacy of R-(-)-deprenyl as adjuvant therapy in advanced parkinsonism. J Neural Transm Suppl 1987; 25:137–147.

55. Golbe LI, Duvoisin RC. Double-blind trial of R-(-)-deprenyl for the "on-off" effect complicating Parkinson's disease. J Neural Transm Suppl. 1987; 25:123–129.

56. Lieberman AN, Gopinathan G, Neophytides A, Foo SH. Deprenyl versus placebo in Parkinson disease: a double-blind study. NY State J Med. 1987; 87(12):646–649.

57. Rascol O, Montastruc JL, Senard JM, Demonet JF, Simonetta M, Rascol A. Two weeks of treatment with deprenyl (selegiline) does not prolong L-dopa effect in Parkinsonian patients: a double-blind cross-over placebo-controlled trial. Neurology 1988; 38(9):1387–1391.

58. Heinonen EH, Rinne UK, Tuominen J. Selegiline in the treatment of daily fluctuations in disability of parkinsonian patients with long-term levodopa treatment. Acta Neurol Scand Suppl 1989; 126:113–118.

59. Teychenne PF, Parker S. Double-blind, crossover placebo controlled trial of selegiline in Parkinson's disease—an interim analysis. Acta Neurol Scand Suppl 1989; 126:119–125.

60. Sivertsen B, Dupont E, Mikkelsen B, Mogensen P, Rasmussen C, Boesen F, Heinonen E. Selegiline and levodopa in early or moderately advanced Parkinson's disease: a double-blind controlled short- and long-term study. Acta Neurol Scand Suppl 1989; 126:147–152.

61. CD Chouza C, Aljanati R, Scaramelli A, De Medina O, Caamano JL, Buzo R, Fernandez A, Romero S. Combination of selegiline and controlled release levodopa in the treatment of fluctuations of clinical disability in parkinsonian patients. Acta Neurol Scand Suppl. 1989; 126:127–137.

62. Golbe LI. Deprenyl as symptomatic therapy in Parkinson's disease. Clin Neuropharmacol 1988; 11(5):387–400.

63. The Parkinson Study Group. Effect of deprenyl on the progression of disability in early Parkinson's disease. N Engl J Med. 1989; 321(20):1364–1371.

64. Parkinson Study Group DATATOP: a multicenter controlled clinical trial in early Parkinson's disease. Arch Neurol. 1989; 46(10):1052–1060.

65. Tetrud JW, Langston JW. The effect of deprenyl (selegiline) on the natural history of Parkinson's disease. Science 1989; 245(4917):519–522.

66. Myllyla VV, Sotaniemi KA, Vuorinen JA, Heinonen EH. Selegiline as a primary treatment of Parkinson's disease. Acta Neurol Scand Suppl. 1991; 136:70–72.

67. Myllyla VV, Sotaniemi KA, Vuorinen JA, Heinonen EH. Selegiline as initial treatment in de novo parkinsonian patients. Neurology. 1992; 42(2):339–343.

68. Olanow CW, Hauser RA, Gauger L, Malapira T, Koller W, Hubble J, Bushenbark K, Lilienfeld D, Esterlitz J. The effect of deprenyl and levodopa on the progression of Parkinson's disease. Ann Neurol. 1995; 38(5):771–777.

69. LeWitt PA. Deprenyl's effect at slowing progression of parkinsonian disability: the DATATOP study. The Parkinson Study Group. Acta Neurol Scand Suppl. 1991; 136:79–86.

70. Shoulson I. An interim report of the effect of selegiline (L-deprenyl) on the progression of disability in early Parkinson's disease. The Parkinson Study Group. Eur Neurol. 1992; 32(suppl 1):46–53.

71. Schulzer M, Mak E, Calne DB. The antiparkinson efficacy of deprenyl derives from transient improvement that is likely to be symptomatic. Ann Neurol. 1992; 32(6):795–798.

72. Brannan T, Yahr MD. Comparative study of selegiline plus L-dopa-carbidopa versus L-dopa-carbidopa alone in the treatment of Parkinson's disease. Ann Neurol. 1995; 37(1):95–98.

73. Olanow CW, Mytilineou C, Tatton W. Current status of selegiline as a neuroprotective agent in Parkinson's disease. Mov Disord. 1998; 13(suppl 1):55–58.

74. Giladi N, McDermott MP, Fahn S, Przedborski S, Jankovic J, Stern M, Tanner C. Freezing of gait in PD: prospective assessment in the DATATOP cohort. Neurology. 2001; 56(12):1712–1721.

75. Shoulson I, Oakes D, Fahn S, Lang A, Langston JW, LeWitt P, Olanow CW, Penney JB, Tanner C, Kieburtz K, Rudolph A. Impact of sustained deprenyl (selegiline) in levodopa-treated Parkinson's-disease: a randomized placebo-controlled extension of the deprenyl and tocopherol antioxidative therapy of parkinsonism trial. Ann Neurol. 2002; 51(5):604–612.

76. Palhagen S, Heinonen EH, Hagglund J, Kaugesaar T, Kontants H, Maki-Ikola O, Palm R, Turunen J. Selegiline delays the onset of disability in de novo parkinsonian patients. Swedish Parkinson Study Group. Neurology. 1998; 51(2):520–525.

77. Lees AJ. Comparison of therapeutic effects and mortality data of levodopa and levodopa combined with selegiline in patients with early, mild Parkinson's disease. Parkinson's Disease Research Group of the United Kingdom. BMJ. 1995; 311(7020):1602–1607.

78. Olanow CW, Myllyla VV, Sotaniemi KA, Larsen JP, Palhagen S, Przuntek H, Heinonen EH, Kilkku O, Lammintausta R, Maki-Ikola O, Rinne UK. Effect of selegiline on mortality in patients with Parkinson's disease: a meta-analysis. Neurology. 1998; 51(3):825–830.

79. Lees AJ, Head J, Shlomo YB. Selegiline and mortality in Parkinson's disease: another view. Ann Neurol 1997; 41(2):282–283.

80. Parkinson Study Group. Mortality in DATATOP: a multicenter trial in early Parkinson's disease. Ann Neurol. 1998; 43(3):318–325.

81. Oakes D. Selegiline and excess mortality. Clin Neuropharmacol 1997; 20(6):542.

82. Ben-Shlomo Y, Churchyard A, Head J, Hurwitz B, Overstall P, Ockelford J, Lees AJ. Investigation by Parkinson's Disease Research Group of United Kingdom into excess mortality seen with combined levodopa and selegiline treatment in patients with early, mild Parkinson's disease: further results of randomized trial and confidential inquiry. BMJ 1998; 316(7139):1191–1196.

83. Donnan PT, Steinke DT, Stubbings C, Davey PG, MacDonald TM. Selegiline and mortality in subjects with Parkinson's disease: a longitudinal community study. Neurology 2000; 55(12):1785–1789.

84. Lees AJ, Katzenschlager R, Head J, Ben-Shlomo Y. Ten-year follow-up of three different initial treatments in de-novo PD: a randomized trial. Neurology 2001; 57(9):1687–1694.

85. Myllyl VV, Sotaniemi KA, Hakulinen P, Maki-Ikol O, Heinonen EH. Selegiline as the primary treatment of Parkinson's disease—a long-term double-blind study. Acta Neurol Scand 1997; 95:211–218.

86. Przuntek H, Conrad B, Dichgans J, Kraus PH, Krauseneck P, Pergande G, Rinne U, Schimrigk K, Schnitker J, Vogel HP. SELEDO: a 5-year long-term trial on the effect of selegiline in early parkinsonian patients treated with levodopa. Eur J Neurol. 1999; 6(2):141–150.

87. Parkinson Study Group. A controlled trial of rasagiline in early Parkinson disease: the TEMPO study. Arch Neurol 2002; 59(12):1937–1943.

88. Parkinson Study Group. A randomized placebo controlled trial of rasagiline in Parkinson's disease patients with levodopa-related motor fluctuations. JAMA, submitted.

89. Shellenberger MK, Clarke A, Donoghue S. Zydis selegiline reduces "off" time and improves symptoms in patients with Parkinson's disease. Mov Disord 2000; 15(suppl 3):116.

18
Amantadine

Jaime Kulisevsky
Autonomous University of Barcelona, Barcelona, Spain
Eduardo Tolosa
University of Barcelona, Barcelona, Spain

I. INTRODUCTION

Since amantadine was first reported to be useful in the treatment of Parkinson's disease (PD) by Schwab et al. (1) in 1969, several clinical trials have tested the efficacy of amantadine alone or in combination with levodopa. Amantadine is a useful, well-tolerated but second-line drug without the dramatic symptomatic effect of levodopa on the cardinal features of PD. It has been observed that discontinuation of amantadine in patients with PD may result in a dramatic worsening of the clinical state (2). Amantadine is a noncompetitive antagonist of the N-methyl-D-aspartate (NMDA) receptor and can have a putative antidyskinetic effect, which has led to renewed clinical and theoretical interest in amantadine.

II. PHARMACOLOGY AND MECHANISM OF ACTION

Amantadine hydrochloride was originally introduced as an antiviral agent effective against A2 Asian influenza (3) and was fortuitously noted to be useful in relieving clinical symptoms in a patient with PD (1). Amantadine hydrochloride is 1-amino-adamantanamine, the salt of a symmetrical 10-carbon primary amine. The drug is readily absorbed (blood levels peak 1–4 h after an oral dose of 2.5 mg/kg) and poorly metabolized in humans (more than 90% of an ingested dose can be recovered unchanged in the urine) (4). Amantadine hydrochloride is available as 100 mg capsules and as a syrup containing 50 mg/50 mL. The recommended dosage for both prophylaxis and treatment of influenza and for PD is 200 mg/d in two divided doses (5,6). Chronic administration has resulted in accumulation of the drug in patients with impaired renal function, in whom it causes concomitant toxicity (7,8).

There are several possible mechanisms of action of amantadine in PD, but the exact mechanism still remains unclear. Most of the behavioral and neurochemical studies indicate that amantadine can interact with catecholamines, especially dopamine. It is apparent from basic pharmacological studies that amantadine may act presynaptically and postsynaptically. Presynaptically, it functions as follows:

1. By enhancing the release of stored catecholamines from intact dopaminergic terminals (9–12).
2. By inhibiting catecholamine reuptake at the presynaptic terminal, which requires high concentrations of the drug to be achieved in vitro and is probably not verified in vivo at therapeutic dosages (13–15).

Postsynaptically, it functions as follows:

1. By direct agonism on dopamine receptors (16,17).
2. By changes in the dopamine receptor conformations that fix the receptor in a high-affinity configuration (17,18). An increase in dopamine receptor binding with long-term amantadine treatment in the mouse has been reported (17), which would not be expected from a drug acting as a receptor agonist but is more characteristic of a dopamine agonist. A recent positron emission tomographic (PET) study (19) suggested that therapeutic doses of amantadine (200 mg/d) do not produce an increase in extracellular levels of dopamine sufficiently to inhibit raclopride binding or that, if present, it is masked by a concurrent increase in receptor availability (17).
3. By a possible combined presynaptic and postsynaptic action causing simultaneous interference with reuptake, release, and receptor interaction not necessarily in a direction favoring increased dopamine stimulation (17).

In addition to its effects on dopamine systems, nondopaminergic properties of amantadine have been proposed, including an anticholinergic action (20,21). There is evidence that the beneficial effects of amantadine may be mediated in part by NMDA receptor blockade (22).

Modulation of the activity of the major excitatory neurotransmitter, glutamate, may be beneficial in PD. The use of antagonists of the NMDA subtype of glutamate receptors can (a) produce a pharmacological blockade of the abnormally increased activity of the subthalamic nucleus, which is thought to play a crucial role in PD, (b) enhance the release and turnover of striatal dopamine in vivo, (c) reverse the akinesia and rigidity associated with monoamine depletion or neuroleptic-induced catalepsy, (d) synergize with dopaminergic agonists and anticholinergic drugs, and (e) protect nigral neurons from death in animal models of PD (22).

The therapeutic benefit of amantadine in PD may be mediated in part by the blockade of glutamate receptors. It has been shown that amantadine displays a considerable affinity for the NMDA receptor and is able to displace the noncompetitive NMDA receptor antagonist MK-801 from the NMDA receptor complex with inhibition constant in the low micromolar range (23). Amantadine also modulates the sensitivity of NMDA receptor ion channel binding sites as measured by phencyclidine binding (24). Importantly, this NMDA receptor antagonistic action is exerted at therapeutic levels (25).

On the other hand, an overactive glutaminergic system has been implicated in the pathogenesis of PD and other chronic neurodegenerative disorders in which neurons compromised by some other processes would be rendered more vulnerable to NMDA receptor–mediated toxicity (22). In such compromised neurons, normal concentrations of glutamate may become lethal, and excitotoxicity might simply be the final common pathway to cell death. It was demonstrated that amantadine is able to inhibit NMDA-induced cell death in neuronal cultures, and synergistic effects of the combination of amantadine and deprenyl have been suggested in the MPTP model of parkinsonism (22–26).

Thus, the role of amantadine as an NMDA antagonist may not only be considered at the symptomatic level, but may prove useful to slow the progression of the disease. Activities of amantadine other than antiviral or antiparkinsonian have been described (27,28). The mechanism that results in improvement in some patients with essential tremor remains elusive (29,30).

III. SIDE EFFECTS

Side effects of amantadine are generally mild, transient, and reversible (6). Its potential toxicity has been studied extensively in controlled situations. In healthy college students taking 200 mg/d for influenza prophylaxis, mild impairment in performance on tests of maximal and sustained attention occurred in some, but no other problems were detected (31). Mild side effects such as difficulty with concentration and lightheadedness occurred in 20–40% of subjects using dosages above 300 mg/d (32–34). More toxic effects, mostly neuropsychiatric in nature, have been reported with higher dosages (6,35) or in patients with renal impairment (7,8). Other side effects that are not clearly dosage-related involve the cardiovascular system and have occurred with long-term use of amantadine. These include livedo reticularis, peripheral edema, congestive heart failure, and orthostatic hypotension (36,37). In all instances, symptoms disappear after discontinuation of the drug or, in extreme circumstances, after hemodialysis (6–8). A death from malignant cardiac arrhythmia induced by amantadine poisoning (suicide attempt) has also been described (38).

Neurological manifestations of amantadine overdosage have been shown to be reversed with physostigmine (39). In psychotic patients, amantadine may cause severe mental symptoms (6). In these patients, amantadine is used to prevent parkinsonism caused by neuroleptics (40). It has been reported that amantadine administration is not associated with the deleterious effects that the anticholinergics produce on memory function, especially in the elderly (41). Nevertheless, combined treatment with anticholinergics and amantadine makes the occurrence of some mental side effects more common (6). Discontinuation of amantadine in neuroleptic-treated patients may precipitate or exacerbate the neuroleptic malignant syndrome (40).

Frequency of side effects with amantadine varies depending on, among other factors, the daily dosage of the drug. In Schwab et al.'s (1) original report on a group of 163 patients treated with maximal daily dosages of 200 mg/d, 22% experienced some type of side effect. The most common side effects are livedo reticularis and ankle edema, dryness of mouth, and difficulty focusing. More uncommon but more troublesome are mental aberrations such as confusion, depression, nightmares, insomnia, agitation, and visual hallucinations. Objective neurological findings can include ataxia, slurred speech, and, rarely, convulsion.

Persistent bilateral ankle edema occurred in 22% of patients in one study and tends to occur within 2–8 weeks of starting amantadine (42). Livedo reticularis is a common undesirable side effect at therapeutic dosages (36) and is probably related to the vasoconstrictor effect of catecholamines released by amantadine (37). It generally appears on the leg and occasionally on the buttocks. Patients usually do not complain about livedo reticularis, and it is generally found on routine inspection of the skin (43). Parkes et al. described livedo reticularis in 90% of their patients (42). Other less common side effects of amantadine in patients with PD are constipation, anorexia, giddiness, and lightheadedness. An evidence-based review of the literature (44) concluded that amantadine for PD "has an acceptable risk, without specialized monitoring."

IV. CLINICAL EFFICACY

In the first uncontrolled study (1), 107 (66%) of 163 patients treated with a maximum daily dosage of 200 mg showed improvement in akinesia and rigidity and some lessening of tremor. One third of the patients who experienced initial reduction of symptoms, particularly akinesia and rigidity, showed a slow but steady reduction of benefit after 4–8 weeks. In another 58%, benefit was sustained from 3 to 8 months of treatment. Twenty-two percent of the patients showed mild side effects that consisted of jitteriness, insomnia, abdominal uneasiness, slight dizziness, and a feeling of depression. These side effects resolved within 36 hours after amantadine was discontinued. In a subsequent publication, Schwab et al. (45) commented that the beneficial effect of amantadine usually occurred within the first 24 hours, following the first 100 mg capsule. A wearing off was generally seen if the patients did not take another 100 mg dose, but further increases in daily dosage usually did not result in a significant increase in benefit. When treatment with the drug was stopped, there was a prompt reappearance of symptoms within 24 hours.

A. Amantadine Versus Placebo as Monotherapy or in Patients Receiving Anticholinergics

In a double-blind study of 13 patients evaluating the effect of amantadine, Mann et al. (46) discontinued use of all previous conventional antiparkinsonian medications. They reported a beneficial effect of amantadine, superior to placebo, in reducing functional disability, but the duration of the trial was only 4 days of either amantadine or placebo. Walker et al. (47) discontinued previous medication in 36 of 42 patients and claimed that amantadine was effective in these patients. Quantitative measurements revealed significant improvement after amantadine in 10 of 19 tests of strength and posture and in all tests of coordination and gait. When amantadine was compared with placebo, an average improvement of 29% occurred in activities of daily living, 14% in tests of coordination, 11% in gait, and 3% in strength. Bauer and McHenry (43) evaluated the efficacy of amantadine monotherapy during a 3-week period. The drug produced a 21% improvement over baseline in PD scores, but this part of their study was not blinded. Butzer et al. (48) conducted a double-blind, placebo-controlled, crossover study in 26 patients. Amantadine provided a 12% improvement over placebo and a 13% improvement over baseline disability. Twenty of the 26 patients selected amantadine for long-term usage.

In a double-blind crossover trial of amantadine and placebo, each given for 2 weeks, Parkes et al. (49) found a significant improvement in PD scores in patients receiving amantadine. The degree of improvement was not related to age, sex, duration, or severity of disease nor to previous thalamotomy. There was no difference in the degree of reduction of total scores with amantadine in patients taking anticholinergics and in those not receiving such drugs. Side effects were more common with placebo treatment than with amantadine.

Parkes et al. (50) also published a study of amantadine dosage in the treatment of PD symptoms. Results of this trial confirmed the benefit seen with amantadine in previous trials and showed considerable individual variation in optimal dosage, with the response being greatest in the most disabled patients.

Hunter et al. (51), in a double-blind, placebo-controlled study of amantadine versus placebo in 17 patients, showed a small beneficial effect of amantadine on physical signs but no significant effect on functional disabilities. Improvement in physical signs was maintained for 8 weeks. Most of the patients studied were receiving anticholinergics throughout the study. In the report by Dallos et al. (52), which involved 62 patients taking anticholinergics in a 4-week double-blind trial, 29 were treated with amantadine and 33 with placebo. Modest but statistically significant improvement was observed in the amantadine-treated patients and patients' reaction to the drug was favorable in 70% of cases. Optimal benefit occurred after the first 2 weeks of treatment, and side effects were insignificant.

Appleton et al. (53) found amantadine superior to placebo among patients receiving anticholinergics both in the patients' own assessments of their abilities to carry out activities of daily living and in the observers' assessments of rigidity, tremor, and akinesia. In time-performance tests, average performance was better while patients were taking amantadine than while taking placebo, but only in some instances were the differences statistically significant. Side effects were few and minor; 19 of the 20 patients studied indicated their preference for amantadine over placebo. Gilligan et al. (54) gave placebo and amantadine to 33 patients with PD, each for a period of 3 weeks. Patients were receiving no concomitant anticholinergic drugs. It was the impression of Gilligan et al. that approximately two thirds of the group showed varying degrees of improvement while taking amantadine. Improvement for the majority of patients was of a subjective nature, but objective improvement in observations of tremor was statistically significant. In three of the patients, improvement was dramatic. Jorgensen et al. (55) assessed the effectiveness of amantadine in 149 patients in a multicenter double-blind trial. Objective improvement was seen in 56% of patients (moderate to marked in 32%), which was more prominent in severely affected patients. In this study, functional improvement reported by patients while on amantadine was frequently greater than that observed clinically. Side effects were generally mild.

B. Amantadine Versus Anticholinergics or Levodopa

A few clinical trials have compared amantadine as monotherapy to anticholinergic drugs and also to levodopa alone. Walker et al. (47), in a double-blind study, were able to compare baseline PD scores on anticholinergics in 30 patients with scores on amantadine as single therapy. Patients performed as well or better on amantadine than on standard optimal anticholinergic therapy in almost every qualitative or quantitative measure assessed. However, very few of the comparisons reached statistical significance.

Parkes et al. (56) compared the effects of benzhexol and amantadine given separately and later combined in 40 previously untreated, mildly disabled patients. In this study, patients received benzhexol, 2 mg four times daily, amantadine, 200 mg twice daily, or amantadine combined with benzhexol in a randomly assigned double-blind crossover trial. They found that benzhexol and amantadine each produced a 15% reduction in functional disability. However, the combination of benzhexol and amantadine produced a 40% reduction in total disability.

Koller (57) compared the efficacy of amantadine with that of trihexyphenidyl and also levodopa in reducing parkinsonian tremor. Each drug was administered for 2 weeks in a double-blind manner. Patients were selected because they were experiencing unilateral tremor without other signs. Amantadine significantly decreased tremor, but mean tremor amplitude reduction from baseline was 59% for trihexyphenidyl compared with 23% for amantadine. Amantadine did not cause more tremor reduction than the anticholinergic in any of the nine patients. At the end of the trial, five patients preferred trihexyphenidyl, whereas none preferred amantadine.

Fieschi et al. (58) gave amantadine to 31 patients for 2 weeks, placebo for one week, and subsequently levodopa. The optimal maintenance dosage for levodopa was reached in 6–12 weeks. Improvement with amantadine was significantly lower than the improvement with levodopa by a factor of 2. These investigators found a strong correlation between the improvements with the two drugs.

Parkes et al. (42,56) compared the effect of amantadine given for 4 weeks with that of levodopa administered during 6 months in individually determined doses and 30 mg a day of metoclopramide to minimize nausea. The efficacy of levodopa was evaluated in a nonblind manner. In this study, 9 of 12 patients preferred levodopa to their previous therapy. Amantadine produced a reduction in mean total disability scores of 17% compared to pretreatment scores ($p < 0.005$ in each case). Levodopa, on the other hand, reduced the total disability score by 36% after 6 months in the nine patients given this drug. Seven of the patients who improved with amantadine later responded to levodopa. Both amantadine and levodopa improved all symptoms of parkinsonism, but the effects of amantadine were slight on akinesia and rigidity and moderate on tremor and posture.

Hunter et al. (51) noted that the effect of amantadine on physical signs was minimal in 17 patients with PD and compared this effect with that obtained with maximal tolerated dosages of levodopa in a previous study in which an identical scoring system was used. Levodopa gave an average improvement of 8 units in a total initial score of 17 of 44, whereas the amantadine effect was only on the order of one unit. In addition, levodopa produced a significant improvement in functional disability that could not be detected in patients taking amantadine.

Barbeau et al. (59) administered amantadine to 53 patients in a double-blind, placebo-controlled study and compared its effects with those of levodopa administered in an open manner to 100 patients. According to the authors, "levodopa appeared to be over-whelmingly the winner except in a very few patients who could not tolerate optimal levodopa." In this study, the degree of response to levodopa could not be predicted from patients' previous responses while using amantadine. Some of the patients in whom amantadine failed were among those experiencing the best results with levodopa.

In summary, the short-term clinical trials in which amantadine was compared with placebo either as single therapy or in patients on anticholinergics indicate that this agent has a useful but modest antiparkinsonian effect. The antiparkinsonian potency of amantadine is clearly inferior to that of levodopa but at least similar to that of the anti-cholinergics. The degree of improvement achieved tends to be similar whether or not the patients are taking anticholinergic drugs. In one study, however, the combination of amantadine and anticholinergics (benzhexol) improved all symptoms by more than the sum of the improvement provided by each drug separately.

C. Long-Term Efficacy of Amantadine

One of the major drawbacks in the treatment of PD with amantadine is the apparent loss of therapeutic efficacy of the drug with time. Several investigators have observed this decline in efficacy, but others have not. Schwab et al. (1) observed that among 163 patients treated continuously with amantadine, benefits were sustained in 58% of patients for a period of 3–8 months. Twenty-six percent continued treatment with decreased benefit, which occurred after 4–8 weeks of treatment. This reduction in improvement usually leveled off and left the patient with moderate symptomatic control. In these patients, withdrawing amantadine entirely induced a prompt exacerbation of their symptoms. When amantadine was reintroduced, the benefit returned. Schwab et al. (45), in a subsequent report on 430 patients, also reports that a demonstrable fall-off in efficacy occurred after 30–60 days of treatment, although a positive response persisted at 60 days in 48% of patients taking amantadine alone or with anticholinergics. In the study by Hunter et al. (51), improvement in physical signs was maintained for 8 weeks, but three of the four patients noted deterioration in functional performance after 2–5 weeks of treatment.

Schwieger and Jenkins (60) observed that in seven patients (29%) an initial improvement was not maintained. These patients reverted to their pretreatment state after 4–8 weeks of therapy. Increasing the dosage of amantadine from 200 to 300 mg/d did not produce any change in the patients' conditions.

Butzer et al. (48) evaluated amantadine in 26 patients. After the initial 4-week double-blind phase, 10 patients chose to continue treatment for 10–12 months. Improvement in tremor and rigidity remained relatively constant, while there was a drop-off in efficacy in the timed tests. These investigators concluded that amantadine appears effective in the long-term treatment of some patients with PD.

Other investigators have not detected a decline in the efficacy of amantadine in long-term clinical trials. Parkes et al. (42) treated 26 patients with amantadine for 12 months. The improvement after 3 months (17% in total disability scores) was not significantly different from that at the end of one year. Zeldowicz and Huberman (61) obtained 25% improvement in a total of 77 patients on amantadine. In 19 patients, the investigators did not observe any decline in therapeutic effect during a mean follow-up of 21 months.

D. Amantadine Plus Levodopa

Several investigators have studied the effects of combining levodopa and amantadine. In these studies investigators have addressed several issues: Is the amantadine response a predictor of the levodopa response? Does previous treatment with amantadine modify the response to levodopa? Can amantadine potentiate the effects of levodopa? Is the administration of amantadine to patients receiving optimal dosages of levodopa of any additional therapeutic value? Can amantadine improve levodopa-related motor fluctuations? Placebo-controlled studies have shown that amantadine is efficacious in reducing levodopa-induced dyskinesias (62–66).

E. Levodopa Added to Amantadine

Godwin-Austin et al. (67) compared levodopa with placebo in 12 patients who had been taking amantadine for 3–6 months and had responded favorably. Ten of the 12 patients showed a distinct improvement with levodopa administered during a 4-week period. Barbeau et al. (59) added levodopa to the treatment of 25 patients receiving steady dosages of amantadine and noted that the dosage level of levodopa necessary to produce optimal results in this subgroup of patients was not essentially different from that in patients not on amantadine and that the degree of response to levodopa could not be predicted in these patients from their previous response to amantadine. In fact, some of the patients who experienced amantadine failure had the best results with levodopa. Parkes et al. (42)

administered amantadine for 3 months to 40 patients and later added levodopa. No significant change was noted in total score or in functional disability at 3 or 9 months, but after one year of levodopa both total and functional disability scores were improved. Substitution of amantadine for placebo at this point in three patients, under double-blind conditions, resulted in worsening of parkinsonism, particularly akinesia. In this group of patients, 45% developed involuntary movements. Bauer et al. (43) observed that levodopa, when added to the treatment of patients on amantadine induced after 6–9 weeks a modest (7%) improvement in disability scores. They concluded that amantadine and levodopa may be an effective combination therapy.

F. Amantadine Added to Levodopa

Trials to determine additional benefits from amantadine in patients already taking levodopa have yielded insufficient or conflicting results. Fieschi et al. (58) found amantadine effective in 11 of 20 patients on levodopa. That trial was not double-blind and lasted only 2 weeks. Godwin-Austin et al. (67) found an additional effect of amantadine in only one of 12 patients who were taking levodopa and anticholinergics on a stable regimen. They suggest that combined treatment with both drugs is only indicated when the maximum tolerated dosage of levodopa is very low. Barbeau et al. (59) added amantadine (200 mg/d) to the previous levodopa regimen in eight patients who had not reached optimal drug levels because of side effects. They observed improvement in seven patients without an increase in side effects, but in one patient involuntary movements worsened. Walker et al. (47) carried out a double-blind crossover trial of 3 weeks duration of amantadine versus placebo in 28 patients. Patients were treated with levodopa for at least 6 months and then randomly started on amantadine or placebo. On average, all parkinsonian scores were better in patients receiving the combination of drugs, with improved tremor, gait, and hand and feet coordination. Nevertheless, functional disability scores of the patients on levodopa and amantadine were similar to those of patients on levodopa alone.

Zeldowicz and Huberman (61), in a nonblind study, gave amantadine to 17 patients previously stabilized on varying dosages of levodopa and detected marked improvement in 15 patients and slight improvement in 2 patients. No increase in the side effects common to levodopa occurred with the addition of amantadine.

Fehling (68) also studied the effect of amantadine versus placebo in a double-blind, one-month crossover study in 21 patients receiving an optimal levodopa dosage. Amantadine was superior to placebo in its effect on total PD scores and postural and limb hypokinesia. Involuntary movements did not change appreciably during the study. From a functional point of view, the improvement noticed was only marginal in most patients and more noticeable in those receiving low dosages of levodopa. Withdrawal of amantadine resulted in worsening of parkinsonian symptoms.

Three studies tried to answer the question of whether levodopa can prevent the usual fall-off in the therapeutic effectiveness of amantadine (61,69,70). Zeldowicz and Huberman (61) administered combined amantadine and levodopa therapy for approximately 11 months to patients with PD receiving standard antiparkinsonian medication. Amantadine was substituted for placebo nonblindly during a 2-week period 3 and 5 months after the onset of combined therapy. In 80% of patients, parkinsonian signs deteriorated while they were taking placebo and in 70% functional disability also worsened. Fahn et al. (69) evaluated the effect of amantadine in patients with PD. After one year of levodopa, 50% of patients responded favorably to amantadine compared to placebo. However, response to amantadine was not consistent throughout the study. Of the eight patients who benefited from amantadine before and after 5 months of levodopa treatment, only four continued to show a significant response after one year of levodopa treatment. Some of the amantadine responders had previously been nonresponders and vice versa.

In Shannon et al.'s long-term study (70), patients with PD and motor fluctuations received open-label amantadine in addition to levodopa and other antiparkinsonian medication. One patient had unpredictable motor fluctuations, and the others experienced end-of-dose deterioration. In this study, moderate improvement in motor fluctuations occurred in 55% of the patients at 2 months and in 65% of patients after 3 months of treatment. There was also significant improvement in parkinsonian disability. The effect of amantadine was transient. The duration of improvement averaged 5.7 months, and all patients deteriorated to their baseline levels of function within 12 months. Patients who responded to the addition of amantadine did not differ from nonresponders in the severity or duration of PD or with respect to treatment, levodopa dosage, or agonist treatment. Adverse effects were mild during amantadine treatment. Two patients reported confusion, one an increase in chorea, and two worsening of foot dystonia. De Devütis et al. (71) studied the effect of 300 mg of amantadine on predictable postprandial afternoon motor fluctuations in 19 patients. In 9 patients, the motor fluctuations disappeared, in 3 patients it was shortened, and in 4 patients the severity of parkinsonism lessened.

The addition of amantadine in patients with levodopa-related motor fluctuations suggests that the addition of this drug may be useful. However, appropriately controlled studies using assessments of motor fluctuations as the primary outcome variable are needed to confirm these clinical impressions. Two studies assessing the antidyskinetic potential of amantadine also assessed motor fluctuations as a secondary outcome variable (62,63). Verhagen Metman et al. (62) performed a crossover, double-blind, placebo-controlled study to evaluate the effects of amantadine on levodopa-induced dyskinesias in 18 patients. Duration of daily "off" time was used to assess effects of amantadine on motor fluctuations. All patients received amantadine or placebo during each 3-week treatment period. The maximum dose of amantadine was 400 mg. Scores for duration of daily "off" decreased significantly in the amantadine group over placebo.

Luginger et al. (63) assessed the effect of amantadine (100 mg t.i.d.) on levodopa-induced dyskinesia in a 5-week, double-blind, crossover trial in 11 patients with advanced PD complicated by motor fluctuations. Daily "on" and "off" times were recorded in diaries over the last 3 days of each 2-week period. Ten patients completed the study. There were no statistically significant differences in hours "on" or "off" in standard home diary recordings between amantadine and placebo.

G. Amantadine as an Antidyskinetic Drug

The most recent lesson (72) from amantadine in the last years has been the finding of a possible antidyskinetic effect of the drug. Verhagen Metman et al. (62) performed a crossover, double-blind, placebo-controlled study to evaluate the effects of amantadine on levodopa-induced dyskinesias and motor fluctuations using an intravenous acute challenge paradigm in 18 patients with advanced PD. All patients received amantadine or placebo during each 3-week treatment period (maximum dose 400 mg). At the end of each 3-week study period, patients were hospitalized and parkinsonian and dyskinesia scores were obtained during a steady-state intravenous levodopa infusion for 7 hours at individually determined optimal rates (the lowest rate producing a maximal antiparkinsonian effect). Secondary outcome measures were motor fluctuations and dyskinesias documented with patient diaries and Unified Parkinson's Disease Rating Scale (UPDRS) interviews. In the 14 patients completing this trial, amantadine significantly reduced dyskinesia severity by 60% compared to placebo without altering the antiparkinsonian effect of levodopa. Motor fluctuations also significantly improved according to UPDRS scores and patient diaries. Four patients withdrew from the study due to adverse reactions (confusion 1, increasing hallucinations 1, recurrence of preexisting palpitations 1, and nausea 1).

To determine the duration of the antidyskinetic effect of amantadine Metman et al. (64) reevaluated the patients participating in their previous study (62) after one year using a nonrandomized, double-blind, placebo-controlled follow-up. Seventeen of the original 18 patients who remained on amantadine participated in this study (13 had remained on amantadine therapy for the entire year) and 4 additional new patients were included. Ten days prior to the follow-up assessment, amantadine was discontinued and replaced with either placebo or 100 mg amantadine. The main outcome measures were parkinsonian symptoms and dyskinesia severity while subjects were receiving steady-state intravenous levodopa infusions. Results showed that amantadine treated patients continued to have significantly reduced dyskinesias, with mean scores 50% lower as compared to the placebo group recorded at the start of the study.

A double-blind, placebo-controlled, crossover trial was performed by Snow et al. (65) comparing amantadine 200 mg/d to placebo in 24 PD patients. After each treatment arm, the patients received an acute challenge of 1.5 times their usual levodopa dose. The primary outcome of the study was the total dyskinesia score evaluated every 30 minutes in a 3-hour period. There was a significant 24% reduction in the total dyskinesia score (from 29.0 with placebo to 22.0 with amantadine; $p = 0.004$). The UPDRS dyskinesia scores were also significantly improved. This improvement was achieved without any influence on the severity of "on" period parkinsonism.

Luginger et al. (63) assessed the effect of amantadine on levodopa-induced dyskinesia in 11 advanced PD patients using a 5-week, double-blind, crossover trial. Amantadine was administered as 300 mg/d in treatment periods of 2 weeks separated by one week wash-out. Dyskinesia severity was assessed following oral levodopa challenges before the first and on the last day of each treatment period and subjective dyskinesia intensity as well as daily "on" and "off" times were recorded by self-scoring diaries. Ten patients completed the study. Dyskinesia severity following oral levodopa challenges was significantly reduced by 52% and the cumulative dyskinesia score by 53% after amantadine treatment compared with baseline and placebo phases. The magnitude of levodopa motor response to oral challenges, as measured by percent reduction in UPDRS motor scores was not different after amantadine or placebo treatment, and there was no significant reduction in daily "off"-time when patients received amantadine.

Instead of studying the acute effect of levodopa on patients previously treated with amantadine, Del Dotto et al. (66) investigated the acute effect of intravenous amantadine on patients with levodopa-induced dyskinesias using a randomized, double-blind, placebo-controlled design. In this study, nine PD patients with motor fluctuations and disabling peak dose dyskinesias received the first morning levodopa dose, followed by a 2-hour 200 mg intravenous amantadine or placebo infusion. Dyskinesias (by means of a modified Abnormal Involuntary Movement Scale) and parkinsonian symptoms (by the UPDRS, motor examination) were evaluated for 5 hours (every 15 minutes during the infusion and for 3 hours thereafter) on 2 different days while patients were taking their usual antiparkinsonian medications. The average dyskinesia scores during the 5-hour evaluation period were significantly lower with amantadine than with placebo infusion. The acute improvement in levodopa-induced dyskinesias (by 50%) was produced without any loss of the antiparkinsonian benefit from levodopa (a trend towards an improvement in UPDRS was observed with amantadine). Two patients reported mild and transient nausea with amantadine.

V. CONCLUSIONS

Amantadine hydrochloride is useful in the treatment of the symptoms of PD. Its therapeutic effectiveness in patients with PD is thought to be mediated through an effect on the nigrostriatal dopaminergic system. It has an antiparkinsonian profile similar to levodopa and leads to an improvement in all cardinal symptoms of the disease. Almost all trials of amantadine have found evidence of at least some improvement in patients with PD. The incidence of significant side effects is low when administered in the 200–300 mg/d range. The results of double-blind studies show that amantadine is useful in reducing levodopa-induced dyskinesias and support the antidyskinetic potential of NMDA antagonism as a possibility of modifying dyskinesias.

REFERENCES

1. Schwab RS, England AC, Poskanzer DC, Young RR. Amantadine in the treatment of Parkinson's disease. JAMA 1969; 208:1168–1170.
2. Berger JR, Weiner WJ. Exacerbation of Parkinson's disease following the withdrawal of amantadine. Neurology 1985; 35(suppl 1):200.
3. Davies WL, Grunert RR, Haff RF, et al. Antiviral activity of 1-adamantamine (amantadine). Science 1964; 144:862–863.
4. Bleidner WE, Harman JB, Hewes WE, Lynes TE, Hermann EC. Absorption, distribution and excretion of amantadine hydrochloride. J Pharmacol Exp Ther 1965; 150:484–490.
5. Amantadine: Does it have a role in the prevention and treatment of influenza? A National Institute of Health Consensus Development Conference. Ann Intern Med 1980; 92(pt 1):256–258.
6. Standaert DG, Young AB. Treatment of central nervous system disorders. In: Hardman JG, Limbird LE, eds. Goodman & Gilman's The Pharmacological Basis of Therapeutics. New York: McGraw-Hill. 1996:503–519.
7. Ing TS, Rahn AC, Armbruster KFS, Oyama JH, Klawans HL. Accumulation of amantadine hydrochloride in renal insufficiency. N Engl J Med 1974; 291:1257.
8. Ing TS, Daugirdas JT, Soung LS, et al. Toxic effects of amantadine in patients with renal failure. Can Med Assoc J 1979; 120:695–698.
9. Grelak RP, Clarek R, Stump JM, Vernier VG. Amantadine-dopamine interaction: possible mode of action in parkinsonism. Science 1970; 169:203–204.
10. Farnebo LO, Fuxe K, Goldstein M, Hamberger B, Ungerstedt U. Dopamine and noradrenaline releasing action of amantadine in the central and peripheral nervous system: a possible mode of action in Parkinson's disease. Eur J Pharmacol 1971; 16:27–38.
11. Stromberg U, Svensson TH. Further studies on the mode of action of amantadine. Acta Pharmacol Toxicol 1971; 30:161–171.
12. Von Voigtlander PF, Moore KE. Dopamine release from the brain in vivo by amantadine. Science 1973; 174:408–410.
13. Heikkila RE, Cohen G. Evaluation of amantadine as a releasing agent or uptake blocker for 3H-dopamine in rat brain slices. Eur J Pharmacol 1972; 20:156–160.
14. Heimans RL, Rand MJ, Fennesy MR. Effects of amantadine on uptake and release of dopamine by a particulate fraction of rat basal ganglia. J Pharm Pharmacol 1972; 24:875–879.
15. Bailey EV, Stone TW. The mechanism of action of amantadine in parkinsonism: a review. Arch Int Pharmacodyn 1975; 216:246–262.
16. Allen RM. Evidence for direct receptor effect of amantadine. Neurosci Abstr 1981; 7:11.
17. Gianutsos G, Chute S, Dunn JP. Pharmacological changes in dopaminergic systems induced by long-term administration of amantadine. Eur J Pharmacol 1985; 110:357–361.

18. Allen RM. Role of amantadine in the management of neuroleptic-induced extrapyramidal syndromes: overview and pharmacology. Clin Neuropharmacol 1983; 6(suppl 1):64–73.
19. Volonte MA, Moresco RM, Gobbo C, et al. A PET study with (11-C) raclopride in Parkinson's disease: preliminary results on the effect of amantadine on the dopaminergic system. Neurol Sci 2001; 22:107–108.
20. Stone TW. Evidence for a nondopaminergic action of amantadine. Neurosci Lett 1977; 4:343–346.
21. Nastuck WC, Su PC, Doubilet P. Anticholinergic and membrane activities of amantadine in neuromuscular transmission. Nature 1976; 264:76–79.
22. Greenamyre JT, O'Brien CF. N-Methyl-D-aspartate antagonists in the treatment of Parkinson's disease. Arch Neurol 1991; 48:977–981.
23. Kornhuber J, Bormann J, Hubers M, Rusche K, Riederer P. Effects of the 1-amino-adamantanes at the MK-801-binding site of the NMDA-receptor-gated ion channel: a human postmortem brain study. Eur J Pharmacol 1991; 206:297–300.
24. Quirion R, Pert CB. Amantadine modulates phencyclidine binding site sensitivity in rat brain. Experientia 1982; 38:955–956.
25. Stoof JC, Booij J, Drukarch B. Amantadine as N-methyl-D-aspartic acid receptor antagonist: new possibilities for therapeutic applications?. Clin Neurol Neurosurg 1992; 94(suppl):S4–S6.
26. Rausch WD, Schallauer E, Chan WW, Riederer P, Weiser M. Effects of L-deprenyl and amantadine in an MPTP-model of parkinsonism. J Neural Transm 1990; 32:269–275.
27. Wandinger KP, Hagenah JM, Kluter H, Rothermundt M, Peters M, Vieregge P. Effects of amantadine treatment on in vitro production of interleukin-2 in de-novo patients with idiopathic Parkinson's disease. J Neuroinmunol 1999; 98:214–220.
28. Tribl GG, Wober C, Schnborn V, Brucke T, Deecke L, Panzer S. Amantadine in Parkinson's disease: lymphocyte subsets and IL-2 secreting T cell precursor frquencies. Exp Gerontol 2001; 36:1761–1771.
29. Manyam BV. Amantadine in essential tremor. Ann Neurol 1981; 9:198–199.
30. Obeso JA, Luquin MR, Artieda J, Martínez Lage JM. Amantadine may be useful in essential tremor. Ann Neurol 1986; 19:99–100.
31. Bryson YJ, Monahan C, Pollack M, Shields WD. A prospective double blind study of amantadine for influenza A virus prophylaxis. J Infect Dis 1980; 141:543–547.
32. Dolin R, Reichman RC, Madore HP, Maynard R, Linton PN, Webber-Jones J. A controlled trial of a amantadine and rimantadine in the prophylaxis of influenza A infection. N Engl J Med 1982; 307:580–584.
33. Hayden FG, Gwattney JM, Van de Castle RL, Adams KF, Giordani B. Comparative toxicity of amantadine HCl in healthy adults. Antimicrob Agents Chemother 1981; 19:226–233.
34. Editorial. The posology of amantadine: A note of caution. JAMA 1980; 243:1 844–845.
35. Fahn S, Craddock G, Kumin G. Acute toxic psychosis from suicidal overdose of amantadine. Arch Neurol 1971; 25:458.
36. Shealy CN, Weath JB, Mercier DA. Livedo reticularis in patients with Parkinson's receiving amantadine. JAMA 1970; 212:1522–1523.
37. Pearce LA, Waterbury LD, Green HD. Amantadine hydrochloride: alteration in peripheral circulation. Neurology 1974; 24:468.
38. Sartori M, Pratt CM, Yound JB. Torsade de pointe. Malignant cardiac arrhythmia induced by amantadine poisoning. Am J Med 1984; 77:388–391.
39. Casey DE. Amantadine intoxication reversed by physostigmine. N Engl J Med 1978; 298:516.
40. Simpson DM, Davis GC. Case report of neuroleptic malignant syndrome associated with withdrawal from amantadine. Am J Psychiatry 1984; 141:796–797.
41. McEvoy JP, McCue M, Spring B, Mohs RC, Lavori PN, Farr RM. Effects of amantadine and trihexyphenidyl on memory in elderly normal volunteers. Am J Psychiatry 1987; 144:573–577.
42. Parkes JD, Baxter RCH, Curzon G, et al. Treatment of Parkinson's disease with amantadine and levodopa. Lancet 1970; 1:1083–1087.
43. Bauer RB, McHenry JT. Comparison of amantadine, placebo, and levodopa in Parkinson's disease. Neurology 1974; 24:715–720.
44. Goetz CG, Koller WC, Poewe W, Rascol O, Sampaio C. Amantadine and other antiglutamate agents. Mov Disord 2002; 17(suppl 4):S13–S22.
45. Schwab RS, Poskanzer DC, England AC, Young RR. Amantadine in Parkinson's disease. Review of more than two years of experience. JAMA 1972; 222:792–795.
46. Mann DC, Pearce LA, Waterbury LD. Amantadine for Parkinson's disease. Neurology 1971; 21:958–962.
47. Walker JE, Albers JW, Tourtellotte WW, et al. A qualitative and quantitative evaluation of amantadine in the treatment of Parkinson's disease. J Chron Dis 1972; 25:149–182.

48. Butzer JF, Silver DE, Sahs AL. Amantadine in Parkinson's disease. A double blind, placebo-controlled cross-over study with long-term follow-up. Neurology 1975; 25:603–606.
49. Parkes JD, Zilkha KJ, Calver DM, Knill-Jones RP. Controlled trial of amantadine hydrochloride in Parkinson's disease. Lancet 1970; 1:259–262.
50. Parkes JD, Zilkha KJ, Marsden CD, Baxter RCH, Knill-Jones RP. Amantadine dosage in treatment of Parkinson's disease. Lancet 1970; 1:1130–1133.
51. Hunter KR, Stern GM, Laurence DR, Armitage P. Amantadine in parkinsonism. Lancet 1970; 1:1127–1129.
52. Danos V, Heatherfield K, Stone P, Allen FAD. Use of amantadine in Parkinson's disease. Results of a double blind trial. Br Med J 1970; 4:24–36.
53. Appleton DB, Eadie MJ, Sutherland JM. Amantadine hydrochloride in the treatment of parkinsonism: a controlled trial. Med J Aust 1970; 2:626–629.
54. Gilligan BS, Veale J, Wodak J. Amantadine hydrochloride in the treatment of Parkinson's disease. Med J Aust 1970; 2:634–637.
55. Jorgensen PB, Bergin JI, Haas L, et al. Controlled trial of amantadine hydrochloride in Parkinson's disease. NZ Med J 1971; 73:26–269.
56. Parkes JD, Baxter RC, Marsden CD, Rees JE. Comparative trial of benzhexol, amantadine and levodopa in the treatment of Parkinson's disease. J Neurol Neurosurg Psychiatry 1974; 37:42226.
57. Koller WC. Pharmacologic treatment of parkinsonian tremor. Arch Neurol 1986; 43:126–127.
58. Fieschi L, Nardini M, Casacchia M, Tedone ME. Amantadine for Parkinson's disease. Lancet 1970; 1:945–946.
59. Barbeau A, Mars H, Botez MI, et al. Amantadine-HCl (Symmetrel) in the management of Parkinson's disease: a double-blind cross-over study. Can Med Assoc J 1971; 105:42–46.
60. Schwieger AL, Jenkins AC. Observations on the effect of amantadine hydrochloride in the treatment of parkinsonism. Med J Aust 1970; 2:630–632.
61. Zeldowicz LR, Huberman J. Long-term therapy of Parkinson's disease with amantadine, alone and combined with levodopa. Can Med Assoc J 1973; 109:588–593.
62. Verhagen Metman L, Del Dotto P, van den Munckhof P, et al. Amantadine as treatment for dyskinesias and motor fluctuations in Parkinson's disease. Neurology 1998; 50:1323–1326.
63. Luginger E, Wenning GK, Bosch S, Poewe W. Beneficial effects of amantadine on L-dopa-induced dyskinesias in Parkinson's disease. Mov Disord 2000; 15:873–878.
64. Metman LV, Del Dotto P, LePoole K, Konitsiotis S, Fang J, Chase TN. Amantadine for levodopa-induced dyskinesias. A 1-year follow-up study. Arch Neurol 1999; 56:1383–1386.
65. Snow BJ, Macdonald L, McAuley D, Wallis W. The effect of amantadine on levodopa-induced dyskinesias in Parkinson's disease: a double-blind, placebo-controlled study. Clin Neuropharmacol 2000; 23:82–85.
66. Del Dotto P, Pavese N, Gambaccini G, et al. Intravenous amantadine improves levodopa-induced dyskinesias: an acute double-blind placebo-controlled study. Mov Disord 2001; 16:515–520.
67. Godwin-Austen RB, Frears CC, Bergmann S, Parkes JD, Knill-Jones RP. Combined treatment of parkinsonism with L-dopa and amantadine. Lancet 1970; 2:383–385.
68. Fehling C. The effect of adding amantadine to optimum L-dopa dosage in Parkinson's syndrome. Acta Neurol Scand 1973; 49:245–251.
69. Fahn S, Isgreen WP. Long term evaluation of amantadine and levodopa combination in parkinsonism by double-blind cross-over analyses. Neurology 1975; 25:695–700.
70. Shannon KM, Goetz CG, Carroll VS, Tanner CM, Klawans HL. Amantadine and motor fluctuations in chronic Parkinson's disease. Clin Neuropharmacol 1987; 6:522–526.
71. De Devütis E, D'Andrea F, Signorelli CD, Cerillo A. L'amantadine nel trattamento dell'ipokinesia transitoria di pazienti parkinsoniani in corso di terapia con L-dopa. Minerva Med 1972; 409: 4007–4008.
72. Goetz CG. New lessons from old drugs: amantadine and Parkinson's disease. Neurology 1998; 50:1211–1212.

19
Thalamotomy

Nicholas M. Boulis and Ali R. Rezai
Cleveland Clinic Foundation, Cleveland, Ohio, U.S.A.
Debbie K. Song
University of Michigan, Ann Arbor, Michigan, U.S.A.

For over 50 years, ablative thalamotomy has been recognized as an effective treatment for tremor of varying etiologies, including the tremor of Parkinson's disease (PD), essential tremor (ET), cerebellar tremors, posttraumatic and postischemic tremors, as well as for other movement disorders including dystonia and hemiballism. Recently, deep brain stimulation (DBS) has emerged as an appealing surgical option for the treatment of tremor. Thalamic DBS has been shown to be equally effective as ablative thalamotomy in the abolition of tremor with fewer complications. DBS provides a degree of flexibility over a permanent lesion since the stimulator can be adjusted or turned off if intolerable side effects arise. Although DBS is widely regarded as the surgical treatment of choice for tremor, thalamotomy still has a therapeutic advantage in patients who cannot tolerate an implantable stimulator with its attendant risks and requirements for close follow-up. This chapter will consider the history of thalamic surgery for movement disorders, the neuroanatomy and pathophysiology of tremor, indications for thalamotomy, techniques involved in thalamotomy, postoperative management and complications, outcomes, and the evolving role of thalamotomy in the treatment of tremor.

I. HISTORICAL ASPECTS

Surgical lesioning techniques were among the first effective treatments for PD and were based on disrupting the corticobasal ganglia-thalamocortical motor loop. Empirical attempts at targeting different structures such as the deep nuclei of the basal ganglia, thalamus, and ansa lenticularis occurred in concert with advances in neurosurgical imaging and localization techniques and the development of stereotactic surgery in the mid-twentieth century.

Surgical approaches for PD were pioneered by Russell Meyers, who first performed an open resection of the head of the caudate nucleus in 1939 and a transventricular sectioning of the ansa lenticularis in 1942 (1). Although these open procedures resulted in effective amelioration of tremor and rigidity, they were associated with unacceptably high mortality and morbidity rates, approaching 15.7% in cases of open ansotomy (2). In 1950, Fénelon targeted the ansa lenticularis with good results in a procedure, which applied stereotactic techniques at open craniotomy (3). Following a subfrontal exposure of the optic tract, an electrode was inserted by hand and the ansa lenticularis was lesioned by electrocautery. Additional evidence that interruption of the pallidofugal pathway could improve the symptoms of PD was provided by a "surgical accident" in 1952, during which Irving Cooper accidentally tore and ligated the anterior choroidal artery of a patient with PD while attempting a mesencephalic pedunculotomy (4). The procedure was aborted after ligation of the artery, but postoperatively the patient was free of his tremor and rigidity, presumably from infarction of the globus pallidus. Cooper subsequently performed anterior choroidal artery ligations for parkinsonism in over 50 patients, but with a prohibitively high mortality rate of 10% (5). Despite good postoperative tremor control, there was a significant risk of hemiparesis due to the variable contribution to the vascular supply of the internal capsule and ventrolateral thalamus from the anterior choroidal artery.

With the development of the first human stereotactic frame by Ernest Speigel and Henry Wycis in 1947, the focus on treating movement disorders such as tremor with stereotactic techniques continued to intensify (2). Anatomical studies of pallidofugal projections from the globus pallidus to the lateral ventral motor thalamus led Hassler and Riechert to theorize that lesions in the motor thalamus could have similar effects to lesions of the globus pallidus (6). In 1951, the duo reported successfully treating tremor and rigidity in a patient with PD by ventrolateral thalamotomy (7). By 1954, they had refined their thalamic targets and recommended the ventralis oralis posterior (Vop) as a lesion target for tremor and the ventralis oralis anterior (Voa) as a target for rigidity (7).

In 1955, Cooper successfully treated a PD patient by alcohol injection into the globus pallidus (8). Instead of using stereotactic guidance, he used a device that he designed to utilize craniocerebral landmarks. Postmortem examination of the lesion revealed it to be located in the ventral lateral thalamus rather than the pallidum as intended. By 1958, Cooper also recommended the ventrolateral thalamus as the preferred target for amelioration of resting tremor and rigidity in patients with PD (2). By the early 1960s, the ventralis intermedius (Vim) nucleus of the thalamus was generally accepted as the optimal target for tremor (2). In 1964, microelectrode recording was introduced as an intraoperative tool for thalamic mapping. This technique improved the precision of lesion placement.

There was a sharp decline in the number of surgical operations performed for parkinsonism following the introduction of levodopa medical therapy in 1968. However, the limitations in pharmacological dopamine replacement therapy eventually became apparent. Within 5 years of levodopa use, the drug's effectiveness against the progressive symptoms of PD wanes in more than 50% of patients requiring increased dosages (9). Prolonged levodopa administration is also associated with unpredictable motor fluctuations and drug-induced dyskinesias (9).

As a result of the limitations of levodopa, by the 1980s there was renewed interest in surgical therapies for PD. Since that time, the techniques of stereotactic thalamotomy have continued to be refined with improvements in stereotactic computed tomography (CT) and magnetic resonance (MR) imaging and neurophysiological target localization, while also providing the surgical foundations for DBS.

II. FUNCTIONAL NEUROANATOMY

Abnormalities of the extrapyramidal system have been implicated in the pathophysiology of movement disorders. Several components of the extrapyramidal system, including regions of the thalamus and globus pallidus, have been targets for ablative therapies in the treatment of movement disorders. Components of the basal ganglia include (a) the striatum, which includes the caudate nucleus and the putamen; (b) the globus pallidus externa (GPe) and globus pallidus interna (GPi); (c) the substantia nigra, which includes the dopaminergic neurons in the substantia nigra pars compacta (SNc) and the gamma-aminobutyric acid (GABAergic) neurons of the substantia nigra pars reticulata (SNr); and (d) the subthalamic nucleus. The principal basal ganglia motor circuit, the basal ganglia-thalamocortical motor loop, consists of inputs from the pre- and postcentral sensorimotor cortex, SNc, and intralaminar thalamic nuclei, which project to the striatum. Specifically, excitatory glutamatergic corticostriatal afferents are arranged in a topographic fashion such that most of the sensorimotor cortical afferents project to the putamen (9–11). These corticostriatal fibers are modulated by extrinsic dopaminergic projections from the SNc as well as serotonergic projections from the dorsal raphe and intrinsic inputs from GABAergic and cholinergic interneurons (10,12). There are two distinct populations of nigrostriatal dopaminergic neurons, which provide inputs to the striatum. Dopa A neurons from the SNc provide direct excitatory input via activation of D1 receptors, while Dopa B neurons provide direct inhibitory input via activation of D2 receptors (9,10). Additional excitatory glutamatergic afferents to the putamen originate from the centromedial (CM) and parafascicular (PF) nuclei of the caudal intralaminar thalamic nuclear group (13).

Information processed in the putamen can be sent to the output nuclei of the basal ganglia, the GPi and SNr, via either the direct or indirect pathway (Fig. 1). Efferent fibers of the direct and indirect pathways arising from the medium-sized spiny striatal neurons are both GABAergic, but neuronal subpopulations can be differentiated morphologically on the basis of neuropeptide and dopamine receptor subtype expression. Striatal neurons that are involved in the direct pathway preferentially express substance P, dynorphin, and the D1 dopamine receptor subtype (10). Such neurons project directly to the GPi and SNr. In contrast, striatal neurons of the indirect pathway preferentially express enkephalin and the D2 dopamine receptor subtype (14,15). Striatal neurons of the indirect pathway project to the GPe, which in turn sends information via inhibitory GABAergic fibers to the subthalamic nucleus (STN). From the STN, excitatory glutamatergic projections are sent to the GPi and SNr.

The inhibitory GABAergic fibers of the GPi and SNr project to various thalamic and brainstem nuclei including the ventral anterior/ventrolateral (VA/VL) thalamus, lateral habenular nucleus, tegmental pedunculopontine nucleus (PPN), and reticular formation (10). From the motor thalamus, excitatory glutamatergic efferent fibers are sent to the premotor, motor, and supplementary motor cortex. In addition to the thalamocortical projections, the corticostriatal, thalamostriatal, Dopa A nigrostriatal, and STN fibers are excitatory. All other intrinsic and output neurons of the basal ganglia network utilize GABA as their principal neurotransmitter and are inhibitory. Hence, activation of the direct pathway results in increased GABAergic transmission to the output nuclei of the basal ganglia. Overall, the resulting reduction in firing of the GPi and SNr basal ganglia outputs causes disinhibition of the thalamus. In contrast, activation of the indirect pathway results in increased inhibitory GABAergic transmission to the GPe with

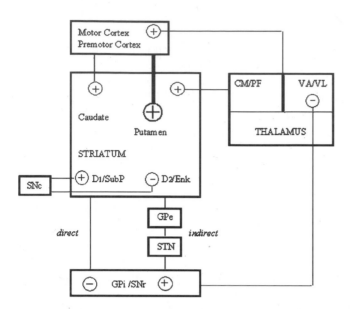

Figure 1 CM, centromedian nucleus; PF, parafascicular nucleus; D1, type I dopamine receptors; D2, type II dopamine receptors; SubP, substance P; Enk, enkephalin; GPi, globus pallidus interna; GPe, Globus pallidus externa; STN, subthalamic nucleus; SNr, substantia nigra pars reticulata; SNc, substantia nigra pars compacta; VA, ventral anterior nucleus; VL, ventrolateral nucleus.

subsequent reduction in GABAergic transmission from the GPe to the STN. Consequently, the firing rate of glutamatergic neurons of the STN is increased, with increased activation of the GPi and SNr. This activation increases inhibition of glutamatergic thalamocortical outputs. Thus, the overall effect of striatal dopamine release is to reduce basal ganglia output from the GPi/SNr, leading to increased activity of thalamocortical projection neurons (Fig. 1).

Several specific components of the ventrolateral nuclei of the thalamus are involved in the functional circuitry of movement disorders. Discourse on thalamic anatomy has been complicated by the use of two main classification schemes: the Hassler scheme and the Anglo-American terminology. In the Anglo-American terminology system, the nuclei of the ventrolateral thalamic mass are classified from anterior to posterior as the ventralis anterior (VA), ventralis lateralis (VL), and the ventralis posterior (VP). In the Hassler scheme, the nuclei are divided into the lateralis polaris, ventralis oralis anterior (Voa), ventralis oralis posterior (Vop), ventralis intermedius (Vim), and the ventralis caudalis (Vc) (9,16). The Vc nucleus, which is populated by neurons that respond to tactile stimulation, is the primary thalamic relay center for the medial lemniscal and spinothalamic tracts and projects to the somatosensory cortex. The posterior portion of the motor nucleus of the thalamus, VL, corresponds to Vop and Vim in the Hassler scheme (Fig. 2). While the neuronal populations of Vim and Vop are histologically and structurally distinct from each other, the boundary between Vim and Vc is less distinct (9,17). The Hassler scheme correlates better with the relevant anatomy and pathophysiology and is used more often in the clinical literature. Nevertheless, problems with defining and classifying human thalamic anatomy persist because the nomenclature

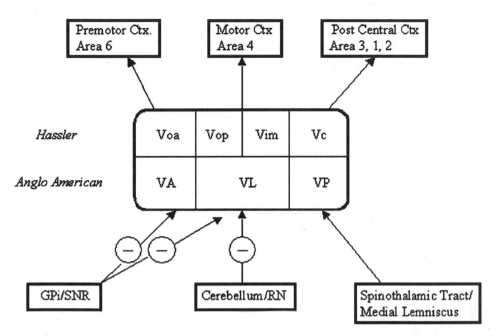

Figure 2 Diagram of the structures projecting to the nuclei of the ventral thalamus, and sites to which these nuclei project. The Hassler nomenclature for thalamic nuclei is listed above the Anglo-American nomenclature. Ctx, cortex; Voa, ventralis oralis anterior; Vop, ventralis oralis posterior; Vim, ventralis intermedius; Vc, ventralis candis; VA, ventralis anterior; VL ventralis lateralis; VP, ventralis posterior; GPi, globus pallidus interna; SNR, substantia nigra pars reticulata; RN, red nucleus.

is based on cytoarchitectonic subdivisions and the transfer of knowledge by analogy from the monkey to human (18). Systems of thalamic nomenclature are limited by the lack of anatomical tracer studies in humans and the discrepancies between thalamic nuclear territories defined by cytoarchitecture versus electrophysiological characteristics.

According to Hassler's original scheme, Voa receives pallidal afferents from the globus pallidus interna pars lateralis, Vop receives afferents from the contralateral cerebellum, and Vim receives sensory information arising from Ia spindle afferents (16,18). This scheme has subsequently been revised as a result of histological analysis and neuroanatomical tracer studies in monkeys that more clearly define the subcortical afferent connections to the thalamic nuclei (17,19–21). While thalamic relay areas that receive cerebellar, pallidal, and nigral afferents do not overlap, the boundaries between such areas in the thalamus do appear to interdigitate (18). Thus, according to more recent schemes, Voa and Vop receive pallidal inputs via the ansa lenticularis and lenticular fasciculus and send efferent projections to the supplementary motor cortex, premotor cortex, and motor cortex (9,18,22). Moreover, Vim is now recognized as the cerebellar receiving center; however, the electrophysiologically defined Vim often encroaches on the anatomical boundaries of Vop as defined by Hassler (18). Vim and Vop receive outflow fibers from the contralateral cerebellum directly via the brachium conjunctivum and thalamic peduncle (9). Indirect cerebellar projections to these nuclei go through the red nucleus (9). From the cerebellar relay areas, fibers project to area 4 of the motor cortex (9).

III. PATHOPHYSIOLOGICAL CONSIDERATIONS

Vim thalamotomy is widely recognized to be an effective treatment for tremor. Parkinsonism is a hypokinetic movement disorder that results from the functional or structural loss of nigrostriatal dopaminergic neurons. The reduction in striatal dopaminergic transmission is associated with increased basal ganglia output from GPi neurons through both the direct and indirect pathways, with the subsequent inhibition of thalamocortical neurons. There are three cardinal motor symptoms of PD: resting tremor, akinesia or bradykinesia, and rigidity. Variation in the severity of each of these parkinsonian motor symptoms and in the response of each of the symptoms to specific lesions suggest that tremor, akinesia, and rigidity are either mediated by independent pathophysiological mechanisms or involve different motor subcircuits. For example, a posteroventral pallidotomy disrupts the pallidofugal pathway and presumably reduces the otherwise increased basal ganglia output in parkinsonism. Such a procedure has been shown to improve each of the motor symptoms of PD, but not to the same extent (11,23). On the other hand, thalamotomy, while effective in patients with tremor, does not improve the akinesia or bradykinesia of PD (11,24). In particular, the efficacy of lesioning the Vim nucleus, the area in the motor thalamus that receives input from the contralateral cerebellum, suggests that cerebellar pathways are also involved in the genesis of certain parkinsonian symptoms such as tremor.

There have been various theories regarding the generation of the resting tremor of PD. One such theory holds that there is a central oscillatory discharge center that acts as a pacemaker in driving the tremor (6,25,26). However, the anatomical location of this center remains in debate. Intraoperative studies have confirmed the presence of "tremor cells" in the Vim and Vop nuclei of the motor thalamus that exhibit calcium spike–associated burst discharge patterns with a frequency equal to the patient's tremor frequency. Alternatively, increased tonic output from the basal ganglia, which occurs in hypokinetic movement disorders such as PD, can lead to hyperpolarization of thalamic cells. Neuronal hyperpolarization and high-frequency, calcium spike–associated burst discharges that occur during recovery from hyperpolarization are associated with oscillatory thalamic behavior. It is unclear whether the tremor cells in the motor thalamus are themselves the source of the tremor or part of a more extensive feedback-loop–mediating tremor (6).

In addition to areas in the motor thalamus, there are sites in the basal ganglia, specifically the GPi in human patients with PD and the STN in monkey models of PD, that exhibit burst activity, thereby implicating the basal ganglia as another possible oscillatory center giving rise to tremor. Pallidal lesions that target tremor cells in the GPi and lesions affecting pallidal efferents in the ansa lenticularis are also effective in relieving tremor in parkinsonian patients (11,27–29). If the GPi were indeed the oscillatory center, the pallidal relay centers, Voa and Vop, would be expected to be the thalamic nuclei with the greatest tremor-related activity and the highest signal-to-noise ratio at the tremor frequency. Maximal tremor-related activity occurs, however, in the cerebellar receiving center, the Vim nucleus, not in the Vop or Voa (25).

Unstable oscillating sensory feedback pathways to the central nervous system have been proposed as an alternative to the central oscillatory discharge center theory. Certain cells in the somatosensory relay center of the thalamus (Vc) respond to passive joint movement. The discharge patterns from such cells have been observed to lag behind electromyographic (EMG) signals that correspond to limb tremor. The lag presumably occurs because of a conduction delay between somatosensory input associated with the tremor and the transmission to the thalamus. These cells, then, fire passively in response to sensory feedback. Other tremor cells in the thalamus, however, have peak discharges that both precede the EMG signal before any active movement and follow in response to movement (30). It is thought that such cells may be involved in generating tremor by an abnormal feedback system generated by extrathalamic circuitry.

While evidence to support a single model for parkinsonian tremor is lacking, each of the existing theories may contribute to the generation of tremor. Empirical observation confirms the presence of tremor cells in the Vim nucleus, and ablative lesions in the Vim are thought to abolish tremor by destroying the synchronized-burst firing activity of such cells. In addition, because cerebellar pathways converge in the Vim nucleus, Vim thalamotomy is also an effective treatment for cerebellar outflow and intention tremors of varying etiologies.

IV. INDICATIONS FOR THALAMOTOMY FOR TREMOR AND PATIENT SELECTION

Vim thalamotomy is indicated for the treatment of medically refractory tremor regardless of etiology. The best candidates, however, are patients with tremor-dominant PD or ET (31). In patients with PD, thalamotomy is most effective for tremor. Thalamotomy should not be considered for patients whose primary motor problem is akinesia or bradykinesia. A resting, pill-rolling tremor with a frequency of 4–6 Hz is most commonly associated with PD (11). Severely affected patients, however, may exhibit a combination of resting, kinetic, and postural tremor and can be treated with thalamotomy as well.

In cases of unilateral or asymmetrical tremor, thalamotomy should be performed on the more severely affected side. In patients with symmetrical, bilateral tremor, thalamotomy should be performed on the dominant side to optimize functional recovery. A single procedure bilateral thalamotomy is generally contraindicated. It is also preferable to avoid a second-side procedure because of the increased morbidity associated with bilateral lesions. A second-side procedure should only be pursued if there has been progression of motor symptoms to the nonoperated side and if the first operation provided immediate and long-term postoperative improvement in tremor. When symptom severity mandates a second-side procedure following unilateral thalamotomy, it is best to wait as long as possible (and a minimum of 6 months) before operating on the second side. Alternative procedures other than a thalamotomy such as the implantation of a deep brain stimulator on the other side is preferable and should be considered. If a second-side ablative procedure must be done, the lesions should be small and asymmetrical to minimize the risk of cognitive and speech impairment (32).

DBS in the Vim thalamus, subthalamic nucleus, or GPi can treat tremor as effectively as a Vim thalamotomy and carries a reduced risk of adverse effects when compared to the risk of an irreversible, ablative lesion. Although DBS has supplanted thalamotomy as the treatment of choice in tremor, thalamotomy still has a role in a population of patients in whom DBS is contraindicated. Vim thalamotomy may be preferred in patients who cannot tolerate a stimulator and its associated potential complications such as hardware malfunction, infection, or electrode breakage. Patients who do not have the means or access to follow-up may be better served by a definitive, single intervention such as Vim thalamotomy.

V. PREOPERATIVE CONSIDERATIONS

Prior to undergoing thalamotomy, the patient should undergo a comprehensive evaluation of his or her movement disorder by a specialized team of neurologists and neurosurgeons. A clinical diagnosis of PD or ET must be confirmed since atypical syndromes with parkinsonian features such as striatonigral degeneration, Shy-Drager syndrome, progressive supranuclear palsy, or toxic and drug-induced disorders have a poorer prognosis for improvement following Vim thalamotomy. Patients with significant cognitive, swallowing, or speech problems should be excluded from consideration for thalamotomy. Stereotactic thalamotomy should be reserved for patients with tremor who have failed adequate medical therapy or who are intolerant of medical therapy. Therapeutic goals and expectations should be tailored to the individual patient.

Patients should undergo standard blood tests to ensure a normal coagulation status in the immediate preoperative period. Aspirin, nonsteroidal anti-inflammatory drugs, and other antiplatelet agents should be stopped 7–14 days prior to surgery. Patients who are on chronic oral anticoagulation should switch to intravenous or subcutaneous heparin administration 5 days prior to surgery, and heparin should be held 6 hours prior to the procedure. Preoperative MR imaging is warranted to identify the extent and location of any intracranial pathology. Patients should remain on any previously prescribed antihypertensive medications, as poorly controlled hypertension can predispose to intra- and postoperative hemorrhage. Antiparkinsonian and antitremor medications should be stopped 6 hours prior to the procedure. Moreover, it is desirable for the tremor to be evident during intraoperative testing so that the effects of test lesions can be assessed. Intravenous dexamethasone may be administered preoperatively and continued on a rapid taper postoperatively; however, there is no definitive evidence that perioperative steroid use is beneficial (9,32). Likewise, prophylactic antibiotics are considered to be optional in view of the low infection rate.

VI. FRAME PLACEMENT

With the patient seated, a MR- and CT-compatible stereotactic head frame is applied. Pin sites are numbed with 1% lidocaine with epinephrine. Commonly used frames for functional stereotactic neurosurgery are the Leksell frame and the Cosman-Roberts-Wells frame. The frame is placed on the head as symmetrically as possible, minimizing rotation (yaw) or lateral tilt (roll). In order for the frame base to be placed parallel to the line connecting the anterior commissure and the posterior commissure (AC-PC line), the frame should be angled approximately 6 degrees from the horizontal. Deviation from this plane (pitch) complicates stereotactic planning.

VII. STEREOTACTIC IMAGING AND ANATOMIC LOCALIZATION

Following placement of the stereotactic head frame, imaging is performed for direct (anatomical) and indirect target localization. Imaging modalities available include stereotactic CT, stereotactic MR imaging, and ventriculography. MR imaging provides excellent spatial resolution, but it is subject to spatial distortion caused by inhomogeneities in the magnetic field and chemical shift artifact. Gadolinium-enhanced spoiled-grass volume coronal and axial volume acquisitions are divided into 1 mm section slices. The anterior and posterior commissures, basal ganglia nuclei, and optic tract are visualized.

Coronal fast spin echo inversion recovery (FSEIR) images can also be obtained in order to distinguish the gray-white borders of the thalamus and, specifically, to identify the spatial relationship between the thalamus and internal capsule. While axial CT imaging provides less resolution of anatomical landmarks (AC and PC) and poorer definition of the gray-white interface surrounding deep nuclear structures, its geometric accuracy is superior to MRI. In many centers, stereotactic MR and CT imaging are utilized in tandem for anatomical target localization. Certain landmarks such as the anterior commissure (AC), posterior commissure (PC), basal ganglia nuclei, third ventricle, and internal capsule are identified on stereotactic MR and CT images. Direct targeting of the Vim alone is insufficient since the divisions between individual thalamic nuclei are not visible.

Together with a stereotactic atlas, the coordinates of the Vim thalamic target can be approximated. Several stereotactic atlases are available, each of which consists of cadaveric brain sections sliced in relationship to known landmarks in the axial, coronal, and sagittal planes. Four commonly used stereotactic atlases are the Schaltenbrand and Bailey, Andrew and Watkins, Van Buren and Borke, and Schaltenbrand and Wahren atlases (33–36). Several of the atlases are part of computer-resident atlas systems, which can superimpose target overlays on a patient's digital CT or MR images. Due to individual patient variation in the spatial relationships between deep subcortical structures and radiographically defined landmarks, there is an inherent degree of inaccuracy when calculating the target coordinates using any of the atlases. Thus, anatomical localization using neuroimaging and stereotactic atlases is only a first estimate of the target. Precise localization and confirmation of the target is achieved by neurophysiological testing.

A combination of direct and indirect imaging can be used. Sagittal T1-weighted MR (1.5 Tesla) images with fat suppression can be used to locate the AC and PC (Fig. 3A). Axial T1-weighted MR slices parallel to the AC-PC line through the basal ganglia are used to check frame placement and to measure the fiducial markers for confirmation of known measurements. The stereotactic MR can be fused to a stereotactic CT. This fusion limits the potential for spatial image distortion. Using the AC and PC as anatomical landmarks,

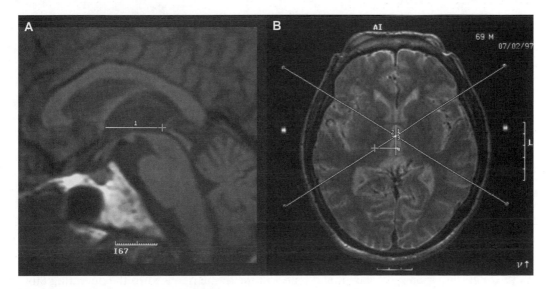

Figure 3 Indirect targeting of the Vim.

the thalamic Vim target is usually 4–5 mm posterior to the midpoint of the AC-PC line, 0–1 mm below the level of the intercommissural plane, and 12–14 mm lateral to the midline (37). If the third ventricle is enlarged, 1–2 mm can be added to the lateral coordinate, or a point 11.5 mm from the lateral border of the third ventricle can be targeted (Fig. 3B) (9). Alternatively, the coordinates of the thalamic target can be approximated by their distance along or orthogonal to the AC-PC line. The Vim nucleus is located 30% of the AC-PC length anterior to the PC, 50% of the AC-PC distance from the midline, and in or slightly inferior to the AC-PC plane (38). Many surgeons rely on macroelectrode stimulation to confirm localization of the appropriate Vim target. The use of microelectrode recording, microstimulation, and macrostimulation prior to lesioning is warranted given the importance of physiological confirmation and the irreversibility of this approach.

As will be discussed below, the Vim is not generally targeted with the initial electrode tract. Rather, the "tactile border" (TB) between Vim and Vc is targeted in order to obtain necessary electrophysiological landmarks. To find the tactile border the method of Guiot is often used. The initial electrode trajectory is often planned to pass from Vim into Vc, hence defining the TB. The termination of this tract is at the level of the AC-PC line, 11.5 mm lateral to the third ventricular border, and 1/8 the distance of the AC-PC line anterior to the PC. This targeting can be confirmed by morphing the Schaltenbrand and Wahren atlas to the individual patient's brain using Framelink software (Sophamor Danek).

Stereotactic ventriculography provides excellent anatomical accuracy and was commonly used in stereotactic procedures prior to the advent of CT and MR imaging. It is considered to be the gold standard for anatomical localization. However, ventriculography is an invasive procedure with potential complications that include cerebrospinal fluid (CSF) leakage, intraoperative brain shift, and the adverse effects associated with the introduction of air or contrast media into the ventricle (39,40). Stereotactic ventriculography is not commonly used today, as stereotactic CT has been shown to be just as accurate as ventriculography for Vim thalamotomy (40).

VIII. ANESTHESIA

Ablative thalamotomy is performed under local anesthesia. An awake patient is necessary for thalamic mapping with both macrostimulation as well as microelectrode recording (MER). General anesthetic significantly alters the physiological activity of these neurons, rendering MER mapping virtually impossible. Preoperative sedation with benzodiazepines or anxiolytics is avoided. Short-acting sedating agents such as propofol or midazolam and analgesics such as sufentanil are used only sparingly and as needed if significant head movement or patient discomfort jeopardizes the reliability and accuracy of the stereotactic procedure.

Standard intraoperative monitors should be placed and intravenous access ipsilateral to the planned thalamotomy should be established. No lines or monitors should be placed on the contralateral limb of interest, which needs to be freely accessed and tested intraoperatively. Normotensive blood pressure should be maintained during the perioperative and intraoperative period.

IX. SURGICAL TECHNIQUE

In the operating room, the patient is supine and the frame is affixed to the operating table via an adapter so that the patient's head is elevated slightly above the level of the chest.

The patient's tremor, strength, and speech should be tested after the patient has been positioned in the operating room. The frontal scalp is prepped, and the intended incision is infiltrated with local anesthetic such as 0.25% marcaine with epinephrine, 1:200,000. The field is draped, and the stereotactic arc is assembled and set to the desired coordinates. A 3 cm linear or curvilinear incision is carried sharply down to bone in the frontal area, approximately 3 cm off the midline and 12–13 cm posterior to the nasion, anterior to the coronal suture. A self-retraining retractor is placed and a burr hole of approximately 14/mm is made. The dura, arachnoid, and pia are coagulated and opened serially. The patient's tremor, strength, and speech should be assessed before the probe is passed. A cannula that holds the microelectrode is introduced stereotactically through the burr hole to a point 15 mm above target. Continuous impedance monitoring may be used to detect CSF and/or pulsatile flow indicative of blood vessels. If encountered, an alternative entry site may alter the trajectory sufficiently to avoid such vessels.

X. PHYSIOLOGICAL LOCALIZATION OF THE VIM THALAMIC TARGET

Since imaging cannot demonstrate individual thalamic nuclei or their borders, intra-operative neurophysiological localization of the Vim thalamic nucleus must be done to refine and confirm the target. Physiological corroboration of the target involves advancing a microelectrode through to the deep subcortical nuclei and white matter. The characteristic set of cell recordings obtained can be used to localize the Vim nucleus. High impedance microelectrodes made from either tungsten or a platinum-iridium alloy are used to record extracellular action potentials from single cells.

The microelectrode is secured into a stainless steel guide tube that is fixed to a calibrated hydraulic microdrive. The microelectrode carrier assembly is mounted onto the head frame. The hydraulic microdrive allows for submillimeter advancements over a total distance of 20–30 mm. Electrical activity from individual cells is conducted through the electrode, amplified, and filtered. A window discriminator can be employed to isolate single cell discharges above background noise. These spikes can be displayed on an oscilloscope and fed into an audioamplifier.

There is a specific organization of the sensory modalities in the ventral tier region within the thalamus, with neurons responsive to light touch (tactile) stimulation situated posteriorly. Anterior to this tactile-responsive region (tactile Vc) is an area responsive to proprioception through stimulation of joint capsule receptors. Further anterior is a collection of neurons in the Vim that is driven by passive movement and activation of muscle spindles. These neurons are often found to fire in synchrony with the patient's tremor. Electrode passage through this area (microthalamotomy) or microstimulation can arrest the tremor. This region is the target for the ablative lesion. Further anterior to the Vim is the Vop, whose neurons are preferentially activated by active rather than passive movements (Fig. 4).

The ventral tier nuclei display a fairly robust somatotopy, with the major anatomical regions represented in concentric lamina analogous to the layers of an onion. In general, neuronal activity related to the lower extremity can be found superiorly, laterally, and inferiorly to the upper extremity, which itself can be found superiorly, laterally, and inferiorly to the head and face. In addition to providing information as to the relative laterality of a given trajectory, this organization should be considered in relation to the

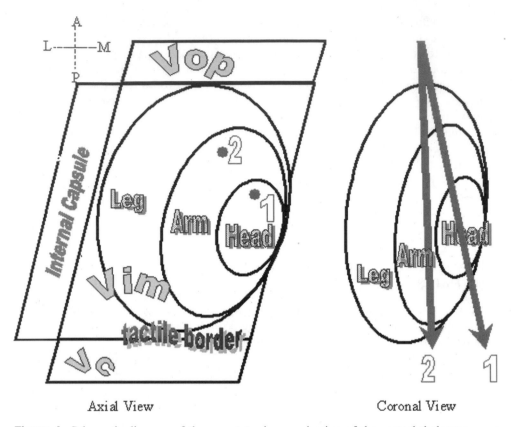

Axial View   Coronal View

Figure 4 Schematic diagram of the somatotopic organization of the ventral thalamus.

type of tremor being treated. Given its concentric organization, however, it is not uncommon for the optimal trajectory to traverse the targeted region (i.e., the upper extremity) in addition to regions that show activity responsive to lower extremity driving. Thus, encountering units with leg proprioceptive fields superficially and deep in the penetration, in addition to upper extremity–related units, does not necessarily indicate that the trajectory is too lateral. In all cases, a tract that encounters units related to the head or face are considered to be too medial, and this area should be avoided in order to minimize the risk of speech and swallowing complications (Fig. 4).

One approach to targeting Vim typically involves a minimum of three penetrations, with the major movement occurring in the anteroposterior plane. It is important to understand the effect of such movement on the somatotopy. In parallel with the thalamus-internal capsule border, the homonculus of the ventral tier nuclei shifts medially as the trajectories move anteriorly. The common rule of thumb is that for each movement 5 mm anteriorly, the homonculus shifts medially 1 mm. As such, it is recommended that tracts be corrected medially as mapping proceeds from the posterior border of Vim forward.

In targeting the Vim nucleus, the goal of microelectrode recording is to identify the anatomical boundaries of the structures to be avoided, including the tactile sensory relay of the Vc and the internal capsule. A lesion too close to the tactile Vc may result in intolerable paresthesias for the patient. In order to delineate the tactile border between Vc and Vim, the trajectory typically begins 15 mm above the anatomically targeted ventral border of the thalamus, generally placing the tip of the guide cannula in the dorsal thalamus. Dorsal thalamic neurons typically discharge in low-frequency bursts, have a lower density, and their action potentials have a lower signal-to-noise ratio. The transition from dorsal to ventral tier nuclei is marked by changes in neuronal frequency, density, and signal-to-noise ratio of extracellular action potentials. Sensorimotor testing and microstimulation are often carried out at 0.5–1.0 mm intervals once the microelectrode has passed from the dorsal to the ventral nuclei.

The initial trajectory is continued until units responsive to light touch, characteristic of tactile Vc, have been identified. Neurons in the Vc have a characteristic electrophysiological profile consisting of very noisy spontaneous cellular activity with many high-voltage (150 μV) discharges. If the tactile Vc has been identified on the first trajectory, the next penetration is usually placed 2 mm anteriorly. If no tactile Vc is encountered on this tract, the tactile border between the two tracts has been isolated. The third trajectory is typically planned for 3–4 mm anterior to where the anterior border of the tactile Vc is thought to be. If the first trajectory fails to encounter the tactile region, the trajectory is moved 2 mm posterior until Vc is encountered. Characterization of neuronal activity in response to sensorimotor driving must also be done to verify the position of the electrode in the Vim. In the Vim, kinesthetic neurons respond to contralateral joint movement, squeezing of muscle bellies, or deep tendon pressure.

Microstimulation helps to verify the position of the trajectory relative to the tactile Vc and internal capsule, thus refining the optimal lesion location. Microstimulation is carried out with biphasic, square wave pulse trains of 0.1–0.3 ms pulses for up to 800 ms at a frequency of 330 Hz and a maximum current of 90 μA. High-frequency stimulation in Vc will evoke somatic sensations consisting of contralateral paresthesias or numbness. At each stimulation site, the patient should be instructed to report any change in sensation that occurs. Sensory thresholds are obtained by progressively reducing the current intensity until stimulation no longer elicits a sensory response. Although paresthesias can also be felt during Vim microstimulation in a patient with tremor, the threshold for inducing paresthesias in the Vc is much lower than that in the Vim. Thus, low-threshold paresthesias indicate that the electrode is positioned posterior to Vim in the Vc. Stimulation of kinesthetic tremor cells in the Vim can have variable effects on tremor and may cause dystonia. A low-frequency (2 Hz) stimulus will typically drive the tremor, while high-frequency (> 50 Hz) stimulation should abolish or reduce the tremor. Suppression of the tremor with 0.5–2.0 V usually indicates accurate targeting. Stimulation of Vim may result in the proprioceptive sensation of movement in the contralateral limb in the absence of any actual joint movement. Less frequently, sensations of vertigo, dread, and fainting can also accompany Vim microstimulation. In the correct location, any paresthesias that occur should be transient and the patient should not experience unpleasant side effects. In some circumstances, the introduction of an electrode into the purported target will ameliorate the patient's tremor, thereby confirming an accurate and appropriate electrode position. In some cases, however, minor adjustments must be made to reposition the electrode given the individual variation and small size of the Vim.

Alternative options to microelectrode stimulation and recording for localization include macrostimulation and semimicroelectrode stimulation with recording. Typically, if microstimulation and microelectrode recording are not used, macrostimulation and semimicroelectrode recordings are employed. Semimicroelectrodes are low-impedance

$(100\,k\Omega)$ bipolar electrodes that are easier to navigate in the electrically hostile environment of the operating room, but cannot record from single cells. Instead, neural background noise and EEG-like field potentials from a cluster of cells is obtained. While semimicroelectrodes are adequate for locating and differentiating neurons that compose thalamic subnuclei, microelectrode techniques are more accurate and precise in the localization of a target area within a given nucleus.

XI. LESION PARAMETERS

Following target confirmation, radiofrequency lesions are made with a temperature-monitored electrode. A reversible test lesion is made by heating the electrode tip to 42–45°C for 30–60 seconds. The patient is then assessed neurologically to determine the effects of the lesion on tremor, strength, coordination, sensation, and verbal skills. If there is improvement in tremor without any untoward neurological side effects, a permanent lesion is made at 70–80°C for 60 seconds. The patient undergoes continuous neurological monitoring during the lesioning, and the process is halted if any neurological impairment is noted. The electrode is kept in position until it has cooled down to below 37°C for 20 seconds, after which it is withdrawn 2–3 mm. Two to three additional lesions can be performed as the electrode is sequentially withdrawn, as guided by intraoperative physiological recordings. Lesions are usually 3–4 mm in diameter and 4–6 mm in the superior-inferior dimension. For PD and ET, the typical lesion volume is 40–60 mm^3 (9,41,42).

Following lesioning and withdrawal of the electrode, the incision is copiously irrigated. The burr hole may be filled with Gelfoam, bone chips, or fibrin glue. The galea is closed with a layer of inverted 3.0 Vicryl sutures, and the skin is closed with 4.0 nylon sutures. The frame is removed and a sterile dressing is applied.

XII. POSTOPERATIVE CARE AND FOLLOW-UP IMAGING

Since intracranial hemorrhage can be a serious cause of morbidity after thalamotomy, blood pressure should be maintained in the normotensive range for 24–72 hours postoperatively, even if pharmacological intervention is required. Patients can be restarted on their preoperative medications, and dexamethasone, if used, can be rapidly tapered. In uncomplicated cases, hospital discharge can occur on postoperative day 1. For maximum rehabilitation, patients may undergo outpatient physical and occupational therapy.

The location and extent of thalamic lesions can be assessed postoperatively by MR imaging. Postoperative MR imaging at 24 hours shows signal changes consistent with tissue destruction and local edema. Lesions typically undergo progressive shrinkage, with the lesion size stabilizing approximately 7 months postoperatively (43). Lesions typically display coagulation necrosis and hemosiderin deposition (Fig. 5) (9).

Although thalamic lesions in the immediate postoperative period may appear as hypodensities on CT imaging, in other cases there may be no detectable change on CT imaging in the acute stage. Immediate postoperative CT imaging is usually done only if the patient experiences neurological deterioration and one is attempting to determine whether the changes are due to an acute hemorrhage or edema.

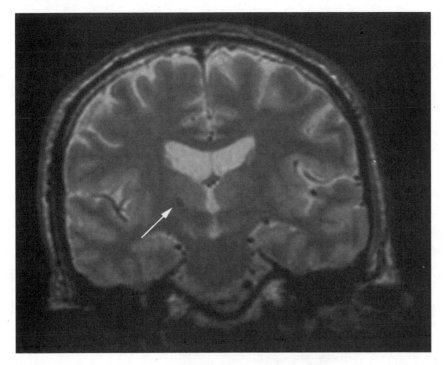

Figure 5 Coronal T2 MRI of a Vim thalamic lesion (arrow).

XIII. COMPLICATIONS

The true complication and outcome rates of thalamotomy are difficult to determine since stereotactic neurosurgery has evolved in recent years with regards to techniques and technology. Improvements in localization by combined radiological and physiological techniques have led to more accurate and precisely targeted ablative lesions, which translates to smaller lesions and reduced risks for injury to surrounding structures. The overall mortality rate is estimated to range from 0.3 to 1.0% (44–47). Advanced age, severe preexisting disease, hypertension, and bilateral lesions are factors associated with increased mortality (9).

The most common source of morbidity is hemorrhage. Thermal injury during lesion generation can damage the walls of nearby blood vessels. Less commonly, hemorrhage may be associated with probe insertion and movement along the thalamotomy tract. In such cases, cortical blood vessel injury can lead to subdural hematoma formation. Hemorrhages may be apparent immediately postoperatively, or they may present 1–2 days after surgery (32).

Serious complications such as hemiparesis, cognitive dysfunction, language and speech difficulties, and sensory abnormalities occur due to imperfect lesion placement or lesions that are too large. Transient limb weakness can occur in 2.5–30% of cases, presumably from electrode placement in or near the internal capsule (Fig. 6) (48–51). Transient hemifacial weakness can occur in 8–25% of patients (49,52). Weakness or hemiparesis can persist in up to 15% of patients (49–51,53,54).

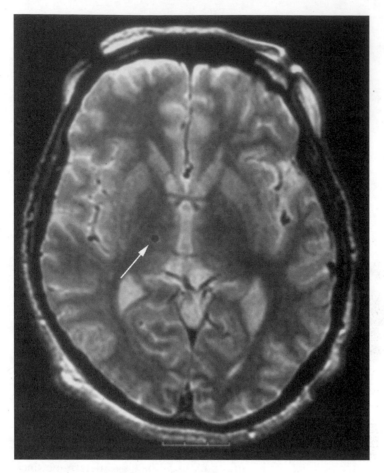

Figure 6 Axial T2 MRI of a thalamic Vim lesion.

Left-sided lesions are more often associated with learning problems, deficits in verbal learning, and dysarthria, whereas right-sided lesions are more often associated with impairments in visuospatial learning and nonverbal performance (55). Memory and language problems can also occur. Transient confusion occurs in the postoperative period in 10–30% of patients, and cognitive deficits have been reported to persist in 1–5% of patients (52,56,57). Risk factors for cognitive impairment following thalamotomy include preoperative cognitive dysfunction, brain atrophy or injury, elderly age, a dominant hemisphere lesion, and bilateral procedures (56). Cognitive dysfunction has been reported in 35% of patients who underwent bilateral thalamotomies (9),(58). Following unilateral thalamotomy, problems with dysarthria or dysphasia can affect 1–25% of patients and persist in approximately 10% of patients (49,50,57,59). Risk factors for dysarthria include bilateral procedures and the presence of dysarthria preoperatively. Hypophonia has also been anecdotally reported following thalamotomy (60).

Injury to the tactile Vc and lesions placed too posteriorly can result in hemisensory deficits and paresthesias. Although paresthesias are usually transient, they have been reported to persist in 19–27% of patients (24,48), and the paresthesias or numbness most often occur in the digits or mouth.

XIV. OUTCOME

Vim thalamotomy is a highly effective treatment for tremor. In patients with PD or ET, thalamotomy is successful in completely or markedly abolishing tremor in 62–100% of cases (46–50,61–64). Thalamotomy significantly improves cerebellar outflow tremors in 60–80% of patients (50,65,66). Although thalamotomy improves tremor and rigidity, the procedure has no beneficial effect on preexisting bradykinesia or akinesia, gait disturbance, speech difficulties, or ataxia (24). Moreover, surgical treatment in PD patients does not halt progression of the disease. The long-term efficacy of thalamotomy has been reported in multiple studies. Forty-eight percent of patients who have undergone unilateral thalamotomy report no worsening of tremor in comparison with their preoperative condition, and up to 40% of patients continue to report improvement in their tremor (52,67). Among 57 patients, Kelly found that 90% of patients were free of tremor 2 years after undergoing unilateral thalamotomy, 86% of patients remained tremor-free 4 years later, and 57% remained tremor-free 10 years later (46). In most PD patients, levodopa therapy is continued postoperatively (42).

Several studies have confirmed the similar efficacies of DBS and thalamotomy for tremor control in patients with PD or ET (24,47,68). The effort required to achieve such control, however, varies among the interventions. In one study of 19 DBS cases and 26 thalamotomy cases for tremor, 23% of the thalamotomies were repeated because of ineffective suppression following the initial operation, whereas none of the DBS procedures had to be repeated (24). Others have reported the need for repeat thalamotomy procedures in 7–12.5% of cases in order to achieve a therapeutic effect (50,69).

XV. CONCLUSION

The appropriate application of thalamotomy for movement disorders in the early twenty-first century remains controversial. Unilateral thalamotomy remains an effective treatment for a variety of tremors, including tremor-predominant PD. However, most practitioners favor the use of stimulation when available given its inherent reversibility and flexibility. In addition, most practitioners prefer GPi and STN as targets for the treatment of PD even when the symptoms are tremor dominant as parkinsonian neurodegeneration is progressive and bradykinesia and rigidity may develop at a later date. Consequently, Vim is currently the favored target for nonparkinsonian tremor. Thus, the major contemporary application of Vim lesions is for nonparkinsonian tremor in cases where stimulation is either contraindicated or not feasible.

REFERENCES

1. Meyers R. The modification of alternating tremor, rigidity, and festination by surgery of the basal ganglia. Res Publ Assoc Res Nerv Ment Dis 1942; 1:602–665.
2. Gildenberg PL. The history of surgery for movement disorders. Neurosurg Clin North Am 1998; 9:283–293.
3. Fénelon F. Essais de traitment neurochirurgical du syndrome parkinsonien par intervention directe sur les voies extrapyramidales immediatement sousstriopallides (anse lenticulaire). Communication suivie de projection du firm d'un des operes pris avant et apres l'intervention. Rev Neurol (Paris) 1950; 83:437–440.
4. Cooper IS. Ligation of the anterior choroidal artery for involuntary movements of parkinsonism. Psychiatr Q 1953; 27:317–319.

5. Cooper IS. Parkinsonism: Its Medical and Surgical Therapy. Springfield, IL: Charles C Thomas, 1961.
6. Perry VL, Lenz FA. Ablative therapy for movement disorders: thalamotomy for Parkinson's disease. Neurosurg Clin North Am 1998; 9:317–323.
7. Hassler R, Riechert T. Indikationen und Lokalisationsmethode der gezielten Hirnoperationen. Nervenarzt 1954; 25:441–447.
8. Cooper IS. Chemopallidectomy: an investigative technique in geriatric parkinsonians. Science 1955; 121:217–218.
9. Burchiel KJ. Thalamotomy for movement disorders. Neurosurg Clin North Am 1995; 6:55–71.
10. Smith Y, Shink E, Sidibé M. Neuronal circuitry and synaptic connectivity of the basal ganglia. Neurosurg Clin North Am 1998; 9:203–222.
11. Wichmann T, DeLong MR. Models of basal ganglia functions and pathophysiology of movement disorders. Neurosurg Clin North Am 1998; 9:223–236.
12. Calabresi P, De Murtas M, Bernardi G. The neostriatum beyond the motor function: experimental and clinical evidence. Neuroscience 1997; 78:39–60.
13. Parent A. Extrinsic connections of the basal ganglia. Trends Neurosci 1990; 13:254–258.
14. Gerfen CR. The neostriatal mosaic: multiple levels of compartmental organization in the basal ganglia. Annu Rev Neurosci 1992; 15:285–320.
15. Gerfen CR, Wilson CJ. The basal ganglia. Björklund A, Hökfelt T, Swanson L, eds. Handbook of Chemical Neuroanatomy: Integrated Systems of the CNS, Part III.. Amsterdam: Elsevier, 1996:369.
16. Hassler R. Architectonic organization of the thalamic nuclei. Schaltenbrand G, Walker AE, eds. Stereotaxy of the Human Brain: Anatomical, Physiological, and Clinical Applications. Stuttgart: Thieme1982:140–180.
17. Jones EG. A description of the human thalamus. Steriade M, Jones EG, McCormick DA, eds. Thalamus. Amsterdam: Elsevier1997:II:425–499.
18. Krack P, Dostrovsky J, Ilinsky I, Kultas-Ilinsky K, Lenz F, Lozano A, Vitek J. Surgery of the motor thalamus: problems with the present nomenclatures. Mov Disord 2002; 17(suppl 3):S2–S8.
19. Hirai T, Jones EG. A new parcellation of the human thalamus on the basis of histochemical staining. Brain Res Rev 1989; 14:1–34.
20. Sidibé M, Bevan MD, Bolam JP, Smith Y. Efferent connections of the internal globus pallidus in the squirrel monkey: I. Topography and synaptic organization of the pallidothalamic projection. J Comp Neurol 1997; 382:323–347.
21. Ilinsky IA, Kultas-Ilinsky K. Neuroanatomical organization and connections of the motor thalamus in primates. Kultas-Ilinsky K, Ilinsky IA, eds. Basal Ganglia and Thalamus in Health and Movement Disorders.. New York: Plenum, 2001:77–91.
22. Hoover JE, Strick PL. Multiple output channels in the basal ganglia. Science 1993; 259:819–821.
23. Baron MS, Vitek JL, Bakay RA, Green J, Kaneoke Y, Hashimoto T, Turner RS, Woodard JL, Cole SA, McDonald WM, DeLong MR. Treatment of advanced Parkinson's disease by posterior GPi pallidotomy: 1-year results of a pilot study. Ann Neurol 1996; 40:355–366.
24. Tasker RR. Deep brain stimulation is preferable to thalamotomy for tremor suppression. Surg Neurol 1998; 49:145–154.
25. Lenz FA, Kwan HC, Martin RL, Tasker RR, Dostrovsky JO, Lenz YE. Single unit analysis of the human ventral thalamic nuclear group: tremor-related activity in functionally identified cells. Brain 1994; 117:531–543.
26. Koller WC, Wilkinson S, Pahwa R, Miyawaki EK. Surgical treatment options in Parkinson's disease. Neurosurg Clin North Am 1998; 9:295–306.
27. Spiegel EA, Wycis HT. Ansotomy in paralysis agitans. Arch Neurol Psychiatry 1954; 71: 598–614.
28. Hassler R, Reichert T, Mundinger F, Umbach W, Ganglegerger JA. Physiological observations in stereotaxic operations in extrapyramidal motor disturbances. Brain 1960; 83:337–350.
29. Svennilson E, Torvik A, Lowe R, Leksell L. Treatment of parkinsonism by sterotactic thermolesions in the pallidal region. Acta Psychiatr Neurol Scand 1960; 35:358–377.
30. Lenz FA, Kwan HC, Dostrovsky JO, Tasker RR, Murphy JT, Lenz YE. Single unit analysis of the human ventral thalamic nuclear group: activity correlated with movement. Brain 1990; 113: 1795–1821.
31. Lou LS, Jankovic J. Essential tremor: clinical correlates in 350 patients. Neurology 1991; 41: 234–238.
32. Bakay RA, Vitek JL, DeLong MR. Thalamotomy for tremor. Rengachary SS, Wilkins RH, eds. Neurosurgery Operative Atlas.. Baltimore: Williams and Wilkins1998:2:299–312.

33. Schaltenbrand G, Bailey P. Introduction to Stereotaxis with an Atlas of the Human Brain. Stuttgart: Thieme, 1959.

34. Andrew J, Watkins ES. A Stereotaxic Atlas of the Human Thalamus and Adjacent Structures: A Variability Study. Baltimore: Williams and Wilkins, 1969.

35. Van Buren JM, Borke RC. Variations and Connections of the Human Thalamus. New York: Springer, 1972.

36. Schaltenbrand G, Wahren W. Atlas for Stereotaxy of the Human Brain. Stuttgart: Thieme, 1977.

37. Francel PC, Coffman D. Three-dimensional volumetric imaging for stereotactic lesional and deep brain stimulation surgery. Rengachary SS, Wilkins RH, eds. Neurosurgery Operative Atlas. Baltimore: Williams and Wilkins, 2000:135–154.

38. Spiegelmann R, Friedman WA. Rapid determination of thalamic CT-stereotactic coordinates: a method. Acta Neurochir (Wien) 1991; 110:77–81.

39. Papadakis N, Mark VH. Intermittent decortication and progressive hyperthermia, hypertension, and tachycardia following methylglucamine iothalamate ventriculogram. Appl Neurophysiol 1980; 43:59–66.

40. Tasker RR, Dostrovsky JO, Dolan EJ. Computerized tomography (CT) is just as accurate as ventriculography for functional stereotactic thalamotomy. Stereotact Funct Neurosurg 1991; 57: 157–166.

41. Hirai T, Miyazaki M, Nakajima H, Shibazaki T, Ohye C. The correlation between tremor characteristics and the predicted volume of effective lesions in stereotaxic nucleus ventralis intermedius thalamotomy. Brain 1983; 106:1001–1018.

42. Quiñones-Molina R, Molina H, Ohye C, Macias R, Alaminos A, Alvarez L, Teijeiro J, Muñoz, Ortega I, Piedra J, Torres A, Morales F, Soler W. CT-oriented microrecording guided selective thalamotomy. Stereotact Funct Neurosurg 1994; 62:200–203.

43. Tomlinson FH, Jack CR, Kelly PJ. Sequential magnetic resonance imaging following stereotactic radiofrequency ventralis lateralis thalamotomy. J Neurosurg 1991; 74:579–584.

44. Heikkinen ER. Stereotactic neurosurgery: new aspects of an old method. Ann Clin Res 1986; 47(suppl 18):73–83.

45. Selby G. Stereotaxic surgery. Koller WCHandbook of Parkinson's Disease. New York: Marcel Dekker, 1987:421–435.

46. Kelly PJ, Gillingham FJ. The long-term results of stereotaxic surgery and L-dopa therapy in patients with Parkinson's disease: a 10-year follow-up study. J Neurosurg 1980; 53:332–337.

47. Schuurman PR, Bosch DA, Bossuyt PM, Bonsel GJ, van Someren EJ, de Bie RM, Merkus MP, Speelman JD. A comparison of continuous thalamic stimulation and thalamotomy for suppression of severe tremor. N Engl J Med 2000; 342:461–468.

48. Linhares MN, Tasker RR. Microelectrode-guided thalamotomy for Parkinson's disease. Neurosurgery 2000; 46:390–398.

49. Fox MW, Ahlskog JE, Kelly PJ. Stereotactic ventrolateralis thalamotomy for medically refractory tremor in post-levodopa era Parkinson's disease patients. J Neurosurg 1991; 75:723–730.

50. Jankovic J, Cardoso F, Grossman RG, Hamilton WJ. Outcome after stereotactic thalamotomy for parkinsonian, essential, and other types of tremor. Neurosurgery 1995; 37:680–687.

51. Selby G. Stereotactic surgery for the relief of Parkinson's disease. Part 2: an analysis of results in a series of 303 patients. J Neurol Sci 1967; 5:343–375.

52. Matsumoto K. Reappraisal of ventrolateral thalamotomy for Parkinson's disease. In: Tasker RR, ed. Neurosurgery: State of the Art Reviews, Vol. 2, No. 1, Stereotactic Surgery. Philadelphia: Hanley and Belfus1987:209–234.

53. Ohye C, Hirai T, Miyazaki M, et al. VIM thalamotomy for the treatment of various kinds of tremor. Appl Neurophysiol 1982; 45:275–280..

54. Matsumoto K, Shichijo F, Fukami T. Long-term follow-up review of cases of Parkinson's disease after unilateral or bilateral thalamotomy. J Neurosurg 1984; 60:1033–1044.

55. Vilkki J, Laitinen LV. Effects of pulvinotomy and ventrolateral thalamotomy on some cognitive functions. Neuropsychologia 1976; 14:67–78.

56. Louw DF, Burchiel KJ. Ablative therapy for movement disorders: complications in the treatment of movement disorders. Neurosurg Clin North Am 1998; 9:367–373.

57. Tasker RR. Surgical aspects. Symposium on extrapyramidal disease. . Appl Ther 1967; 9:454.

58. Krayenbuhl H, Wyss OAM, Yasargil MG. Bilateral thalamotomy and pallidotomy as treatment for bilateral parkinsonism. J Neurosurg 1961; 18:429–444.

59. Van Manen J, Speelman JD, Tans RJ. Indications for surgical treatment of Parkinson's disease after levodopa therapy. Clin Neurol Neurosurg 1984; 86:207–218.

60. Bell DS. Speech functions of the thalamus inferred from the effects of thalamotomy. Brain 1968; 106:981–1000.
61. Nagaseki Y, Shibazaki T, Hirai T, Kawashima Y, Hiato M, Wada H, Miyazaki M, Ohye C. Long-term follow-up results of selective VIM-thalamotomy. J Neurosurg 1986; 65:296–302.
62. Kelly PJ, Ahlskog JE, Goerss SJ, Daube JR, Duffy JR, Kall BA. Computer-assisted stereotactic ventralis lateralis thalamotomy with microelectrode recording control in patients with Parkinson's disease. Mayo Clin Proc 1987; 62:655–664.
63. Shahzadi S, Tasker RR, Lozano A. Thalamotomy for essential and cerebellar tremor. Stereotact Funct Neurosurg 1995; 65:11–17.
64. Giller CA, Dewey RB, Ginsburg MI, Mendelsohn DB, Berk AM. Stereotactic pallidotomy and thalamotomy using individual variations of anatomic landmarks for localization. Neurosurgery 1998; 42:56–65.
65. Goldman MS, Kelly PJ. Symptomatic and functional outcome of stereotactic ventralis lateralis thalamotomy for intention tremor. J Neurosurg 1992; 77:223–229.
66. Marks PV. Stereotactic surgery for post-traumatic cerebellar syndrome: an analysis of seven cases. Stereotact Funct Neurosurg 1993; 60:157–167.
67. Broggi G, Giorgi C, Servello D. Stereotactic neurosurgery in the treatment of tremor. Acta Neurochir Suppl (Wien) 1987; 39:73–76.
68. Pahwa R, Lyons KE, Wilkinson SB, Tröster AI, Overmann J, Kieltyka J, Koller WC. Comparison of thalamotomy to deep brain stimulation of the thalamus in essential tremor. Mov Disord 2001; 16:140–143.
69. Narabayashi H. Lessons from stereotaxic surgery using microelectrode techniques in understanding Parkinsonism. Mount Sinai J Med 1988; 55:50–57.

20
Pallidotomy

Nestor Galvez-Jimenez
Cleveland Clinic Florida, Weston, Florida, U.S.A.

Maurice R. Hanson
Cleveland Clinic Naples, Naples, Florida, U.S.A.

I. HISTORICAL PERSPECTIVE

During the twentieth century many surgical procedures, were developed for the treatment of Parkinson's disease (PD) and other movement disorders (Fig. 1). Cortical excisions, capsulotomies, caudotomies, ansotomics, pedunculotomies, pyramidotomies, and ramicectomies were performed with variable results, and most procedures were fraught with complications (1–3), especially hemiparesis. In 1952 Cooper accidentally ligated the anterior choroidal artery in a patient with postencephalitic parkinsonism with severe rigidity, tremor, and retrocollis who was scheduled for a left cerebral peduncolotomy. In the postoperative period, tremor and rigidity improved on his right side and no hemiparesis was present (3,4). These findings resulted in a surgical target shift to the pallidum and outflow tracts (4,5). Cooper did not use stereotactic techniques for his procedures as developed by Spiegel and Wycis (6). In 1953 Narabayashi and Okuma published their first case of "chemical" pallidotomy in a PD patient (7). About the same time, Guiot and Brion reported the use of electrical coagulation of the anterodorsal pallidum (8). Leksell performed anterodorsal pallidotomies with poor results until he moved his target to the posteroventral pallidal area, which is the point where the ansa lenticularis begins (9). Of the 19 patients operated on by Leksell in the posteroventral pallidum, 95% experienced improvements in tremor, rigidity, and bradykinesia for up to 5 years. About the same time, ventrolateral thalamotomies, spearheaded by Hassler and Richert, proved to be extremely effective for the suppression of tremor. During that period, thalamotomies became a well-established surgical treatment for medically refractory PD tremor. During the latter part of the 1960s, levodopa became an established form of medical therapy and the use of surgical procedures dramatically diminished. Motor complications resulting from the long-term use of levodopa soon became evident.

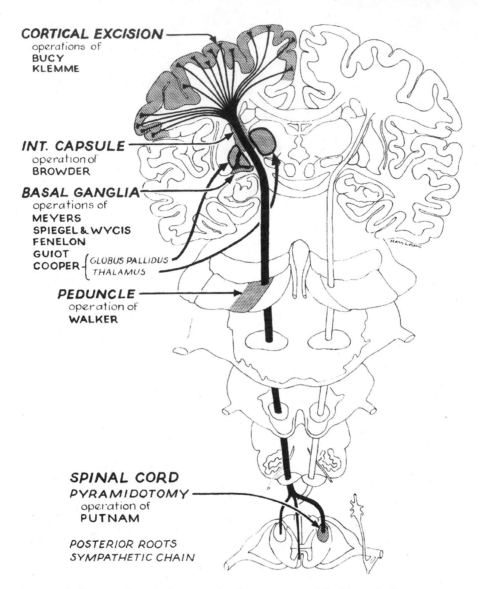

Figure 1 Proposed surgical targets for the treatment of Parkinson's disease.

These complications, coupled with advances in intraoperative recording devices and neuroimaging techniques, led to a resurgence of surgical treatments for disabling motor complications during the 1980s and 1990s.

II. PATHOPHYSIOLOGICAL BACKGROUND

In the normal physiological state, cortically mediated impulses are driven by the interaction between the direct striato-pallido-thalamocortical loop and the indirect striato-subthalamic-pallido-thalamocortical loop (Fig. 2). The direct pathway is a monosynaptic pathway that utilizes GABA, substance P, and dynorphin as neurotransmitters. The indirect

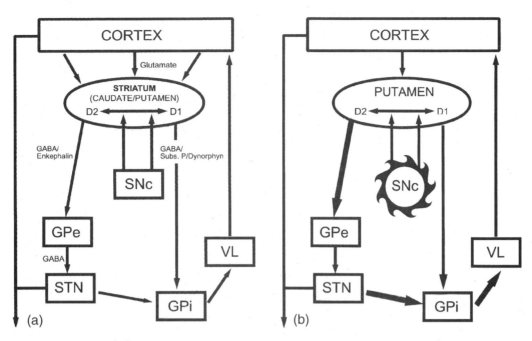

Figure 2 (a) Normal motor circuitry. (b) Motor circuitry in Parkinson's disease. SNc, substantia nigra pars compaeta; GPe, globus pallidus externa; STN, subthalamic nucleus; GPi, globus pallidus interna; VL, ventral lateral thalamus; GABA, gamma amino butyric acid; Subs. P - substance P.

pathway projecting to the lateral globus pallidus utilizes GABA and enkephalins as neurotransmitters. During the dopamine deficiency state there is underactivity of the direct pathway with concomitant overactivity of the indirect pathway. The inhibitory GABAergic output from the globus pallidus externa (GPe) to the subthalamic nucleus (STN), globus pallidus interna (GPi), and substantia nigra pars reticulata (SNr) results in an excitatory drive from the sensorimotor portion of the STN into the thalamocortical loop via the GPi (Fig. 2b). The net result is the inhibition of cortically mediated impulses, leading to bradykinesia and rigidity. The main structure driving this system is the STN via the GPi, making them suitable surgical targets for PD. A strategically placed lesion in the GPi results in improvements in bradykinesia and rigidity. The more ventrally located the lesion, the better the bradykinesia response. This response is probably related to destruction of the neurons and axons comprising the ansa lenticularis, which represents the major pallidofugal pathway projecting to the ventral anterior and ventrolateral thalamic nuclei. It is important to note that worsening of dyskinesias such as drug-induced chorea or dystonia are not observed after pallidotomy. Parkinsonian tremor has a different pathophysiological basis. Synchronization of oscillatory discharges within the basal ganglia-thalamo-cortical loop may be the cause of tremor. Modulation of these oscillatory discharges using dopaminergic pharmacological manipulation or disruption of these oscillations with destructive or neuro-modulatory surgical techniques such as deep brain stimulation (DBS) may result in improvements of tremor. In advanced PD, akinesia and gait disturbances may be due to involvement of the pedunculopontine nuclei (PPN), and other brainstem and cortical areas may be responsible for the development of autonomic dysfunction and cognitive decline (10).

In patients with PD there is inhibition of the dorsolateral prefrontal, supplementary motor, and primary motor areas. Ceballos-Baumann et al. demonstrated correction of these alterations after surgery using positron emission tomography (PET). Others (12–14) have supported these findings. In addition, using transcranial magnetic cortical stimulation (TMS), correction of excessive movement-related cortical neuronal discharges was demonstrated in PD patients after pallidotomy (15). Young et al. (16), using TMS, demonstrated lengthening of the cortical stimulation silent period in PD patients after pallidotomy, suggesting a decrease in the activation of cortical motor inhibitory circuits.

III. PATIENT SELECTION

There are no age restrictions for pallidotomy. It has been documented to be safe and well tolerated in patients in their eighties (17). Patients should have levodopa-responsive idiopathic PD with motor fluctuations and drug-induced dyskinesia despite maximum optimal medical therapy. Patients undergoing pallidotomy should not have dementia, other cognitive or psychiatric disturbances, or any medical conditions that would preclude surgery, compromise assessments, or increase surgical risk.

IV. COMPLICATIONS/RISKS

A review of multiple pallidotomy reports indicated an average mortality rate of 8% and the occurrence of serious complications in 15% of patients (17–21,25,29,30,32–36,39,42,43). Complications included dysarthria, dysphagia, hemiparesis, transient relief or worsening of PD symptoms, visual disturbances, seizures, transient hiccups, square wave jerks, and eye lid apraxia. Neuropsychological complications included depression, confusion, hallucinations, disinhibition, compulsions, apathy, and abulia.

V. METHODOLOGY

The main goal during pallidotomy for PD is the strategic location of the target and precise placement of the lesion. In pallidotomy, the optimal site for the lesion is the postero-ventral portion of the GPi. Prior to pallidotomy the preoperative assessment of the patient should include (a) a careful history and physical examination, performed by a movement disorders specialist, (b) an assessment of the surgical risk by a neuro-surgeon with expertise in stereotactic and lesioning procedures, (c) a neuropsychological assessment, (d) neuroimaging, and (e) a Unified Parkinson's Disease Rating Scale (UPDRS) and dyskinesia scale in the practically defined worst off and best on.

The surgical methodology proceeds as follows. Neuroimaging with selection of the target area involves magnetic resonance imaging (MRI) and/or brain computed tomography (CT) performed for careful localization of the target. The use of MRI and CT fusion technique may provide the best correction for the distortion that may coexist with the use of MRI alone. It has been determined that using brain MRI alone may lead to a 2–3 mm error in target localization. To determine the coordinates for the pallidum, the anterior and posterior commissures (AC/PC) should be identified. After the AC/PC line is obtained, the mid AC/PC point is determined. The posteroventral portion of the pallidum is approximately 18–22 mm lateral to the AC/PC line, 3–6 mm inferior to the AC/PC line, and 2–3 mm anterior to the mid AC/PC line. A burr hole is created, usually in the frontal area,

Table 1 Commonly Observed Properties of GPe, GPi, and Border Neurons in the Globus Pallidus of Patients with Parkinson's Disease

	GPe	GPi	Border
Discharge pattern	Burst and pauses	Irregular	Regular
Discharge rate, Hz	10–20 or 40–60	60–300 (mean 90)	10–40
Response to movement	Excited, inhibited, or unaffected	Excited, inhibited, or unaffected	No
Position relative to optic tract	10–17 mm dorsal	2–10 mm dorsal	Variable

Source: Ref. 57.

anterior to the coronal suture and lateral to the sagittal plane. It has been estimated that there is an additional brain shift in the anteroventral plane due to air entry via the burr hole, adding further distortion to the initial stereotactic imaging coordinates. Microelectrode recording helps refine the surgical target and is performed while the patient is awake.

In many centers, functional mapping of the target area has become an integral part of the surgical procedure for localization. Recording begins above the target to allow identification of the GPe, border zone, GPi, optic tract, and internal capsule. The different segments of the globus pallidus are identified based on their differential responses to stimulation and firing pattern. The neurons in the GPe have a firing rate of 40–60 Hz and those in the GPi of 67–86 Hz (Table 1) (22–24).

Once the target has been localized, a reversible radio-frequency lesion is performed using a probe delivering a temperature of 45°C for 30 seconds to detect any potential side effects. A permanent lesion is created delivering a temperature of 75°C for 60 seconds. Using this technique a cylindrical lesion will typically measure 3–4 mm in diameter and 5–6 mm in its longitudinal plane (25).

VI. PALLIDOTOMY OUTCOMES

In 1992 Laitinen et al. (9) reported their experience with posteroventral pallidotomy in 38 PD patients with follow-up for up to 71 months (mean 28 months). Patients included in the study had PD with severe tremor, rigidity, bradykinesia, dyskinesias, gait difficulties, and muscle pain. In most the predominant symptom was bradykinesia with or without tremor. There were 20 men and 18 women with a mean age of 60.3 years (30–80 years) and a mean duration of PD of 9.4 years (2–20 years). All patients had been treated with conventional medical therapy without success. The surgery was unilateral in 34 patients and bilateral in 4. Eight patients had a prior unilateral thalamotomy, and two had bilateral thalamotomies. Unfortunately, these patients were assessed at a time when standardized scales such as the UPDRS were not routinely used. Instead, Laitinen and colleagues used nonvalidated writing, drawing, and gait scales to record their observations making comparison of surgical outcomes difficult to compare with current studies. This seminal study provided the impetus for the resurgence of the use of pallidotomy for the treatment of PD. In this study, tremor improved in 81% and rigidity and hypokinesia in 92% of patients (9). Drug-induced dyskinesias, painful muscle cramps, speech volume, and gait were improved in most patients. In 2 patients anxiety was also improved. With regard to lesion location, they felt that the lesion should be located as close as possible to the optic tract and just dorsal to the amygdala complex. The mean size of the pallidal lesion was 95 mm^3. Due to the proximity of this lesion to the optic tract, homonymous hemianopsia may result.

Dogali et al. reported their experience in 18 patients with advanced PD who underwent ventroposterior pallidotomy. The mean age of the surgical group was 59.8 years (range 42–79 years); there were 11 men and 7 women with a mean duration of illness of 10 years. All patients were assessed using the Core Assessment Program for Intracerebral Transplantation (CAPIT) protocol (26–28). The patients were assessed at baseline after being off medications for 12 hours (practically defined off), within 2 weeks after surgery, and every 3 months thereafter for one year. Patients were also assessed on medications (best on state) after the administration of antiparkinsonian medications. All patients had their visual fields assessed using Goldman computer-assisted perimetry and MRI pre- and postoperatively. No immediate postoperative morbidity was noted, although one patient developed transient (24 hours) sexual disinhibition and another patient had a contralateral infarct 7 months after the initial procedure. The patient recovered and became ambulatory in 3 months but was left with hemiparesis and was excluded from the analysis. Sustained improvements were noted in rigidity, bradykinesia, resting tremor, gait, balance, and dyskinesias up to 12 months. The postoperative UPDRS scores improved by 65% in the off state, ipsilateral limb scores by 24.2%, and contralateral limb scores by 38.2%.

In 1995 Lozano et al. (29) reported the first study attempting to circumvent some of the methodological flaws that permeated the medical and surgical literature up to that time ("... assessments have often been uncritical, uncontrolled, unblinded, and lacking in accepted clinical rating methodologies"). Fourteen patients (8 men, 6 women) with severe motor fluctuations, dyskinesias, and a level of disability that interfered with self-care and activities of daily living (ADL) were included in the study. Patients were evaluated using the CAPIT protocol. The patients were assessed after a "practically defined worst off state" defined as a drug-free interval of at least 12 hours followed by the best on state when patients were assessed one hour after taking their usual morning anti PD medications. Detailed visual field testing and neuropsychological testing were performed. The lesion was placed in the posteroventromedial pallidum. In addition, using intraoperative neuronal cell recording with microstimulation to identify the optic tract and internal capsule further refined the localization of the surgical target. All patients had a unilateral pallidotomy to the side contralateral to their worst symptoms. If patients had symmetrical symptoms, the side contralateral to the dominant hand was lesioned. The size of the lesion was approximately 6–8 mm in diameter. In the postoperative state no patients were found to have visual loss or hemiparesis. Three patients had mild transient facial weakness for 2–3 weeks. Four patients developed transient euphoria. In all patients with facial weakness, marked edema was found along the internal capsule. One significant finding during the operative period was transient dystonia or choreoathetosis on the operated side. Patients having these movements were more likely to have a better outcome in motor functioning postoperatively. In the off state the total motor UPDRS scores improved by 30%, akinesia by 33%, postural instability/gait disturbance by 23%, rigidity by 36%, and UPDRS ADL scores by 30%. In the on state drug-induced dyskinesias improved by 92% in the contralateral lesioned side and by 32% in the ipsilateral side. There was a nonsignificant reduction of total dosage of medication postoperatively. Tremor, was also found to be significantly reduced on the side contralateral to the lesion.

Lang et al. (30) followed this cohort of patients for up to 2 years. All patients were examined preoperatively and reexamined at 6 months (39 patients), one year (27 patients), and 2 years (11 patients). The percent improvements at 6 months were as follows: off-period motor function 28%, with the most improvement in the contralateral limb, ADLs 29%, contralateral dyskinesias 82%, ipsilateral dyskinesias 44%, and rigidity 44%. The improvement in ipsilateral dyskinesias was lost at one year, and the improvements in postural stability and gait lasted only 3–6 months. Overall there were no significant changes in the use of medications postoperatively. The authors concluded that at 2 years pallidotomy continues to control dyskinesias and off-period disability. In a follow-up study (31), the same cohort of 40 patients was followed for a median of 52 months (range 41–64 months). Of the 40 patients only 20 were included in this study and were assessed during both the on and off states. The combined ADL and motor function on the UPDRS was 18% better at the last evaluation compared to baseline. The same was noted for contralateral off-period symptoms such as contralateral tremor (66% improvement), contralateral rigidity (43%), and bradykinesia (18%) and for the on period contralateral dyskinesias (71%). The authors concluded that in patients with advanced PD, pallidotomy controls contralateral off-period symptoms and on-period contralateral dyskinesias for up to 5.5 years.

Another study (32) reported 15 patients who underwent posterior GPi pallidotomy one year after surgery. Their findings included almost complete resolution of contralateral on-period dyskinesias and off-period contralateral tremor, rigidity, and bradykinesia for up to one year after surgery.

Samuel et al. (33) studied the effects of unilateral ventral medial pallidotomy in 26 patients with medically intractable PD with marked drug-induced dyskinesias. Contralateral dyskinesias improved by 67%, ipsilateral dyskinesias by 45%, axial dyskinesias by 50%, off motor scores by 27%, contralateral rigidity by 25%, ipsilateral rigidity by 22%, contralateral tremor by 33%, contralateral bradykinesia by 24%, gait and postural instability by 7%, and off walking time by 29%. An incidence of 7.7% for fatal complications was noted in the study. This included one patient who died from complications of a cerebral hemorrhage and a woman with PD for 7 years who sustained a massive hemorrhagic infarction in the middle cerebral territory with edema and midline shift. The authors noted that with experience the incidence of complications diminished. They concluded that drug-induced dyskinesias are the main indication for this procedure.

Measures of postural stability using computerized posturography, sway and sensory integration, and the UPDRS were not better after surgery, although 56% of patients (9/16) who were able to stand before surgery showed improvement in the average stability score or a decrease in the number of falls after surgery. The authors concluded that pallidotomy results in improved postural stability (34).

Variations in surgical technique, especially intraneuronal cell recordings, continues to be a topic of much debate. Two studies examined the outcome of posteroventral pallidotomy in 61 patients having surgery without intraneuronal cell recordings. De Bie et al. (35) enrolled 37 patients with advanced PD who, despite adequate medical therapy, continued to have severe motor fluctuations, painful dystonias, dyskinesias, and rigidity. Patients were randomly assigned to unilateral pallidotomy within one month or to pallidotomy after at least 6 months. The authors found an improvement in the off motor UPDRS scores in the pallidotomy group (47 to 32.5) as compared to the control group, which worsened from 52.5 to 56.5. Drug-induced dyskinesias improved by 50% when compared with the control group, and the UPDRS ADL scores improved by a median of 7 in the pallidotomy group.

In a similar study, Kishore et al. (36) enrolled 24 patients with advanced PD with motor fluctuations and dyskinesias who had a CT-guided posteroventral pallidotomy without the use of intraneuronal cell recordings. The aim of the authors was to mimic as much as possible the "average" surgical environment most likely encountered. They also found significant improvements in PD patients' off-period motor scores, especially in the contralateral side with ameliorations of medication-related contralateral and ipsilateral abnormal involuntary movements. Side effects were minimal except for transient facial weakness in five and permanent weakness in one. The authors concluded that their results were similar to those who use microelectrode recording, suggesting that this part of the procedure can be safely omitted. The authors also commented on time of surgery. Using their simplified method, the actual surgical procedure took an average of 2.5 hours when compared with over 8 hours for those cases where intraoperative neuronal cell recordings were performed.

Some have criticized the findings of some of these studies on the basis of the placebo effect. Obeso et al. (37) argued that in trials of novel antiparkinsonian medications, the placebo effect has been estimated to be as high as 30%. He argued that the rating scales used to evaluate the benefits of surgery make it difficult to avoid the placebo effect. They demonstrated that by using more sophisticated analyses of movement at the shoulder, arm, wrist, finger, and knee, the benefits of surgery were amplified. They concluded that when using the current clinical rating scales such as the UPDRS, large changes in motor function may be concealed and difficult to demonstrate. Shannon et al. (38) reported in 26 PD patients an overall improvement in total motor UPDRS of 18%. This improvement was transient and was attributable to improvements in tremor, rigidity, and bradykinesia scores. They observed declining efficacy over time in midline or global measures such as gait and postural instability, proposing that the short-lived benefit in these symptoms was due to misplacement or shrinkage of the lesion, progression of PD, or a transient placebo effect.

Many neurosurgeons are reluctant to perform bilateral destructive lesions due to major morbidity, such as cognitive, memory, language, swallowing, and speech disturbances, after a bilateral procedure (39). Similar concerns have been raised for staged bilateral pallidotomies. Therefore, staged bilateral pallidotomies are not routinely performed (40). Sutton et al. (40) performed bilateral pallidotomies in a total of four patients. They concluded that overall functional improvement in patients with advanced PD was not remarkable except for improvement in drug-induced dyskinesias or dystonia in the side contralateral to the lesion. Patient 1 had a subdural hematoma, worsening speech, and balance difficulties after a right pallidotomy. His gait difficulties were related to an ipsilateral (right foot) dystonia. He underwent a second contralateral procedure (left pallidotomy), resulting in improved dystonia but no improvement in gait or freezing. He developed severe depression with suicidal ideation after the second procedure. Patient 4 had a staged bilateral pallidotomy, developing depression after the second surgery. The authors concluded that ventroposterolateral pallidotomy may reduce contralateral medication-related dyskinesias or dystonia. In 14 patients with staged bilateral pallidotomy (41), gait or postural stability did not improve and there was a high incidence of bulbar symptoms. Siegel and Metman (42) argued that bilateral posteroventral pallidotomy may improve gait. Others (43) have challenged those findings. The American Academy of Neurology Task Force on the Evaluation of Surgery for Parkinson's Disease recommended against bilateral pallidotomies due to the high incidence of speech complications (44).

Implanting contralateral pallidal DBS electrodes in patients with a prior unilateral pallidotomy is a reasonable alternative to a bilateral lesioning procedure. In a pilot study Galvez-Jimenez et al. (45) showed that contralateral GPi stimulation in patients who already had a unilateral pallidotomy may improve ipsilateral PD symptoms. The authors argued that patients who had a unilateral pallidotomy may experience increasing disability due to persistent and progressive symptoms on the unoperated side. The reversible nature of the stimulation allows flexibility, as stimulation can be adjusted depending on the patients need and response. In addition, if complications such as swallowing or speech difficulties ensue, the patient has the flexibility of turning off the stimulation or the physician can adjust the stimulation parameters to obviate these complicating symptoms. Gamma knife pallidotomy has proven to be risky and fraught with many side effects and is rarely recommended for the treatment of advanced PD. Poor anatomical localization, lack of target confirmation, and perhaps a larger tissue destruction have all contributed to the poor outcomes seen with this procedure (46,47).

Findings on neuropsychological evaluations after posteroventral pallidotomy have been variable. In most patients there are no recognizable alterations (48–50), but decline in verbal learning and fluency has been reported with left-sided lesions and visuospatial dysfunction with right-sided lesions. Most of these alterations are transient and improve 6–12 months after surgery. In some patients, behavioral changes due to frontal lobe dysfunction may be seen in up to 25–30% of patients after surgery (51,52). Alegret et al. (53) reported that in patients with PD, there is a transient worsening of prefrontal and visuospatial functions at 3 months but improvement up to 4 years after surgery. The authors concluded that there are no permanent neuropsychological effects after surgery. Hayashi et al. (54) recently demonstrated improved attention resulting in enhanced motor function and reaction time in 12 PD patients after unilateral pallidotomy.

Vitek et al. (55) studied 36 PD patients who were randomized to either medical therapy ($n = 18$) or unilateral pallidotomy ($n = 18$). The authors used the change in total UPDRS score at 6 months as the primary outcome variable. Secondary outcome variables included the UPDRS motor subcore and independent scores for tremor, rigidity, bradykinesia, gait, and postural instability. Patients included in the study had motor fluctuations or dyskinesias, Hoehn and Yahr stage III or greater when off, and unsatisfactory clinical response to maximal medical management. All patients with atypical parkinsonism, abnormal brain MRI, poor response to levodopa, and unstable associated medical conditions (such as hypertension, heart failure, or dementia) were excluded. All antiparkinsonian medications were left unchanged. Twenty patients were followed for 2 years and the remainder for 6 months. The total UPDRS score improved by 32% after 6 months in the pallidotomy group as compared with the medical treatment group, who deteriorated by 5% in 6 months. The total motor UPDRS OFF improved by 32% in the pallidotomy group. Tremor was completely abolished in the pallidotomy but not in the medical treatment group. Off state rigidity improved by 55% contralaterally and 41% ipsilaterally 6 months after surgery. Similarly, contralateral bradykinesia improved by 39% in the off state and 27% in the on state. Compared to baseline, off-state gait and postural instability improved by 32% and on-state by 34% in the surgical group. Contralateral drug-induced dyskinesias were almost completely ameliorated and were reduced by 36% on the ipsilateral side. The medical group had an 8% worsening of dyskinesias during the 6-month period. There were no differences between the surgical and medical group in neuropsychological measures except for a slight decline in letter fluency in the surgical group. The authors concluded that unilateral pallidotomy offers significant improvement in the cardinal symptoms of PD when compared with those treated with best medical therapy.

VII. SUMMARY

The importance and long-term future of lesioning procedures such as pallidotomy in the era of neuromodulation and DBS appears to be limited. Notwithstanding, pallidotomy has been shown to be safe and effective for the amelioration of medication-related abnormal involuntary movements on the side contralateral to the lesion, as well as rigidity, bradykinesia, and tremor (56). Because of the potential increased incidence of speech, swallowing, and behavioral disturbances with bilateral procedures, bilateral pallidotomies cannot be recommended. Contralateral pallidal DBS in patients with a prior pallidotomy appears to be a safer alternative.

REFERENCES

1. Krauss JK, Grossman RG, Jankovic J. Pallidal Surgery for the Treatment of Parkinson's Disease and Movement Disorders. Philadelphia: Lippincott-Raven, 1998.
2. Cooper IS. Parkinsonism. Its Medical and Surgical Therapy. Springfield, IL: Charles C Thomas, 1961.
3. Cooper IS. Involuntary Movement Disorders. Hoeber Medical Division. New York: Harper & Row, 1969.
4. Meyers R. Surgical procedure for postencephalitic tremor, with notes on the physiology of the premotor fibers. Arch Neurol Psychiatr 1940; 44:455-459.
5. Meyers R. Surgical experiments in the therapy of certain extrapyramidal disease: a current evaluation. Acta Psych Neurol 1951; 67:1-39.
6. Spiegel EA, Wycis HT, Marks M, et al. Stereotaxic apparatus for operations on the human brain. Science 1947; 106:349-350.
7. Narabayashi H, Okuma T. Procaine-oil blocking of the globus pallidum for the treatment of rigidity and tremor of parkinsonism. Proc Jpn Acad 1953; 29:134-137.
8. Guiot G, Brion S. Traitement des mouments anormaux par la coagulation pallidale. Technique et resultants. Rev Neurol 1953; 89:578-580.
9. Laitinen LV, Bergenheim AT, Hariz MI. Leksell's posteroventral pallidotomy in the treatment of Parkinson's disease. J. Neurosurgery 1992; 76:53-61.
10. Pahapill PA, Lozano AM. The pedunculopontine nucleus and Parkinson's disease. Brain 2000; 123:1767-1783.
11. Ceballos-Baumann AO, Obeso JA, Vitek JL, Delong MR, Bakay R, Linazasoro G, Brooks DJ. Restoration of thalamocortical activity after posteroventral pallidotomy in Parkinson's disease. Lancet 1994; 344:814.
12. Samuel M, Ceballos-Baumann AO, Turjanski N, Boecker H, Gorospe A, Lizazasoro G, Homes AP, DeLong MR, Vitek JL, Thomas DG, Quinn NP, Obeso JA, Brooks DJ. Pallitodotomy in Parkinson's disease increases supplementary motor area and prefrontal activation during performance of volitional movements an H2(15)O PET study. Brain 1997; 120:1301-1313.
13. Ceballos-Baumann AO, Brooks DJ. Basal ganglia function and dysfunction revealed by PET activation studies. Adv Neurol 1997; 74:127-139.
14. Brooks DJ, Samuel M. The effects of surgical treatment of Parkinson's disease on brain function: PET findings. Neurology 2000; 55(6):S52-59.
15. Strafella A, Ashby P, Lozano A, Lang AE. Pallidotomy increases cortical inhibition in Parkinson's disease. Can J Neurol Sci. 1997; 24:133-136.
16. Young MS, Triggs WJ, Bowers D, Greer M, Friedman WA. Stereotactic pallidotomy lengthens the transcranial magnetic cortical stimulation silent period in Parkinson's disease. Neurology 1997; 49:1278-1283.
17. Uitti RJ, Wharen RE, Turk MF, Lucas JA, Finton MJ, Graff-Radford NR, Boylan KB, Goerss SJ, Kall BA, Adler CH, Caviness JN, Atkinson EJ. Unilateral pallidotomy for Parkinson's disease: comparison of outcome in younger versus elderly patients. Neurology 1997; 49:1072-1077.
18. Obeso JA, Guridi J, M DeLong. Surgery for Parkinson's disease. J Neurol Neurosurg Psychiatry 1997; 62:2-8.
19. Biousse V, Newman NJ, Carroll C, Mewes K, Vitek JL, Bakay RAE, Baron MS, DeLong MR. Visual fields in patients with posterior GPi pallidotomy. Neurology 1998; 50:258-265.

20. Averbuch-Heller L, Stahl JS, Hlavin ML, Leigh RJ. Square-wave jerks induced by pallidotomy in parkinsonian patients. Neurology 1999; 52:185–188.
21. de Bie RMA, Speelman JD, Schuurman PR, Bosch DA. Transient hiccups after posteroventral pallidotomy for Parkinson's disease. J Neurol Neurosurg Psychiatry 1999; 67:124–125.
22. Hutchinson WD, Lozano AM, Davis KD, Saint-Cyr JA, Lang AE, Dostrovsky JO. Differential neuronal activity in segments of globus pallidus in Parkinson's disease patients. Neuroreport 1994; 5:1533–1537.
23. Beric A, Sterio D, Dogali M, Fazzini E, Eidelberg D, Kolodny E. Characteristics of pallidal neuronal discharges in Parkinson's disease patients. Adv Neurol. 1996; 69:123–128.
24. Filion M, Tremblay L. Abnormal spontaneous activity of globus pallidus neurons in monkeys with MPTP-induced parkinsonism. Brain Research 1991; 547:142–151.
25. Dogali M, Fazzini E, Kolodny E, Eidelbeg D, Sterio D, Devinsky O, Beric A. Stereotactic ventral pallidotomy for Parkinson's disease. Neurology 1995; 45:753–761.
26. Langston JW, Widner H, Goetz C, et al. Core Assessment Program for Intracerebral Transplantation (CAPIT). Mov Disord 1992; 7:2–13.
27. Defer GL, Widner H, Marie RM, Remy P, Levivier M. Core Assessment Program for Surgical Interventional Therapies in Parkinson's Disease (CAPSIT-PD). Mov Disord 1999; 14:572–584.
28. Goetz CG, Stebbins GT, Shale HM, Lang AE, Chernik DA, Chmura TA, Ahlskog JE, Ddorflinger EE. Utility of an objective dyskinesia rating scale for Parkinson's disease: inter- and intrarater reliability assessment. Mov Disord 1994; 9:390–394.
29. Lozano AM, Lang AE, Galvez-Jimenez N, Miyasaki J, Duff J, Hutchinson D. Effect of GPi pallidotomy on motor function in Parkinson's disease. Lancet 1995; 346:1383–1387.
30. Lang AE, Lozano AM, Montogomery E, Duff J, Tasker R, Hutchison W. Posteroventral medial pallidotomy in advaced Parkinson's disease. N Engl J Med 1997; 337:1036–1042.
31. Fine J, Duff J, Chen R, Hutchison W, Lozano A, Lang AE. Long-term follow-up of unilateral pallidotomy in advanced Parkinson's disease. N Engl J Med 2000; 342:1708–1714.
32. Baron MS, Vitek JL, Bakay RAE, Green J, Kaneoke Y, Hashimoto T, Turner RS, Woodward JL, Cole SA, McDonal WM, Delong MR. Treatment of advanced Parkinson's disease by posterior GPi pallidotomy: 1-year results of a pilot study. Ann Neurol 1996; 40:355–366.
33. Samuel M, Caputo E, Brooks DJ, Schrag A, Scaravilli T, Branston NM, Rothwell JC, Marsden CD, Thomas DGT, Lees AJ, Quinn NP. A study of medial pallidotomy for Parkinson's disease: clinical outcome, MRI location and complications. Brain 1998; 121:59–75.
34. Melnick ME, Dowling GA, Aminoff MJ, Barbaro NM. Effect of pallidotomy on postural control and motor function in Parkinson disease. Arch Neurol 1999; 56:1361–1365.
35. de Bie RMA, de Haan RJ, Nijssen PCG, Wijnand A, Beute GN, Bosch DA, Haaxma R, Schmand B, Schuurman PR, Staal MJ, Speelman D. Unilateral pallidotomy in Parkinson's disease: a randomized, single-blind, multicentre trial. Lancet 1999; 354:1665–1669.
36. Kishore A, Turnbull IM, Snow BJ, de la Fuente-Hernandez R, Schulzer M, Mak E, Yardley S, Calne DB. Efficacy, stability and predictors of outcome of pallidotomy for Parkinson's disease. Six-month follow-up with additional 1-year observations. Brain 1997; 120:729–737.
37. Obeso JA, Linazasoro G, Rothwell JC, Jahanshahi M, Brown R. Assessing the effects of pallidotomy in Parkinson's disease. Lancet 1996; 347:1490.
38. Shannon KM, Penn RD, Kroin JS, Adler CH, Janko KA, York M, Cox SJ. Stereotactic pallidotomy for the treatment of Parkinson's disease. Efficacy and adverse effects at 6 months in 26 patients. Neurology 1998; 50:434–438.
39. Burchiel KJ. Thalamotomy for movement disorders. In: Gildenberg PLGE, ed. Neurosurgery Clinics of North America-Functional Neurosurgery. Philadelphia: W.B. Saunders Company, 1995: 55–72.
40. Sutton JP, Couldwell W, Lew M, Mallory L, Grafton S, DeGiorgio C, Welsh M, Apuzzo M, Jamshid A, Waters CH. Ventroposterior medial pallidotomy in patients with advanced Parkinson's disease technique and applications. Neurosurgery 1995; 36:1112–1116.
41. Counihan TJ, Shinobu LA, Eskandar EN, Cosgrove GR, Penney JB. Outcomes following staged bilateral pallidotomy in advanced Parkinson's disease. Neurology 2001; 56:799–802.
42. Siegel KL, Metman LV. Effects of bilateral posteroventral pallidotomy on gait of subjects with Parkinson's disease. Arch Neurol 2000; 57:198–204.
43. Pincus MM. Beneficial effect of bilateral pallidotomy on gait is unproven. Arch Neurol 2000; 57:1231.
44. Hallett M, Litvan I, et al. Evaluation of surgery for Parkinson's disease. A report on the Therapeutics and Technology Assessment Subcommittee of the American Academy of Neurology. Neurology 1999; 53:1910–1921.

45. Galvez-Jimenez N, Lozano A, Tasker R, Duff J, Hutchison W, Lang AE. Pallidal stimulation in Parkinson's disease patients with a prior unilateral pallidotomy. Can J Neurol Sci 1998; 25: 300–305.

46. Friedman JH, Epstein M, Sanes JN, Lieberman P, Cullen K, Linquist C, Daamen M. Gamma knife pallidotomy in advanced Parkinson's disease. Ann Neurol 1996; 39:535–538.

47. Bonnen JG, Iacono RP, Lulu B, Mohamed AS, Gonzalez A, Schoonenberg T. Gamma knife pallidotomy: case report. Acta Neurochir 1997; 139:442–445.

48. Perrine K, Dogali M, Fazzini E, Sterio D, Kolodny E, Eidelberg D, Devinsky O, Beric A. Cognitive functioning after pallidotomy for refractory Parkinson's disease. J Neurol Neurosurg Psychiatry 1998; 65:150–154.

49. Scott R, Gregory R, Hines N, Carroll C, Hyman N, et al. Neuropsychological, neurological and functional outcome following pallidotomy for Parkinson's disease. A consecutive series of eight simultaneous bilateral and twelve unilateral procedures. Brain 1998; 121:659–675.

50. Greem J, Barnhart H. The impact of lesion laterality on neuropsychological change following posterior pallidotomy: a review of current findings. Brain Cognition 2000; 42:379–398.

51. Trepanier LL, Saint-Cyr JA, Lozano AM, Lang AE. Neuropsychological consequences of postero-ventral pallidotomy for the treatment of Parkinson's disease. Neurology 1998; 51:207–215.

52. Stebbins GT, Gabrieli JDE, Shannon KM, Penn RD, et al. Impaired frontostriatal cognitive functioning following posteroventral pallidotomy in advanced Parkinson's disease. Brain Cognition 2000; 42:348–363.

53. Alegret M, Valldeoriola F, Tolosa E, Vendrell P, Junque C, Martinez J, Rumia J. Cognitive effects of unilateral posteroventral pallidotomy: a 4 year follow-up study. Mov Disord 2003; 18:323–328.

54. Hayashi R, Hashimoto T, Tada T, Ikeda S. Effects of unilateral pallidotomy on voluntary movement, and simple and choice reaction times in Parkinson's disease. Mov Disord 2003; 18:515–523.

55. Vitek J, Bakay RAE, Freeman A, et al. Randomized trial of pallidotomy versus medical therapy for Parkinson's disease. Ann Neurol 2003; 53:558–569.

56. Lang AE. Surgery for Parkinson's disease. A critical evaluation of the state of the art. Arch Neurol 2000; 57:1118–1125.

57. Lozano AM, Hutchinson WD, Tasker RR, Lang AE, Junn F, Dostrorsky JO. Microelectrode recordings define the ventral posteromedal pallidotomy target. Stereotact Funct Neuro Surg 1998; 71:153–163.

21
Subthalamotomy

J. Guridi, M. C. Rodríguez-Oroz, J. Arbizu, M. Manrique, and J. A. Obeso
Universidad de Navarra, Pamplona, Spain

L. Alvarez, R. Macias, and G. Lopez-Flores
Centro de Restauración Neurologica, Havana, Cuba

Surgery for Parkinson's disease (PD) was revitalized some 10 years ago when pallidotomy was shown to improve the cardinal features on the side contralateral to the lesion and drastically reduce levodopa-induced dyskinesias (1). Axial motor features such as gait initiation and freezing problems, flexor posture of the trunk, and postural reflexes do not respond to pallidotomy (2,3). Bilateral pallidotomy is associated with a large incidence of cognitive and speech problems, and consequently this surgical procedure is rarely performed (4–6). Deep brain stimulation (DBS) of the globus pallidus internus (GPi) and subthalamic nucleus (STN) may be performed bilaterally without a similar rate and severity of complications and are the current therapies for surgical treatment of advanced PD. However, DBS is an expensive technique and, therefore, is not available worldwide. Subthalamotomy could be an alternative for specific patients under special circumstances.

The STN is currently recognized as one of the targets for the surgical treatment of PD. This is in accordance with the current pathophysiological model in which the STN plays a critical role in the output of the basal ganglia (BG) (7). Until recently, STN clinical importance was only recognized in relation to hemiballism after stroke. The decision to target the STN for PD was the consequence of experimental studies in the 1-methyl-4-phenyl-1,2,3,6-tetrahydropyridine (MPTP) (8,9) monkey model.

I. ANATOMICAL CONSIDERATIONS

The STN is a small and ovoidal nuclear structure in the mesencephalon that receives inputs from the cortex (glutamatergic), globus pallidus externus (GPe) (GABAergic), centromedian-parafascicular complex (CMPf) of the thalamus (glutamatergic), substantia nigra pars compacta (SNc) (dopaminergic), and pedunculo pontine nucleus (PPN) (GABAergic and acetylcholinergic). The main efferences of the STN are sent to the GPi, GPe, substantia nigra pars reticulata (SNr), and striatum. STN output is excitatory (glutamatergic) (8,9). Microstimulation of STN produces excitation of the SNr and GPe (10) and entopeduncular nucleus in rats (11).

The organization of BG has been explained in the animal model for hypokinetic and hyperkinetic conditions (8,12,13). In this model, the main afferent structure of the BG, the striatum (caudate and putamen), receives information from the cortex (glutamatergic), which is sent to the GPi and SNr, the main efferent pathways to the thalamus and brainstem (GABAergic). Two main circuits in the BG work in parallel, the direct pathway (putamen-GPi) that is mediated by GABA (inhibitory) and peptide substance P and the indirect pathway from the putamen to the GPe (GABA with enkephalin) that projects to the STN. The STN projects with glutamate (excitatory), and consequently this structure is the hallmark of conditions of the BG (14,15). In the dyskinetic model, subthalamic hypoactivity is sent to the GPi/SNr and the GABAergic activity to the thalamus is decreased, leading to excessive movement (hyperkinetic condition). The parkinsonian state is associated with STN hyperactivity that overactivates the GPi/SNr, leading to hyper-inhibition (GABAergic) of the thalamocortical and brainstem motor system, leading to a greater difficulty to move (bradykinesia). The pathophysiological basis of rigidity and tremor has not been well defined (8,12,16).

Subthalamic hyperactivity was indicated by in situ hybridization studies showing that messenger ribonucleic acid (mRNA) expression of cytochrome oxidase I (enzyme of the mitochondrial respiratory chain) and glutamic acid decarboxylase (GAD) was increased (17–19) as was the neuronal firing rate in MPTP monkeys compared to normal animals (20–22). Bergman et al. reported an improvement in the side contralateral to the surgery in two parkinsonian monkeys after ibotenic acid lesion in the STN (23). Contralateral tremor, rigidity, and bradykinesia were improved and persisted until sacrifice. Hemichorea was present in both animals resolving in 24 hours in one animal and persisting in the other (23). Aziz et al. also reported successful alleviation of parkinsonism in six parkinsonian monkeys after a thermolytic STN lesion (24,25). The surgical procedure was bilateral in two and unilateral in four monkeys. Tremor, rigidity, posture, spontaneous movement and facial expression in the animals were improved. Hemichorea after the surgical lesioning was not a problem, appearing only in three monkeys and with mild intensity (24,25). Guridi et al. also reported a similar experience after chemical lesion (kainic acid) in the STN (26,27). Symptom alleviation was bilateral but mainly contralateral during the long-term follow-up of the animals. Manual motor tests performed in the monkeys showed a significant improvement after surgery. All animals developed a moderate and persistent hemichorea (26,27). The motor improvement was paralleled by functional changes. These STN lesions reversed the elevation of markers of metabolic hyperactivity in the GPi of the monkeys (19,27) and the entopeduncular nucleus of the rat (28,29) as well as decreasing the firing rate in these output nuclei. Parkinsonian patients with a vascular stroke in the basal ganglia with involvement of the STN had improvements in their parkinsonism contralateral to the stroke (30,31). The studies suggest that the hyperactivity of the STN-GPi/SNr plays a crucial role in the pathophysiology of parkinsonism. Subthalamic lesions induce an improvement in contralateral symptoms, and the impact of the surgery is correlated with behavioral and metabolic changes.

II. SUBTHALAMOTOMY IN CLASSIC NEUROSURGERY

The subthalamotomy described in classic surgery was not a lesion within the STN (Luysii nucleus) because it may induce hemichorea/hemiballism (HCB) in patients. The lesion described in the literature was the disruption of the pallidothalamic and the cerebellorubrothalamic pathway (campotomy by the lesion in the Forel field) similar to a medial pallidotomy. The lesion in this area induced beneficial effects as reported by Andy et al. (32) in 16 out of 20 patients for rigidity and in 15 out of 25 of tremor cases. The target was placed in the posterior subthalamic area (field H2 of Forel, zona incerta, and the prerubral field medial to STN). The authors reported that the lesion in the posterior subthalamic area did not induce HCB even if the lesion involved the STN (32). Campotomy may have the advantage of interrupting nearly all pallidofugal fibers with a relatively small lesion (33) (Fig. 1).

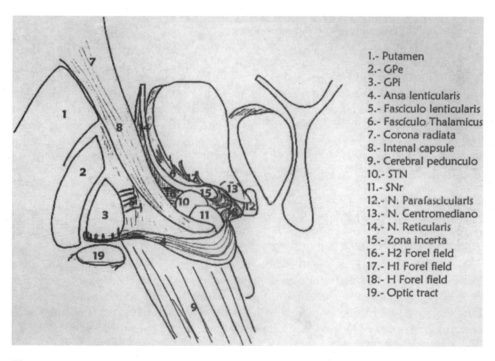

1.- Putamen
2.- GPe
3.- GPi
4.- Ansa lenticularis
5.- Fasciculo lenticularis
6.- Fascículo Thalamicus
7.- Corona radiata
8.- Intenal capsule
9.- Cerebral pedunculo
10.- STN
11.- SNr
12.- N. Parafascicularis
13.- N. Centromediano
14.- N. Reticularis
15.- Zona incerta
16.- H2 Forel field
17.- H1 Forel field
18.- H Forel field
19.- Optic tract

Figure 1 The pallidothalamic pathway is one of the basal ganglia outputs to the thalamus. The anatomical loop includes the ansa lenticularis and the fasciculus lenticularis. The ansa lenticularis arises from the lateral portion (sensorimotor) of the globus pallidus interna (GPi) forming a bundle ventral to the nucleus and dorsal to the optic tract. The fibers run ventral and medially around the posterior limb of the internal capsule and anterior to the substantia nigra (SN) and subthalamic nucleus (STN). The ansa lenticularis extends posteriorly to enter in Forel field H near the centromedian nucleus of the thalamus and zona incerta. The fasciculus lenticularis arises from the inner portion of the GPi and emerges from the dorsomedial area of the nucleus. It traverses the internal capsule surrounding the STN and SN. Between the STN and zona incerta, this bundle is called the Forel H2 field. Fibers of the fasciculus lenticularis in H2 and the ansa lenticularis in H Forel form the thalamic fasciculus located medial to the zona incerta (Forel field H1). Campotomies during "classic" neurosurgery placed this target reaching the ansa lenticularis and fasciculus lenticularis in H or H2 of Forel. (From Ref. 58.)

Hassler performed the first thalamotomy in the ventralis oralis anterior (Voa), which is the pallidal projection pathway in the thalamus, and later moved his target to the ventralis oralis posterior (Vop), which he described as a cerebellar thalamic field (34). Hassler considered ventralis intermedius (Vim) thalamotomy less effective than Vop thalamotomies. He suggested that the bundle from the cerebellum to the Vop was below Vim. According to this theory, the Vop thalamotomy reaching this bundle should have an excellent tremor response. Hassler's lesion in the subthalamic area was followed by lesions in the Voa and the Vop to destroy not only the zona incerta, but also the pathway from the pallidum to Voa and from the cerebellum to the Vop (35). Mundinger chose a different target in the zona incerta in 156 patients. According to his report, the majority of patients had 100% alleviation of symptoms versus 86% of those with a Vop lesion only (36). The zona incerta for Mundinger was the lesion that included the H1 and H2 Forel fields (Fig. 1). Contrary to previous reports, Fager described that the lesions performed in the subthalamic area were less effective and more hazardous than larger lesions in the thalamus (37). Other surgeons performed lesions in different subthalamic regions for tremor control, reporting different results (38,39).

In conclusion, subthalamotomies performed in "classic" neurosurgery, called campotomies, were lesions of different pathways surrounding the STN: anterior and dorsal STN region (zona incerta), medial (H2 bundle of Forel), or posterior and dorsal to the nucleus (area prelemniscus) (Fig. 1). The surgical procedures destroyed the pallido-thalamic projections (fasciculo lenticularis or the ansa lenticularis) and the cerebello-rubro-thalamic pathway below the ventrolateralis nucleus of the thalamus in their projection to the Voa, Vop, and Vim respectively. This is substantially different from currently performed subthalamotomy, that is aimed to lesion the nucleus proper with the hypothetical objective of decreasing STN hyperactivity.

III. SURGICAL PROCEDURE

A. Surgical Candidates

Patients selected for bilateral subthalamotomy are similar to those chosen for DBS of the STN. This includes, patients with PD who have a good response to levodopa, no atypical features, no dementia, and motor fluctuations and dyskinesias that are not well controlled with pharmacological therapies. Occasionally, patients with very asymmetrical but severe tremor, bradykinesia, and rigidity on one hemibody may also be considered candidates for unilateral subthalamotomy.

Patients who are not able to travel to and regularly return to the center for programming may be good candidates for subthalamotomy. Other candidates may include patients with a high risk of chronic infection in whom the DBS device may increase the risk of infection. In addition, subthalamotomy may be an option in countries in which DBS is not available.

B. Imaging Procedure

Magnetic resonance imaging (MRI) is performed 24–48 hours before surgery. The sequences used are T1 and T2, 2 mm thick with no interspace. On the day of surgery after placement of the stereotactic frame using local anesthesia and after withdrawal of antiparkinsonian medication, a computed tomography (CT) scan is performed. The slices are 2 mm thick with no interspaces and the information from the CT and MRI is sent to a neuronavigation computer where the fusion image is made, assuming errors less than 2 mm.

There are two methods to choose the target: indirect and direct. In *indirect targeting*; the anterior and posterior commissures are identified in T2 sequence and the intercommissural line (IL) is measured. A theorical target 3 mm posterior to the midpoint, 12 mm lateral, and 4 mm below the IL is selected. *In direct targeting*, the STN in axial section is viewed in correlation with the red nucleus (RN) and the mamillothalamic tractus. The RN is a medial anatomical structure in the midbrain. In the slice of the RN with the maximun diameter in the anterior part of the nucleus, the STN is found lateral to the structure (40). The STN is in the posterior and medial portion of the internal capsule. The target coordinates are correlated with the Schaltenbrand-Wharen atlas (41). The use of indirect and direct targeting produces a greater accuracy in the image procedure.

C. Electrophysiology

The use of anatomical imaging is not always enough to target the STN and locate the sensorimotor portion of the nucleus. Consequently, electrophysiological recording is recommended. The precise methodology employed for the recordings varies among centers. For instance, semi-micro-electrode recording or single unit extracellular potentials are two possible options.

Recording tracts are made on a parasagittal plane with a 45–60° angle with respect to the IL. Neuronal activity corresponds to the striatum followed by a low-amplitude fiber activity that corresponds to the internal capsule. Thalamic activity (generally 10 mm above the target) is recorded with discharge in burst related to the thalamic reticular nucleus. After the thalamus, there is approximately 1–3 mm with discharges corresponding to the zona incerta and fibers (fasciculus lenticularis). The electrical activity suddenly increases with multiple units discharging at a relatively high frequency with firing rates of approximately 33 Hz (42). Such activity is very abrupt and corresponds to the dorsal portion of the STN. The activity is recorded for 1–5 mm depending on the angle and portion of the nucleus. There are neurons in the sensorimotor area of the nucleus that correlate with active and passive movement of the limbs (Table 1). The units that respond to a single joint are often grouped in clusters that may be identified in the different tracts. In tremor patients, tremor units are also recorded in the lateral region of the STN (42).

D. Lesioning

The electrode probe is advanced as far as the dorsal border of the STN, and macro-stimulation (300 Hz, pulse width 0.2 ms, 0.3–0.7 mA) is performed at intervals of 2 mm until the ventral border of the nucleus is reached. These parameters allow the lesion to be performed approximately 2 mm away from the internal capsule to avoid adverse

Table 1 STN Characteristics of Microelectrode Recordings

High spontaneous firing rate (approx 33 Hz)
Responsive to passive/active manipulations (kinesthetic units)
Discharging correlated with tremor
Tremor suppression with microstimulation
No capsular or lemniscal response to microstimulation

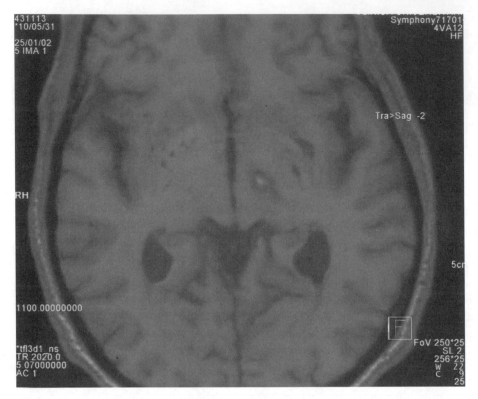

Figure 2 Postoperative magnetic resonance imaging (MRI) performed 24 hours after surgery showing subthalamic nucleus (STN) lesion. The lesion (inner zone) and the edema (outer zone) is shown. The edema also reaches the internal capsule. The MRI is a T1 sequence and the lesioning tip of the electrode is 1.1 mm in diameter, 3 mm in length, and a temperature of 80°C for 60 seconds. The diameter of the lesion is 3 mm.

effects. The temperature of the probe is 60, 70, and then 80°C for 60 seconds. The lesion is made in the sensorimotor portion of the STN after mapping the nucleus. In tremor patients the lesion is placed where microstimulation induces tremor arrest. During the procedure tremor and rigidity are closely assessed and are alleviated or abolished. In some patients a mild dyskinesia is induced during the lesion period but resolves in hours. Rarely, dyskinesia may persist for weeks. Volume of the lesion is calculated in the operating room and confirmed by MRI postoperatively (Fig. 2).

IV. CLINICAL OUTCOME

The experience with STN surgery for patients with advanced PD is limited. Alvarez et al. (43) reported 11 patients followed for 12 months after surgery. A significant reduction in the motor Unified Parkinson's Disease Rating Scale (UPDRS) scores was observed at 12 months postoperatively (50%; $p < 0.01$). The UPDRS motor score in the on state was also reduced by 39% ($p < 0.01$). Facial expression, postural instability, bradykinesia, rigidity, freezing, gait disturbance, and tremor were improved at 12 months. Dyskinesias were observed in the side contralateral to the surgery in six patients, and they were mild, resolving spontaneously in 24 hours except in one, in whom dyskinesias lasted for 5 days. One patient had an excellent immediate postoperative response but developed severe HCB on the seventh day postsurgery due to a large infarct in the subthalamic region. This patient required a pallidotomy one year later in order to control the HCB.

Seven of the 11 patients treated with unilateral subthalamotomy between October 1995 and July 1997 had progressive disability from the nonoperated side and aggravation of some axial features. In those patients, a lesion in the contralateral STN was performed 12–24 months following the first operation. The second lesion was not associated with any noticeable cognitive deficit or worsening of speech.

An open-label, pilot study of the viability and efficacy of bilateral simultaneous subthalamotomy was performed between 1998 and 2000. Eleven patients were followed for several years. Subthalamotomy produced a significant reduction in the off UPDRS motor score 1, 2, and 3 years after surgery compared to preoperative scores. Sixteen patients assessed at 3 years showed a 49% reduction ($p < 0.003$) in the off UPDRS motor score. All cardinal features (bradykinesia, rigidity, tremor, gait, and postural instability) were substantially improved, as were activities of daily living. The on medication assessment also showed a significant improvement at 12 months, but this effect deteriorated ($p < 0.03$) at the 3-year evaluation. These effects were associated with a substantial reduction ($> 50\%$) in daily levodopa dose 3 years postoperatively. Ten patients developed dyskinesias during or immediately after surgery that were very severe in 3 patients but evolved toward spontaneous attenuation. Dyskinesias had resolved at 3 months in 7 patients and at 12 months in one patient. At 12 months, dyskinesias were present with mild intensity in 2 patients.

There was no evidence of cognitive deficit after extensive neuropsychological assessesment (Litvan et al., unpublished). Adverse events that were judged clinically relevant consisted of dyskinesias and ataxia in 3 of the 11 patients. Dyskinesias resolved in all 3 patients and ataxia resolved in 2. One patient remained disabled because of ataxia and disequilibrium. Lesions in these patients were larger than usual. Speech deterioration was the second major adverse event, and dysarthria was severe in 7 patients. Dysarthria was present in these patients prior to surgery.

Guridi et al. (44) reported five patients. Three showed asymmetrical tremor-predominant disease with moderate motor disability when off (mean UPDRS 25) and relatively short disease duration of 6 years. The two other patients showed bilateral and severe disability with off UPDRS scores of 50 and 55 and disease durations of 10 and 14 years. Unilateral subthalamotomy was performed in four patients (Table 2). One of the patients with severe bilateral disease had surgery on only one side due to an adverse event. Shortly after the surgery this patient developed a brain abscess along the trajectory of the cannula used during the surgery. The abcess was stereotactically drained and resolved subsequently with antibiotic therapy. Six months after surgery the patient developed heart failure and could not be operated on the contralateral side.

The three patients in whom a unilateral lesion was planned and undertaken had a dramatic response. Tremor was abolished on the contralateral side and was completely controlled up to a maximum of 3 years. Bradykinesia and rigidity also improved markedly. The remaning patient with severe bilateral PD had complex motor fluctuations and severe dyskinesias. Mild chorea on the side contralateral to the largest lesion was seen for 2 weeks postoperatively. These did not increase with levodopa and subsided spontaneously over the next weeks.

Table 2 Subthalamotomy in Parkinson's Disease

Case	Age, y (disease duration)	H-Y	UPDRS preop, off/on	Main symptoms	Side	Follow-up (months)	UPDRS postop	Dyskinesias
1	50(6)	I	19/12	Tremor	R	39	0 (100%)	
2	70(5)	I	18/11	Tremor	L	16	7(60%)	
3	75(7)	II	32/15	Tremor, rigidity	R	23	15(53%)	
4	47(10)	IV-V	55/23	Axial, tremor, dyskinesias	Bilateral	14	12/6 (78%)	Mild (2 week)
5	72(14)	IV-V	50/22	Motor fluctuations	R	Lost	30(40% 6 m)	

H-Y, Hoehn and Yahr; UPDRS, Unified Parkinson's Disease Rating Scale.
Source: Ref. 44.

Gill and Heywood (45,46) reported 13 cases of unilateral subthalamotomy and 10 bilateral surgeries. All patients showed a contralateral alleviation of tremor, rigidity, and bradykinesia, but the report did not include any formal evaluation scale. Levodopa was reduced by 50% with a reduction in dyskinesias of approximately 70%. Only one patient developed a contralateral HCB lasting 3 weeks. Complications included one infarct and one case of worsened dysarthria (45,46). They also reported discrete cognitive changes in some patients, but neuropsychological testing did not show any statistically significant changes after surgery (47).

Barlas et al. described nine patients with unilateral subthalamotomy. Apparently there was marked motor improvement (evaluation scales were not reported), and only one patient developed HCB (48). Su et al. (49) described eight patients with advanced PD and subthalamotomy. All cases had improvements in bradykinesia (37%), rigidity (56%), and tremor (63%), and the benefits were mantained throughout 18 months follow-up except for a decline in tremor. Axial motor signs like speech, facial expression, and rising from a chair were also improved with unilateral subthalamotomy (48%; $p < 0.04$) at 18 months. UPDRS activities of daily living and motor scores improved 35% in the off state ($p < 0.02$). Dyskinesias were reduced 75% at 18 months ($p < 0.03$). They reported three patients with HCB, and one patient died from this complication. They suggested that the volume of the lesion in the cases with dyskinesia was increased compared to the cases without HCB (49).

V. PATHOPHYSIOLOGICAL CONSIDERATIONS: DYSKINESIAS AND SUBTHALAMOTOMY

Lesion of the STN induces marked changes in the metabolic state of the BG, thalamus, and cortex. Su et al reported in six patients a significant reduction in glucose (FDG) utilization in the vicinity of SNr, GPi, ventral thalamus, and pons (50). Our limited experience supports such findings and extends them to a marked restoration of the thalamo-cortical projection (Fig. 3). Carbon and Eidelberg described the effect of subthalamotomy as the largest of all surgical approaches for PD (51). Subthalamotomy

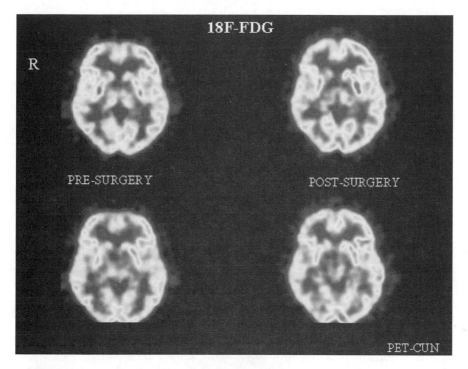

Figure 3 Positron emission tomography (PET) with 18-F fluorodeoxyglucose (FDG) in a patient with unilateral subthalamotomy of the right hemisphere (left). Six months after surgery FDG uptake in the pallidal and thalamic regions is reduced. This is compatible with reduced activity in the pallido-thalamic projection following reduced excitatory drive from the subthalamic nucleus (STN). There is also hypometabolism in the frontal cortex, probably secondary to surgery. In the left hemisphere there is hypermetabolism in the lenticular nucleus that may be due to the lack of antiparkinsonian medication for several months.

is capable of drastically reducing the abnormal and excessive inhibitory BG output to the thalamus and cortex in parallel with clinical improvement (51).

Lesion of the STN is typically associated with HCB. This has been demonstrated in both monkeys and humans (52–55). However, the severity and ease to trigger HCB was found to be lower in parkinsonian than in normal monkeys (56). In addition, HCB following stroke in humans has a tendency to subside spontaneously over weeks or months. HCB is produced following lesion of the STN in PD patients, but in the majority of cases dyskinesia is of mild intensity and short-lasting.

It is not known why subthalamotomy does not lead to severe HCB in PD. Lozano suggested that the lesion extends dorsally to damage the pallidothalamic projection, producing a pallidotomy-like effect that prevents the development of HCB (57). However, many patients do develop transient dyskinesias during surgery. Those with severe and persistent HCB had the largest lesions, extending more dorsally than the smallest lesions. One example was a patient with PD in whom an STN lesion was performed with excellent immediate response but with a delayed stroke involving a large thalamo-subthalamic area dorsally and substantia nigra ventrally 7 days after the surgery (43). He developed HCB of the lower limb that was not controlled with drugs, and a

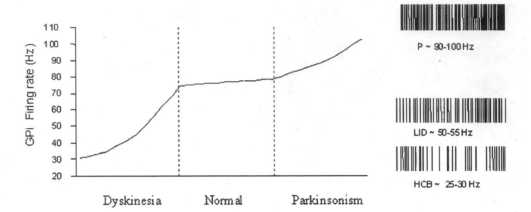

Figure 4 Representation of the subthalamic nucleus (STN) activity in three different motor conditions and globus pallidus interna (GPi) output. In the normal condition STN lesions induce a reduction in GPi activity to the thalamus. A similar lesion in a parkinsonian brain does not decrease GPi activity and the threshold for the appearance of dyskinesias is higher than in the normal condition. (Modified from Ref. 56.)

pallidotomy was performed a year later. These combined lesions left the patient without BG output, but his motor ability in the affected side was minimally impaired. This argues against the hypothesis that interruption of pallidofugal fibers is responsible for the reduced frequency and severity of dyskinesia with subthalamotomy. Rather, this may be due to functional adaptive changes occurring in the BG that are more overt and readily occurring in the parkinsonian brain (56). Lesion or blockade of the STN reduces the excitatory drives to the GPi and should lead to pallidal hypoactivity and, therefore, according to the model, dyskinesia facilitation (Fig. 4). In the dopamine-depleted brain, however, the GABA inhibitory effect on the "direct" striato-pallidal projection is reduced, compensating in part for the lack of excitatory subthalamic drive after subthalamotomy. In addition, STN lesion also leads to hypoactivity of the GPe, which in turn disinhibits the GPi, again shifting the predominant neuronal activity in the GPi toward the nondyskinetic range (56).

VI. CONCLUSIONS

Subthalamic lesion induces a marked improvement in the cardinal signs of PD on the side contralateral to the surgery. The effects are almost instantaneous after the lesion and the benefit is mantained up to 3 years. However, a recurrence of tremor has been observed in some patients. Bilateral subthalamotomy is associated with improvement of axial motor features. It also reduces daily levodopa doses, and dyskinesia. Hemichorea/ballism is the most serious complication after subthalamic lesioning. This particular aspect is closely related to the volume of the lesion. This complication is transitory in most patients but in some cases might require a pallidotomy to obtain complete control.

ACKNOWLEDGMENT

Maria Puy Obanos and James Allwood corrected and prepared the review for publication.

REFERENCES

1. Laitinen LV, Bergenheim AT, Hariz MI. Leksell's posteroventral pallidotomy in the treatment of Parkinson's disease. J Neurosurg 1992; 76:52–59.
2. Hallett M, Litvan I. and the Members of the Task Force on Surgery for Parkinson's disease of the American Academy of Neurology. Therapeutic and Technological Assessment Committee. Mov Disord 2000; 15:436–438.
3. Alkhani A, Lozano AM. Pallidotomy for Parkinson's disease: a review of contemporary literature. J Neurosurg 2001; 94:43–49.
4. Favre J, Burchiel KJ, Taha JM, Hammerstad J. Outcome of unilateral and bilateral pallidotomy for Parkinson's disease: patient assessment. Neurosurgery 2000; 46:344–355.
5. Merello M, Starkstein S, Nouzeilles MI, Kuzis G, Leiguarda R. Bilateral pallidotomy for treatment of Parkinson's disease induced corticobulbar syndrome and psychic akinesia avoidable by globus pallidus lesion combined with contralateral stimulation. J Neurol Neurosurg Psychiatry 2001; 71: 611–614.
6. Intermann PM, Masterman D, Subamaniam I, DeSalles A, Behnke E, Frysinger R, Bronstein JM. Staged bilateral pallidotomy for treatment of Parkinson's disease. J Neurosurg 2001; 94:437–444.
7. Guridi J, Luquin MR, Herrero MT, Obeso JA. The subthalamic nucleus: a possible target for stereotaxic surgery in Parkinson's disease. Mov Disord 1993; 8:421–429.
8. Albin R, Young AB, Penney JB. The functional anatomy of the basal ganglia disorders. Trend Neurosci 1989; 12:366–375.
9. Parent A, Hazrati L-N. Functional anatomy of the basal ganglia. II. The place of subthalamic nucleus and external pallidum in basal ganglia circuitry. Brain Res Revi 1995; 20:128–154.
10. Kita H, Kitai ST. Efferent projections of the subthalamic nucleus in the rat: light and electron microscopic analysis with the PHA-L method. J Comp Neurol 1987; 260:435–452.
11. Robledo P, Feger J. Excitatory influence of the rat subthalamic nucleus to substantia nigra pars reticulata and pallidal complex: electrophysiological data. Brain Res 1990; 518:47–54.
12. DeLong MR. Primate models of movement disorders of basal ganglia origin. Trends Neurosci 1990; 13:281–285.
13. Alexander GE, Crutcher MD. Functional architecture of the basal ganglia circuits: neural substrates of parallel processing. Trends Neurosci 1990; 13:266–271.
14. Parent A, Hazrati L-N. Functional anatomy of the basal ganglia. I. The cortico-basal ganglia-thalamo-cortical loop. Brain Res Revi 1995; 20:91–127.
15. Kitai ST, Kita H. Anatomy and physiology of the subthalamic nucleus: a driving force of the basal ganglia. In: Carpenter MB, Jarayaman, eds. The Basal Ganglia II. Structure and functions. Current Concepts. New York: Plenun Press, 1987:357–373.
16. Mitchell IJ, Clarke CE, Boyce S, Robertson RG, Peggs D, Sambrook MA, Crossman AR. Neural mechanisms underlying parkinsonian symptoms based upon regional uptake of 2-deoxy-glucose in monkeys exposed to 1-methyl-4-phenyl-1,2,3,6-tetrahydropyridine. Neuroscience 1989; 32:213–226.
17. Vila M, Levy R, Herrero MT, Ruberg M, Faucheux B, Obeso JA, Agyd Y, Hirch EC. Consequences of nigrostriatal denervation on the functioning of the basal ganglia in human and nonhuman primates: on in situ hybridization study of the cytocrome oxidase subunit I mRNA. J Neurosci 1997; 17:765–773.
18. Vila M, Herrero MT, Levy R, Faucheux B, Ruberg M, Guillen J, Luquin MR, Guridi J, Javoy-Agyd F, Agyd Y, Obeso JA, Hirch EC. Consequences of nigrostriatal denervation on the gamma-aminobutiric acidic neurons of subststantia nigra pars reticulata and superior colliculus in parkinsonian syndromes. Neurology 1996; 46:802–809.
19. Herrero MT, Levy R, Ruberg M, Vila M, et al. Consequence of nigrostriatal messenger RNA in the pallidum. Neurology 1996; 47:219–224.
20. Bergman H, Wichmann T, Karmon B, DeLong MR. The primate subthalamic nucleus. II. Neuronal activity in thr MPTP model of parkinsonism. J Neurophysiol 1994; 72:507–519.
21. Filion M, Tremblay L. Abnormal spontaneous activity of the globus pallidus neurons in monkeys with MPTP induced parkinsonism. Brain Res 1991; 547:142–151.
22. Wichmann T, Bergman H, DeLong MR. The primate subthalamic nucleus. III. Changes in motor behaviour and neuronal activity in the internal pallidum induced by subthalamic inactivation in the MPTP model of parkinsonism. J Neurophysiol 1994; 72:521–529.
23. Bergman H, Whichmann T, DeLong MR. Reversal of experimental parkinsonism by lesions of the subthalamic nucleus. Science 1990; 249:1436–1438.

24. Aziz TZ, Peggs D, Sambrook MA, Crosmman AR. Lesion of the subthalamic nucleus for the alleviation of 1-methyl-4-phenyl-1,2,3,6-tetrahydropyridine (MPTP)-induced parkinsonism in the primate. Mov Disord 1991; 6:288–292.
25. Aziz TZ, Peggs D, Agarwal E, Sambrook MA, Crosmman AR. Subthalamic nucleotomy alleviates parkinsonism in the 1-methyl-4-phenyl-1,2,3,6-tetrahydropyridine (MPTP)-exposed primates. Br J Neurosurg 1992; 6:575–582.
26. Guridi J, Herrero MT, Luquin MR, Guillén J, Obeso JA. Subthalamotomy improves MPTP-induced parkinsonism in monkeys. Stereotact Funct Neurosurg 1994; 62:98–102.
27. Guridi J, Herrero MT, Luquin MR, Guillén J, Ruberg M, Laguna J, Obeso JA. Subthalamotomy in parkinsonian monkeys. Behavioural and biochemical analysis. Brain 1996; 119:1717–1727.
28. Blandini F, García-Osuna M, Greenamyre JT. Subthalamic ablation reverses changes in basal ganglia oxidative metabolism and motor response to apomorphine induced by nigrostriatal lesion in rats. Eur J Neurosci 1997; 9:1407–1413.
29. Delfs JM, Ciaramitaro VM, Parry TJ, Chesselet MF. Subthalamic nucleus lesions: widespread effects on changes in gene expression induced by nigrostriatal dopamine depletion in rats. J Neurosci 1995; 15:6562–6575.
30. Sellal F, Hirsch E, Lisovosky F, Mutchler V, Collard M, Marescaux C. Contralateral disappearance of parkinsonian signs after subthalamic hematoma. Neurology 1992; 42:255–256.
31. Vidakovic A, Dragasevic N, Kostic JS. Hemiballism: report of 25 cases. J Neurol Neurosurg Psychiatry 1994; 57:945–949.
32. Andy OJ, Jurko MF, Sias FR. Subthalamotomy in treatment of parkinsonian tremor. J Neurosurg 1963; 20:860–870.
33. Spiegel EA, Wycis HT, Szekely EG, Adams J, Flanagan M, Baird HW. Campotomy in various extrapiramidal disorders. J Neurosurg 1963; 20:871–884.
34. Hassler R, Riechert T. Indikationen und Lokalizations in Methode der gezielten Hirnoperationen. Nervenarzt 1954; 25:441–447.
35. Hassler R, Mundinger F, Riechert G. Pathophysiology of tremor at rest derived from the correlation of anatomical and clinical data. Confin Neurol 1970; 32:79–87.
36. Mundinger F. Stereotaxic interventions on the zona incerta area for treatment of extrapyramidal motor disturbances and their results. Confin Neurol 1965; 26:222–230.
37. Fager ChA. Evaluation of thalamic and subthalamic surgical lesions in the alleviations of Parkinson's disease. J Neurosurg 1968; 28:145–149.
38. Velasco FC, Molina-Negro P, Bertrand C, Hardy J. Futher definition of the subthalamic target for arrest of tremor. J Neurosurg 1972; 36:184–191.
39. Houdart R, Mamo H, Dondey M, Cophignon J. Résultats des coagulations sous-thalamiques dans la maladie de Parkinson. Rev Neurol Paris 1965; 112:521–529.
40. Bejjani B-P, Dormont D, Yelnik J, Damier Ph, Arnulf I, Bonnet A-M, Marsault C, Agid Y, Philippon J, Cornu P. Bilateral subthalamic stimulation for Parkinson's disease by using three-dimensional stereotactic magnetic resonance imaging and electrphysiological guidance. J Neurosurg 2000; 92:615–625.
41. Schaltenbrand G, Wahren W. Atlas for Stereotaxy of the Human Brain. 2d ed. Stuttgart: Thieme, 1977.
42. Rodriguez-Oroz MC, Rodriguez M, Guridi J, Mewes K, Chockkman V, Vitek JL, DeLong MR, Obeso JA. The subthalamic nucleus in Parkinson's disease: somatotopic organization and physiological characteristics. Brain 2001; 124:1777–1790.
43. Alvarez L, Macias R, Guridi J, Lopez G, Alvarez E, Maragoto C, Teijeiro J, Torres A, Pavon N, Rodrigez-Oroz MC, Ochoa L, et al. Dorsal subthalamotomy for Parkinson's disease. Mov Disorders 2001; 16:72–78.
44. Guridi J, Rodriguez-Oroz MC, Manrique M, Obeso JA. Subthalamotomy for Parkinson's disease. Acta Neurochir 2002; 144:1068 A.
45. Gill SS, Heywood P. Bilateral dorsolateral subthalamotomy for advanced Parkinson's disease. Lancet 1997; 350:1224.
46. Gill SS, Heywood P. Subthalamic nucleus lesions. Lozano AM, ed. Movement Disorders Surgery. Basel: Karger, 2000:188–195.
47. McCarter R, Walton NH, Rowan A, Gill S, Palomo M. Cognitive functioning after subthalamic nucleotomy for refractory Parkinson's disease. J Neurol Neurosurg Psychiatry 2000; 69:60–66.
48. Barlas O, Hanagasi HA, Imer M, Sahin HA, Sencer S, Emre M. Do unilateral ablative lesions of the subthalamic nucleus in parkinsonian patients lead to hemiballism? Mov Disord 2001; 16:306–310.

49. Su PC, Tseng H-M, Liu H-M, Yen R-F, Liou H-H. Subthalamotomy for advanced Parkinson disease. J Neurosurg 2002; 97:598–606.
50. Su PC, Ma YM, Fukuda, Mentis M, Tseng H-M, Yen R-F, Liu H-M, Moeller JR, Eidelberg D. Metabolic changes following subthalamotomy for advanced Parkinson's disease. Ann Neurol 2001; 50:514–520.
51. Carbon M, Eidelberg D. Modulation of regional brain function by deep brain stimulation: studies with positron emission tomography. Curr Opin Neurol 2002; 15:451–455.
52. Lee MS, Marsden CD. Movement disorders following lesions of the thalamus or subthalamic region. Mov Disord 1994; 9:493–507.
53. Shannon KR. Ballism. Jankovic J, Tolosa E "Parkinson's Disease and Movement Disorders". 3rd ed. Baltimore: Williams and Wilkins, 1998:365–375.
54. Dierssen G, Gioino G. Correlación anatómica del hemibalismo. Rev Clin Española 1961; 82: 283–305.
55. Hamada I, DeLong MR. Excitotoxic acid lesions of the primate suthalamic nucleus result in transient dyskinesias of the contralateral limbs. J Neurophysiol 1992; 68:1850–1858.
56. Guridi J, Obeso JA. The subthalamic nucleus, hemiballismus and Parkinson's disease: reappraisal of a neurosurgical dogma. Brain 2001; 124:5–19.
57. Lozano AM. The subthalamic nucleus: myth and opportunities. Mov Disord. 2001; 16:183–184.
58. Nieuwenhuys R, Voogd J, Van Huijen J, Huijzen Chr van. The Human Central Nervous System: A Synopsis and Atlas. New York: Springer-Verlag, 1978.

22
Thalamic Deep Brain Stimulation

Daniel Tarsy and Thorkild V. Norregaard

*Harvard Medical School and Beth Israel Deaconess Medical Center,
Boston, Massachusetts, U.S.A.*

I. INTRODUCTION

Discussion of thalamic surgery for treatment of tremor begins with an understanding of current thalamic anatomical terminology. Several nomenclatures have been used for the nuclei of the motor thalamus (1–4). Hassler's terminology (1) in the Schaltenbrand atlas (5) is most commonly used in the current movement disorders literature and will be used in this chapter. The motor thalamus lies ventrally and from front to back and consists of the lateral polaris (Lpo), lying most anteriorly, receiving input from the globus pallidus interna (GPi) and the substantia nigra reticulata (SNr); the ventralis oralis anterior (Voa) and the ventral oralis posterior (Vpo) receiving input from the GPi; and the ventral intermediate nucleus (Vim) receiving input from the cerebellum and the lemniscal system (6). The relative contribution of cerebellar and lemniscal input to the Vim is a subject of debate and depends at least in part on whether human clinical or monkey anatomical data are used (6). The ventralis caudalis (Vc) lies posterior to the motor thalamus and receives lemniscal and spinothalamic sensory input. In the Anglo-American nomenclature, the ventral anterior nucleus (VA) includes the Lpo and the Voa, the ventrolateral nucleus (VL) includes the Vop and the Vim, and the ventral posterior nucleus is equivalent to the Vc. Hassler proposed that the Voa was a good target for treatment of rigidity while the Vop was more suitable for treatment of tremor (7).

Microelectrode recordings obtained during stereotactic surgery have identified thalamic neurons which burst spontaneously with a frequency identical to the tremor frequency (8). These are located in the ventral motor thalamus but have also been identified in other thalamic nuclei, the medial GPi, putamen, caudate, and subthalamic nucleus (STN). In the thalamus these have been particularly well studied in the Vc, Vim, Voa, and Vop, where they correlate with electromyographic recordings of tremor (9). The Vim has been demonstrated to be the target of choice for treatment of tremor (7). Neuronal bursts also occur in response to active or passive movement of small joints

(10,11). Intraoperative identification of these movement-sensitive neurons with microelectrode recording is helpful in locating thalamic sites for optimal placement of lesions or stimulating electrodes for treatment of tremor. Surgical ablation and high-frequency stimulation of areas in the Vim nucleus that contain "tremor cells" successfully abolish tremor. However, the pathophysiological role of these "tremor cells" in the generation of tremor is uncertain since similar tremor bursts can be identified in the GPi (12) and STN (13) and lesions in these areas also abolish tremor.

Thalamotomy was introduced for treatment of tremor in the late 1950's and proved to be very effective. Prior to the introduction of levodopa therapy, thalamotomy was the most commonly performed surgical procedure for the treatment of parkinsonian tremor. This occurred because of its reduced morbidity compared with pallidotomy and its striking benefit for tremor. However, evaluation of surgical results was typically qualitative rather than quantitative, and controlled studies comparing the procedures were not done in that era. The surgical target for thalamotomy was usually the Vim but sometimes included the Vop immediately anterior for control of rigidity or levodopa-induced dyskinesia. Following the availability of pharmacological treatments for parkinsonian and essential tremor, medication-resistant tremors continued to provide an indication for thalamotomy (14). Unilateral thalamotomy produces long-term effective treatment of contralateral tremor in up to 85% of patients, but there is a high incidence of transient complications lasting up to 3 months in as many as 60% of patients and a lower but substantial incidence of permanent complications, especially involving speech, in up to 23% of treated patients (15).

II. DEEP BRAIN STIMULATION

A. Background

Deep brain stimulation (DBS) is a novel and rapidly expanding treatment for PD (16,17). Three targets have been used in PD: the Vim nucleus of the thalamus, GPi, and STN. In the 1960s, the use of intraoperative stimulation of brain targets in preparation for ablative surgery had established the concept that low-frequency Vim stimulation activated or "drove" tremor while high-frequency stimulation suppressed tremor (18–20) This technique was used at the time of surgery to identify the proper site for thalamic lesioning (20–22). The high frequency of adverse effects associated with bilateral thalamotomy motivated Benabid to carry out the first permanent implantations of thalamic stimulators for the treatment of parkinsonian and essential tremor (22,23).

B. Vim DBS Surgical Procedure

Details of the surgical procedure vary across surgical centers. One procedure for Vim thalamic stimulator implantation is as follows: patients are admitted to the hospital on the morning of surgery. A stereotactic frame is attached to the skull under local anesthesia in the operating room. A localizing computed tomographic scan (CT) or magnetic resonance image (MRI) is performed. Axial cuts are made through the region of the third ventricle parallel to the anterior commissure/posterior commissure (AC/PC) plane. A target in the Vim is selected at or just above the level of the AC/PC line, 25% of the AC/PC distance anterior to PC, and 11.5 mm lateral to the wall of the third ventricle. The target and the fiducial points for the localizing frame are recorded from the scanner and processed to determine the x, y, and z coordinates for the calculated target. In the operating room a coronal burr hole is placed 3.0 cm lateral to the midline under local anesthesia. A stylet containing a guide cannula is inserted through the burr hole to within 10 mm of the Vim target.

Microelectrode recording is not always routinely used to identify tremor cells in the Vim or to define the relationship of the Vim to the Vc since the response of tremor to intraoperative stimulation provides such a clear endpoint, which predicts a good therapeutic outcome (24–28). The electrode implantation site can be determined by the effects of macrostimulation using a quadripolar DBS lead. This lead with four platinum-iridium contacts is introduced through the guide cannula and advanced towards the target. Stimulation is performed using a hand-held test stimulator with electrode 0 (most distal electrode) negative, electrode 1 positive, and electrodes 2 and 3 off (−,+,off,off). Voltage is increased at each stimulation site by 1.0 V increments to a maximum of 6–8 V while tremor and presence or absence of contralateral face, hand, or leg paresthesia or upper limb dysmetria are evaluated. Persistent or excessive paresthesia indicates that the location is too posterior. In some cases, dysmetria indicates that the location is too anterior. The electrode tip is implanted at a point where maximal tremor suppression is consistently achieved in several trials with a voltage of 4.0 V or less while producing no more than transient paresthesia (< 15 s) in the face and/or arm.

When there is inadequate tremor suppression, excessive paresthesia, or limb dysmetria, the electrode is repositioned and additional electrode insertions are done. When tremor control is satisfactory, the DBS lead is anchored to the burr hole using a plastic burr hole ring and cap. Following this, stimulation is repeated to assure that no movement of the lead has occurred. The lead is coiled under the galea. In some centers, lead position is also verified by fluoroscopy at this point. Postoperative MRI is done after surgery to exclude hemorrhage and evaluate lead position.

Under general anesthesia, the implantable pulse generator (IPG) is implanted in an infraclavicular pouch and connected to the intracerebral electrode with a subcutaneously tunneled extension lead. A dual channel IPG is available in Europe, which allows two DBS leads to be connected to a single IPG, each of which can be separately programmed. The pulse generator is turned on several days to weeks after implantation depending on the surgical center. It is programmed to yield maximal tremor suppression with minimal paresthesia. Stimulation parameters programmed by telemetry are voltage, pulse width, stimulation frequency, and contact selection. Patients may exhibit a microthalamotomy effect, which is a temporary reduction or disappearance of tremor even with the stimulator off due to the trauma of electrode placement. This usually indicates good electrode position (29).

C. Postoperative Programming

Postoperative programming of patients with Vim DBS is much simpler and less time consuming than for either GPi or STN DBS. This is because in most cases effective electrode settings and stimulation parameters have been established at the time of surgery. In addition, responses of tremor to changes in stimulator parameters have an immediate and obvious effect. If the stimulator is activated immediately after surgery there is usually a gradual change in stimulator response over the next several weeks. If there is a significant postoperative microthalamotomy effect, programming should be delayed until the reappearance of significant tremor. In very rare instances there may be a sufficiently persistent microthalamotomy effect such that stimulator activation may not be required.

Most centers begin programming 2–6 weeks following surgery. Once tremor control is established, the patient returns as needed for programming adjustments. Programming methods for Vim DBS have been reviewed in detail (30–32). Assessment of benefit requires evaluation of the patient's tremor with the involved limb at rest, in specific postures known to maximize tremor in that particular patient, and during voluntary activity such as drinking from a glass or writing. Paresthesia is routinely encountered with Vim DBS. More posterior lying distal electrodes which lie closer to Vc produce this effect. Paresthesia is typically mild and occurs for only several seconds after the stimulator is turned on. If it is persistent, uncomfortable, or involves a large area, the voltage should be lowered or a different electrode contact should be used. Paresthesia threshold may increase with time so that at a given voltage it is prominent shortly following surgery and diminishes later on. If cerebellar signs (limb ataxia, dysmetria, gait disturbance) or dysarthria occur, appropriate adjustments must be made in the stimulator parameters. These effects are much more common with bilateral than unilateral Vim DBS and, unlike tremor, do not always appear immediately after stimulator adjustments. Once effective tremor control has been established, it should be possible to reduce or discontinue tremor medications, although most PD patients selected for Vim DBS are medication resistant and are not taking medications.

During programming, the IPG is reassessed for all stimulation parameters including voltage, pulse width, frequency, and electrode settings. It is important to first establish the most effective electrode contacts and to decide whether monopolar or bipolar stimulation will be used. Monopolar stimulation is initially tested with the IPG case as anode (+) and one electrode contact as cathode (−). Monopolar stimulation creates a broad field of current of about 1–1.5 mm (33). Activation of two adjacent contacts will provide an even broader field of current spread. Bipolar stimulation may be established between two contacts, one of which is the anode and the other the cathode. This produces a narrower field of current with a more focused effect. Monopolar stimulation is usually used since increased current spread allows for lower voltage stimulation, which conserves battery life. Bipolar stimulation is useful when adverse effects such as persistent paresthesia (posterior spread) or ataxia (anterior spread) limit optimal tremor control. Each electrode setting should be assessed by increasing voltage by 0.5 V increments until there is satisfactory tremor suppression. Voltage should be kept under 3.7 V when using the Itrel II or the Soletra IPG since battery consumption increases abruptly above 3.6 V. If needed, stronger effects should be obtained by increasing pulse width or exploring other electrode combinations. The usual effective pulse width for Vim DBS is between 60 and 120 μs. The most effective stimulation frequency is 130 Hz, with higher frequencies producing little additional benefit for Vim tremor control.

The patient is instructed on how to turn the device on or off with a hand-held magnet or with the Access Review Therapy Controller (Medtronic Inc., Model 7438), which can also indicate whether the device is on or off. Where tolerated, the patient is encouraged to turn the device off before sleep to conserve battery life and to reduce the likelihood of tolerance. Most patients with PD tremor prefer to keep the IPG on when they retire in order to avoid interference with sleep by severe rest tremor. However, in some patients, tremor may recur after turning off the IPG in exaggerated fashion as a temporary "rebound tremor," which can last for as long as one hour and may require 24-hour stimulation for prevention (34–36). Patients should be instructed that common magnet-containing devices, such as cordless telephones, refrigerator doors, and metal detectors, may inadvertently turn the IPG on or off. Patients with severe tremor typically have little difficulty determining whether the IPG is on or off. When in doubt, a small, portable AM radio tuned to 530 kHz can be held over the IPG. If the IPG is on it will cause interference and create a buzzing noise. The Access Review Therapy Controller provides a more reliable method of determining the status of the IPG. The controller device currently available in the United States does not allow for adjustments in voltage or other stimulation parameters.

D. Safety of Vim DBS

Initially MRI was considered to be contraindicated in patients with DBS. A full-body radiofrequency coil or head transmit coil that extends over the chest area should be avoided. However, using certain precautions, the safety of MRI in this setting has been demonstrated, and 0.2–2.0 Tesla MRI can be carried out in patients with the Itrel II IPG without risk of discomfort or injury to the patient at either the IPG or electrode end of the system, provided that the cerebral electrodes lie outside of the examined brain region (37,38). MRI may turn the IPG on or off during scanning or induce voltages in the IPG or electrodes, causing sudden uncomfortable levels of stimulation. The IPG amplitude should be set to zero and should be turned off prior to entering the scanner. Therapeutic shortwave, ultrasound, or microwave applied anywhere on the body is strictly contraindicated with DBS. Two patients with bilateral DBS implants suffered coma and death following shortwave treatment of the jaw region in one case and the thoracolumbar area in the second due to heating of the cerebral electrodes and tissue destruction (39,40). There has been little reported experience concerning the safety and function of cardiac pacemakers or implanted defibrillators in patients with DBS. Potential risks include interference by the IPG of cardiac pacemaker or defibrillator function, inadvertent activation or deactivation of the cardiac pacemaker by the IPG programmer, and other potentially hazardous interactions between the two devices. Although more experience is necessary, the experience of a single published case indicates that treatment with concomitant DBS and cardiac pacemaker and defibrillator devices may be safe and effective if precautions concerning positioning of the devices in the chest are undertaken (41).

E. Thalamotomy Versus Vim DBS

There are several potential advantages of thalamic DBS over thalamotomy. DBS is reversible and unassociated with significant long-term tissue reaction or damage (42). In contrast to a surgical lesion, DBS therapy is adjustable. Several stimulation parameters can be changed as needed following implantation including frequency, amplitude, pulse width, and locus of stimulation. Unilateral and bilateral DBS have both been associated with fewer adverse effects than ablation. Bilateral stimulation allows for treatment of bilateral and midline motor symptoms not treatable with ablation without risk of permanent adverse effects on speech and cognitive function. Finally, future interventions remain available to a patient following DBS, while ablation surgery may limit these interventions. Disadvantages of DBS relate to greater cost, need for battery replacement, device-related complications such as skin breakdown, infection, electrode breakage, or pulse generator failure, and the need for regular follow-up at a center capable of programming the IPG.

F. Mechanism of Action of Vim DBS

The mechanism of action of high-frequency DBS remains poorly understood, but it has been assumed to parallel the effects of an ablative lesion. The clinical effects of stimulation and lesioning in the same structure are very similar, suggesting that stimulation produces a "physiological lesion." Benabid et al. suggested that this effect may be due to "jamming" of the targeted nucleus, thereby preventing the relay of excessive or abnormal patterns of neuronal firing originating from that structure (43). They later suggested the term "electrical neuroinhibition" to describe the effect of high-frequency stimulation (44).

Although it is assumed that Vim high-frequency stimulation mimics ablation by suppressing abnormal neuronal activity, the situation in GPi and STN, where neurons fire at higher than normal frequency in PD, may be more complex than in the thalamus. Whereas Vim DBS suppresses tremor immediately, the effect of GPi and STN DBS in reducing bradykinesia in PD requires minutes or longer, suggesting a different mechanism of action (45). In this situation, rather than exerting a direct inhibitory effect on neurons, there may be an indirect effect through a synaptic mechanism involving enhanced synaptic transmission (46). Vitek (47) has suggested that high-frequency stimulation may both inhibit neuronal activity within the nucleus and activate distant neurons by increasing efferent output. Excitability of axons is higher than neuronal cell bodies, and large myelinated axons are more excitable than unmyelinated axons (48). Moreover, neurophysiological studies indicate that high-frequency stimulation can either activate or inactivate neurons and nerve fibers (49,50). Effects on nerve fibers may also differ anatomically with fiber activation, being either orthodromic on cortical structures or antidromic on cerebellar structures (51).

Effective tremor suppression in PD by Vim DBS is associated with reduced cerebellar blood flow, suggesting that cerebellar deactivation may be a mechanism of action of Vim DBS (51). Several effects of Vim DBS on cortical blood flow have also been described, including increased blood flow in the dorsolateral prefrontal cortex and reduced blood flow in sensory association, cingulate, and supplementary motor cortex (52). Whether these cortical responses are important for clinical effects or are nonspecific consequences of Vim DBS is uncertain (52). An additional level of complexity is suggested by observations that Vim DBS activates ipsilateral regional motor cortical cerebral blood flow (rCBF) in essential tremor (53), whereas thalamotomy reduces ipsilateral motor cortical rCBF in tremor-dominant PD (54), suggesting that DBS and lesioning may have different mechanisms of action (53). It has also been suggested that thalamic DBS may suppress tremor by activating the thalamic reticular nucleus, which in turn inhibits thalamic relay nuclei such as the Vim nucleus (55). Finally, it is also possible that DBS exerts its effect by causing release of neurotransmitters either locally or in other brain regions receiving input from the targeted nucleus (45).

III. THALAMIC STIMULATION FOR PARKINSONIAN TREMOR

A. Background

Although tremor is often a major and visible feature of PD, in most patients it is not the most disabling symptom of the disease. The results of thalamotomy indicated that even after successful alleviation of tremor, many patients were left with functional disability due to bradykinesia that was unrelieved by this procedure. Some particularly disabling postural tremors in PD such as reemergent tremor (56) are easily overlooked as they may not reappear until a new position of the hand has been assumed for several seconds.

Adverse effects on speech and cognitive function which were sometimes associated with thalamotomy, especially when carried out bilaterally, led to alternative approaches for surgical treatment of tremor. Historically, chronic thalamic stimulation had already been used for the treatment of chronic pain. Andy (21) suggested that chronic thalamic stimulation might be preferable to lesioning for treatment of tremor, especially in elderly, poor-risk patients. He implanted chronic electrodes and stimulated at 50–125 Hz in several thalamic nuclei in nine patients with a variety of motor disorders. He treated five patients with parkinsonian tremor, three of whom were targeted in Vim (21). In most cases, stimulation was limited to 30–60 minutes, three or four times daily, but three patients underwent continuous stimulation. Results in parkinsonian tremor were "fair to excellent," but duration of follow-up was unstated. Siegfried and Lippitz (57) carried out Vim DBS in 40 patients with PD tremor, most of whom had previous contralateral thalamotomies, and 29 experienced complete tremor control. Tasker (58) also reported on chronic thalamic stimulation at 60 Hz in a small number of patients, one of whom had parkinsonian tremor, but with poor and short-lived results.

Benabid et al. (23) pursued Vim stimulation further and concluded that it could be used as chronic therapy in patients with parkinsonian or essential tremor who had previously undergone contralateral thalamotomy to avoid the adverse effects of bilateral thalamotomy. In his initial report, six patients with PD with previous thalamotomy were implanted in the contralateral Vim (23) and stimulated at up to 130 Hz. Three patients were greatly improved and were connected to permanent stimulators, thereby inaugurating the era of DBS for the long-term treatment of movement disorders. Numerous studies have documented the effect of Vim DBS in essential tremor involving the extremities, head, and voice (22,24–28,43,59–65).

B. Patient Selection

Proper patient selection is crucial for the successful surgical treatment of movement disorders. General requirements for stereotactic surgery in PD include good general health, ability to undergo and cooperate with the demands of stereotactic neurosurgery while awake, no uncontrolled psychiatric disorder, and no dementia. In the case of DBS, patients must be willing and able to return for follow-up visits for reprogramming of the IPG. Vim DBS should therefore be considered for treatment of parkinsonian tremor only if it stands out as the major disabling feature of the disease and has been refractory to pharmacological treatment. Bradykinesia, rigidity, and postural instability should be minor or absent. The effect of thalamotomy on bradykinesia is disappointing, and patients dramatically relieved of tremor were not functionally improved following surgery. Similar to thalamotomy, Vim DBS improves rigidity only slightly and has no effect on bradykinesia or gait disorder. An advantage of Vim DBS is that advanced age is not a contraindication.

Since GPi and STN DBS effectively suppress parkinsonian tremor, the role of Vim DBS for this indication is questionable (65,66). It may be appropriate to consider unilateral Vim DBS for patients with tremor-dominant PD without significant or disabling bradykinesia, rigidity, or gait disturbance. In a study of 12 PD patients followed for a mean of 40 months after Vim DBS, Unified Parkinson's Disease Rating Scale (UPDRS) motor scores did not change from baseline while tremor control was maintained (66a). In a 2-year follow-up study in which most patients had tremor-dominant PD, tremor suppression remained stable for 2 years without a significant increase in akinesia, rigidity, gait disturbance, or dose requirement for antiparkinsonian medication (67). Although bilateral Vim DBS has been effective for head and voice tremor associated with essential tremor (62,68), it appears less effective in PD due at least in part to increased susceptibility to adverse effects on speech and balance in PD patients compared to patients with essential tremor (59).

Although it was initially reported that Vim DBS is more effective in relieving distal than proximal tremor (22,44), two studies have shown uniform and equal benefit of Vim DBS on rest, kinetic, distal postural, and proximal postural tremor in PD (25,69). Lower limb, midline, and even ipsilateral resting tremor may also be relieved in some patients (25). If lower extremity tremor is the principal indication for Vim DBS, a more lateral site in Vim may need to be chosen for electrode implantation (70). Severity, distribution, and type of tremor should be documented by standard tremor rating scales such as the UPDRS motor scale (71) or the Tremor Rating Scale (72).

C.   Results of Vim DBS in Parkinsonian Tremor

In Benabid et al.'s early report (22) of Vim DBS for tremor, a total of 26 patients with disabling parkinsonian tremor were implanted, 21 of whom had undergone no previous neurosurgery. Eight patients underwent bilateral Vim DBS implanted simultaneously. Contralateral upper limb tremor was totally suppressed in 23 and markedly improved in 9 out of 34 patients receiving thalamic stimulation. Similar to the effects of thalamotomy, rigidity was slightly improved, but there was no effect on akinesia. A micro-thalamotomy effect lasting for 1–10 days occurred in some patients. Adverse effects were mild and stimulation related, including limb or face paresthesia, limb dystonia, and dysmetria. Dysarthria and gait disequilibrium occurred in six patients, five of whom had either bilateral DBS or a previous thalamotomy, and could be controlled by reducing the intensity of one or both stimulators.

Subsequent studies by Benabid et al. (43,60,73) involving up to 91 patients with PD documented this improvement for up to at least 3–6 months. There was good to excellent tremor suppression in 88% of PD patients. In their experience, resting tremor was better controlled than postural or action tremor, distal better than proximal or axial tremor, and upper better than lower extremity tremor (44). Stimulation voltage had to be increased over the first several weeks following surgery, likely due to increases in tissue impedance. Tolerance evidenced by reduced clinical effect or need for increased stimulus voltage has been reported in some (34) but not all studies (23,74,75).

Subsequent studies with more prolonged follow-up have confirmed the therapeutic effect of Vim DBS on parkinsonian tremor, which has been effective in approximately 90% of patients (Table 1) (24–27,36,69,75–77). There have been few published long-term follow-up efficacy studies concerning Vim DBS for tremor. Pollak et al. reported continued good tremor control in 80 patients with PD over 3 years (78). Lyons et al. reported continued good tremor control in 12 patients over 40 months (66a). In a North American prospective multicenter trial (five sites), 24 PD patients were implanted with Vim thalamic stimulators and were evaluated using a double-blind assessment at 3 months and open follow-up assessments at 6, 9, and 12 months following surgery (24). There was a significant decrease in contralateral tremor compared to baseline with total resolution of tremor in 14 of 24 PD patients. However, by contrast with essential tremor patients in the same study, functional activities of daily living (ADLs) such as handwriting, dressing, and cutting food were not improved, likely due to lack of improvement in parkinsonian bradykinesia. A single center study of 19 patients using similar methodology and examiner-blinded assessment at 3 months produced similar results with regard to both

Table 1 Published Results of VIM DBS for Parkinsonian Tremor

Study (Ref.)	No. of patients	Duration of follow-up	Tremor reduction
Benabid et al., 1996 (60)	80	6 months	Total or marked 88%
Blond et al., 1992 (26)	10	Mean 19.4 months	Major 80%
Alesch et al., 1995 (74)	23	12 months	Total or major 82%
Koller et al., 1997 (24)	24	12 months	Total 58%; significantly reduced tremor scores
Hubble et al., 1997 (69)	10	3 months[a]	Significantly reduced tremor scores
Ondo et al., 1998 (27)	19	3 months[a]	83–88% improved
Tasker, 1998 (70)	16	?	Total or almost total 88%
Limousin et al.,1999 (28)	73	12 months	Significantly reduced tremor scores
Kumar et al., 1999 (36)	11	Mean 16 months	Significantly reduced tremor scores
Hariz et al., 1999 (34)	22	Mean 21 months	Good tremor control 70%
Albanese et al., 1999 (77)	27	11 months	Improved tremor scores 73%
Schuurman et al., 2000 (99)	22	24 months	Total or marked 95%
Krauss et al., 2001 (29)	45	Mean 11.9 months	Excellent or marked 89%
Obwegeser et al., 2001 (25)	10	3 months	Significantly reduced tremor scores
Lyons et al., 2001 (66a)	12	Mean 40 months	Significantly reduced tremor scores

[a]Blinded evaluation at 3 months.

tremor and ADLs (27). A European prospective multicenter trial (13 sites) in 73 PD patients assessed patients in an unblinded fashion for 12 months following surgery (28). There was a statistically significant decrease in contralateral tremor, which was similar in magnitude to the North American trial. In contrast to the North American trial, ADLs were improved in the European study. Other studies have confirmed that subjective global disability ratings improve similarly in PD patients compared with essential tremor patients (69,79). Although tremor is clearly improved and most studies have shown improved ADLs following Vim DBS, quality-of-life measures have not been extensively studied following Vim DBS (80) in contrast to other surgical treatments of PD (81).

In one multicenter trial, Vim nucleus stimulation appeared to improve contralateral akinesia in addition to tremor (28). However, akinesia was mild preoperatively, may have been difficult to assess in the presence of severe tremor, and likely improved postoperatively due to improved tremor. In other studies, akinesia has shown little or no change following Vim DBS (25,26,60). Gait and balance in PD patients have shown only minor and inconsistent improvement (82–84). In one study, levodopa-induced dyskinesias were improved following thalamic DBS in five affected patients (26,85), but this has not been a universal finding (86). A subsequent analysis concluded that effects on dyskinesia in this study may have been due to more medial and deeper electrode placement closer to centromedian and parafascicular nuclei (86).

D. Adverse Effects of Vim DBS

Adverse effects associated with Vim DBS have been infrequent in short-term studies and related to (a) regional effects of stimulation, (b) hardware-related complications, and (c) neurological consequences of intracerebral electrode implantation.

1. Regional Effects of Stimulation

In Benabid et al.'s early reports (22), adverse effects were mild and limited to stimulation effects such as contralateral paresthesia, limb dystonia, and cerebellar dysmetria. These could all be controlled by stimulation adjustments. Dysarthria and gait disequilibrium were uncommon and typically limited to patients receiving bilateral stimulation or who had undergone previous contralateral thalamotomy. Paresthesia is a very common and expected adverse effect. Although it occurs in approximately 70% of patients (87), it is commonly limited to only several seconds after the IPG is turned on. Paresthesia is due to spread of DBS effect on Vc, the thalamic sensory receiving nucleus immediately posterior to Vim. Dysmetria and gait disequilibrium is attributable to DBS effects on Vop, the pallidal receiving nucleus immediately anterior to Vim. The incidence of serious paresthesia was only 2.5% in the Medtronic clinical investigation of DBS for tremor (87). The higher frequency of dysarthria, dysmetria, and disequilibrium in patients undergoing bilateral Vim DBS has been documented (59,75,88). Although these adverse effects can usually be managed by adjustments in stimulation voltage and pulse width, tremor suppression on at least one side of the body is sometimes compromised (59).

2. Hardware-Related Complications

Long-term studies of DBS have shown a higher incidence of adverse effects related to hardware complications than reported in the short-term studies (88–90). Lyons et al. reported their experience over 6 years in 206 patients undergoing 275 implants, 169 of which were in the Vim (88). There were a total of 135 hardware complications in the group, including lead revisions or replacements, extension wire replacements, and IPG replacements. The incidence of these complications was unusually high, especially the large number of IPG replacements, but other long-term studies have recently reported similar results. Oh et al. (89) reported a 33-month retrospective study of 79 patients with 124 electrode implants, 38 of which were in the thalamus. Overall, 25.3% of patients had hardware-related complications, including lead fractures, lead migrations, open circuits, erosions and/or infections, foreign body reactions, and cerebrospinal fluid leaks. The hardware-related complication rate per electrode year was 8.4%, and many occurred as late complications, possibly explaining the lower rates of hardware complications reported in short-term studies. Joint et al. (90) studied their experience over 3 years and reported a 20% occurrence rate of hardware-related problems in 49 operated patients with 79 implants, 14 of which were in the thalamus. These included lead fractures, lead erosion, IPG malfunction, and lead misplacement. DBS technology is rapidly evolving, and it is likely that procedural and equipment modifications such as moving the electrode connector away from the cervical region to the scalp, the use of low profile connectors, and the use of microplate and screw fixation at the burr hole instead of a silicone burr ring and cap will reduce hardware complications (25). In an autopsy study of six PD patients with thalamic DBS, pathological examination up to 70 months following electrode implantation showed only a thin inner capsule of connective tissue and mild fibrillary gliosis around the lead track and active contact electrode (42). Thus, there is no evidence that chronic thalamic stimulation or the implanted device produce significant or progressive tissue damage. Explantation of the intracerebral electrode is rarely necessary and is indicated only in the presence of active infection or skin erosion unresponsive to medical management or skin grafting. If explantation should be required and reimplantation is not feasible, it may be possible to generate a permanent thalamotomy using the DBS electrode to create a lesion prior to its removal (91,92).

3. Neurological Adverse Effects

Transient mild postoperative headache attributable to the stereotaxic frame and skull fixation bolts is common. Intraoperative focal or generalized seizures are uncommon and not more frequent than for other stereotactic neurosurgical procedures. Permanent neurological deficits from Vim DBS are uncommon. The most potentially serious neurological adverse effect is intracranial hemorrhage. Benabid et al. (60) reported six intracerebral microhematomas in 177 operations, 3 of which were symptomatic. The incidence of documented intracranial hemorrhage was 2% in the North American and 5% in the European trials (24,28). The incidence of intracranial hemorrhage among 266 patients in the Medtronic clinical investigation of DBS treatment of tremor was 2.6% (87). Hemorrhages include subdural and intracerbral hematomas. Many intracerebral hematomas are asymptomatic, limited to the region of the electrode tract, and discovered only by postoperative brain imaging. For example, Lyons et al. (88) reported a 9.8% rate of asymptomatic intracranial bleeding detected by postoperative imaging compared with a 2.2% rate of symptomatic intracranial bleeding. There was only one immediate postoperative death among 266 patients enrolled in the Medtronic clinical trial of DBS for treatment of tremor (87). Detailed neuropsychological testing has shown no significant change in cognitive function following thalamic stimulation (80,93,94), although mild deficits in verbal fluency have been documented (60,94).

E. Vim DBS Compared with Thalamotomy

Speech and cognitive deficits following unilateral and bilateral thalamotomy and tremor recurrence rates of 4–22% (95) motivated Benabid to consider Vim DBS (60). Increasing thalamotomy size to prevent recurrence of tremor only served to increase the frequency of neurological morbidity (96). It has been suggested that Vim DBS is less helpful for rigidity and levodopa-induced dyskinesia than thalamotomy (97). This is likely because historically ablative lesions often included the Vop in addition to the Vim. There is universal agreement that neither procedure improves akinesia.

There have been relatively few studies directly comparing Vim DBS and thalamotomy. In a retrospective, nonrandomized study Tasker (70) compared 16 PD patients who underwent Vim DBS with 23 PD patients who underwent thalamotomy (this study also included six patients with essential tremor whose outcomes were not separated from the PD patients). Follow-up was greater than one year in 60% of patients. Clinical outcome was assessed in an unblinded fashion using a semiquantitative scale. Outcomes were similar in the two groups with complete abolition of contralateral tremor in 42% of both groups and "virtually" complete abolition of tremor in 79% of Vim DBS patients and 69% of thalamotomy patients. Tremor recurred in 5% of Vim DBS cases and 15% of thalamotomy cases. No Vim DBS case required repeat surgery, while 23% of thalamotomy cases had to be repeated in order to achieve a satisfactory response. The major difference between the two groups was in complication rates. Intracerebral hemorrhage occurred in 4% of thalamotomy cases and in none of the Vim DBS cases. Permanent ataxia occurred in 15% and permanent paresthesia in 34% of thalamotomy cases. By contrast, stimulation-induced ataxia and paresthesia occurred in 5% and 47% of Vim DBS cases, respectively, but could be alleviated by stimulation adjustment in all cases. Modern studies of unilateral thalamotomy have shown little postoperative cognitive change (98).

There is only one published prospective, randomized study comparing Vim and thalamotomy in patients with PD (99). In this study, which also included patients with essential tremor and multiple sclerosis, 22 patients with PD were assigned to Vim DBS and 23 to thalamotomy. The follow-up period was 2 years, but the main analyses were carried out using 6-month outcomes. Outcomes were assessed in an unblinded fashion using an ADL scale, a subjective patient assessment of functional status, and several tremor-rating scales. In PD patients improvement in ADL scores was significantly greater following Vim DBS than thalamotomy. Improvement in PD tremor was similar in the two treatment groups, but adverse events were much more common in the thalamotomy group. Tremor was suppressed completely in 20 of 21 Vim DBS cases compared with 20 of 23 thalamotomy cases. Adverse effects were primarily stimulator related in the Vim DBS cases except for one case each of hematoma, infection at the pulse generator site, and intracerebral hemorrhage. By contrast, permanent adverse effects occurred in 16 of 23 PD patients undergoing thalamotomy, including cognitive deterioration, dysarthria, gait or balance disturbance, and ataxia. Neuropsychological outcomes were not reported in this study.

F. Summary

Vim DBS is highly effective for treatment of tremor in PD. It is safer (70,99) than thalamotomy and can be carried out bilaterally in either one or two sessions with less risk for speech or gait impairment than thalamotomy (59). Nearly all adverse effects such as paresthesia, dysmetria, gait disturbance, and dysarthria are directly related to stimulation and can be managed by altering stimulus parameters. Serious infectious complications such as meningitis and brain abcess are exceedingly rare, and there is no long-term tissue damage around the electrodes (42). Hardware problems such as lead fractures, skin erosions, scalp infection, infection at the IPG site, and IPG failure have been reported in several long-term studies (88–90). New procedural and technical advances should reduce the frequency of these hardware complications.

In PD patients, the only indication for thalamic DBS is control of unilateral, functionally disabling tremor that has failed medical management. Patients with disabling tremor-dominant PD with stable or very slowly progressive akinesia are potentially good candidates for thalamic DBS. If PD appears to be more progressive and disability is due to bradykinesia, gait disturbance, motor fluctuations, or levodopa-induced dyskinesia, either GPi or STN DBS may be more appropriate.

ACKNOWLEDGMENTS

We appreciate the support of the Olender Foundation and the assistance of Patricia Ryan, Lisa Scollins, Dawn Mechanic, and Kristin Corapi.

REFERENCES

1. Hassler R. Introduction to Stereotaxis with an Atlas of the Human Brain. Stuttgart: Thieme, 1959.
2. Walker AE. Normal and pathological physiology of the human thalamus. In: Schaltenbrand G, Walker AE, eds. Stereotaxy of the Human Brain: Anatomical, Physiological, and Clinical Applications. Stuttgart: Thieme, 1982:181–217.
3. Jones EG. Correlation and revised nomenclature of ventral nuclei in the thalamus of human and monkey. Stereotact Funct Neurosurg 1990; 54/55:1–20.
4. Hirai T, Jones EG. A new parcellation of the human thalamus on the basis of histochemical staining. Brain Res Rev 1989; 14:1–34.

5. Schaltenbrand G, Wahren W. Atlas for Stereotaxy of the Human Brain. Stuttgart: Thieme, 1977.

6. Krack P, Dostrovsky J, Ilinsky I, Kultas-Ilinsky K, Lenz F, Lozano A, Vitek J. Surgery of the motor thalamus: problems with the present nomenclatures. Mov Disord 2002; 17(suppl 3): S2–S8.

7. Hua SE, Garonzik IM, Lee JI, Lenz FA. Thalamotomy for tremor. Tarsy D, Lozano AM, Vitek JL, eds. Surgical Treatment of Parkinson's Disease and Other Movement Disorders. Totowa, NJ: Humana Press, 2003:99–113.

8. Albe-Fessard D, Arfel G, Guiot G. Activities electriques characteristiques de quelques structures cerebrales chez l'homme. Ann Chir 1962; 17:1185–1214.

9. Lenz FA, Tasker RR, Kwan HC, et al. Single unit analysis of the human ventral thalamic nuclear group: correlation of thalamic "tremor cells" with the 3-6 Hz component of parkinsonian tremor. J Neuroscience 1988; 8:754–764.

10. Ohye C, Narabayashi H. Physiological study of presumed ventralis intermedius neurons in the human thalamus. J Neurosurg 1979; 50:290–297.

11. Lenz FA, Kwan HC, Dostrovsky JO, Tasker RR, Murphy JT, Lenz YE. Single unit analysis of the human ventral thalamic nuclear group. Brain 1990; 113:1795–1821.

12. Hutchison WD, Lozano AM, Tasker RR, Lang AE, Dostrovsky JO. Identification and characterization of neurons with tremor-frequency activity in human globus pallidus. Exp Brain Res 1997; 113:557–563.

13. Bergman NH, Wichmann T, Karmon B, DeLong MR. The primate subthalamic nucleus: II. Neuronal activity in the MPTP model of parkinsonism. J Neurophysiol 1994; 72:507–520.

14. Kelly PJ, Gillingham FJ. The long-term results of stereotaxic surgery and L-dopa therapy in patients with Parkinson's disease. J Neurosurg 1980; 53:332–337.

15. Hallett M, Litvan I. A Task Force on Surgery for Parkinson's Disease. Evaluation of surgery for Parkinson's disease. Neurology 1999; 53:1910–1921.

16. Starr PA, Vitak JL, Bakay RAE. Deep brain stimulation for movement disorders. Neurosurg Clin North Am 1998; 9:381–402.

17. Obeso JA, Benabid AL, Koller WC. Deep brain stimulation for Parkinson's disease and tremor. Neurology 2000; 55(suppl 6):S1–S66.

18. Hassler R, Riechart T, Munginer F, et al. Physiological observations in stereotaxic operations in extrapyramidal motor disturbances. Brain 1960; 83:337–350.

19. Ohye C, Kubota K, Hooper HE, et al. Ventrolateral and subventrolateral thalamic stimulation. Arch Neurol 1964; 11:427–434.

20. Cooper IS, Upton ARM, Amin I. Reversibility of chronic neurologic deficits. Some effects of electrical stimulation of the thalamus and internal capsule in man. Appl Neurophysiol 1980; 43:244–258.

21. Andy OJ. Thalamic stimulation for control of movement disorders. Appl Neurophysiol 1983; 46:107–111.

22. Benabid AL, Pollak P, Gervason C, et al. Long-term suppression of tremor by chronic stimulation of the ventral intermediate thalamic nucleus. Lancet 1991; 337:403–406.

23. Benabid AL, Pollak P, Loveau A, Henry S, Rougemont J. Combined (thalamotomy and stimulation) stereotactic surgery of the VIM thalamic nucleus for bilateral Parkinson disease. Appl Neurophysiol 1987; 50:344–346.

24. Koller W, Pahwa R, Busenbark K, Hubble J, Wilkinson S, Lang A, Tuite P, Sime E, Lozano A, Hauser R, Malapira T, Smith D, Tarsy D, Miyawaki E, Norregaard T, Kormos T, Olanow CW. High-frequency unilateral thalamic stimulation in the treatment of essential and parkinsonian tremor. Ann Neurol 1997; 42:292–299.

25. Obwegeser AA, Uitti RJ, Witte RJ, Lucas JA, Turk MF, Wharen Jr. RE. Quantitative and qualitative outcome measures after thalamic deep brain stimulation to treat disabling tremors. Neurosurgery 2001; 48:274–284.

26. Blond S, Caparros-Lefebvre D, Parker F, et al. Control of tremor and involuntary movement disorders by chronic stereotactic stimulation of the ventral intermediate thalamic nucleus. J Neurosurg 1992; 77:62–68.

27. Ondo W, Jankovic J, Schwartz K, et al. Unilateral thalamic deep brain stimulation for refractory essential tremor and Parkinson's disease tremor. Neurology 1998; 51:1063–1069.

28. Limousin P, Speelman JD, Gielen F, et al. Multicentre European study of thalamic stimulation in parkinsonian and essential tremor. J Neurol Neurosurg Psychiatry 1999; 66:289–296.

29. Krauss JK, Simpson Jr. RK, Ondo WG, Pohle T, Burgunder JM, Jankovic J. Concepts and methods in chronic thalamic stimulation for treatment of tremor: technique and application. Neurosurgery 2001; 48:535–543.

30. Kumar R. Methods of programming and patient management with deep brain stimulation. Tarsy D, Lozano AM, Vitek JL, eds. Surgical Treatment of Parkinson's Disease and Other Movement Disorders. Totowa, NJ: Humana Press, 2003:189–212.
31. Volkmann J, Herzog J, Kopper F, Deuschl G. Introduction to the programming of deep brain stimulators. Mov Disord 2002; 17(suppl 3):S181–S187.
32. Dowsey-Limousin P. Postoperative management of Vim DBS for tremor. Mov Disord 2002; 17(suppl 3):S208–S211.
33. Ashby P. What does stimulation in the brain really do?. Prog Neurol Neurosurg 2000; 15:236–245.
34. Hariz MI, Shamsgovara P, Johansson F, Hariz GM, Fodstad H. Tolerance and tremor rebound following long-term chronic thalamic stimulation for parkinsonian and essential tremor. Stereotact Funct Neurosurg 1999; 72:208–218.
35. Fogel W, Kronenbuerger M, Tronnier VM, Eifert B, Meinck HM. Tremor rebound as a side-effect of thalamic stimulation for suppression of tremor. Mov Disord 1998; 13(suppl 3):139–140.
36. Kumar K, Kelly M, Toth C. Deep brain stimulation of the ventral intermediate nucleus of the thalamus for control of tremors in Parkinson's disease and essential tremor. Stereotact Funct Neurosurg 1999; 72:47–61.
37. Tronnier VM, Staubert A, Hahnel S, Sarem-Aslani A. Magnetic resonance imaging with implanted neurstimulators: an in vitro and in vivo study. Neurosurgery 1999; 44:118–126.
38. Rezai AR, Lozano AM, Crawley AP, Joy MLG, Davis KD, Kwan CL, Dostrovsky JO, Tasker RR, Mikulis DJ. Thalamic stimulation and functional magnetic resonance imaging: localization of cortical and subcortical activation with implanted electrodes. J Neurosurg 1999; 90:583–590.
39. Nutt JG, Anderson VC, Peacock JH, Hammerstad JP, Burchiel KJ. DBS and diathermy interaction induces severe CNS damage. Neurology 2001; 56:1384–1386.
40. Department of Health and Human Services. Two cases of coma due to adverse interaction between therapeutic shortwave devices and deep brain stimulators. August 30, 2001.
41. Obwegeser AA, Uitti RJ, Turk MF, Wszolek UM, Flipse TR, Smallridge RC, Witte RJ, Wharen Jr. RE. Simultaneous thalamic deep brain stimulator and implantable cardioverter-defibrillator. Mayo Clin Proc 2001; 76:87–89.
42. Haberler C, Alesch F, Mazal PR, et al. No tissue damage by chronic deep brain stimulation in Parkinson's disease. Ann Neurol 2000; 48:372–376.
43. Benabid AL, Pollak P, Siegneuret E, Hoffmann D, Gay E, Perret J. Chronic VIM thalamic stimulation in Parkinson's disease, essential tremor, and extrapyramidal dyskinesias. Acta Neurochir 1993; 58(suppl):39–44.
44. Benabid AL, Benazzouz A, Hoffmann D, Limousin P, Krack P, Pollak P. Long-term electrical inhibition of deep brain targets in movement disorders. Mov Disord 1998; 13(suppl 3):119–125.
45. Benazzouz A, Hallett M. Mechanism of action of deep brain stimulation. Neurology 2000; 55(suppl 6):S13–S16.
46. Lozano AM. Deep brain stimulation for Parkinson's disease. Parkinsonism and related disorders 2001; 7:199–203.
47. Vitek JL. Mechanisms of deep brain stimulation: excitation or inhibition. Mov Disord 2002; 17(suppl 3):S69–S72.
48. Dostrovsky JO, Lozano AM. Mechanisms of deep brain stimulation. Mov Disord 2002; 17(suppl 3):S63–S68.
49. Ranck JB. Which elements are excited in electrical stimulation of the mammalian central nervous system: a review. Brain Res 1975; 98:417–440.
50. Schlag J, Villablanca J. A quantitative study of temporal and spatial response patterns in a thalamic cell population electrically stimulated. Brain Res 1967; 8:255–270.
51. Deiber MP, Pollak P, Passingham R, et al. Thalamic stimulation and suppression of parkinsonism tremor. Evidence of cerebellar de-activation using positron emission tomography. Brain 1993; 116:267–279.
52. Fukuda M, Edwards C, Eidelberg D. Positron emission tomography in surgery for movement disorders. In: Tarsy D, Lozano AM, Vitek JL, eds. Surgical Treatment of Parkinson's Disease and Other Movement Disorders.. Totowa, NJ: Humana Press, 2003:301–311.
53. Ceballos–Baumann AO, Boecker H, Fogel W, et al. Thalamic stimulation for essential tremor activates motor and deactivates vestibular cortex. Neurology 2001; 56:1347–1354.
54. Boecker H, Wills A, Ceballos-Baumann AO, et al. Stereotactic thalamotomy in tremor dominant Parkinson's disease: a H215O PET study of motor activation. Ann Neurol 1997; 41:108–111.
55. Ashby P, Rothwell JC. Neurophysiologic aspects of deep brain stimulation. Neurology 2000; 55(suppl 6):S17–S20.

56. Jankovic J, Schwartz KS, Ondo W. Re-emergent tremor of Parkinson's disease. J Neurol Neurosurg Psychiatry 1999; 67:646–650.
57. Siegfried J, Lippitz B. Chronic electrical stimulation of the VL-VPL complex and of the pallidum in the treatment of movement disorders: personal experience since 1982. Stereotact Funct Neurosurg 1994; 62:71–75.
58. Tasker RR. Effets sensitifs et moteurs de la stimulation thalamique chez l'homme. Applications cliniques. Rev Neurol 1986; 142:316–326.
59. Ondo W, Almaguer M, Jankovic J, Simpson RK. Thalamic deep brain stimulation. Comparison between unilateral and bilateral placement. Arch Neurol 2001; 58:218–232.
60. Benabid AL, Pollak P, Gao D, et al. Chronic electrical stimulation of the ventralis intermedius nucleus of the thalamus as a treatment of movement disorders. J Neurosurg 1996; 84:203–214.
61. Hubble JP, Busenbark KL, Wilkinson S, Penn RD, Lyons K, Koller WC. Deep brain stimulation for essential tremor. Neurology 1996; 46:1150–1153.
62. Taha JM, Janszen MA, Favre J. Thalamic deep brain stimulation for the treatment of head, voice, and bilateral limb tremor. J Neurosurg 1999; 91:68–72.
63. Carpenter MA, Pahwa R, Miyawaki KL, Wilkinson SB, Seral JP, Koller WC. Reduction in voice tremor under thalamic stimulation. Neurology 1998; 50:796–798.
64. Deuschl G, Bain P. Deep brain stimulation for tremor: patient selection and evaluation. Mov Disord 2002; 17(suppl 3):S102–S111.
65. Tarsy D, Norregaard T, Hubble J. Thalamic deep brain stimulation for Parkinson's disease and essential tremor. Tarsy D, Lozano Am, Vitek JL, eds. Surgical Treatment of Parkinson's Disease and Other Movement Disorders. Totowa, NJ: Humana Press, 2003:153–161.
66. Krack P, Benazzouz A, Pollak P, Limousin P, Piallat B, Hoffmann D, Xie J, Benabid AL. Treatment of tremor in Parkinson's disease by subthalamic nucleus stimulation. Mov Disord 1998; 13:907–914.
66a. Lyons KE, Koller WC, Wilkinson SB, Pahwa R. Long term safety and efficacy of unilateral deep brain stimulation of the thalamus for Parkinson tremor. J Neurol Neurosurg Psychiatry 2001; 71:682–684.
67. Apetauerova D, Ryan P, Mechanic D, Norregaard T, Tarsy D. Parkinson's disease remains stable for two years following thalamic deep brain stimulation for tremor. Mov Dis 2001; 16:990–991.
68. Obwegeser AA, Uitti RJ, Turk MF, Strongosky AJ, Wharen RE. Thalamic stimulation for the treatment of midline tremors in essential tremor patients. Neurology 2000; 54:2342–2344.
69. Hubble JP, Busenbark KL, Wilkinson S, et al. Effects of thalamic deep brain stimulation based on tremor type and diagnosis. Mov Disord 1997; 12:337–341.
70. Tasker RR. Deep brain stimulation is preferable to thalamotomy for tremor suppression. Surg Neurol 1998; 49:145–154.
71. Fahn S, Elton RL. Unified rating scale for Parkinson's disease. Fahn S, Marsden CD, eds. Recent Developments in Parkinson's Disease. Florham Park, NY: Macmillan, 1987:153–163, 293–304.
72. Fahn S, Tolosa E, Marin C. Clinical rating scale for tremor. Jankovic J, Tolosa E, eds. Parkinson's Disease and Movement Disorders. 2nd ed. Baltimore: Williams & Wilkins 1993:225–234.
73. Benabid AL, Benazzouz A, Gao D, et al. Chronic electrical stimulation of the ventralis intermedius nucleus of the thalamus and of other nuclei as a treatment for Parkinson's disease. Techni Neurosurg 1999; 5:5–30.
74. Alesch F, Pinter MM, Helscher RJ, Fertl L, Benabid AL, Koos WT. Stimulation of the ventral intermediate thalamic nucleus in tremor dominated Parkinson's disease and essential tremor. Acta Neurochir 1995; 136:75–81.
75. Tarsy D, Ryan P, Mechanic D, Norregaard T. Thalamic deep brain stimulation for Parkinson's and essential tremor. Parkinsonism Rel Disord 1999; 5(suppl):S112.
76. Blond S, Siegfried J. Thalamic stimulation for the treatment of tremor and other movement disorders. Acta Neurochir1991(suppl 52):109–111.
77. Albanese A, Nordera GP, Caraceni T, et al. Longterm ventralis intermedius thalamic stimulation for parkinsonian tremor. Italian Registry for Neuromodulation in Movement disorders. Adv Neurol 1999; 80:631–634.
78. Pollak P, Benabid AL, Limousin P, Benazzouz A. Chronic intracerebral stimulation in Parkinson's disease. Adv. Neurol 1997; 74:213–220.
79. Hariz GM, Bergenheim AT, Hariz MI, Lindberg M. Assessment of ability/disability in patients treated with chronic thalamic stimulation for tremor. Mov Disord 1998; 13:78–83.
80. Troster AI, Fields JA. The role of neuropsychological evaluation in the neurosurgical treatment of movement disorders. Tarsy D, Lozano AM, Vitek JL, eds. Surgical Treatment of Parkinson's Disease and Other Movement Disorders. Totowa, NJ: Humana Press, 2003:213–240.

81. Gray A, McNamara I, Aziz T, Gregory R, Bain P, Wilson J, Scott R. Quality of life outcomes following surgical treatment of Parkinson's disease. Mov Disord 2002; 17:68–75.

82. Burleigh AL, Horak FB, Burchiel JK, Nutt JG. Effects of thalamic stimulation on tremor, balance, and step initiation. A single subject study. Mov Disord 1993; 8:519–524.

83. Defebvre L, Blatt JL, Blond S, et al. Effect of thalamic stimulation in Parkinson disease. Arch Neurol 1996; 53:898–903..

84. Pinter MM, Murg M, Alesch F, et al. Does deep brain stimulation of the nucleus ventralis intermedius affect postural control and locomotion in Parkinson's disease? Mov Disord 1999; 14:958–963.

85. Caparros-Lefebvre D, Blond S, Vermersch P, et al. Chronic thalamic stimulation improves tremor and levodopa-induced dyskinesias in Parkinson's disease. J Neurol Neurosurg Psychiatry 1993; 56:268–273.

86. Caparros-Lefebvre D, Blond S, Feltin MP, Pollak P, Benabid AL. Improvement of levodopa induced dyskinesias by thalamic deep brain stimulation as related to slight variation in electrode placement: possible involvement of the centre median and parafascicularis complex. J Neurol Neurosurg Psychiatry 1999; 67:308–314.

87. Medtronic, Inc. Deep brain stimulation for the treatment of tremor using the Medtronic Model 3387 DBS™ lead and the Itrel® II Model 7424 implantable pulse generator. Final Report. 2002.

88. Lyons KE, Koller WC, Wilkinson SB, Pahwa R. Surgical and device-related events with deep brain stimulation. Neurology 2001; 55(suppl 3):A147.

89. Oh MY, Abosch A, Kim SH, Lang AE, Lozano AM. Long-term hardware-related complications of deep brain stimulation. Neurosurgery 2002; 50:1268–1276.

90. Joint C, Nandi D, Parkin S, Gregory R, Aziz T. Hardware-related problems of deep brain stimulation. Mov Disord 2002; 17(suppl 3):S175–S180.

91. Oh MY, Hodaie M, Kim SH, Alkhani A, Lang AE, Lozano AM. Deep brain stimulator electrodes used for lesioning: proof of principle. Neurosurgery 2001; 49:363–369.

92. Kumar R, McVicker JM. Radiofrequency lesioning through an implanted deep brain stimulating electrode: treatment of tolerance to thalamic stimulation in essential tremor. Mov Disord 2000; 15(suppl 3):69.

93. Caparros-Lefebre D, Blond S, Pecheux N, Pasquier F, Petit H. Evaluation neuropsychologique avant et après stimulation thalamique chez 9 parkinsoniens. Rev Neurol 1992; 148:117–122.

94. Troster AI, Fields JA, Pahwa R, et al. Neuropsychological and quality of life outcome after thalamic stimulation for essential tremor. Neurology 1999; 53:1174–1780.

95. Hirai T, Miyazaki M, Nakajima H, et al. The correlation between tremor characteristics and the predicted volume of effective lesions in stereotaxic nucleus ventralis intermedius thalamotomy. Brain 1983; 106:1001–1018.

96. Stellar S, Cooper IS. Mortality and morbidity in cryothalamectomy for parkinsonism. A statistical study of 2,868 consecutive operations. J Neurosurg 1968; 28:459–467.

97. Pollak P, Fraix V, Krack P, Moro E, Mendes A, Chabardes S, Koudsie A, Benabid AL. Treatment results: Parkinson's disease. Mov Disord 2002; 17(suppl 3):S75–S83.

98. Lund-Johansen M, Hugdahl K, Wester K. Cognitive function in patients with Parkinson's disease undergoing stereotaxic thalamotomy. J Neurol Neurosurg Psychiatry 1996; 60:564–571.

99. Schuurman PR, Bosch DA, Bossuyt PMN, et al. A comparison of continuous thalamic stimulation and thalamotomy for suppression of severe tremor. N Engl J Med 2000; 342:461–468.

23

Globus Pallidal Deep Brain Stimulation

Joshua M. Rosenow*, Jaimie M. Henderson, and Ali R. Rezai

Cleveland Clinic Foundation, Cleveland, Ohio, U.S.A.

The globus pallidus has long been the focus of attention for surgeons treating Parkinson's disease (PD). Spiegel and Wycis, credited with ushering in human stereotactic surgery (1), are also responsible for initiating pallidal surgery. Their 1954 publication (2) reporting six patients treated with electrolytic pallidotomy described improvements in contralateral tremor and rigidity. Their target was the pallidofugal fibers of the ansa lenticularis emerging from the ventral aspect of the nucleus, making the operation more appropriately termed "ansotomy." This was followed by Narabayashi's (3) series of patients treated using a stereotactic device of his own design. However, he created lesions using a mixture of procaine oil, which tended to wear off and lead to the reappearance of tremor within several weeks.

Pallidotomy continued to gain popularity as a treatment for PD in the pre-levodopa era. Fenelon (4), Leksell (5), Guiot (6), and Cooper (7) all advocated creating pallidal lesions that specifically targeted the posteroventrolateral aspect of the nucleus so that the mesial pallidum and emerging fibers of the ansa lenticularis were both included in the lesion. This produced significant reductions in rigidity as well as tremor. Both stereotactic and nonstereotactic methods were used to introduce devices for lesioning the pallidum. One technique, described by Cooper, was the deliberate occlusion of the anterior choroidal artery to produce ischemia of the medial pallidum (8). However, the artery irrigated too variable a territory to produce consistent results and he abandoned the procedure.

Once Hassler (9) introduced thalamotomy, it proceeded to supplant pallidotomy by virtue of its dramatic effects on tremor. Some investigators continued to perform pallidal surgery, the most prominent being Lars Leksell, whose experience with pallidotomy was reviewed in 1959 by Svennilson et al. (5) and revived in 1992 by Laitinen et al. (10,11). The reemergence of the pallidum as a target for the surgical treatment of PD is due to the ability of pallidal lesions to alleviate all the cardinal features of the disorder. After thalamic deep brain stimulation (DBS) was introduced in 1987, it gained acceptance for

---

**Current affiliation*: Northwestern University, Chicago, Illinois, U.S.A.

tremor control and grew in popularity because bilateral procedures could be performed without the adverse effects associated with bilateral lesions (12). Given these results and the modern results of pallidotomies performed by Laitinen et al. (10,11) and others (13–16), the pallidum became the next logical target for chronic electrical stimulation.

I. RATIONALE FOR THE PALLIDUM AS A TARGET

The discovery of the effects of 1-methyl-4-phenyl-1,2,3,6-tetrahydropyridine (MPTP) in inducing a parkinsonian state in humans as well as in primate models has allowed for dramatic advances in our understanding of normal and pathological basal ganglia functional anatomy (17,18). The current models of basal ganglia physiology hold that the globus pallidus interna (GPi) serves as the major outflow relay nucleus for the basal ganglia along with the substantia nigra pars reticulata (SNr). The direct and indirect basal ganglia circuits converge on these structures. Cortical efferents synapse in the putamen. Subsequently, the indirect pathway reaches GPi from the putamen via the external segment of the globus pallidus (GPe) and the subthalamic nucleus (STN), which provides excitatory glutaminergic input to the GPi. The direct pathway consists of inhibitory GABAergic input directly from the putamen. The GABAergic outflow of GPi projects to the ventrolateral thalamus (VA/VL) via the ansa lenticularis and fasciculus lenticularis. Mesencephalic nuclei such as the pedunculopontine nucleus (PPN) receive projections as well, but these are of uncertain significance.

Dopaminergic efferents from the substantia nigra pars compacta (SNc) synapse in the putamen and serve to inhibit the overall output of GPi, thus reducing thalamic inhibition. Loss of nigral dopamine in PD leads to hyperactivity of the STN and GPi with overinhibition of downstream targets such as the thalamus and cortex. Thus, according to this model, inactivation of the GPi should ameliorate PD symptomatology.

Functional imaging studies of PD patients have demonstrated hyperactivity of the lentiform nucleus, consistent with these assumptions (19). Improvement following pallidotomy has been correlated with a postoperative decrease in lentiform hypermetabolism, as well as increases in supplementary motor and dorsolateral prefrontal cortex (DLPFC) activity (20–22). A position emission tomography (PET) study of GPi stimulation in nine patients demonstrated increased regional cerebral blood flow (rCBF) to the ipsilateral supplementary motor area and putamen/GPe, consistent with a restoration of cortical motor activity following deactivation of the overly inhibitory GPi (23). Low-intensity stimulation did not produce these changes. Other studies have shown either direct excitatory or facilitatory effects on the motor cortex with effective GPi stimulation (24,25).

II. MECHANISM OF ACTION

The similarity between the clinical effects of chronic stimulation and traditional lesioning procedures, particularly for thalamic and pallidal targets, has led many to suggest that DBS exerts its effect by inhibiting neuronal activity of the target structure, thus creating a temporary, reversible "functional" lesion (26). In an in vitro study in the rat, high-frequency (100–250 Hz) stimulation of the STN resulted in a transient blockade of the persistent sodium current as well as L- and T-type calcium currents. There results are consistent with an inhibitory effect of stimulation (27). Straightforward inhibition, however, cannot explain the efficacy of high-frequency stimulation (HFS) in the treatment of dystonia via pallidal stimulation, as pallidal activity in dystonia is hypoactive, in sharp contrast to the hyperactivity present in PD. It has therefore been suggested that HFS, rather than simply inhibiting a hyperactive structure, acts via a resynchronization of abnormal output patterns present in disease or via a "jamming" of these abnormal patterns by HFS (28–30). There is some suggestion that activation of fibers of passage may also play a large role in the efficacy of HFS. For example, it has been suggested that the optimal target for STN stimulation may be outside the actual nucleus, possibly affecting the passing fibers in the zona incerta (31–33).

There is emerging evidence to suggest that activation, rather than inhibition, of either neurons or axons is at least partially responsible for the effects of DBS (34). Pallidal stimulation in parkinsonian monkeys reduces, but does not block, neuronal firing, leading some investigators (35) to presume a role for activation of GABAergic neurons. This preferential activation of presynaptic fibers over postsynaptic fibers is supported by the lower threshold for presynaptic activation (36).

DBS clearly has effects on systems beyond the basal ganglia. The supplementary motor area, cingulate cortex, and DLPFC are all activated during clinically effective DBS of either the STN or GPi. The effect on the DLPFC is significantly more pronounced during STN stimulation than with pallidal stimulation (37). The precise mechanisms underlying the efficacy of DBS are still strongly debated (38,39). It is probable that DBS exerts its effects via a number of differing but interrelated mechanisms, which come into play depending on the site being stimulated, the disease entity being treated, and the stimulation parameters used.

III. INTRAOPERATIVE NEUROPHYSIOLOGY

Accurate targeting of the GPi requires a thorough understanding of the anatomy and neurophysiology of the basal ganglia. The optimal target in GPi is bordered by the internal capsule medially and anteriorly, GPe laterally and superiorly, and the optic tract ventrally. Magnetic resonance imaging (MRI) usually demonstrates the anatomy of this region quite well. Initial targeting is carried out with a stereotactic frame and localizer in place in order to derive the three-dimensional coordinates of the target. Although MRI can be used alone, many centers acquire a computed tomography (CT) scan with the stereotactic localizer in place and perform image fusion to an MRI scan obtained without the localizer. In this way the advantages of each imaging modality are exploited: the anatomical specificity of MRI and the accuracy and resistance to artifact of CT.

Standard stereotactic formulas are used to locate the posteroventral lateral GPi target in relation to the midcommissural point (MCP). For those patients with standard size skulls and no ventriculomegaly, the target is typically 18–22 mm from the midline, 3 mm anterior to the MCP, and 6 mm below the intercommissural line. The coordinates are adjusted based on the MRI appearance of the GPi. A typical trajectory will pass through the striatum, the GPe, the internal (GPii) and external (GPie) segments of the GPi, and end near the optic tract. The distinct electrical signatures of each are used to determine the final target.

Detailed reviews of the neurophysiological localization of the pallidal target have been published elsewhere (15,16,40–45). Briefly, the optimal microelectrode track passes through the striatum, GPe, both the GPie and GPii segments of GPi, and terminates ventral to the pallidum so that the location of the optic tract may be determined. The pallidofugal fibers of the ansa lenticularis lie at the ventral border of the pallidum. As previously stated, the initial target is usually selected between 18 and 22 mm lateral to the midline (with compensation for an enlarged third ventricle, if required), 3 mm anterior to the midpoint of the AC-PC line, and 6 mm below the AC-PC line.

The striatum is usually quiet, marked by only a few cells with slow firing rates (4–6 Hz). The GPe exhibits bursting cells as well as cells with high-amplitude discharges punctuated by pauses. Once through the electrically silent medial pallidal lamina, GPie is encountered. At this time, the hyperactivity of the parkinsonian pallidum is evident, as high-amplitude high frequency discharges are seen. Lower-amplitude discharges mark the border cells present in the lamina between GPie and GPii. Once the microelectrode is in GPi, cells that fire in synchrony with the patient's tremor may be noted. Importantly, GPi contains a population of neurons that respond to kinesthetic movements with either increased or decreased firing rate. Areas of pallidal neurons that correspond to the upper and lower limbs or face may be mapped.

Moving the electrode track posteriorly and conducting microstimulation helps to determine the location of the internal capsule by noting muscle contractions. The optic tract is localized with microstimulation 1–2 mm after penetrating the ventral border of GPi. Stimulation too close to these fibers produces phosphenes in the contralateral visual field. It is important that the final electrode position take into account the position of these structures to avoid unintended stimulation effects.

Once an appropriate track is identified, the permanent electrode is placed to the prescribed depth, typically using fluoroscopy for confirmation. Macrostimulation is performed with the hand-held stimulator. Stimulation is begun with gradually escalating voltages. At each level, the patient is assessed for both therapeutic effects and adverse side effects. Worrisome effects include sustained paresthesias, dysarthria, forced gaze deviation, muscle contractions, and phosphenes. The results of macrostimulation are not intended to predict a patient's final outcome, but only to verify that an acceptable therapeutic window exists between effective stimulation and unacceptable side effects. A CT scan may be obtained soon after the operation to assess electrode position and to rule out intracranial hemorrhage. Patients often undergo postoperative MRI scanning for the purposes of electrode position confirmation and functional imaging studies. Guidelines have been published regarding the safety of implanted neurostimulation systems in the MRI environment (46).

IV. CLINICAL RESULTS

A. Parkinson's Disease

Laitinen et al.'s articles published in 1992 (10,11) revived pallidotomy as a method of addressing all the cardinal features of PD. Shortly thereafter, Siegfried and Lippitz (47) described their results in three patients who underwent implantation of bilateral GPi DBS systems using Leksell's target. All three achieved significant reduction in medication-induced side effects and on-off fluctuations. Bradykinesia, freezing, and speech also improved. The patients' Webster rating scale scores improved between 32 and 54%. No complications were noted. Medication was reduced in one patient, unchanged in one patient, and increased in one patient.

Published series of patients undergoing pallidal stimulation have been proliferating. Loher et al.'s (48) one-year results in 16 patients showed a 38% improvement in medication-off Unified Parkinson's Disease Rating Scale (UPDRS) motor scores and a 33% improvement in activities of daily living (ADL) scores in those patients receiving unilateral stimulation. Bilateral stimulation led to a slight improvement in these results.

Some improvement in the medication-on state was also noted. In a larger series of 36 patients (49), bilateral pallidal stimulation resulted in a median motor improvement of 37% and an increase from 28 to 64% of time during the day without disabling involuntary movements. Kumar et al. (50) reported 6-month follow-up on 22 patients (17 implanted bilaterally). Their total UPDRS motor scores improved 31% and ADL scores improved 39%. Medication-induced dyskinesias decreased by two thirds. Multiple reports have continued to demonstrate the beneficial effects of GPi stimulation on dyskinesias, on-off fluctuations, and tremor (51–56). Chronic pallidal stimulation has also been validated in the setting of prior pallidotomy (53). In a cohort of four patients who underwent GPi stimulation contralateral to a prior pallidotomy, motor scores improved by almost 50%, while bradykinesia was decreased by 37% and tremor by 93% without serious adverse cognitive or motor effects (53).

A few direct comparisons of GPi and STN stimulation for PD have been published. Most groups have suggested that the STN target is preferable, although considerable debate remains. The largest multicenter study (49) found that STN stimulation was more efficacious and enabled patients to reduce their medication while GPi stimulation did not. The series published by Krause et al. (57) and Krack et al. (58) both suggested that STN was the preferable target due to better symptomatic improvement, lower stimulation voltages, and the ability to decrease medication dose. Burchiel et al. (59) conducted a randomized trial of pallidal versus STN stimulation. While the results off medication were similar for the two groups (44% improvement with STN stimulation and 39% with GPi), GPi, but not STN, stimulation improved parkinsonian symptoms while patients were in the medication-on state. Moreover, while both targets provided equal improvements in rigidity (37–47%), bradykinesia (25%), and tremor (74%), axial symptomatology was relieved only by GPi stimulation. However, only STN stimulation allowed patients to reduce their medication dosage, in this case by 51%, while levodopa-induced dyskinesias decreased by 67%. Other reports also favored the STN (60,61). Using the results of their comparison between the two targets, Volkmann et al. (62) argued that a trade-off existed. STN stimulation allowed patients to reduce their medication by 63% while using one third of the power required for effective GPi stimulation. However, the incidence of stimulation-induced side effects such as dysarthria, hypophonia, and eyelid opening apraxia, while low, was greater when the STN was used rather than GPi. Clearly, larger randomized studies are needed to settle this debate. Table 1 shows the results of selected series of GPi DBS for PD.

Table 1 Selected Results of Deep Brain Stimulation of the Globus Pallidus Interna (GPi) for Parkinson's Disease

Study (Ref.)	Patients	Follow-up (months)	Results
Gross et al., 1997 (55)	7	12–36	UPDRS off motor—60%
Krack et al., 1998 (58)	5	1–12	UPDRS off motor—39%, 29% increased
Burchiel et al., 1999 (59)	4	12	UPDRS off motor—40%, no change in meds
Siegfried et al., 1999 (88)	26	5–51	Webster scale—41%, decreased meds
Kumar et al., 2000 (50)	22	6	UPDRS off motor—31%; dyskinesias—66%
DBS Study Group, 2001 (49)	38	6	UPDRS off motor—37%
Loher et al., 2002 (48)	16	12	UPDRS off motor—41%

Compared to the STN, GPi is larger and contains a "target within the target" since the entire GPi is not covered by stimulation, as may be the case with the STN. Finding the optimal site within GPi may be a challenge. Changing the target within the pallidum may evoke different clinical effects. For example, several studies have suggested that stimulation of the posteroventral target of Leksell's pallidotomy is most effective for treating tremor and especially for relieving dyskinesias (52,63,64). One study based on MRI (65) suggested that both the ansa lenticularis and the lenticular fasciculus lie within the accepted coordinate range of Leksell's target. However, moving the target to the dorsal pallidum has been reported to produce a more pronounced effect on akinesia (63). In fact, dorsal pallidal stimulation (possibly including the GPe) may induce dyskinesias and may oppose the effects of dopaminergic medication (64,66). Yelnik et al. (67) found similar results without discovering a definite somatotopic arrangement of the pallidum. Bejjani et al. (63) noted that akinesia and gait worsened significantly as increasing voltage was applied to the ventral contacts (postulated to be within the Leksell target). This occurred whether the patient was in the on or off state. In the on state, enough of a therapeutic window existed between suppression of medication-induced dyskinesias and worsening of akinesia to make chronic stimulation viable. Stimulation through the more dorsal contacts significantly improved gait, akinesia, and rigidity in the off state, but had no significant effect when applied while the patient was in the on state.

Other investigators have suggested moving the target anteriorly within the pallidum (68). Iacono et al. (68) believed that this adjustment has the same effect as placing the effective contacts within GPe. They theorized that this would be desirable since GPe is just upstream from the STN and usually exerts an inhibitory influence. However, if stimulation creates a "functional lesion," then it should not enhance the output of the pallidum. Others have utilized the older, originally described anterior pallidotomy target, medial, dorsal, and anterior to Leksell's target (69). Iacono's target, while anterior and dosal to the Leksell target, was not much more medial (19.5 mm lateral to the AC-PC line). Essentially, the electrode is directed to the medial apex of GPi, where it meets the internal capsule. This is intended to affect the ansa lenticularis and lenticular fasciculus as they traverse the internal capsule in close proximity to one another. Both of these strategies have demonstrated encouraging results in limited series, but have not been proven in substantial patient populations.

Unfortunately, most of these papers fail to specifically define the target area. Bejjani et al. (63) states that they aimed for "the posteroventral part of the GPi." Burchiel et al. (59) and Krack et al. (58) do not mention any details of their pallidal targets. Krack utilized monopolar stimulation of the most ventral contacts, while Burchiel used bipolar stimulation between the two middle contacts. These factors all prevent accurate comparisons from being made both between GPi and STN stimulation groups within each study and, more importantly, between the GPi stimulation groups in different studies.

B. Dystonia

Dystonia has a long history of neurosurgical treatment, and reports continue to emerge describing the use of DBS in dystonia with a variety of subcortical targets. However, the disorder is extremely heterogeneous, with a widely varying clinical spectrum and multiple etiologies (idiopathic, genetic, posttraumatic, poststroke, etc.), making the assembly of large patient populations problematic (70).

In reviewing their experience with thalamic (Vim) stimulation, the Grenoble group commented that the results in their five patients with dystonia were unimpressive (71).

Table 2   Selected Results of Deep Brain Stimulation of the Globus Pallidus Interna (GPi) for Dystonia

Study (Ref.)	Patients	Follow-up (months)	Results
Kumar et al., 1999 (73)	1	12	67% improvement
Islekel et al., 1999 (74)	1	1	Patient symptom-free
Coubes et al., 2000 (75)	7	3	Burke-Fahn-Marsden (BFM) scores—90%
Loher et al., 2000 (82)	1	48	Sustained "marked improvement"
Vercueil et al., 2001 (81)	8	6–24	> 50% improvement in BFM motor/ disability scores
Bereznai et al., 2002 (78)	6	3–12	BFM scores—72.5%
Krauss et al., 2002 (77)	8	20	Toronto Western scale Severity—63%, Disability—69%
Vesper et al., 2002 (79)	2	6	BFM scores—80–95%

Multiple papers demonstrate that stimulation of the GPi is the most efficacious surgical treatment for this disorder. Multiple small series have documented improvement in Burke-Fahn-Marsden (BFM) dystonia scores (72–80). Vercueil et al. (81) found that eight patients maintained a greater than 50% improvement in the motor and disability portions of the BFM score as long as 24 months postoperatively. In addition, GPi stimulation has been found to maintain a robust effect 4 years after implantation (82). The best results are noted in those patients with familial idiopathic generalized dystonia secondary to the DYT1 gene mutation (79,83,84). These patients may achieve improvements of up to 95% in the BFM score.

Several small series focusing on patients with cervical dystonia have been reported (72,84,85). The two patients reported by Kulisevsky et al. (86) reported significant improvement in pain (55% and 64%). However, one patient's motor score improved by only 21% and the other's returned to baseline after improving by only 7%. Among the three patients reported by Krauss et al. (72) and followed 6–15 months, total severity scores improved 41–53%, pain improved 33–57%, and disability improved 50–80%. The procedure is complicated in these patients by their very disease in that cervical torsion complicates frame placement, imaging, and image fusion. Moreover, patient tolerance of the procedure is limited, as they are restrained in a fixed frame for several hours. In addition, cervical torsion puts these patients at high risk for such complications as lead fracture and other wound-related complications (77). Table 2 shows the results of selected series of GPi stimulation for dystonia.

Trottenberg et al. (87) reported a single patient with severe medically intractable tardive dystonia treated with bilateral DBS systems in both GPi and Vim. Stimulation of the GPi electrodes led to a 73% improvement in the BFM rating score. There was also a 54% improvement in the patient's abnormal involuntary movement scale score. A rebound phenomenon was noted within 1–2 hours of the discontinuation of stimulation. Vim stimulation produced no significant clinical benefit.

V. CONCLUSIONS

Stimulation of the globus pallidus is emerging as an effective treatment for PD and dystonia. Published studies suggest that pallidal stimulation may compare favorably to

STN stimulation for the treatment of PD, although the ideal target remains uncertain. A large, randomized trial comparing pallidal stimulation with STN stimulation in PD patients is currently underway. In the treatment of childhood dystonias, pallidal stimulation may offer dramatic improvements for a patient population in whom effective treatments are few.

REFERENCES

1. Spiegel EA, Wycis HT, Marks M, Lee AJ. Stereotaxic apparatus for operations on the human brain. Science 1947; 106:349–350.
2. Spiegel EA, Wycis HT. Ansotomy in paralysis agitans. Arch Neurol Psychiatry 1954; 71:598–614.
3. Narabayashi H, Okuma T. Procaine oil blocking of the globus pallidus for the treatment of rigidity and tremor of parkinsonism. Proc Jpn Acad 1953; 29:310–318.
4. Fenelon F. Neurosurgery of ansa lenticularis in dyskinesias and in parkinson's disease: review of principles and techniques of a personal operation. Semaine Hop Paris 1955; 31:1835–1837.
5. Svennilson E, Torvik A, Lowe R, Leksell L. Treatment of parkinsonism by stereotactic thermolesions in the pallidal region. A clinical evaluation of 81 cases. Acta Psychiatr Neurol Scand 1960; 35:358–377.
6. Guiot G, Brion S. Traitment des mouvements anormaux par la coagulation pallidale: technique et resultats. Rev Neurol 1953; 89:578–580.
7. Cooper IS. Chemopallidectomy and chemothalamectomy. Cooper IS, ed. Parkinsonism: Its Medical and Surgical Therapy. Vol. 1. Springfield, IL: Charles C Thomas, 1961:57–129.
8. Cooper IS. Surgical occlusion of the anterior choroidal artery. In: Cooper IS, ed. Parkinsonism: Its Medical and Surgical Therapy. Vol. 1. Springfield, IL: Charles C Thomas, 1961:38–56.
9. Hassler R, Riechert T. Indikationen und Lokalisationsmethode der Geziel Hirnoperationnen. Nervenarzt 1954; 25:441–447.
10. Laitinen LV, Bergenheim AT, Hariz MI. Leksell's posteroventral pallidotomy in the treatment of Parkinson's disease. J Neurosurg 1992; 76:53–61.
11. Laitinen LV, Bergenheim AT, Hariz MI. Ventroposterolateral pallidotomy can abolish all parkinsonian symptoms. Stereotact Funct Neurosurg 1992; 58:14–21.
12. Tasker RR. Deep brain stimulation is preferable to thalamotomy for tremor suppression. Surg Neurol 1998; 49:145–154.
13. Alterman RL, Kelly PJ. Pallidotomy technique and results: The New York University experience. Neurosurg Clin North Am 1998; 9:337–344.
14. Iacono RP, Shima F, Lonser RR, Kuniyoshi S, Maeda G, Yamada S. The results, indications, and physiology of posteroventral pallidotomy for patients with Parkinson's disease. Neurosurgery 1995; 36:1118–1127.
15. Lozano A, Hutchison W, Kiss ZH, Tasker R, Davis K, Dostrovsky JO. Methods for microelectrode-guided posteroventral pallidotomy. J Neurosurg 1996; 84:194–202.
16. Guridi J, Gorospe A, Ramos E, Linazasoro G, Rodriguez MC, Obeso JA. Stereotactic targeting of the globus pallidus internus in Parkinson's disease: Imaging versus electrophysiological mapping. Neurosurgery 1999; 45:278–289.
17. Wichmann T, DeLong MR. Models of basal ganglia function and pathophysiology of movement disorders. Neurosurg Clin North Am 1998; 9:223–236.
18. Lozano AM, Lang AE. Pallidotomy for Parkinson's disease. Neurosurg Clin North Am 1998; 9: 325–336.
19. Brooks DJ. Positron emission tomography studies in movement disorders. Neurosurg Clin North Am 1998; 9:263–282.
20. Eidelberg D, Moeller JR, Ishikawa T, et al. Regional metabolic correlates of surgical outcome following unilateral pallidotomy for Parkinson's disease. Ann Neurol 1996; 39:450–459.
21. Eidelberg D, Moeller JR, Kazumata K, et al. Metabolic correlates of pallidal neuronal activity in Parkinson's disease. Brain 1997; 120:1315–1324.
22. Samuel M, Ceballos-Baumann AO, Turjanski N, et al. Pallidotomy in Parkinson's disease increases supplementary motor area and prefrontal activation during performance of volitional movements an H2(15)O PET study. Brain 1997; 120:1301–1313.
23. Davis KD, Taub E, Houle S, et al. Globus pallidus stimulation activates the cortical motor system during alleviation of parkinsonian symptoms. Nat Med 1997; 3:671–674.

24. Chen R, Garg RR, Lozano AM, Lang AE. Effects of internal globus pallidus stimulation on motor cortex excitability. Neurology 2001; 56:716–723.
25. Devos D, Derambure P, Bourriez JL, et al. Influence of internal globus pallidus stimulation on motor cortex activation pattern in Parkinson's disease. Clin Neurophysiol 2002; 113:1110–1120.
26. Benabid AL, Benazzouz A, Hoffmann D, Limousin P, Krack P, Pollak P. Long-term electrical inhibition of deep brain targets in movement disorders. Mov Disord 1998; 13:119–125.
27. Beurrier C, Bioulac B, Audin J, Hammond C. High-frequency stimulation produces a transient blockade of voltage-gated currents in subthalamic neurons. J Neurophysiol 2001; 85:1351–1356.
28. Montgomery EBJ, Baker KB. Mechanisms of deep brain stimulation and future technical developments. Neurol Res 2000; 22:259–266.
29. Vitek JL. Surgery for dystonia. Neurosurg Clin North Am 1998; 9:345–366.
30. Hammond C, Garcia L, Beurrier C, Audin J, Bioulac B. Activity of subthalamic nucleus neurons during high frequency stimulation in vitro. Neuromodulation 2002: Defining the Future, Aix-les-bains, France, 2002.
31. Voges J, Volkmann J, Allert N, et al. Bilateral high-frequency stimulation in the subthalamic nucleus for the treatment of Parkinson disease: correlation of therapeutic effect with anatomical electrode position. J Neurosurg 2002; 96:269–279.
32. Lanotte MM, Rizzone M, Bergamasco B, Faccani G, Melcarne A, Lopiano L. Deep brain stimulation of the subthalamic nucleus: anatomical, neurophysiological, and outcome correlations with the effects of stimulation. J Neurol Neurosurg Psychiatry 2002; 72:53–58.
33. Nandi D, Chir M, Liu X, et al. Electrophysiological confirmation of the zona incerta as a target for surgical treatment of disabling involuntary arm movements in multiple sclerosis: use of local field potentials. J Clin Neurosci 2002; 9:64–68.
34. Ashby P, Kim YJ, Kumar R, Lang AE, Lozano AM. Neurophysiological effects of stimulation through electrodes in the human subthalamic nucleus. Brain 1999; 122:1919–1931.
35. Boraud T, Bezard E, Bioulac B, Gross C. High frequency stimulation of the internal globus pallidus (GPi) simultaneously improves parkinsonian symptoms and reduces the firing frequency of GPi neurons in the MPTP-treated monkey. Neurosci Lett 1996; 215:17–20.
36. Grill WM, McIntyre CC. Extracellular excitation of central neurons: implications for the mechanisms of deep brain stimulation. Thal Rel Sys 2001; 1:269–277.
37. Limousin P, Greene J, Pollak P, Rothwell J, Benabid AL, Frackowiak R. Changes in cerebral activity pattern due to subthalamic nucleus or internal pallidum stimulation in Parkinson's disease. Ann Neurol 1997; 42:283–291.
38. Vitek JL. Mechanisms of deep brain stimulation: excitation or inhibition. Mov Disord 2002; 17: S69–S72.
39. Dostrovsky JO, Lozano A. Mechanisms of deep brain stimulation. Mov Disord 2002; 17(suppl 3): S63–S68.
40. Lozano AM, Hutchison WD. Microelectrode recordings in the pallidum. Mov Disord 2002; 17: S150–S154.
41. Lozano AM, Hutchison WD, Tasker RR, Lang AE, Junn F, Dostrovsky JO. Microelectrode recordings define the ventral posteromedial pallidotomy target. Stereotact Funct Neurosurg 1998; 71:153–163.
42. Vitek JL, Bakay RA, Hashimoto T, et al. Microelectrode-guided pallidotomy: technical approach and its application in medically intractable Parkinson's disease. J Neurosurg 1998; 88:1027–1043.
43. Lenz FA, Dostrovsky JO, Kwan HC, Tasker RR, Yamashiro K, Murphy JT. Methods for microstimulation and recording of single neurons and evoked potentials in the human central nervous system. J Neurosurg 1988; 68:630–634.
44. Alterman RL, Sterio D, Beric A, Kelly PJ. Microelectrode recording during posteroventral pallidotomy: impact on target selection and complications. Neurosurgery 1999; 44:315–323.
45. Alterman RL, Reiter GT, Shils J, et al. Targeting for thalamic deep brain stimulator implantation without computer guidance: assessment of targeting accuracy. Stereotact Funct Neurosurg 1999; 72:150–153.
46. Rezai AR, Finelli D, Nyenhuis JA, et al. Neurostimulation systems for deep brain stimulation: in vitro evaluation of magnetic resonance imaging-related heating at 1.5 tesla. J Magn Reson Imaging 2002; 15:241–250.
47. Siegfried J, Lippitz B. Bilateral chronic electrostimulation of ventroposterolateral pallidum: a new therapeutic approach for alleviating all parkinsonian symptoms. Technique and application. Neurosurgery 1994; 35:1126–1130.

48. Loher TJ, Burgunder JM, Pohle T, Weber S, Sommerhalder R, Krauss JK. Long-term pallidal deep brain stimulation in patients with advanced Parkinson disease: 1-year follow-up study. J Neurosurg 2002; 96:844–853.

49. DBS Study Group. Deep-brain stimulation of the subthalamic nucleus or the pars interna of the globus pallidus in Parkinson's disease. N Engl J Med 2001; 345:956–963.

50. Kumar R, Lang AE, Rodriguez-Oroz MC, et al. Deep brain stimulation of the globus pallidus pars interna in advanced Parkinson's disease. Neurology 2000; 55(12):S34–S39.

51. Ghika J, Villemure JG, Fankhauser H, Favre J, Assal G, Ghika-Schmid F. Efficiency and safety of bilateral contemporaneous pallidal stimulation (deep brain stimulation] in levodopa-responsive patients with Parkinson's disease with severe motor fluctuations: a 2-year follow-up review. J Neurosurg 1998; 89:713–718.

52. Peppe A, Pierantozzi M, Altibrandi MG, et al. Bilateral GPi DBS is useful to reduce abnormal involuntary movements in advanced Parkinson's disease patients, but its action is related to modality and site of stimulation. Eur J Neurol 2001; 8:579–586.

53. Galvez-Jimenez N, Lozano A, Tasker R, Duff J, Hutchison W, Lang AE. Pallidal stimulation in Parkinson's disease patients with a prior unilateral pallidotomy. Can J Neurol Sci 1998; 25:300–305.

54. Pahwa R, Wilkinson S, Smith D, Lyons K, Miyawaki E, Koller WC. High-frequency stimulation of the globus pallidus for the treatment of Parkinson's disease. Neurology 1997; 49:249–253.

55. Gross C, Rougier A, Guehl D, Boraud T, Julien J, Bioulac B. High-frequency stimulation of the globus pallidus internalis in Parkinson's disease: a study of seven cases. J Neurosurg 1997; 87: 491–498.

56. Volkmann J, Sturm V, Weiss P, et al. Bilateral high-frequency stimulation of the internal globus pallidus in advanced Parkinson's disease. Ann Neurol 1998; 44:953–961.

57. Krause M, Fogel W, Heck A, et al. Deep brain stimulation for the treatment of Parkinson's disease: subthalamic nucleus versus globus pallidus internus. J Neurol Neurosurg Psychiatry 2001; 70:464–470.

58. Krack P, Pollak P, Limousin P, et al. Subthalamic nucleus or internal pallidal stimulation in young onset Parkinson's disease. Brain 1998; 121:451–457.

59. Burchiel KJ, Anderson VC, Favre J, Hammerstad JP. Comparison of pallidal and subthalamic nucleus deep brain stimulation for advanced Parkinson's disease: results of a randomized, blinded pilot study. Neurosurgery 1999; 45:1375–1384.

60. Krack P, Poepping M, Weinert D, Schrader B, Deuschl G. Thalamic, pallidal, or subthalamic surgery for Parkinson's disease?. J Neurol 2000; 247(suppl 2):II122–34.

61. Allert N, Volkmann J, Dotse S, Hefter H, Sturm V, Freund HJ. Effects of bilateral pallidal or subthalamic stimulation on gait in advanced Parkinson's disease. Mov Disord 2001; 16:1076–1085.

62. Volkmann J, Allert N, Voges J, Weiss PH, Freund HJ, Sturm V. Safety and efficacy of pallidal or subthalamic nucleus stimulation in advanced PD. Neurology 2001; 56:548–551.

63. Bejjani B, Damier P, Arnulf I, et al. Pallidal stimulation for Parkinson's disease. Two targets? Neurology 1997; 49:1564–1569.

64. Krack P, Pollak P, Limousin P, et al. Opposite motor effects of pallidal stimulation in Parkinson's disease. Ann Neurol 1998; 43:180–192.

65. Patil A-A, Hahn F, Sierra-Rodriguez J, Traverse J, Wang S. Anatomical structures in the Leksell pallidotomy target. Stereotact Funct Neurosurg 1998; 70:32–37.

66. Krack P, Pollak P, Limousin P, Hoffmann D, Benazzouz A, Benabid AL. Inhibition of levodopa effects by internal pallidal stimulation. Mov Disord 1998; 13:648–652.

67. Yelnik J, Damier P, Bejjani BP, et al. Functional mapping of the human globus pallidus: contrasting effects of stimulation in the internal and external pallidum in Parkinson's disease. Neuroscience 2000; 101:77–87.

68. Iacono RP, Lonser RR, Maeda G, et al. Chronic anterior pallidal stimulation for Parkinson's disease. Acta Neurochir 1995; 137:106–112.

69. Durif F, Lemaire JJ, Debilly B, Dordain G. Acute and chronic effects of anteromedial globus pallidus stimulation in Parkinson's disease. J Neurol Neurosurg Psychiatry 1999; 67:315–322.

70. Rosenow J, Das K, Rovit RL, Couldwell WT. Irving S. Cooper and the genesis of intracranial stimulation for movement disorders and epilepsy. Stereotact Funct Neurosurg 2002; 78:95–112.

71. Benabid AL, Pollak P, Gao D, et al. Chronic electrical stimulation of the ventralis intermedius nucleus of the thalamus as a treatment of movement disorders. J Neurosurg 1996; 84:203–214.

72. Krauss JK, Pohle T, Weber S, Ozdoba C, Burgunder JM. Bilateral stimulation of globus pallidus internus for treatment of cervical dystonia. Lancet 1999; 354:837–838.

73. Kumar R, Dagher A, Hutchison WD, Lang AE, Lozano AM. Globus pallidus deep brain stimulation for generalized dystonia: clinical and PET investigation. Neurology 1999; 53:871–874.

74. Islekel S, Zileli M, Zileli B. Unilateral pallidal stimulation in cervical dystonia. Stereotact Funct Neurosurg 1999; 72:248–252.

75. Coubes P, Roubertie A, Vayssiere N, Hemm S, Echenne B. Treatment of DYT1-generalised dystonia by stimulation of the internal globus pallidus. Lancet 2000; 355:2220–2221.

76. Vayssiere N, Hemm S, Zanca M, et al. Magnetic resonance imaging stereotactic target localization for deep brain stimulation in dystonic children. J Neurosurg 2000; 93:784–790.

77. Krauss JK, Loher TJ, Pohle T, et al. Pallidal deep brain stimulation in patients with cervical dystonia and severe cervical dyskinesias with cervical myelopathy. J Neurol Neurosurg Psychiatry 2002; 72:249–256.

78. Bereznai B, Steude U, Seelos K, Botzel K. Chronic high-frequency globus pallidus internus stimulation in different types of dystonia: a clinical, video, and MRI report of six patients presenting with segmental, cervical, and generalized dystonia. Mov Disord 2002; 17:138–144.

79. Vesper J, Klostermann F, Funk T, Stockhammer F, Brock M. Deep brain stimulation of the globus pallidus internus (GPI) for torsion dystonia—a report of two cases. Acta Neurochir Suppl 2002; 79:83–88.

80. Tronnier VM, Fogel W. Pallidal stimulation for generalized dystonia. Report of three cases. J Neurosurg 2000; 92:453–456.

81. Vercueil L, Pollak P, Fraix V, et al. Deep brain stimulation in the treatment of severe dystonia. J Neurol 2001; 248:695–700.

82. Loher TJ, Hasdemir MG, Burgunder JM, Krauss JK. Long-term follow-up study of chronic globus pallidus internus stimulation for posttraumatic hemidystonia. J Neurosurg 2000; 92:457–460.

83. Krack P, Vercueil L. Review of the functional surgical treatment of dystonia. Eur J Neurol 2001; 8:389–399.

84. Vercueil L, Krack P, Pollak P. Results of deep brain stimulation for dystonia: a critical reappraisal. Mov Disord 2002; 17(suppl 3):S89–S93.

85. Andaluz N, Taha JM, Dalvi A. Bilateral pallidal deep brain stimulation for cervical and truncal dystonia. Neurology 2001; 57:557–558.

86. Kulisevsky J, Lleo A, Gironell A, Molet J, Pascual-Sedano B, Parcs P. Bilateral pallidal stimulation for cervical dystonia: dissociated pain and motor improvement. Neurology 2000; 55:1754–1755.

87. Trottenberg T, Paul G, Meissner W, Maier-Hauff K, Taschner C, Kupsch A. Pallidal and thalamic neurostimulation in severe tardive dystonia. J Neurol Neurosurg Psychiatry 2001; 70:557–559.

88. Siegfried J, Taub E, Wellis GN. Long-term electrostimulation of the ventroposterolateral pallidum in the treatment of Parkinson's disease. Adv Neurol 1999; 80:623–626.

24

Subthalamic Nucleus Deep Brain Stimulation

Drew S. Kern and Rajeev Kumar

Colorado Neurological Institute, Englewood, Colorado, U.S.A.

I. INTRODUCTION

Surgical treatment of movement disorders has markedly expanded in the past decade because of our enhanced understanding of basal ganglia circuitry and pathophysiology of Parkinson's disease (PD). Advancements in neuroimaging [especially magnetic resonance imaging (MRI)] and intraoperative electrophysiological recordings have increased stereotaxic surgical targeting accuracy. Abnormal subthalamic nucleus (STN) activity has been implicated to be important in the genesis of the clinical features of PD. Altering this aberrant activity using STN deep brain stimulation (DBS) has been effective for moderate to advanced PD with sustained benefit for several years.

II. ANATOMY AND PHYSIOLOGY OF THE SUBTHALAMIC NUCLEUS

The STN is a small biconvex-shaped structure of approximately $315 \, \text{mm}^3$ located inferior to the zona incerta (Zi), superior to the substantia nigra reticulata (SNr), lateral to the red nucleus and fields of Forel (H_1 and H_2), and medial to the internal capsule (Fig. 1) (1–4). The human STN contains approximately 300,000 neurons (1–3,5). The STN is somatotopically organized into three functional areas: the dorsolateral area devoted to sensorimotor function, the ventromedial portion involved in association processing, and the most medial portion (the tip of the STN) involved in the limbic system (6). Movement-related cells are somatotopically arranged within the sensorimotor area with the medial and central portion of the STN responsive to leg movements and the lateral portion responsive to arm movements (7).

In the classic model of basal ganglia circuitry, the STN receives GABAergic inhibitory afferent projections from the globus pallidus externa (GPe) and sends the only glutamatergic excitatory outputs in the basal ganglia to the globus pallidus interna (GPi) and the SNr (the main inhibitory outputs of the basal ganglia). Afferents from the GPe project to the lateral and rostral portion of the STN. Efferents to the GPi originate principally in the medial and caudal region while efferents to the SNr originate more diffusely within

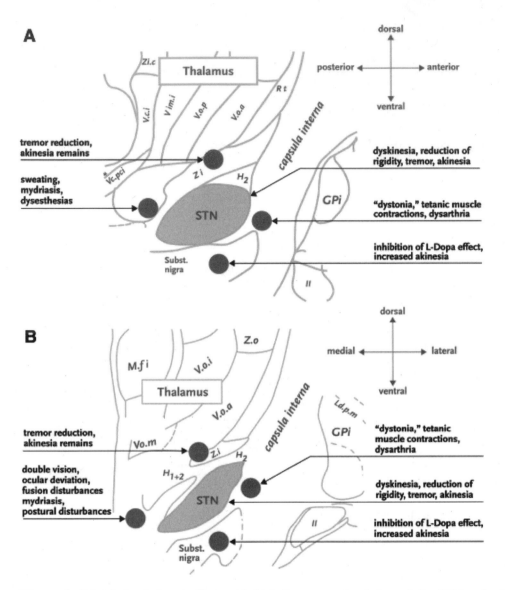

Figure 1 Stimulation-induced effects with high-frequency stimulation of the STN and adjacent structures. (A) Sagittal section 12 mm lateral to anterior commissure–posterior (AC-PC) commissure line; (B) frontal section 1.5 mm behind the midcommissural point (MCP). (From Ref. 107.)

the STN (6). In PD, striatal dopaminergic deficiency is thought to lead to overactivity of the indirect pathway (involving the STN) and underactivity of the direct pathway. Consequently, there is increased inhibition of the GPe with resultant hyperactivity of the STN causing increased excitation of the GPi/ SNr, increased thalamic inhibition, and finally reduced thalamocortical facilitation of movement. Animal and human studies have elucidated that the STN also sends projections to a wide range of additional structures including the GPe, the substantia nigra pars compacta (SNc), the pedunculo-pontine nucleus (PPN), the substantia innominata, and the mesencephalic and pontine reticular formation. The STN also receives many afferent projections from regions other than the GPe including the cortex (specifically the primary motor cortex, the premotor cortex, the sensorimotor cortex), the dorsal raphe nucleus, the PPN, the centromedian-parafascicularis nucleus of the thalamus (CM/Pf), GABAergic and cholinergic afferents from the PPN, as well as dopaminergic inputs from the SNc (4,6,8). GPe lesioning in rodent models of parkinsonism results in only a 20% increase in STN neuronal firing, although response to cortical afferents is modified compared to normal, intact rodents (9). Hence, STN activity is modulated by a complex network, and the STN influences a large number of structures.

A. Subthalamic Nucleus in Parkinson's Disease

STN neurons in normal nonhuman primates fire at a mean of 18–20 Hz, with 75% of neurons exhibiting stable oscillatory activity (3). After 1-methyl-4-phenyl-1,2,3,6-tetra-hydropyridine (MPTP) administration and the development of stable parkinsonian features, the mean STN neuron firing frequency increases by 29% (3). In animal models of parkinsonism, STN neurons exhibit two patterns of response to cortical excitation: (a) cells located within the central portion of the STN respond with two excitatory peaks (EPSPs) separated by a short inhibitory phase (an IPSP most likely due to afferents from the pallidum); (b) peripherally located cells demonstrate sustained excitation. Following these two different responses to cortical stimulation, a long period of inhibition follows resulting from decreased afferent excitation from the cortex (6,9).

STN neurons in parkinsonian patients discharge at approximately 40 Hz with three different cell types characterized by their firing pattern: tremor cells, cells with high oscillatory frequency of 15–30 Hz, and cells with both tremor and high-frequency oscillations (10–12). Tremor cells are found almost exclusively in patients with visible resting tremor (12). During limb movements, high-frequency oscillations are reduced; however, there is no consistent modification of discharge rate, suggesting that the pattern of cortical input to the STN is modified (10). Acute intraoperative dopaminergic stimulation with apomorphine reduces firing rate as well as high-frequency oscillations of STN neurons (10,11). These studies suggest that STN neuron discharge pattern and frequency are important in determining the clinical manifestations of parkinsonism.

B. Deep Brain Stimulation of the Subthalamic Nucleus and Neuroprotection

The STN sends glutamatergic projections to a wide range of structures (including the SNc), and excessive glutamatergic input from a hyperactive STN could lead to excitotoxic cell death in these targets (4). Furthermore, the SNc sends reciprocal dopaminergic projections to the STN, which may increase the discharge rate of the STN, perpetuating this deadly cycle. Therefore, surgical interventions that reduce STN activity might slow the underlying progression of PD. For example, electrolytic lesions of the STN in rodent models reduce the burst firing of nigral dopaminergic cells by 93% (13).

If DBS reduces STN firing and neuroprotection can be conclusively demonstrated in humans and not just in rodent models of PD, then this intervention may become appropriate in early PD. Currently, there are no convincing clinical data for neuro-protection in humans to justify moving surgery to an earlier stage of the disease; therefore, at present, hope for neuroprotection should not be a factor in the decision for surgery.

III. MECHANISM OF DEEP BRAIN STIMULATION OF THE SUBTHALAMIC NUCLEUS

The mechanism of DBS is currently incompletely understood, with conflicting reports suggesting that stimulation results in either excitation or inhibition of STN neurons. Nevertheless, the effects of STN DBS have been well documented to be frequency dependent, with the greatest relief of symptoms at greater than 100 Hz and no therapeutic relief at less than 50 Hz. Stimulation pulse width determines which neural elements are preferentially affected; longer pulse widths influence the cell soma, while shorter pulse widths mainly affect axons. Furthermore, DBS results in highly localized stimulation because relatively low currents are used, which result in small current spread (about 2–3 mm with intensity of 2 mA) with current decreasing proportionally to the square of the distance (14,15).

Long-term use of DBS does not result in significant neuronal damage. Postmortem examination of patients who have undergone chronic long-term DBS reveals only minimal gliosis surrounding the stimulating electrode (16,17). Most features of PD return within seconds or minutes upon discontinuation of STN stimulation, though some improvement may persist for several hours. The persistence of some of the effects of DBS stimulation after discontinuation suggests that some degree of downstream central nervous system plasticity is induced with chronic stimulation.

Some evidence suggests that stimulation more likely affects axons projecting from the STN rather than cell bodies within the STN. Voges et al. reported that the greatest benefit of STN DBS is most commonly due to stimulation of fiber tracts adjacent to the STN (18). The greatest benefit usually occurs with stimulation using contacts located within the STN, but significant benefit stimulating the zona incerta (Zi) and the fields of Forel has been reported (19). Since the clinical results of DBS are comparable to ablation, direct inhibition of the STN via depolarization blockade of myelinated axons with stimulation has been proposed as the mechanism of action; however, the stimulation rates used clinically for DBS are much lower than that required to create a depolarization blockade in animal models (20). Neuronal inhibition may be more likely to occur via hyperpolarization since after termination of STN stimulation, cellular responsiveness is inhibited for 50 to greater than 500 ms, which is followed by a period of excitation and then further inhibition (21). It is also possible that stimulation may indirectly inhibit the STN by exciting inhibitory interneurons; however, reports on the existence of interneurons within the STN are varied (6). Alternatively stimulation may excite afferent fibers from the GPe, resulting in STN inhibition (20).

The efficacy of DBS may predominantly depend on downstream rather than local effects. Rather than inhibition, DBS might activate fibers and transfer nonphysiological and incomprehensible messages to downstream target nuclei, which are then disregarded ("neuronal jamming"). Alternatively, STN DBS may modify the excitability of downstream connections. STN stimulation might antidromically excite the GPe, and consequently the GABAergic projections from the GPe would inhibit the GPi. This hypothesis is supported by a study that found short-latency excitation of the GPi and GPe following stimulation of the STN in parkinsonian primates (22). There is some evidence that high-frequency stimulation of the STN increases striatal dopamine concentrations, increases extracellular glutamate in the GPe and SNr, and increases SNr extracellular concentrations of GABA (23,24). These neurochemical studies question the hypothesis that STN DBS results in inhibition since downstream targets appear to be activated following STN stimulation.

Several functional imaging and physiological studies have been performed in patients. Positron emission tomography (PET) studies performed in resting patients have found that bilateral STN DBS increases regional cerebral blood flow (rCBF) in the presupplementary motor area, anterior cingulate cortex, dorsolateral prefrontal cortex, and medial frontal gyrus while decreasing primary motor cortex rCBF (25,26). During movement, activation of the anterior cingulate cortex, supplementary motor area, premotor cortex and globus pallidus increases more with bilateral stimulation than with unilateral stimulation (25,27). Increases in supplementary motor area and anterior cingulate cortex rCBF are correlated with improvement in motor performance (27). STN stimulation may result in impaired task performance (prolonged reaction time) of word processing associated with decreased rCBF of the right anterior cingulate cortex and the right ventral striatum and increased rCBF of the left angular gyrus (28). Transcranial magnetic stimulation (TMS) of the motor cortex in PD patients during STN DBS helps to restore intracortical inhibition toward normal levels (29). These studies confirm that STN DBS has widespread cortical effects that influence motor and nonmotor function in PD patients.

IV. SUBTHALAMIC STIMULATION VERSUS SUBTHALAMOTOMY

DBS and lesioning of the STN (subthalamotomy) result in comparable improvement of parkinsonism. Only a few case series with small patient cohorts have been reported detailing the effects of subthalamotomy. Historically, STN lesioning was thought to be associated with a high risk of hemiballism; although transient dyskinesias are common, recent studies indicate that this complication rarely persists (30,31). Unilateral subthalamotomy predominately improves contralateral symptoms, and the beneficial effects may be sustained for at least 2 years (32,33). Bilateral subthalamotomy has been safely performed and may result in greater improvement than unilateral procedures, with 50 60% improvement in motor performance and 50 100% reduction of drug therapy (33–36). There are extremely limited data reported on the adverse effects of subthalamotomy, but left-sided lesions may be more apt to impair verbal cognition than right-sided lesions (37).

In general, DBS electrode implantation causes fewer permanent neurological adverse effects compared with lesioning because minimal brain tissue is destroyed. Radiofrequency lesions might be inadvertently expanded or be misplaced to involve important structures adjacent to the STN. Schuurman et al.(38) directly compared the effects of unilateral thalamotomy and thalamic stimulation in a randomized controlled study of patients with PD, essential tremor, and multiple sclerosis. Efficacy in controlling contralateral limb tremor was similar 6 months postoperatively; however, thalamotomy was associated with a significantly higher complication rate. Although no direct comparison between STN DBS and subthalamotomy has been performed, bilateral stimulation can be safely performed and, based on the experience with GPi and thalamic stimulation and ablation, might have a lower risk of cognitive and bulbar adverse effects (39–44). With DBS, stimulation parameters can be adjusted to maximize beneficial results and minimize adverse effects caused by current spread to adjacent structures. DBS electrodes can also be surgically repositioned if they are initially suboptimally situated, and the hardware can be removed at any time. In contrast, the effects of ablation are irreversible and not adjustable without additional surgery, which may occasionally be required to expand an inadequate lesion.

Compared with subthalamotomy, STN DBS does require an additional surgery performed under general anesthesia to implant the internal pulse generator (IPG) and connector wire. The IPG also needs to be surgically replaced every 3–7 years due to battery depletion. Several visits are typically necessary following electrode implantation to adjust the stimulation parameters, while minimal follow-up is required after subthalamotomy. Approximately 25–30% of patients may experience hardware complications typically involving mechanical hardware breakage or skin erosion, which may be associated with cutaneous infection (45,46). These complications usually require replacement of damaged or infected hardware and sometimes treatment with antibiotics. Migration of the DBS electrode has also been reported (46). In patients with severe postural instability and frequent falls, subthalamotomy may be preferred since falls may damage or displace DBS hardware. STN DBS is also a very expensive procedure compared with subthalamotomy; hence, in many areas of the world, lesioning procedures are the only affordable surgical option.

V. PATIENT SELECTION

A multidisciplinary team consisting of a movement disorders neurologist, a functional neurosurgeon, and a neuropsychologist helps to optimally select patients for surgery. The role of the neurologist is to ensure the correct diagnosis and that all appropriate non-surgical treatments have been employed. The neurosurgeon evaluates the patient's general health with respect to the risks of surgery and discusses with the patient the potential complications of surgery, including a 1–2% chance of intracerebral hemorrhage per operated side, which could result in serious neurological disability or death. The neuropsychologist performs an in-depth cognitive examination to determine if there are any signs of dementia and interviews the patient and caregiver to determine if there are behavioral abnormalities or psychiatric problems such as anxiety, substance abuse, depression, or mania.

Although there are no firmly validated criteria to select patients for surgery, some basic guidelines have been adopted by many surgical centers. STN DBS should be considered for PD patients with medication-refractory motor fluctuations and levodopa-induced dyskinesias, disabling medication-refractory tremor, or marked medication intolerance making medical management unsatisfactory, which results in substantial disability. The patient and the physician should compare the potential for significant improvement and potential adverse effects of more aggressive drug therapy compared with surgery. Many factors must be considered in this decision, including the patient's personal, professional, and social situation. Regardless, surgery should not be unnecessarily delayed until the patient loses his or her job or there is a significant decrease in independence and loss of quality of life (47).

Patients must have the mental and physical stamina to endure a lengthy and demanding procedure and be cognitively healthy with low levels of anxiety in order to provide useful intraoperative feedback and assist with postoperative stimulation adjustments. Demented patients tend to become more confused intraoperatively, being unable to provide reliable reports of adverse effects during intraoperative stimulation, and it may be difficult to optimally program stimulation parameters due to their lack of insight into their own motor status. Furthermore, surgery can potentially worsen preexisting cognitive deficits in PD patients with features suggestive of early neuro-degenerative dementia (48). Cognitive abnormalities that are a result of PD should not be considered exclusion criteria, but significant abnormalities not normally present in the neurological disease (such as impaired lexical and semantic verbal fluency) may be the basis for exclusion (49). Patients who hallucinate or develop other symptoms of psychosis with dopaminergic drugs are often demented or almost universally become demented within the next few years; hence, these patients should generally be excluded from surgery (48,49). However, in highly select cases surgery might be considered for those with the combination of mild preoperative cognitive abnormalities and severe motor disability, where the potential for worsening cognition with surgery is outweighed by the possibility of improvement in motor disability and activities of daily living (ADL) (50).

Previous surgery for PD does not contraindicate additional surgery if the patient is otherwise an appropriate surgical candidate. There are reports of successful bilateral STN DBS performed in patients with prior unilateral thalamotomy, unilateral or bilateral thalamic DBS, unilateral pallidotomy, and unilateral or bilateral GPi DBS (50–52).

Some groups exclude older patients (especially those older than 70 years of age) because in general this group benefits less compared with a younger population due to more levodopa-refractory (and surgery refractory) disability and has a higher risk of cognitive deterioration with surgery (14). However, elderly patients with a very good levodopa response and who are otherwise healthy clearly demonstrate significant improvement.

The degree of improvement obtained with a supramaximal dose of levodopa or apomorphine after overnight withdrawal of antiparkinson medication is highly predictive of the response to STN DBS (53,54). Therefore, the levodopa test is an important part of the evaluation to determine the degree of benefit obtainable with surgery. With the exception of tremor, signs that are not improved with levodopa usually fail to improve with surgery and include cognitive and psychiatric problems, on-period freezing, levodopa-refractory dysarthria, dysphagia, and postural instability. Furthermore, the levodopa test reinforces for the patient and family realistic expectations of the potential maximal results of surgery. Some reports indicate that in select patients, response to levodopa may not predict the potential effectiveness of DBS. STN DBS performed in two levodopa-unresponsive tremor-dominant PD patients (with F-dopa PET-confirmed PD) had marked improvement of all features of PD (55). Lentiform nucleus hypermetabolism on FDG-PET scanning also correlates with the response to levodopa and pallidotomy (56) and may correlate with the response to STN DBS. STN DBS may also be appropriate in select patients who are unable to tolerate adequate doses of antiparkinsonian medication because of somnolence, severe nausea, and vomiting despite domperidone and other antiemetics or psychiatric adverse effects in the absence of cognitive impairment, since this procedure allows marked antiparkinsonian drug reduction (57).

Additional contraindications include severe uncontrolled hypertension, cancer, cardiac, renal, hepatic, or pulmonary diseases and marked cerebral atrophy or extensive white matter T_2 signal changes, which could increase the risk for hemorrhage. Patients with on-period postural instability with frequent falls preoperatively may be considered candidates for surgery with some caution because they are at a higher risk of falls and injury due to reduced bradykinesia and faster gait associated with improvements from STN DBS. Patients must have emotional support available from family or other caregivers; postoperatively, there may be a difficult adjustment period associated with the new role of the patient being less dependent on others. Caregivers must also aid patients in attending multiple DBS programming visits. Finally, patients with unrealistic expectations such as believing that STN DBS is a "cure" should be excluded due to potential psychological difficulties that could ensue postoperatively.

There are very few published data regarding STN DBS for atypical parkinsonian syndromes. STN DBS was ineffective in one case of non–apomorphine-responsive multiple system atrophy (MSA) and one case of levodopa-refractory vascular parkinsonism

(54,58). A small fraction of MSA patients demonstrate a good levodopa response that is complicated by disabling levodopa-induced chorea or, more commonly, dystonia. However, in four patients with levodopa-unresponsive MSA, bilateral STN DBS significantly improved ADL and motor performance, reducing rigidity and akinesia one month postoperatively. In three of these patients followed up to 2 years postoperatively, ADL progressively declined to baseline values, although some mild motor benefit was sustained (59).

A recent cost-effectiveness analysis indicated that DBS for the treatment of PD may be considered cost-effective compared with the best medical treatment, providing that the overall improvement is 18% greater than the best medical treatment (60). This is indeed the case as bilateral STN DBS results in approximately 50% improvement in off-drug parkinsonism and antiparkinsonian medication is reduced by approximately 50%.

VI. CLINICAL RESULTS OF DEEP BRAIN STIMULATION OF THE SUBTHALAMIC NUCLEUS

A. Motor Effects

Table 1 summarizes the beneficial effects of bilateral STN DBS reported by several studies. Off-drug motor and ADL Unified Parkinson's Disease Rating Scale (UPDRS) scores are improved approximately 50% and 40%, respectively, with STN DBS 6–12 months post-operatively (53,61–66). Off-period dystonia is improved by 60–65% with bilateral STN DBS (67,68). On-period UPDRS motor scores are modestly improved with STN stimulation (about 25%) (53,61–66). On-period ADL scores are also improved likely in part due to reduction in dyskinesias. Levodopa-induced dyskinesias are significantly improved by 50–60% due to reduction of antiparkinsonian medication (67,69). After long-term chronic STN DBS and drug reduction, sensitization to the pro-dyskinetic effects of levodopa is markedly reduced (67). Vingerhoets et al. reported that 50% of patients followed 2 years postoperatively were able to stop all drug therapy, with consequent complete elimination of motor fluctuations and dyskinesias (70). The patient cohort who still required antiparkinsonian medication despite optimal adjustment of the DBS parameters had ongoing dyskinesias and motor fluctuations. This study reports an unusually high percentage of patients who were able to cease drug therapy and is not in keeping with the reports of most groups, who have found that only about 10% of patients are able to stop all antiparkinsonian medication. Axial motor features including speech, neck rigidity, rising from a chair, posture, gait, and postural instability are improved by approximately 70% with bilateral STN DBS assessed 6 months postoperatively (71). Nonmotor fluctuations (NMF) are also markedly improved, especially asthenia, irritability, and drenching sweats (72).

Limited long-term follow-up data for bilateral STN DBS are available. However, preliminary data reported by the Grenoble group suggest that patients remain considerably improved 5 years postoperatively compared to baseline. Off-drug motor and ADL scores deteriorated over 5 years but remained much better than baseline, and antiparkinsonian medication requirements also continued to be significantly reduced. By 3 years post-operatively, on-drug motor and ADL scores became worse than baseline, largely reflecting progression of levodopa- and stimulation-refractory axial features of parkinsonism including gait, postural reflexes, and speech (73). In a similar study patients were evaluated up to 3 years postoperatively, and improvements in off-drug motor and ADL scores were maintained over time, while on-drug motor and ADL scores were not sustained (46).

Table 1 Effects of Bilateral Deep Brain Stimulation of the Subthalamic Nucleus in Patients with Parkinson's Disease

Study (Ref.)	Nature of study	Number of patients in study	Mean age of patients (y)	Number of patients analyzed	Postoperative evaluation (months)	Reported outcomes (% improvement)					
						Motor		ADL		Dyskinesia	Medication
						Off	On	Off	On		
Kumar et al., 1998 (61)	Double-blind	7	67	7	6	65	41	30	−18	83	40
The DBS for PD Study Group 2001 (62)	No blind	96	59	96	6	52	25	44	9	58	37
Welter et al., 2002 (53)	No blind	41	56	41	6	64	28	62	37	76	67
Limousin et al., 1998 (63)	Blind	24	56	20	12	~60	~5	—	—	84	50
Burchiel et al., 1999 (64)	Double-blind	6	63	5	12	44	15	—	—	67	51
Volkmann et al., 2001 (65)	No blind	16	60	16	12	67	−9	56	20	90	63
Vesper et al., 2002 (66)	No blind	38	56	38	12	37	48	—	—	72	36
Vingerhoets et al., 2002 (70)	No blind	20	63	20	21 (range 3–24)	45	—	37	—	79	92
Kern et al., 2003 (46)	No blind	28	62	27	22 (range 3–36)	37	11	31	16	—	57
Batir et al., 2002 (73)	No blind	49	—	42	60	54	−48	49	−93	39	63

Reported outcomes represent mean percent reduction in standardized rating scale scores, dyskinesias, and drug dosage at last follow-up compared with preoperative evaluations. Off represents assessments scored after overnight drug withdrawal, and on indicates scores with drug treatment. Postoperative off scores were compared with preoperative off evaluations, and on scores were compared with preoperative on assessments for motor and ADL sections of the Unified Parkinson's Disease Rating Scale (UPDRS) in patients. Various measures were used by each study to assess dyskinesias and calculate levodopa equivalence. Dashed lines indicate no reported data.

Select patients with highly asymmetrical parkinsonism may be candidates for unilateral STN DBS, although this surgery should be undertaken with caution since the need to reduce antiparkinson medication may lead to an uneven effect, with the ipsilateral side of the body being undertreated and becoming excessively parkinsonian. Nevertheless, in very asymmetrical tremor-dominant patients, unilateral STN DBS has been done without problems (55). In a recent report of 23 patients with advanced PD, there was a median 31% improvement in off-drug motor UPDRS scores 4 months after unilateral STN DBS. At one year follow-up, relatively few patients required contralateral STN DBS (74). Formal comparison has demonstrated superior effects of bilateral STN DBS on limb bradykinesia, axial features, and other components of PD compared to unilateral procedures (75).

The majority of adverse effects of bilateral STN DBS are transient, occurring as the stimulation parameters are adjusted. These are dependent on the exact electrode location and include dysarthria, tonic contraction, paresthesias, and diplopia (Fig. 1) (62,70). STN stimulation induces dyskinesias in most patients with optimally placed electrodes; reduction of antiparkinsonian medication usually resolves this problem, allowing stimulation to be increased over weeks to months. Pretarsal blepharospasm (often requiring treatment with botulinum toxin injection) occurs in 10–20% of patients and is an indicator of highly effective stimulation.

B. Psychiatric and Cognitive Effects

The majority of cognitive adverse effects are likely the direct result of electrode implantation, with stimulation only minimally affecting cognitive function. In younger cognitively intact patients, STN DBS is extremely well tolerated without significant impairment on neuropsychological assessments. In a large study examining patients one year postoperatively, there was only minor worsening of lexical fluency on-stimulation versus off-stimulation (76). In older patients (especially those with borderline cognitive function), a number of cognitive processes reliant on intact frontal-striatal circuitry may be significantly impaired with surgery (48). In elderly patients, transient confusion can persist for up to 2 weeks postoperatively, usually managed by general supportive measures as well as reduction of anti-parkinsonian medication. In rare cases, confusion accompanied by psychotic features such as hallucinations can occur and the use of atypical neuroleptics such as clozapine or quetiapine may be useful.

Bilateral STN DBS has positive acute psychotropic effects on motivation, fatigue, tension, and anxiety and may induce amphetamine-like stimulating effects or euphoria, possibly due to inadvertent stimulation of the limbic portion of the STN (77). During the process of DBS programming, levodopa may need to be reduced to control dyskinesias (77). However, excessive levodopa reduction may result in transient depression, anhedonia, abulia, and fatigue (65).

Some patients may have difficulty socially readjusting to their greater independence and difficulty with spouses who have lost their long-term functional role as a caregiver (78). There are also reports that surgery may accentuate preexisting anxiety, depression, or mania, resulting in significant behavioral abnormalities or even suicide (78).

A variety of acute, dramatic psychiatric syndromes have been observed during stimulation of the STN or surrounding region. Current spread to the SNr may result in acute stimulation-induced depression, potentially leading to attempted suicide (78–80). STN stimulation may also induce mania including hypersexuality (81,82). Although predominately due to stimulation, mania can persist even in the absence of stimulation (possibly due to STN lesioning during electrode implantation) but gradually subsides over several months. Stimulation-induced involuntary laughter which subsides immediately upon termination of stimulation has also been elicited, most likely due to inadvertent spread of stimulation to the limbic portion of the STN (the medial tip) (83). Furthermore, stimulation of the posteromedial hypothalamic area, the triangle of Sano, can cause attacks of rage and aggressive behavior (84). In contrast, marked benefit on co-morbid obsessive compulsive disorder (OCD) in PD patients has been achieved with STN DBS likely due to stimulation of the limbic portion of the STN (85). The variety of psychiatric effects observed with STN DBS emphasizes the important nonmotor role of the basal ganglia.

VII. SUBTHALAMIC VERSUS THALAMIC AND PALLIDAL STIMULATION

A. Thalamic Deep Brain Stimulation

DBS of the ventralis intermedius nucleus of the thalamus (Vim) results in 80–90% improvement in contralateral arm tremor and may diminish rigidity, but does not improve other features of PD such as bradykinesia and gait disorders (69,86,87). Contralateral levodopa-induced dyskinesias may also be improved if the DBS electrode is positioned in the centromedian/parafascicularis nucleus (CM/Pf) or anterior to the Vim [in the ventralis oralis anterior (Voa)/ventralis oralis posterior (Vop)]. Overall ADLs are not improved following thalamic DBS since bradykinesia is not improved and is generally the greatest source of disability in PD; however, manual tasks worsened by tremor such as handwriting may be improved (87–89). The beneficial effects of thalamic stimulation on contralateral tremor are sustained at least 3 years postoperatively, although with unilateral Vim DBS the minor improvements in ipsilateral tremor seen postoperatively are lost relatively quickly (86,87,90)

Unilateral Vim DBS usually does not cause clinically significant worsening of cognition, though on formal neuropsychological testing verbal episodic memory may decline (86,91). Common stimulation-induced adverse effects include paresthesias, tonic muscle contraction, dysarthria, and disequilibrium, which resolve with terminating stimulation or adjusting stimulation parameters (38,90,91). Current spread ventrally to cerebellothalamic fibers may also result in stimulation-induced ataxia (69). Stimulation-induced adverse effects are more prevalent with bilateral implantation, especially dysarthria, disequilibrium, and gait disorders (92).

Many patients who initially undergo Vim DBS for treatment of tremor have subsequently required GPi or STN surgery to treat other symptoms, such as bradykinesia, gait disorder, and levodopa-induced dyskinesias, which have become more pronounced with progression of PD. Because STN DBS improves tremor as effectively as thalamic surgery, Vim DBS is rarely recommended as a treatment for patients with PD. Instead GPi or STN surgery should be considered in patients with severe medication-refractory tremor-dominant PD.

B. Deep Brain Stimulation of the Globus Pallidus Interna

Although there has not been a large randomized study comparing GPi and STN DBS, some data suggest that STN DBS may be superior. STN DBS allows marked reduction or discontinuation of antiparkinsonian medication, while with GPi DBS medication is largely unchanged. Furthermore, STN stimulation requires less battery power due to lower stimulation parameters, probably because the STN is a smaller target than the pallidum (93). This results in fewer surgeries in order to replace the battery and, as a result, less cost. The STN may be an easier surgical target because it is more clearly identified by MRI. Despite these advantages, STN DBS requires more frequent follow-up visits with complex postoperative management of medication and stimulation settings. Other problems are also more frequent with STN DBS, including stimulation-induced dyskinesias, mood changes, stimulation-induced dysarthria, and sialorrhea.

There are relatively few data published regarding the long-term effects of bilateral GPi DBS. Some case series suggest a significant deterioration after 1–3 years, with recurrent off-periods and motor fluctuations that subsequently require more aggressive drug therapy; there is no indication that dyskinesias are increased over time (94,95). Some of these patients have subsequently undergone bilateral STN DBS with significant benefit (50).

VIII. SURGICAL METHODOLOGY

Surgery is performed with the patient awake in order to facilitate feedback of the beneficial and adverse effects of microstimulation and macrostimulation. Antiparkinsonian medication is withheld overnight prior to surgery so as to maximize off-period parkinsonism to allow optimal intraoperative assessment of the benefit of stimulation. Patients may become agitated during surgery. If patient reassurance fails, the use of short-acting benzodiazepines (e.g., midazolam) is warranted (96). If the patient becomes combative during surgery, administration of low-dose propafol sedation is generally helpful. It is occasionally possible to later terminate sedation and resume the procedure with improved patient cooperation. During a lengthy operation, patients may complain of back or neck pain and the use of a low-dose, short-acting narcotic (e.g., fentanyl) may be useful if additional padding and adjustment of the relationship between the operating table and stereotactic frame is inadequate. If patient behavior cannot be controlled and cooperation is lacking, terminating the surgery may be the most appropriate option to ensure patient safety and eliminate the probability of a misplaced electrode.

The operative methodology for DBS is similar to ablative stereotactic neurosurgery, excluding the final stage of electrode implantation. First, a stereotactic head frame is fixed to the skull to establish a 3D coordinate system to allow correlation of the preoperative imaging with each point in the brain and to prevent intraoperative head movement. Selection of the initial operative target may be performed indirectly (using a set formula based on the position of the anterior and posterior commissures) or directly using MRI visualization of the STN to account for inter-individual anatomical variations. Computed tomography (CT), MRI, or ventriculography may be used to identify the anterior and posterior commissures (97–102). CT- and MRI image–based fusion may also be performed to compensate for targeting error with MRI alone due to magnetic field inhomogeneity. The planned initial surgical trajectory should have an anterior-posterior angle of 45–60°, with shallower trajectories allowing one to avoid penetrating the anterior thalamus (possibly a source of some of the cognitive complications associated with the procedure). Although traditionally a vertical approach has been used, there has been a shift towards using a medial-lateral angle of 10–30° to avoid penetrating the lateral ventricle (reducing the risk of intraoperative brain shift and DBS electrode deviation) and increase the length of STN penetration by the DBS electrode due to its anatomical position.

There has been considerable debate regarding the advantages and disadvantages of microelectrode recording (MER) used in addition to traditional macrostimulation techniques to functionally identify the most appropriate site for electrode implantation. There has not been a randomized study of different surgical techniques confirming that MER improves outcomes compared with macrostimulation alone. However, the addition of MER should theoretically improve accuracy of the final electrode implantation site, provide assurance that the electrode is placed in the sensorimotor portion of the STN, and allow compensation for intraoperative brain shift or imaging anomalies (97–100,103). The use of MER significantly lengthens operative time. In addition, the number of microelectrode or macroelectrode penetrations in the brain is correlated with the risk of intracranial hemorrhage, and this risk should ideally be minimized while maintaining acceptable clinical outcomes (62). MER may be performed using a single microelectrode, with subsequent tracts performed serially as necessary to map the location of the sensorimotor portion of the STN and identify critical nearby structures (especially the corticospinal tract located along the anterior and lateral borders of the STN). Alternatively, many groups prefer to perform multiple simultaneous MER tracts using a fixed array of microelectrodes, most commonly a central microelectrode and four outer trajectories located 2 mm anteriorly, posteriorly, medially, and laterally. Using a five-electrode fixed array permits extensive mapping of the STN and surrounding region in a relatively short period of time and comparison of the data obtained in each trajectory without the concern about potential brain shift, which might occur in between multiple serial single MER tracts.

The STN can be distinguished from its neighboring structures based upon its irregular discharge rate (mean of 34–47 Hz), large amount of background noise that is characteristic of increased cell density, and the presence of movement-related neurons (100,102,104). The STN is typically recorded over a maximum of 5.3–5.9 mm. Upon exiting the STN, a short, relatively quiet area of approximately 1 mm may precede encountering SNr neurons, which are characterized by their regular, high-frequency firing rate (mean 71–86 Hz).

After recording, microstimulation may be performed at multiple sites along the tract, which often allows identification of nearby structures through induction of adverse effects (see Fig. 1). One may also estimate how close these structures are to the electrode tip by noting the stimulation current required to induce these adverse effects. Many groups perform high-amplitude stimulation through a semi-microelectrode and also perform serial examination of the clinical effects on features of parkinsonism.

Upon identification of the target site, the DBS electrode is implanted. The DBS electrode consists of four platinum-iridium contacts, with each contact 1.5 mm in length and separated by either 0.5 mm (model 3389) or 1.5 mm (model 3387). The DBS electrode is implanted so that it spans the sensorimotor portion of the STN identified by MER or the area of greatest clinical effectiveness and highest threshold for adverse effects identified with stimulation. Macrostimulation may be performed prior to fixation to the skull using a hand-held external stimulator (Medtronic Model 3625 or 3628) or via an electrically isolated constant current stimulator. The threshold for both adverse and beneficial effects should be assessed (see Fig. 1). Intraoperative stimulation-induced dyskinesias and improvement of segmental akinesia with stimulation are correlated with the greatest postoperative improvement of motor performance and reduction of antiparkinsonian medication, reflecting optimal electrode positioning (105). The hardware is finally secured to the skull with a plastic cap, metal plate, or cement. The remainder of the DBS hardware [implantable pulse generator (IPG) and extension cables] may be implanted under general anesthesia the same day or in a subsequent surgery. In the United States two single-channel IPGs, the Itrel II^{TM} and the Soletra^{TM}, are available, while in Canada, Europe, and elsewhere a dual-channel IPG is also available, the Kinetra^{TM}. The Kinetra may be associated with a slightly higher risk of adverse effects, such as infection and cutaneous erosion, possibly related to its greater weight and size (66). Since the Kinetra can independently stimulate two electrodes, bilateral DBS surgical time may be reduced because only one IPG is inserted subclavicularly compared with the need to implant two Soletra devices.

IX. POSTOPERATIVE MANAGEMENT

Postoperative management of PD patients with STN DBS is complex and demands a tremendous amount of time. Detailed guidelines have been published (96,106,107).

A. DBS Equipment and Stimulation Parameters

Stimulation settings are adjusted by means of a programmer placed on the skin overlying the IPG. The following stimulation parameters are adjustable: choice of active stimulation contacts including monopolar vs. bipolar stimulation, frequency, voltage, and pulse width. The Soletra can be turned off or on by the patient using a magnet (Control Magnet Model 7452) or using a hand-held patient programmer (Access Review^{TM} 7438). The Kinetra comes with the Access Therapy Controller^{TM}, which allows the patient to turn the stimulator off and on as well as modify the stimulation amplitude within parameters specified by the physician.

Determining the most effective contact(s) for stimulation is the first and most important task during stimulation programming. Monopolar stimulation is tested first with a single contact on the lead set as the cathode (−) and the pulse generator itself set as the anode (+). The threshold for persistent adverse effects and the degree of clinical benefit obtained stimulating below this threshold with monopolar stimulation of each contact should be determined with initial stimulation parameters of 60 μs and 130 Hz. Although generally one contact is used as the cathode, it is occasionally useful to activate two adjacent contacts for a broader field of current diffusion. Bipolar stimulation (one electrode contact as the anode and an adjacent electrode contact as the cathode) is valuable if adverse effects due to current spread to adjacent structures limits stimulation efficacy.

The IPG produces square wave pulses of 60–450 μs duration. Sixty μs is preferred since energy consumption is conserved and this pulse width results in the greatest therapeutic window (108,109). In the event that greater current spread is necessary for optimal results, then the pulse width may be increased, though rarely above 120 μs for STN DBS.

The Soletra is capable of stimulating at a rate up to 185 Hz and the Kinetra at rates up to 250 Hz. STN DBS has frequency-dependent effects on bradykinesia and rigidity with improvement beginning at approximately 100 Hz and plateauing at 130 Hz, with only minor additional improvement attainable with higher-frequency stimulation (108,109). Higher stimulation frequencies increase the "intensity" and clinical effects of stimulation in a given area, do not increase current spread, but do reduce battery life; hence, the lowest frequency of stimulation should be utilized whenever possible. Therefore, for STN DBS stimulation at 130 Hz should be used and only increased to 185 Hz if suboptimal benefit is achieved and an increase in pulse width or amplitude results in adverse effects due to current spread.

Battery life is largely dependent on the amount of daily usage. Most PD patients require stimulation 24 hours per day in order to maintain nocturnal mobility and because of significant delayed beneficial effects of continuous stimulation on bradykinesia and gait, which would be lost if stimulation were stopped at night. With STN DBS, typical battery lifetime for the Soletra is 4–7 years. In PD patients with STN DBS who have substantially decreased their dosage of antiparkinsonian medication, battery failure may result in severe worsening. Antiparkinsonian medication may need to be transiently increased until battery replacement. IPG failure with battery depletion occurs over several days; therefore, if the patients notice waning of the effects of stimulation, they should contact their physician to have the IPG assessed. For PD patients who live in remote areas, battery replacement may be performed prophylactically according to the predicted battery lifetime.

Battery consumption for the Kinetra is linear across the entire amplitude range (0–10.5 V), while battery consumption for the Soletra increases abruptly when amplitude is increased from 3.6 to 3.7 V due to a "doubling circuit," in which a second capacitor is switched into the system. Therefore, stimulation amplitude ≤ 3.6 V should be used to prolong battery life when using the Soletra. If greater current spread and clinical effects are required with a given electrode combination, stimulation pulse width should be increased rather than stimulation amplitude.

B. Deep Brain Stimulation Programming

Some groups begin chronic stimulation within a day of surgery, while others prefer to wait approximately 2–4 weeks after electrode implantation to begin programming, allowing most of the acute microlesion effect to wane with resolution of peri-electrode edema (which influences stimulation parameters) and wounds over the IPG to heal, making programming more comfortable. A few DBS programming sessions are usually necessary to optimize the stimulation settings, although the actual number of sessions required may be highly variable between individual patients. Figure 2 details the initial programming process, which in the case of bilateral STN DBS is carried out on each side independently. Thereafter, bilateral stimulation is begun and the threshold for stimulation-induced dyskinesias may be reduced compared to unilateral stimulation, necessitating reduction in stimulation amplitude.

Identifying the nature of the adverse effects of stimulating the STN region allows one to determine the relative location of each of the contacts to adjacent structures and appropriate management (Fig. 1). A large number of adverse effects can be induced by current spread outside of the target. Stimulation too far lateral or anterior may stimulate the corticospinal tract and corticobulbar fibers and result in dysarthria and tonic muscle contraction (107,110). Unilateral eye deviation due to stimulation of fascicles of the oculomotor nerve occurs if stimulation is too medial, while stimulating medially in the region of the red nucleus may induce postural disturbances and gait ataxia (107,110). Stimulation of the medial lemniscus, located posterior to the STN, induces paresthesias and dysesthesias (110). Stimulation ventrally in the SNr may increase akinesia or inhibit the effects of levodopa (107). Adverse effects that rapidly habituate (e.g., paresthesias) do not prevent further increase in stimulation if needed, while adverse effects that do not habituate (e.g., tonic muscle contraction) require a reduction or change in stimulation (107).

Most STN programming is initially performed with the patient in the off-drug state after overnight withdrawal of antiparkinsonian medication (14). The clinical effects of any setting should be assessed after approximately 15 minutes of chronic stimulation.

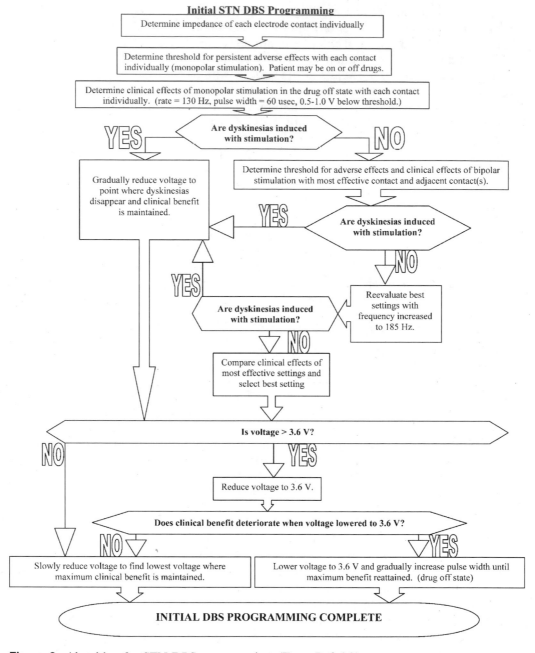

Figure 2   Algorithm for STN DBS programming. (From Ref. 96.)

Rigidity and tremor are generally improved in less than 1 minute, while bradykinesia gradually improves over several minutes and may take several hours to be maximally improved. Off-period dystonia is also markedly improved within minutes of initiating stimulation. Stimulation-induced dyskinesias may occur within minutes to days and suggest that parkinsonism may be maximally improved (14,111). Prior to assessing the effects of another stimulation setting, stimulation should be turned off for at least 10 minutes in order to avoid carry-over effects. If no significant benefit is obtained with any contact, then the electrode is most likely suboptimally positioned and drug therapy should be increased until the electrode can be surgically repositioned.

The effects of STN DBS on drug-induced dyskinesias should be assessed once the patient has taken levodopa, generally in the afternoon, since dyskinesias commonly exhibit a diurnal pattern. Since STN stimulation reduces the threshold for levodopa to induce dyskinesias, antiparkinsonian medication must be reduced in order to reduce dyskinesias. One option is to first reduce and discontinue levodopa while maintaining continuous dopaminergic stimulation, if needed, with long-acting dopamine agonists, which are less likely to induce dyskinesias. With drug reduction and continuous STN stimulation, the threshold for reduction of dyskinesias gradually increases, allowing a corresponding increase in stimulation over the first 3–6 months postoperatively (106). As mentioned earlier, overly aggressive levodopa reduction may result in abulia, anhedonia, and depression due to the withdrawal of its positive psychotropic effects.

Depression related to drug withdrawal must be differentiated from that due to inadvertent stimulation of the SNr, which resolves within minutes of stopping stimulation. Reinstitution of levodopa up to the threshold that produces mild nondisabling dyskinesias usually quickly improves these symptoms. For persistent symptoms or when disabling dyskinesias limit levodopa therapy, the use of serotonin reuptake inhibitors can be helpful (107). Reduction in dopaminergic medication may also unmask symptoms of previously unrecognized restless legs syndrome (RLS). Although STN stimulation itself may improve RLS, additional drug therapy is often necessary. Reintroduction of controlled-release levodopa or dopamine agonists may be very helpful, but may significantly increase dyskinesias. In such cases, use of benzodiazepines or opiates may be preferred (96).

In the first 2–3 months postoperatively, the effects of STN stimulation may seem to wane as the microlesion associated with surgery diminishes. This can be managed by slightly increasing stimulation. If stimulation-induced adverse effects prevent optimal improvement, then changing stimulation to an adjacent contact or bipolar stimulation should be considered. If optimum improvement is still not achievable, the electrode is likely suboptimally positioned and dopaminergic therapy should be increased. By 3 months, stimulation settings remain relatively stable in the majority of patients.

X. FUTURE DEVELOPMENTS

Although STN DBS represents a tremendous advance in the symptomatic therapy of advanced PD, hardware complications and complexity of surgery and postoperative management limit the availability of this therapy. To address these concerns hardware manufacturers are currently developing a rechargeable IPG, which may eliminate the need for battery replacement, and changing the design of other components of the system. The development of a closed-loop system with sensors that detect local neuronal activity, a processing system to interpret these data, and potentially multiple output electrodes might allow more precise and physiological modification of local nuclei and downstream connections, resulting in greater efficacy and applicability of DBS to a greater variety of neurological disorders. The duration of surgery may be shortened by eliminating the need for MER and the precision of surgery improved if the STN could be adequately imaged and surgery guided by new-generation higher field strength intraoperative MRI scanners. These technological advances could move DBS to a first-line therapy.

REFERENCES

1. Abosch A, Lang AE, Hutchison WD, Lozano AM. Subthalamic deep brain stimulation for Parkinson's disease. Tarsy D, Vitek JL, Lozano AM, eds. Surgical Treatment of Parkinson's Disease and Other Movement Disorders. Totowa, NJ: Humana Press Inc., 2003:175–187.

2. Obeso JA, Rodriguez MC, DeLong MR. Basal ganglia pathophysiology: a critical review. Obeso JA, DeLong MR, Ohye C, Marsden CD, eds. Advances in Neurology, The Basal Ganglia and New Surgical Approaches for Parkinson's Disease. Philadelphia: Lippincott-Raven, 1997:74:3–18.

3. Bergman H, Wichmann T, Karmon B, DeLong MR. The primate subthalamic nucleus. II. Neuronal activity in the MPTP model of parkinsonism. J Neurophysiol 1994; 72:507–520.

4. Rodriguez MC, Obeso JA, Olanow CW. Subthalamic nucleus-mediated excitotoxicity in Parkinson's disease: a target for neuroprotection. Ann Neurol 1998; 44(suppl 1):175–188.

5. Lange H, Thorner G, Hopf A. [Morphometric-statistical structure analysis of humanstriatum, pallidum and nucleus subthalamicus. III. Nucleus subthalamicus]. J Hirnforsch 1976; 17:31–41.

6. Parent A, Hazrati LN. Functional anatomy of the basal ganglia. II. The place of subthalamic nucleus and external pallidum in basal ganglia circuitry. Brain Res Brain Res Rev 1995; 20:128–154.

7. Theodosopoulos PV, Marks WJ Jr, Christine C, Starr PA, Locations of movement-related cells in the human subthalamic nucleus in Parkinson's disease. Mov Disord 2003; 18:791–798.

8. Parent A, Cicchetti F. The current model of basal ganglia organization under scrutiny. Mov Disord 1998; 13:199–202.

9. Fujimoto K, Kita H. Response characteristics of subthalamic neurons to the stimulation of the sensorimotor cortex in the rat. Brain Res 1993; 609:185–192.

10. Levy R, Ashby P, Hutchison WD, Lang AE, Lozano AM, Dostrovsky JO. Dependence of subthalamic nucleus oscillations on movement and dopamine in Parkinson's disease. Brain 2002; 125:1196–1209.

11. Brown P, Oliviero A, Mazzone P, Insola A, Tonali P, Di Lazzaro V. Dopamine dependency of oscillations between subthalamic nucleus and pallidum in Parkinson's disease. J Neurosci 2001; 21:1033–1038.

12. Levy R, Hutchison WD, Lozano AM, Dostrovsky JO. High-frequency synchronization of neuronal activity in the subthalamic nucleus of parkinsonian patients with limb tremor. J Neurosci 2000; 20:7766–7775.

13. Smith ID, Grace AA. Role of subthalamic nucleus in the regulation of nigral dopamine neuron activity. Synapse 1992; 12:287–303.

14. Pollak P. Deep brain stimulation. Presented at the 52nd Annual Meeting of the American Academy of Neurology, San Diego, CA, May 1, 2000.

15. Tehovnik EJ. Electrical stimulation of neural tissue to evoke behavioral responses. J Neurosci Methods 1996; 65:1–17.

16. Caparros-Lefebvre D, Ruchoux MM, Blond S, Petit H, Percheron G. Long-term thalamic stimulation in Parkinson's disease: postmortem anatomoclinical study. Neurology 1994; 44:1856–1860.

17. Haberler C, Alesch F, Mazal PR, Pilz P, Jellinger K, Pinter MM, Hainfellner JA, Budka H. No tissue damage by chronic deep brain stimulation in Parkinson's disease. Ann Neurol 2000; 48:372–376.

18. Voges J, Volkmann J, Allert N, Lehrke R, Koulousakis A, Freund HJ, Sturm V. Bilateral high-frequency stimulation in the subthalamic nucleus for the treatment of Parkinson disease: correlation of therapeutic effect with anatomical electrode position. J Neurosurg 2002; 96:269–279.

19. Kumar R, Martin K, McVicker JM. Correlation of electrode location and clinical effects in subthalamic nucleus (STN) deep brain stimulation (DBS) in Parkinson's disease. Neurology 2000; 54(suppl 3):281–282.

20. Ashby P, Rothwell JC. Neurophysiologic aspects of deep brain stimulation. Neurology 2000; 55(suppl 6):17–20.

21. Dostrovsky JO, Lozano AM. Mechanisms of deep brain stimulation. Mov Disord 2002; 17(suppl 3):63–68.

22. Hashimoto T, Elder CM, DeLong MR, Vitek JL. Responses of pallidal neurons to electrical stimulation of the subthalamic nucleus in experimental parkinsonism. Mov Disord 2000; 15(suppl 3):31.

23. Bruet N, Windels F, Poupard A, Savasta M. High frequency stimulation of subthalamic nucleus increases striatal dopamine release in normal and partially dopaminergic denervated rats. Mov Disord 2000; 15(suppl 3):15.

24. Windels F, Bruet N, Poupard A, Savasta M. High frequency stimulation of subthalamic nucleus increases extracellular contents of glutamate in substantia nigra and external pallidum. Mov Disord 2000; 15(suppl 3):15.

25. Ceballos-Baumann AO, Boecker H, Bartenstein P, von Falkenhayn I, Riescher H, Conrad B, Moringlane JR, Alesch F. A positron emission tomographic study of subthalamic nucleus stimulation in Parkinson's disease: enhanced movement-related activity of motor-association cortex and decreased motor cortex resting activity. Arch Neurol 1999; 56:997–1003.
26. Sestini S, Scotto di Luzio A, Ammannati F, De Cristofaro MT, Passeri A, Martini S, Pupi A. Changes in regional cerebral blood flow caused by deep-brain stimulation of the subthalamic nucleus in Parkinson's disease. J Nucl Med 2002; 43:725–732.
27. Strafella AP, Dagher A, Sadikot AF. Cerebral blood flow changes induced by subthalamic stimulation in Parkinson's disease. Neurology 2003; 60:1039–1042.
28. Schroeder U, Kuehler A, Haslinger B, Erhard P, Fogel W, Tronnier VM, Lange KW, Boecker H, Ceballos-Baumann AO. Subthalamic nucleus stimulation affects striato-anterior cingulate cortex circuit in a response conflict task: a PET study. Brain 2002; 125:1995–2004.
29. Cunic D, Roshan L, Khan FI, Lozano AM, Lang AE, Chen R. Effects of subthalamic nucleus stimulation on motor cortex excitability in Parkinson's disease. Neurology 2002; 58:1665–1672.
30. Barlas O, Hanağasi H, İmer M, Sçahin HA, Sencer S, Emre M. Do unilateral ablative lesions of the subthalamic nucleu in parkinsonian patients lead to hemiballism?. Mov Disord 2001; 16:306–310.
31. Guridi J, Obeso JA. The subthalamic nucleus, hemiballismus and Parkinson's disease: reappraisal of a neurosurgical dogma. Brain 2001; 124:5–19.
32. Alvarez L, Macias R, Guridi J, Lopez G, Alvarez E, Maragoto C, Teijeiro J, Torres A, Pavon N, Rodriguez-Oroz MC, Ochoa L, Hetherington H, Juncos J, DeLong MR, Obeso JA. Dorsal subthalamotomy for Parkinson's disease. Mov Disord 2001; 16:72–78.
33. Su PC, Tseng H-M, Liu H-M, Yen R-F, Liou H-H. Treatment of advanced Parkinson's disease by subthalamotomy: one-year results. Mov Disord 2003; 18:531–538.
34. Alvarez L, Macias R, Lopez G, Maragoto C, Teijeiro J, Torres A, Alvarez E, Pavon N, Ochoa L. Bilateral subthalamotomy in Parkinson's disease (PD). Mov Disord 1998; 13(suppl 2):303.
35. Gill SS, Heywood P. Bilateral subthalamic nucleotomy can be accomplished safely. Mov Disord 1998; 13(suppl 2):201.
36. Alvarez L, Macias R, Lopez G, Alvarez E, Maragoto C, Teijeiro J, Garcia I, Villegas A, Piedra J, Leon M, Pavon N, Rodriguez-Oroz MC, Guridi J, Obeso JA. Bilateral subthalamotomy in Parkinson's disease. Mov Disord 2000; 15(suppl 3):65.
37. McCarter RJ, Walton NH, Rowan AF, Gill SS, Palomo M. Cognitive functioning after subthalamic nucleotomy for refractory Parkinson's disease. J Neurol Neurosurg Psychiatry 2000; 69:60–66.
38. Schuurman PR, Bosch DA, Bossuyt PM, Bonsel GJ, van Someren EJ, de Bie RM, Merkus MP, Speelman JD. A comparison of continuous thalamic stimulation and thalamotomy for suppression of severe tremor. N Engl J Med 2000; 342:461–468.
39. Scott R, Gregory R, Hines N, Carroll C, Hyman N, Papanasstasiou V, Leather C, Rowe J, Silburn P, Aziz T. Neuropsychological, neurological and functional outcome following pallidotomy for Parkinson's disease. A consecutive series of eight simultaneous bilateral and twelve unilateral procedures. Brain 1998; 121:659–675.
40. Merello M, Starkstein S, Nouzeilles MI, Kuzis G, Leiguarda R. Bilateral pallidotomy for treatment of Parkinson's disease induced corticobulbar syndrome and psychic akinesia avoidable by globus pallidus lesion combined with contralateral stimulation. J Neuol Neurosurg Psychiatry 2001; 71:611–614.
41. Ghika J, Ghika-Schmid F, Fankhauser H, Assal G, Vingerhoets F, Albanese A, Bogousslavsky J, Favre J. Bilateral contemporaneous posteroventral pallidotomy for the treatment of Parkinson's disease: neuropsychological and neurological side effects. Report of four cases and review of the literature. J Neurosurg 1999; 91:313–321.
42. Favre J, Burchiel KJ, Taha JM, Hammerstad J. Outcome of unilateral and bilateral pallidotomy for Parkinson's disease: patient assessment. Neurosurgery 2000; 46:344–353.
43. Intemann PM, Masterman D, Subramanian I, DeSalles A, Behnke E, Frysinger R, Bronstein JM. Staged bilateral pallidotomy for treatment of Parkinson disease. J Neurosurg 2001; 94:437–444.
44. Hallett M, Litvan I. Task Force on Surgery for Parkinson's Disease. Evaluation of surgery for Parkinson's disease: a report of the therapeutics and technology assessment subcommittee of the American Academy of Neurology. Neurology 1999; 53:1910–1921.
45. Oh MY, Abosch A, Kim SH, Lang AE, Lozano AM. Long-term hardware-related complications of deep brain stimulation. Neursurgery 2002; 50:1268–1274.
46. Kern DS, McVicker JH, Martin K, Kumar R. Sustained long-term benefit and adverse effects of bilateral subthalamic nucleus (STN) deep brain stimulation (DBS) in Parkinson disease (PD). Neurology 2003; 60(suppl 1):120–121.

47. Mesnage V, Houeto JL, Welter ML, Agid Y, Pidoux B, Dormont D, Cornu P. Parkinson's disease: neurosurgery at an earlier stage? J Neurol Neurosurg Psychiatry 2002; 73:778–779.
48. Saint-Cyr JA, Trépanier LL, Kumar R, Lozano AM, Lang AE. Neuropsychological consequences of chronic bilateral stimulation of the subthalamic nucleus in Parkinson's disease. Brain 2000; 123:2091–2108.
49. Saint-Cyr JA, Trépanier LL. Neuropsychologic assessment of patients for movement disorder surgery. Mov Disord 2000; 15:771–783.
50. Houeto JL, Bejjani PB, Damier P, Staedler C, Bonnet AM, Pidoux B, Dormont D, Cornu P, Agid Y. Failure of long-term pallidal stimulation corrected by subthalamic stimulation in PD. Neurology 2000; 55:728–730.
51. Mogilner AY, Sterio D, Rezai AR, Zonenshayn M, Kelly PJ, Beric A. Subthalamic nucleus stimulation in patients with a prior pallidotomy. J Neurosurg 2002; 96:660–665.
52. Yokoyama T, Sugiyama K, Nishizawa S, Yokota N, Ohta S, Uemura K. Subthalamic nucleus stimulation for gait disturbance in Parkinson's disease. Neurosurgery 1999; 45:41–47.
53. Welter ML, Houeto JL, Tezenas du Montcel S, Mesnage V, Bonnet AM, Pillon B, Arnulf I, Pidoux B, Dormont D, Cornu P, Agid Y. Clinical predictive factors of subthalamic stimulation in Parkinson's disease. Brain 2002; 125:575–583.
54. Pinter MM, Alesch F, Murg M, Helscher RJ, Binder H. Apomorphine test: a predictor for motor responsiveness to deep brain stimulation of the subthalamic nucleus. J Neurol 1999; 246:907–913.
55. Kern DS, McVicker JH, Martin K, Kumar R. Effective subthalamic nucleus (STN) deep brain stimulation (DBS) in levodopa-unresponsive parkinsonism. Neurology 2003; 60(suppl 1):125.
56. Kazumata K, Antonini A, Dhawan V, Moeller JR, Alterman RL, Kelly P, Sterio D, Fazzini E, Beric A, Eidelberg D. Preoperative indicators of clinical outcome following stereotaxic pallidotomy. Neurology 1997; 49:1083–1090.
57. Iansek R, Rosenfeld JV, Huxham FE. Deep brain stimulation of the subthalamic nucleus in Parkinson's disease. Med J Aust 2002; 177:142–146.
58. Krack P, Dowsey PL, Benabid AL, Acarin N, Benazzouz A, Künig G, Leenders KL, Obeso JA, Pollak P. Ineffective subthalamic nucleus stimulation in levodopa-resistant postischemic parkinsonism. Neurology 2000; 54:2182–2184.
59. Visser-Vandewalle V, Temel Y, Colle H, van der Linden C. Bilateral high-frequency stimulation of the subthalamic nucleus in patients with multiple system atrophy–parkinsonism. Report of four cases. J Neurosurg 2003; 98:882–887.
60. Tomaszewski KJ, Holloway RG. Deep brain stimulation in the treatment of Parkinson's disease: a cost-effectiveness analysis. Neurology 2001; 57:663–671.
61. Kumar R, Lozano AM, Kim YJ, Hutchison WD, Sime E, Halket E, Lang AE. Double-blind evaluation of subthalamic nucleus deep brain stimulation in advanced Parkinson's disease. Neurology 1998; 51:850–855.
62. The Deep-Brain Stimulation for Parkinson's Disease Study Group. Deep-brain stimulation of the subthalamic nucleus or the pars interna of the globus pallidus in Parkinson's disease. N Engl J Med 2001; 345:956–963.
63. Limousin P, Krack P, Pollak P, Benazzouz A, Ardouin C, Hoffmann D, Benabid AL. Electrical stimulation of the subthalamic nucleus in advanced Parkinson's disease. N Engl J Med 1998; 339:1105–1111.
64. Burchiel KJ, Anderson VC, Favre J, Hammerstad JP. Comparison of pallidal and subthalamic nucleus deep brain stimulation for advanced Parkinson's disease: results of a randomized, blinded pilot study. Neurosurgery 1999; 45:1375–1382.
65. Volkmann J, Allert N, Voges J, Weiss PH, Freund HJ, Sturm V. Safety and efficacy of pallidal or subthalamic nucleus stimulation in advanced PD. Neurology 2001; 56:548–551.
66. Vesper J, Chabardes S, Fraix V, Sunde N, Østergaard K. the Kineta Study Group. Dual channel deep brain stimulation system (Kinetra) for Parkinson's disease and essential tremor: a prospective multicentre open label clinical study. J Neurol Neurosurg Psychiatry 2002; 73:275–280.
67. Bejjani BP, Arnulf I, Demeret S, Damier P, Bonnet AM, Houeto JL, Agid Y. Levodopa-induced dyskinesias in Parkinson's disease: is sensitization reversible?. Ann Neurol 2000; 47:655–658.
68. Pollak P, Fraix V, Krack P, Moro E, Mendes A, Chabardes S, Koudsie A, Benabid AL. Treatment results: Parkinson's disease. Mov Disord 2002; 17(suppl 3):75–83.
69. Kumar R. Deep brain stimulation. Jankovic JJ, Tolosa E, eds. Parkinson's Disease and Movement Disorders. Philadelphia: Lippincott Williams and Wilkins2002:4:674–689.
70. Vingerhoets FJ, Villemure JG, Temperli P, Pollo C, Pralong E, Ghika J. Subthalamic DBS replaces levodopa in Parkinson's disease: two-year follow-up. Neurology 2002; 58:396–401.

71. Bejjani BP, Gervais D, Arnulf I, Papadopoulos S, Demeret S, Bonnet AM, Cornu P, Damier P, Agid Y. Axial parkinsonian symptoms can be improved: the role of levodopa and bilateral subthalamic stimulation. J Neurol Neurosurg Psychiatry 2000; 68:595–600.

72. Witjas T, Kaphan E, Azulay JP, Regis J, Chérif AA, Peragut JC. Effects of subthalamic nucleus (STN) deep brain stimulation (DBS) on non-motor fluctuations (NMF) on Parkinson's disease. Neurology 2001; 56(suppl 3):274.

73. Batir A, Krack P, Fraix V, Koudsie A, Chabardes S, Funkiewiez A. Five-year follow-up of bilateral stimulation of the subthalamic nucleus in advanced Parkinson's disease (PD). Mov Disord 2002; 17(suppl 5):196–197.

74. Arzbaecher JM, Bakay RAE, Sierens D, Verwey NA, Myre B, Verhagen L. Quality of life outcomes in patients with advanced Parkinson's disease treated with unilateral deep brain stimulation of the sub-thalamic nucleus. Neurology 2003; 60(suppl 1):121–122.

75. Kumar R, Lozano AM, Sime E, Halket E, Lang AE. Comparative effects of unilateral and bilateral subthalamic nucleus deep brain stimulation. Neurology 1999; 53:561–566.

76. Pillon B, Ardouin C, Damier P, Krack P, Houeto JL, Klinger H, Bonnet AM, Pollak P, Benabid AL, Agid Y. Neuropsychological changes between "off" and "on" STN or GPi stimulation in Parkinson's disease. Neurology 2000; 55:411–418.

77. Funkiewiez A, Ardouin C, Krack P, Fraix V, Van Blercom N, Xie J, Moro E, Benabid AL, Pollak P. Acute psychotropic effects of bilateral subthalamic nucleus stimulation and levodopa in Parkinson's disease. Mov Disord 2003; 18:524–530.

78. Houeto JL, Mesnage V, Mallet L, Pillon B, Gargiulo M, du Moncel ST, Bonnet AM, Pidoux B, Dormont D, Cornu P, Agid Y. Behavioural disorders, Parkinson's disease and subthalamic stimulation. J Neurol Neurosurg Psychiatry 2002; 72:701–707.

79. Bejjani BP, Damier P, Arnulf I, Thivard L, Bonnet A-M, Dormont D, Cornu P, Pidoux B, Samson Y, Agid Y. Transient acute depression induced by high-frequency deep brain stimulation. N Engl J Med 1999; 340:1476–1480.

80. Doshi PK, Chhaya N, Bhatt MH. Depression leading to attempted suicide after bilateral subthalamic nucleus stimulation for Parkinson's disease. Mov Disord 2002; 17:1084–1085.

81. Kulisevsky J, Berthier ML, Gironell A, Pascual-Sedano B, Molet J, Parés P. Mania following deep brain stimulation for Parkinson's disease. Neurology 2002; 59:1421–1424.

82. Romito LM, Raja M, Daniele A, Contarino MF, Bentivoglio AR, Barbier A, Scerrati M, Albanese A. Transient mania and hypersexuality after surgery for high-frequency stimulation of the subthalamic nucleus in Parkinson's disease. Mov Disord 2002; 17:1371–1374.

83. Krack P, Kumar R, Ardouin C, Dowsey PL, McVicker JM, Benabid AL, Pollak P. Mirthful laughter induced by subthalamic nucleus stimulation. Mov Disord 2001; 16:867–875.

84. Bejjani BP, Houeto JL, Hariz M, Yelnik J, Mesnage V, Bonnet AM, Pidoux B, Dormont D, Cornu P, Agid Y. Aggressive behavior induced by intraoperative stimulation in the triangle of Sano. Neurology 2002; 59:1425–1427.

85. Mallet L, Mesnage V, Houeto JL, Pelissolo A, Yelnik J, Behar C, Gargiulo M, Welter ML, Bonnet A-M, Pillon B, Cornu P, Dormont D, Pidoux B, Allilaire JF, Agid Y. Compulsions, Parkinson's disease, and stimulation. Lancet 2002; 360:1302–1304.

86. Koller W, Pahwa R, Busenbark K, Hubble J, Wilkinson S, Lang A, Tuite P, Sime E, Lazano A, Hauser R, Malapira T, Smith D, Tarsy D, Miyawaki E, Norregaard T, Kormos T, Olanow CW. High-frequency unilateral thalamic stimulation in the treatment of essential and parkinsonian tremor. Ann Neurol 1997; 42:292–299.

87. Limousin P, Speelman JD, Gielen F, Janssens. Multicentre European study of thalamic stimulation in parkinsonian and essential tremor. J Neurol Neurosurg Psychiatry 1999; 66:289–296.

88. Woods SP, Fields JA, Lyons KE, Koller WC, Wilkinson SB, Pahwa R, Tröster AI. Neuropsychological and quality of life changes following unilateral thalamic deep brain stimulation in Parkinson's disease: a one-year follow-up. Acta Neurochir (Wien) 2001; 143:1273–1277.

89. Obwegeser AA, Uitti RJ, Witte RJ, Lucas JA, Turk MF, Wharen RE Jr. Quantitative and qualitative outcome measures after thalamic deep brain stimulation to treat disabling tremors. Neurosurgery 2001; 48:274–281.

90. Lyons KE, Koller WC, Wilkinson SB, Pahwa R. Long term safety and efficacy of unilateral deep brain stimulation of the thalamus for parkinsonian tremor. J Neurol Neurosurg Psychiatry 2001; 71:682–684.

91. Tröster AI, Wilkinson SB, Fields JA, Miyawaki K, Koller WC. Chronic electrical stimulation of the left ventrointermediate (Vim) thalamic nucleus for the treatment of pharmacotherapy-resistant Parkinson's disease: a differential impact on access to semantic and episodic memory?. Brain Cogn 1998; 38:125–149.

92. Krauss JK, Simpson RK Jr, Ondo WG, Pohle T, Burgunder JM, Jankovic J. Concepts and methods in chronic thalamic stimulation for treatment of tremor: technique and application. Neurosurgery 2001; 48:535–541.

93. Krack P, Pollak P, Limousin P, Hoffmann D, Xie J, Benazzouz A, Benabid AL. Subthalamic nucleus or internal pallidal stimulation in young onset Parkinson's disease. Brain 1998; 121:451–457.

94. Ghika J, Villemure JG, Fankhauser H, Favre J, Assal G, Ghika-Schmid F. Efficiency and safety of bilateral contemporaneous pallidal stimulation (deep brain stimulation) in levodopa-responsive patients with Parkinson's disease with severe motor fluctuations: a 2-year follow-up review. J Neurosurg 1998; 89:713–718.

95. Volkmann J, Allert N, Voges J, Koulousakis A, Sturm V, Freund H-J. Long-term results of bilateral pallidal DBS in advanced Parkinson's disease (PD). Mov Disord 2002; 17(suppl 5):203.

96. Kumar R. Methods of programming and patient management with deep brain stimulation. Tarsy D, Vitek JL, Lozano AM, eds. Surgical Treatment of Parkinson's Disease and Other Movement Disordres. Totowa, NJ: Humana Press Inc.2003:189–212.

97. Limousin P, Pollak P, Benazzouz A, Hoffmann D, Le Bas JF, Broussolle E, Perret JE, Benabid AL. Effect of parkinsonian signs and symptoms of bilateral subthalamic nucleus stimulation. Lancet 1995; 345:91–95.

98. Hutchison WD, Allan RJ, Opitz H, Levy R, Dostrovsky JO, Lang AE, Lozano AM. Neurophysiological identification of the subthalamic nucleus in surgery for Parkinson's disease. Ann Neurol 1998; 44:622–628.

99. Lozano A, Hutchison W, Kiss Z, Tasker R, Davis K, Dostrovsky J. Methods for microelectrode-guided posteroventral pallidotomy. J Neurosurg 1996; 84:194–202.

100. Starr PA, Christine CW, Theodosopoulos PV, Lindsey N, Byrd D, Mosley A, Marks WJ Jr. Implantation of deep brain stimulators into the subthalamic nucleus: technical approach and magnetic resonance imaging–verified lead locations. J Neurosurg 2002; 97:370–387.

101. Simuni T, Jaggi JL, Mulholland H, Hurtig HI, Colcher A, Siderowf AD, Ravina B, Skolnick BE, Goldstein R, Stern MB, Baltuch GH. Bilateral stimulation of the subthalamic nucleus in patients with Parkinson disease: a study of efficacy and safety. J Neurosurg 2002; 96:666–672.

102. Sterio D, Zonenshayn M, Mogilner AY, Rezai AR, Kiprovski K, Kelly PJ, Beric A. Neurophysiological refinement of subthalamic nucleus targeting. Neurosurgery 2002; 50:58–67.

103. Bejjani BP, Dormont D, Pidoux B, Yelnik J, Damier P, Arnulf I, Bonnet AM, Marsault C, Agid Y, Philippon J, Cornu P. Bilateral subthalamic stimulation for Parkinson's disease by using three-dimensional stereotactic magnetic resonance imaging and electrophysiological guidance. J Neurosurg 2000; 92:615–625.

104. Pralong E, Ghika J, Temperli P, Pollo C, Vingerhoets F, Villemure JG. Electrophysiological localization of the subthalamic nucleus in parkinsonian patients. Neurosci Lett 2002; 325:144–146.

105. Houeto JL, Welter ML, Bejjani PB, Tezenas du Montcel S, Bonnet AM, Mesnage V, Navarro S, Pidoux B, Dormont D, Cornu P, Agid Y. Subthalamic stimulation in Parkinson's disease: intraoperative predictive factors. Arch Neurol 2003; 60:690–694.

106. Krack P, Fraix V, Mendes A, Benabid AL, Pollak P. Postoperative management of subthalamic nucleus stimulation for Parkinson's disease. Mov Disord 2002; 17(suppl 3):188–197.

107. Volkmann J, Fogel W, Krack P. Postoperative neurological management—stimulation of the subthalamic nucleus. Akt Neurol 2000; 27(suppl 1):23–39.

108. Moro E, Esselink RJ, Xie J, Hommel M, Benabid AL, Pollak P. The impact of Parkinson's disease of electrical parameter settings in STN stimulation. Neurology 2002; 59:706–713.

109. Rizzone M, Lanotte M, Bergamasco B, Tavella A, Torre E, Faccani G, Melcarne A, Lopiano L. Deep brain stimulation of the subthalamic nucleus in Parkinson's disease: effects of variation in stimulation parameters. J Neurol Neurosurg Psychiatry 2001; 71:215–219.

110. Pollak P, Krack P, Fraix V, Mendes A, Moro E, Chabardes S, Benabid AL. Intraoperative micro- and macrostimulation of the subthalamic nucleus in Parkinson's disease. Mov Disord 2002; 17(suppl 3):155–161.

111. Limousin P, Pollak P, Hoffmann D, Benazzouz A, Perret JE, Benabid AL. Abnormal involuntary movements induced by subthalamic nucleus stimulation. Mov Disord 1996; 11:231–235.

25
Cell Transplantation

Robert A. Hauser and Theresa A. Zesiewicz
*Parkinson's Disease and Movement Disorders Center,
University of South Florida, Tampa, Florida, U.S.A.*

I. INTRODUCTION

Medical management of Parkinson's disease (PD) has long-term limitations. Fifty percent of PD patients who are treated with levodopa develop motor complications (fluctuations and dyskinesias) after 5 years of therapy (1). In addition, many patients develop disabling symptoms such as dementia or imbalance, for which medical therapy provides little or no benefit.

Transplantation of cells to replace those that are lost to the disease process provides a rational method to achieve long-term control of symptoms (2). PD is associated with a relatively selective degeneration of dopaminergic nigrostriatal neurons, and patients with disability related to motor fluctuations retain the ability to respond to dopaminergic stimulation. The transplantation of cells that could restore physiological dopamine stimulation might theoretically restore optimal motor function throughout the day. Patients with disability due to nondopaminergic symptoms might still respond to cell transplantation if such cells could migrate to the areas where cells have been lost, integrate into the neuronal circuitry, and function in a physiological fashion. It is hoped that stem cells possess such capabilities.

Attempts at cell transplantation in PD patients to date have focused on improving clinical status in patients with an unsatisfactory response to medical management due to motor fluctuations. Preclinical and open-label studies have suggested considerable promise. However, double-blind studies have largely been negative, and some patients who received human embryonic mesencephalic tranplants developed severe ("runaway") dyskinesias.

The preclinical groundwork for cell transplantation in PD was developed in the late 1970s and early 1980s, when human embryonic mesencephalic cell transplantation was performed in parkinsonian rat models with subsequent improvement in motor behavior (3–5). Grafting studies in animal models demonstrated that mesencephalic grafts survived and reinnervated the striatum while improving motor deficits in parkinsonian rats and monkeys (2). Behavioral improvement depended on the implantation site (6,7) and the age of the grafted tissue (2). Fetal mesencephalon transplants were subsequently performed in human subjects in open-label and double-blind trials (8–27). Because of ethical concerns and the limited supply of human embryonic tissue, alternative cells have been investigated, including porcine embryonic mesencephalic cells and human retinal cells. This chapter will review the current literature on cell transplantation in PD patients.

II. HUMAN FETAL MESENCEPHALIC TRANSPLANTATION IN PD: OPEN-LABEL TRIALS

Several hundred PD patients have received transplanted human mesencephalic tissue, mostly in small, unblinded trials at multiple investigational sites (9–27). Transplanted patients were mostly those who has medication-resistant disability related to motor fluctuations (28). Fetal transplants were prepared as blocks of tissue or suspensions of dissociated cells (28). Donor age varied from 5 to 17 weeks postconception (28), and three to five fetal nigra were generally transplanted per side into the striatum. In some studies patients received immunosuppression.

Many of these studies found that transplanted dopamine neurons survived transplantation and led to clinical motor improvement over several months to years, with reductions in off time, improvement in Unified Parkinson's Disease Rating Scale (UPDRS) scores, decreased dyskinesia, and lowering of levodopa dosages (9–27). Hauser et al. found 32% improvement in UPDRS total off scores 20 months following transplantation in six patients (23). On time without dyskinesia improved from 22 to 60%, and fluorodopa (FD) uptake as measured by positron emission tomography (PET) was significantly increased at 6 (48%) and 12 months (61%). Increases in FD uptake were correlated with improvement on UPDRS. Two subjects died 18 months after surgery from unrelated causes, and autopsies demonstrated apparently healthy transplanted cells numbering 82,000–138,000 per side (19). Wenning et al. found that in six transplanted patients evaluated at 1 year and four patients evaluated at 2 years, off UPDRS scores were improved 18 and 26% and off time was reduced 34 and 44%. FD uptake increased 68% at 8–12 months after transplantation (25).

Although several other open-label trials also found that transplanted patients experienced clinical benefit, there was variable symptom improvement following transplantation in these trials (9–27). Variability in surgical technique, including amount of tissue used and sites transplanted, may have played a role in this variability in clinical outcomes.

Autopsies performed on two transplanted patients demonstrated healthy graft tissue, including large numbers of surviving dopaminergic cells and physiological reinnervation patterns (18,19). Transplanted grafts extended neuritic process 2–7 mm (28). Grafting at 5 mm intervals resulted in reinnervation of up to 78% of the postcommissural putamen, and survival of dopamine neurons following grafting ranged from 5 to 20%. No graft rejection was observed, although immune markers were activated (29).

PET scans following transplantation in many open-label studies demonstrated increased FD uptake in the graft area (9,19,28,30), consistent with graft survival. Grafted mesencephalic tissue was found to better survive in the putamen than the caudate nucleus in short- and long-term follow-up (2), based on FD PET studies (10,16,17,25). More profuse vascularization in the putamen creating a better atmosphere for the graft to survive may explain these findings (2). Piccini et al. demonstrated synaptic dopamine release from embryonic nigral transplants using raclopride PET in a patient who had received a transplant in the right putamen 10 years earlier and experienced sustained, marked clinical benefit (24).

Evidence from open-label studies indicated that transplanted embryonic mesencephalic cells could survive transplantation, uptake FD as seen on PET scans, at least partially reinnervate the striatum, and release dopamine into the synapse. In addition, these studies suggested clinical benefit, especially with regard to improving motor function during the off state and decreasing off time. However, any clinical benefit observed in open-label studies could potentially be due in part or whole to placebo effects. A reliable evaluation of the clinical benefits of fetal cell transplantation required double-blind, sham surgery–controlled studies (31).

III. HUMAN FETAL MESENCEPHALIC TRANSPLANTATION IN PD: DOUBLE-BLIND TRIALS

Freed et al. evaluated transplantation of embryonic dopamine neurons into 40 advanced PD patients in a double-blind, sham surgery–controlled trial (8). Patients (34–75 years of age, mean disease duration 14 years) were randomly assigned to undergo transplantation or sham surgery and were followed in a double-blind manner for one year, after which time those in the sham surgery group were offered transplantation. Mesencephalic tissue from a total of four embryos was transplanted into the putamen bilaterally. All patients had PD for more than 7 years, and had previously responded favorably to levodopa.

The primary outcome measure was a subjective global rating of the change in the disease that was mailed in by patients 12 months following surgery. The global rating was scored on a scale of -3 to $+3$, corresponding to phrases ranging from "parkinsonism markedly worse (-3)" to "parkinsonism markedly improved $(+3)$" compared to baseline. Secondary outcome variables included estimates of transplant growth by ^{18}F-fluorodopa PET and clinical scales including the UPDRS, Schwab and England scoring during off time, and patient diaries.

There was not a significant difference in the primary outcome variable across groups. The mean ($\pm$SD) global rating score was 0.0 ± 2.1 for transplanted patients compared to -0.4 ± 1.7 for sham surgery patients ($p = 0.62$). For patients younger than 60 years of age, subjective global scores were 0.5 ± 2.1 in the transplanted group and -0.3 ± 1.7 in the sham-surgery group ($p = 0.36$). For patients older than 60 years of age, the scores in the transplanted group were -0.7 ± 2.0 and -0.4 ± 1.7 in the sham-surgery group ($p = 0.80$).

Total UPDRS off scores were not different across groups at one year. Younger patients who were transplanted had a 28% improvement in total UPDRS off scores ($p = 0.01$) compared to the sham-surgery group. UPDRS off motor scores decreased 18% for the whole transplantation group ($p = 0.04$), and 34% for the younger patients ($p = 0.005$). There was also improvement in the Schwab and England scores for younger patients in the transplant group compared to the sham-surgery group ($p = 0.006$). ^{18}F-fluorodopa uptake in the putamen on PET increased $40 \pm 42\%$ in the transplanted group compared to a decline of $2 \pm 17\%$ in the sham-surgery group ($p = 0.001$). Changes in PET scans were similar in younger and older patients. There was a positive correlation between PET uptake and clinical improvements in younger patients. Autopsy results in two patients who died from causes unrelated to surgery revealed 2,000–23,000 surviving transplanted dopamine neurons per transplant track.

Although the change in the chosen primary outcome variable, the global rating scale, was not significantly different between groups, various secondary outcome variables suggested that there was some clinical benefit, especially for the younger patients. The choice of the global rating scale as the primary outcome measure has met some criticism in that it has not been validated or tested with regard to sensitivity in this paradigm. Nonetheless, the lack of difference in this rating scale suggests that any benefits observed were not sufficient to meaningfully impact overall function in these patients. The observation that increases in FD uptake on PET scans was similarly increased in younger and older patients, but that clinical benefit as measured by secondary outcome variables was mostly limited to younger patients suggests that survival of transplanted dopamine cells is not affected by recipient age but clinical response to transplantation may be limited by lesser brain plasticity or more diffuse degeneration in older patients. The magnitude of baseline response to levodopa may be predictive of clinical benefit following transplant as younger patients exhibited approximately a 50% greater levodopa response than older patients.

Thirty-three patients in this study ultimately received transplants and were followed for as long as 3 years after surgery. Dystonia and dyskinesia that persisted after elimination or reduction of antiparkinsonian therapy (runaway dyskinesias) occurred in 5 (15%) of the 33 patients more than one year after surgery. All 5 patients were 60 years of age or younger when they received transplantation surgery, and had experienced severe motor fluctuations prior to surgery. Three of the 5 patients received transplants during the initial double-blind phase, while the other 2 received transplants as part of the open-label extension trial.

Ma et al. used FD PET to evaluate alterations in dopamine function after transplantation (32). The transplant patients (age 46.8 ± 8.3 years, disease duration 11.6 ± 2.7 years) who developed runaway dyskinesia with little or no dopaminergic therapy following surgery (DYS+) were compared to transplant patients (48.9 ± 7.6 years, disease duration 12.2 ± 3.8 years) who did not develop dyskinesia (DYS-). All patients evaluated were members of the younger transplant group, i.e., < 60 years old. FD PET values were compared in each set of patients at baseline and at 12 and at 24 months following transplantation. At baseline, there was no significant difference in PET signal in the putamen between the two groups (DYS+ and DYS-). Following transplantation the increase in overall PET signal in the DYS+ group was twice that of the DYS−group at 12 months ($p < 0.03$) and almost three times larger at 24 months ($p < 0.005$). FD uptake was significantly increased in the left putamen in the DYS+ group ($p < 0.0003$), and no significant difference was observed on the right. Increases were primarily localized to two discrete areas, the dorsal putamen extending posteriorly, and the ventral putamen. At 24 months following transplantation, FD PET signal in the dorsal putamen increased from a baseline value of 47% of normal in both groups to 60% of normal in the DYS− group and 80% of normal for the DYS+ group. In the ventral putamen, baseline values in both groups were 57% of normal and increased to 73% of normal in the DYS + group, while there was no significant change in this area in the DYS− group. Of note, FD PET measures did not reach supranormal values over the 24-month follow-up in either group.

These findings suggest that the striata should not be viewed as homogeneous targets for neural transplantation. Supranormal FD uptake is not necessary to produce dyskinesias. There may be a therapeutic window for transplantation, and the degree of optimal reinnervation may vary within the striatum. This may necessitate the development of surgical techniques that allow more localized and better controlled delivery of grafted tissue.

Preliminary results of another prospective double-blind, placebo-controlled trial were presented by Olanow et al. at the Seventh International Congress of Parkinson's Disease and Movement Disorders (33). Thirty-four advanced PD patients were randomized to receive bilateral transplantation with one donor per side, four donors per side, or sham procedures. This study further differed from that of Freed et al. in that tissue was not stored for longer than 48 hours, grafts were implanted into the postcommissural putamen and separated by no more than 5 mm, and immunosuppression was used for 6 months. Patients were followed for 2 years and the primary outcome variable was the change in UPDRS motor score during the "practically defined off" (in the morning after antiparkinsonian medication had been withheld for at least 12 hours). Thirty-one patients completed the trial, 2 died during the trial, and 3 afterward, all from causes unrelated to the surgery. Patients who received transplantation with four donors demonstrated well-innervated striatum on autopsy. PET results demonstrated a significant dose-dependent increase in FD uptake with no change in sham-surgery patients and an approximate one-third increase in patients receiving four donors.

No significant differences were identified in clinical measures following transplantation. Increases (worsening) compared to baseline in UPDRS motor scores while off medication were 9.4 for placebo, 3.5 for one donor, and -0.72 for four donors ($p = 0.096$ for four vs. placebo). Transplanted patients improved for approximately 9 months, suggesting the possibility of a delayed immune response. There were no significant differences in on time without dyskinesias, off time, activities of daily living (ADL) scores, or levodopa dose requirements. Thirteen of 23 transplanted patients developed off-medication dyskinesias, and 3 required surgical treatment to control them. No off-medication dyskinesia was observed in sham-surgery patients.

Double-blind studies confirm that transplanted fetal mesencephalic cells can survive transplantation as evidenced by both autopsy studies and increased FD uptake. These studies have not demonstrated definitive benefit, although they do suggest modest clinical benefit in various measures of parkinsonian severity. Further studies are required to determine why such limited clinical benefit is achieved relative to cell survival and apparent striatal reinnervation. Evaluation of graft dopamine release and postsynaptic stimulation on a microanatomical level may be necessary. The development of off-medication dyskinesia has been identified as a significant adverse event in a substantial proportion of transplanted patients. This represents a critical hurdle that must be overcome if transplantation is to be developed into a useful clinical therapy. Further study is required to learn the etiological basis of off-medication dyskinesia to understand how it might be avoided.

III. PORCINE FETAL MESENCEPHALIC TRANSPLANTATION IN PD

Schumacher et al. evaluated unilateral transplantation of embryonic porcine ventral mesencephalic tissue in advanced PD patients in an open-label study (34). Twelve patients underwent transplantation; 6 received cyclosporine immunosuppression and 6 received tissue treated with a monoclonal antibody directed against major histocompatibility complex class I. The groups were considered together and followed for one year. Off total UPDRS scores improved 19% ($p = 0.01$). FD PET scans failed to show changes on the implanted side. In one transplanted patient in the cyclosporine group who came to autopsy at approximately 8 months, three surviving grafts containing a total of 638 porcine dopamine cells were identified (35).

Hauser et al. reported a double-blind, randomized trial of bilateral transplantation of fetal porcine ventral mesencephalic cells versus imitation surgery in patients with advanced PD (36). Ten patients received a total of 48×10^6 porcine cells implanted into one site in each caudate and five sites in each putamen. Eight control patients underwent imitation surgery. Transplanted patients received cyclosporine throughout the study and prednisone for 75 days postsurgery, and the control group received placebo cyclosporine and prednisone. The primary outcome variable was the change in total UPDRS score in the off state 18 months after surgery. Transplanted patients demonstrated a mean improvement over baseline of $24.6 \pm 25.0\%$, and control patients demonstrated a mean improvement of $21.6 \pm 14.0\%$ ($p = 0.6$). There were no significant differences across groups for off time, on time, or investigator global evaluations. There were no significant differences across groups in FD PET scans at 12 months.

Although an open-label study suggested possible clinical benefit, this double-blind study did not identify significant improvement comparing transplanted to imitation surgery patients. This experience confirms that a substantial placebo effect can be seen in surgical trials in PD and demonstrates the need for definitive, randomized, double-blind, sham-surgery–controlled studies.

IV. RETINAL CELL TRANSPLANTATION

Transplanted cultured human retinal pigment epithelial (RPE) cells are currently being evaluated as a source of dopamine or dopamine precursors that may ameliorate parkinsonian symptoms. RPE cells are harvested from the posterior layer of the retina next to the choroid (37) and have been shown to survive in rodent and nonhuman primate models with minimal host immune response while improving parkinsonian symptoms. Watts et al. evaluated the safety and efficacy of unilateral RPE transplantation in six advanced PD patients in an open-label pilot study (38). RPE cells attached to cross-linked gelatin microcarriers (Spheramine) were implanted into the postcommissural putamen contralateral to the worst affected side and no immunosuppression was used. At 6 and 9 months following surgery, motor UPDRS scores improved 33% and 42%, respectively from preoperative baseline scores. One patient has been followed for 15 months, with a 44% improvement in motor UPDRS from baseline. Half of the patients experienced moderate to marked reductions in off time and had reduced Dyskinesia Rating Scale scores compared to baseline. The procedure was well tolerated. Double-blind studies are required to provide a definitive evaluation.

V. STEM CELLS

The therapeutic potential of stem cells has captured the public imagination like few other scientific endeavors. For brain repair, the great hope is that stem cells will provide an unlimited, self-renewing source of cells that can be transplanted, migrate to areas of injury or degeneration, and replace lost cells by differentiating into the appropriate cell type and integrating into host neuronal circuitry. Nonetheless, the field of stem cell biology is still in its infancy and many hurdles remain.

Embryonic stem (ES) cells are pluripotent cells isolated from the inner cell mass of blastocysts which give rise to all cell types (39). Multipotent stem cells are also capable of self-renewal but have a more restricted potential than ES cells and are often defined by the organ from which they are derived. Neural stem cells (NSC) are multipotent stem cells capable of differentiating into any of the three neural lines: neurons, oligodendrocytes, and astrocytes. NSCs can be isolated from either the developing or adult brain. In the adult brain, NSCs have been derived from the subventricular zone and the subgranular zone of the hippocampal dentate gyrus, areas of high-density cell division. Alternative sources of multipotent stem cells are nonneural tissue including bone marrow or umbilical cord blood.

Obtaining a neural phenotype from ES cells is not difficult. However, it has been surprisingly difficult to achieve a complete and coordinated induction of multipotent stem cells into a single cell type. In the laboratory, ES and NSC cells are exposed to a variety of complex manipulations and exposures to growth factors and other signals to induce differentiation into midbrain dopaminergic neurons (39). However, most of these regimens are plagued by a relatively low yield regarding the proportion of dopaminergic cells or a poor cell survival rate following grafting. It seems likely, though, that further refinements to the differentiation and maintenance regimens will improve this situation over time. The potential for stem cells to cause tumors must be carefully evaluated, and molecular controls may be engineered into stem cells targeted for transplantation.

An alternative or adjunctive approach for stem cell transplantation is the delivery of neurotrophic factors. At this time, most interest is focused on the delivery of glial-derived neurotrophic factor (GDNF). Potential methods of delivery include viral gene transfer, direct infusion, and stem cell delivery. Viral delivery of GDNF in aged monkeys has been demonstrated to increase numbers of dopamine neurons and protect against 1-methyl-4-phenyl-1,2,3,6 tetrahydropyridine (MPTP) toxicity (40). An open-label pilot study of direct infusion of GDNF into the putamen of PD patients has also shown promise (41). GDNF overexpressing NSCs prevented the degeneration of nigral dopamine neurons in mice after intrastriatal injection of 6-hydroxydopamine (6-OHDA) and reduced amphetamine and apomorphine-induced turning (42). Potential advantages of stem cell delivery of GDNF over viral delivery may include more targeted effects, better standardization and quantification, and the potential to include molecular control mechanisms in case the cells need to be shut off.

VI. CONCLUSION

Cell transplantation has the potential of improving function in PD patients by providing dopamine replacement or by replacing lost neurons. After two decades of research, there remains hope, but no transplantation strategy has yet been proven to provide PD patients consistent and meaningful benefit. The obstacles to achieving this goal have become more clearly defined. Experience from human fetal mesencephalic transplantation studies has demonstrated that such cells can survive transplantation and function in the sense that they uptake FD and can release dopamine. But clinical benefit has been modest, and some patients have experienced disabling runaway dyskinesias. Understanding the biological basis of these problems may show the way for the future. It may be critical to avoid considering the striatum as a homogeneous target and study cell transplant effects at the microanatomical level. Is dopamine replacement occurring in a physiological fashion at the right synapses? Before a cell transplantation strategy can play a therapeutic role in the management of PD, greater clinical benefit must be achieved and runaway dyskinesia must be avoided. New cells, including stem cells, are being developed and tested in animal models. Some of these are genetically modified to boost their own survival or to help protect host neurons. Double-blind clinical trials are accepted as a means of clearly defining the safety and efficacy of a transplantation protocol.

REFERENCES

1. Poewe WH, Lees AJ, Stern GM. Low-dose therapy in Parkinson's disease; a 6-year follow-up. Neurology 1986; 36:1528–1530.
2. Lindvall O. Neural Transplantation: can we improve the symptomatic relief?. Adv Neurol 1999; 80:635–640.
3. Ungerstedt U, Arbuthnott GW. Quantitative recording of rotational behavior in rats after 6-hydroxy-dopamine lesions of the nigrostriatal dopamine system. Brain Res 1970; 24(3):485–493.
4. Bjorklund A, Stenevi U. Reconstruction of the nigrostriatal dopamine pathway by intracerebral nigral transplants. Brain Res 1979; 177(3):555–560.
5. Perlow MJ, Freed WJ, Hoffer BJ, et al. Brain grafts reduce motor abnormalities produced by destruction of nigrostriatal dopamine system. Science 1979; 204(4393):643–647.
6. Dunnett SB, Bjorklund A, Schmidt RH, et al. Behavioral recovery in rats with unilateral 6-OHDA lesions following implantation of nigral cell suspensions in different forebrain sites. Acta Physiol Scand Suppl 1983; 522:29–37.
7. Bjorklund A, Stenevi U, Schmidt RH, et al. Intracerebral grafting of neuronal cell suspensions. II. Survival and growth of nigral cell suspensions implanted in different brain sites. Acta Physiol Scand Suppl 1983; 522:9–18.
8. Freed CR, Greene PE, Breeze RE et al. Transplantation of embryonic dopamine neurons for severe Parkinson's disease. N Engl J Med 2001; 344:710–719.
9. Freed CR, Breeze RE, Rosenberg NL, et al. Transplantation of human fetal dopamine cells for Parkinson's disease: results at 1 year. Arch Neurol 1990; 47:505–512.
10. Lindvall O, Brundin P, Widner H, et al. Grafts of fetal dopamine neurons survive and improve motor function in Parkinson's disease. Science 1990; 247:574–577.
11. Freed CR, Breeze RE, Resenberg NL, et al. Fetal neural implants for Parkinson's disease: results at 15 months. In: Lindvall O, Bjorklund A, Winder H, et al. Intracerbral Transplantation in Movement Disorders. Amsterdam: Elsevier, 1991: 69–77.
12. Freed CR, Breeze RE, Rosenberg NL, et al. Survival of implanted fetal dopamine cells and neurologic improvement 12 to 46 months after transplantation for Parkinson's disease. N Engl J Med 1992; 327:1549–1555.
13. Breeze RE, Wells TH Jr, Freed CR. Implantation of fetal tissue for the management of Parkinson's disease: a technical note. Neurosurgery 1995; 36:1044–1047.
14. Freed CR, Breeze RE, Rosenberg NL, Schneck SA. Embryonic dopamine cell implants as a treatment for the second phase of Parkinson's disease: replacing failed nerve terminals. In: Freed CR, Breeze RE, Rosenberg NL, Schneck SA. Embryonic dopamine cell implants as a treatment for the second phase of Parkinson's Disease: replacing failed nerve terminals. In: Narabayaski H, Nagatsu T, Yanagisawa N, Mizuno Y, eds. Advances in Neurology. Vol 60. Parkinson's disease: from Basic Research to Treatment. New York: Raven Press, 1993: 721–728.
15. Spencer DD, Robbins Rj, Naftolin F, et al. Unilateral transplantation of human fetal mesencephalic tissue into the caudate nucleus of patients with Parkinson's disease. N Engl J Med 1992; 327:1541–1548.
16. Widner H, Tetrud J, Rehncrona S, et al. Bilateral fetal mesencephalic grafting in two patients with parkinsonism induced by 1-methyl-4-phenyl-1,2,3,6-tetrahydropyridine (MPTP). N Engl J Med 1992; 327:1556–1563.
17. Lindvall O, Sawle G, Widner H, et al. Evidence for long-term survival and function of dopaminergic grafts in progressive Parkinson's disease. Ann Neurol 1994; 35:172–180.
18. Freeman TB, Olanow CW, Hauser RA, et al. Bilateral fetal nigral transplantation into the post-commissural putamen in Parkinson's disease. Ann Neurol 1995; 38:379–388.
19. Kordower JH, Freeman TB, Snow BJ, et al. Neuropathological evidence of graft survival and striatal reinnervation after the transplantation of fetal mesencephalic tissue in a patient with Parkinson's disease. N Engl J Med 1995; 332:1118–11124.
20. Peschanski M, Deger G, N'Guyuen JP, et al. Bilateral motor improvement and alteration of L-dopa effect in two patients with Parkinson's disease following intrastriatal transplantation of foetal ventral mesencephalon. Brain 1994; 17:487–499.

21. Defer GL, Geny C, Ricolfi F, et al. Long-term outcome of uniliaterally transplanted parkinsonian patients. I. Clinical approach. Brain 1996; 119:41–50.
22. Kopyov OV, Jacques D, Lieberman A, et al. Clinical study of fetal mesencephalic intracerebral transplants for the treatment of Parkinson's disease. Cell Transplant 1996; 5:327–337.
23. Hauser RA, Freeman TB, Snow BJ, et al. Long-term evaluation of bilateral fetal nigral transplantation in Parkinson's disease. Arch Neurol 1999; 56:179–187.
24. Piccini P, Brooks DJ, Bjorklund A, et al. Dopamine release from nigral transplants visualized in vivo in a Parkinson's patient. Nat Neurosci 1999; 12:1137–1140.
25. Wenning GK, Odin P, Morrish P, et al. Short- and long-term survival and function of unilateral intrastriatal dopaminergic grafts in Parkinson's disease. Ann Neurol 1997; 42:95–107.
26. Kordower JH, Freeman TB, Chen EY, et al. Fetal nigral grafts survive and mediate clinical benefit in a patient with Parkinson's disease. Mov Disord 1998; 13:383–393.
27. Lindvall O, Widner H, Rehncrona S, et al. Transplantation of fetal dopamine neurons in Parkinson's disease: one-year clinical and neurophysiological observations in two patients with putaminal implants. Arch Neurol 1992; 31:155–173.
28. Hallett M, Litvan I, and the Task Force on Surgery for Parkinson's disease. Evaluation of surgery for Parkinson's disease. Neurology 1999; 53:1910–1921.
29. Freeman RB, Willing A, Zigova T et al. Neural transplantation in Parkinson's disease. Adv Neurol 2001; 86:435–445.
30. Kordower JH, Rosenstein JM, Collier TJ, et al. Functional fetal nigral grafts in a patient with Parkinson's disease: chemoanatomic, ultrastructural and metabolic studies. J Comp Neurol 1996; 370:203–230.
31. Freeman TB, Vawter DE, Leaverton PE, et al. Use of placebo surgery in controlled trials of a cellular-based therapy for Parkinson's disease. N Engl J Med 1999; 341(13):988–992.
32. Ma Y, Feigin A, Dhawan V, et al. Dyskinesia after fetal cell transplantation for parkinsonism: a PET study. Ann Neurol 2002; 52:628–634.
33. Olanow C. Transplantation for Parkinson's disease: Pros, cons, and where do we go from here? Mov Disord 2002; 17:S15.
34. Schumacher JM, Ellias SA, Palmer EP, et al. Transplantation of embryonic porcine mesencephalic tissue in patients with PD. Neurology 2000; 54(5):1042–1050.
35. Deacon T, Schumacher J, Dinsmore J, et al. Histological evidence of fetal pig neural cell survival after transplantation into a patient with Parkinson's disease. Nat Med 1997; 3(3):350 353.
36. Hauser RA, Watts RL, Freeman TB. A double-blind, randomized, controlled, multicenter clinical trial of the safety and efficacy of transplanted fetal porcine ventral mesencephalic cells versus imitation surgery in patients with Parkinson's disease. Mov Disord 2001; 16:983–984.
37. Subramanian T. Cell transplantation for the treatment of Parkinson's disease. Semin Neurol 2001; 21(1):103–115.
38. Watts RL, Raiser C, Stover N, et al. Stereotaxic intrastriatal implantation of retinal pigment epithelial cells attached to microcarriers in advanced Parkinson disease patients: long-term follow-up. Neurology 2002; 58:A241.
39. Arenas E. Stem cells in the treatment of Parkinson's disease. Brain Res Bull 2002; 57(6):795–808.
40. Kordower JH, Emborg ME, Bloch J, et al. Neurodegeneration prevented by lentiviral vector delivery of GDNF in primate models of Parkinson's disease. Science 2000; 290(5492):767–773.
41. Gill S, Nikunj K, O'Sullivan K, et al. Intraparenchymal putaminal administration of glial-derived neurotrophic factor in treatment of advanced Parkinson's disease. Neurology 2002; 58:A241.
42. Akerud P, Canals JM, Snyder EY, Arenas E. Neuroprotection through delivery of glial cell line-derived neurotrophic factor by neural stem cells in a mouse model of Parkinson's disease. J Neurosci 2001; 21(20):8108–8118.

26

Electroconvulsive Therapy

Raymond Faber

*University of Texas Health Science Center at San Antonio and
South Texas Veterans Health Care Center,
San Antonio, Texas, U.S.A.*

Electroconvulsive therapy (ECT) is an important adjunctive treatment for both the motor difficulties and mood disturbances of Parkinson's disease (PD). The antidepressant effects of ECT are indubitable and very well established. ECT is a highly effective treatment for severe depression. For depression with psychotic or catatonic features, ECT can be life-saving. In addition, there is literature on ECT improving motor function in patients with PD. In official task force reports in 1990 and 2001, the American Psychiatric Association included PD as an indication for ECT (1,2). This chapter provides practical guidelines for using ECT for both the mood and motor symptoms of PD.

I. HISTORICAL REVIEW AND OVERVIEW

The modern origins of convulsive therapy are found in Budapest, where Ladusa Meduna in 1934 first demonstrated the beneficial effects of convulsions on abnormal mental states (3). Meduna postulated an antagonism between seizures and psychosis. He used injections of camphor and then pentylenetetrazol to induce seizures, and subsequent clinical improvement in mood disorders, psychosis, and catatonia result. His successes were replicated, and in 1938 Cerletti and Bini in Rome developed the electrical stimulus as a more predictable and immediate method of seizure induction.

ECT was widely accepted in psychiatry with the empirical observation that its greatest effectiveness was in depression, catatonia, and mania. Its effects in schizophrenia were less robust, and it tended to have adverse effects when given to neurotic patients. Initially seizures were unmodified, and the resulting generalized convulsions frequently caused vertebral compression fractures and less frequently long bone fractures. Succinylcholine was developed in the 1940s and was quickly adopted to minimize orthopedic complications. Treatments begin with a short-acting anesthetic agent, followed by succinylcholine, and then the electrical stimulus. Ventilation with supplemental oxygen became standard along with oximetry and vital sign monitoring.

Numerous randomized controlled trials have confirmed the effectiveness of ECT (2). Further refinements include alternatives to the original bilateral frontotemporal electrode placement such as right unilateral, asymmetrical, and bifrontal placements. There have also been major advances using more optimal dosing of the electrical stimulus. This often involves determining the precise seizure threshold for each patient and dosing slightly above threshold for bilateral placements and dosing severalfold above threshold for unilateral placement (4).

The greatest drawback to ECT is temporary memory impairment. Most depressed patients have impairments of registration, encoding, and spontaneous recall. Performance on memory tests improves after ECT as the mood disorder resolves. However, during an average course of ECT given three times a week up to nine sessions, events occurring shortly before and after treatments are not encoded well, so patients typically have gaps in their memory for events occurring around the time of the treatment series. In almost all instances, new learning is not impaired after a course of ECT. There is a subtle retrograde amnesia for events occurring in the past year or two, which typically resolves within 6 months. Memory complaints when present typically resolve several months after the treatment series. An occasional patient may complain of enduring memory difficulty. When this occurs, it is associated with bilateral frontotemporal electrode placement, persistence or recurrence of depressive symptoms, and sometimes abnormal personality traits (2). It is rare for a patient to be unwilling to consider ECT for the treatment of depression because of concerns about memory.

II. DEPRESSION AND PARKINSON'S DISEASE

Depression occurs frequently in patients with PD (5,6). However, there is considerable variation in the type, frequency, and intensity of depressive symptoms. Most patients with PD and depression do not have symptoms and impairments that meet DSM-IV criteria for major depression. Suicide rates are not increased in PD. Yet lowered mood, loss of interests, and lack of enjoyment can be present intermittently and detract significantly from quality of life. Anxiety symptoms frequently accompany depression. These worries and fears can culminate in panic attacks and cause more distress than sadness (7,8). It is not unusual for the first onset of depression to occur 2–3 years before the diagnosis of PD. There are speculations about depression and PD sharing an overlapping pathophysiology involving serotonin (9). The occurrence of depression and anxiety in PD is only weakly correlated with disease severity and duration. Off periods are often associated with severe anxiety and dysphoria, which resolves once the patient regains an on state (10). Antidepressant medications can be effective treatments for depression in PD. Bupropion with putative noradrenergic and dopaminergic actions, tricyclic antidepressants, and serotonin reuptake inhibitors are all treatment options (6).

ECT should be considered to treat depression in PD when patients have severe dysphoria that has not responded to adequate trials of at least two antidepressants. In particular, if there is high suicide potential, ECT can be rapidly effective to diminish suicidal thinking. The highest efficacy of ECT is in the melancholic subtype, wherein patients have fixed, unremitting dysphoria that is unreactive to what normally would be pleasurable diversions. ECT is also particularly effective in psychotic depressions, which are uncommon in PD.

III. ANTIPARKINSONIAN EFFECTS OF ECT

It is now accepted that ECT has beneficial effects on the motor disabilities of PD, including rigidity, bradykinesia, and tremor. This observation was first made in the 1940s (11). Most publications on ECT in PD concern patients who received ECT for psychiatric indications, primarily depression, and were noted to have considerable motor improvement. In 28 reports (12,13–20) on 80 patients with PD and psychiatric comorbidity, 56 patients improved, yielding a 70% response rate. Because depression and other psychiatric disorders can cause a worsening of PD, the beneficial effects of ECT might simply be due to improvements in mental state. This is unlikely to be a complete explanation since several cases have been reported of a dissociation of motor improvement without amelioration of depression (13,21). One patient who had previously been immobile tried to act on his suicide ideation by attempting to jump out a window after a course of ECT (13).

The most compelling evidence of ECT having anti-PD effects are reports of patients without depression having motor improvements. The only randomized controlled trial of ECT in PD included 11 subjects, 6 of whom initially received "sham" ECT, i.e., after being prepared and anesthetized they did not receive an electrical stimulus. After six "sham" sessions they received a course of real ECT. Cumulatively, 9 of the 11 subjects responded. Overall on time increased from 32% to 71%. Their duration of response ranged from 2 to 6 weeks and averaged about 3 weeks (22).

Twelve open trials of ECT in nondepressed patients with PD have been published. The first such report was in 1959 wherein following ECT, five of eight patients with PD had improvement, in particular with rigidity (23). Ward et al. in 1980 reported a negative study, as none of the five PD patients treated responded (24). Balldin et al. in 1980 and 1981 (25,26) obtained excellent benefits in five of nine PD patients, who had an overall decrease of their off time from 54% to 5%. Berger and de Soto (27) reported transient improvement lasting only hours, but confirming the concept of ECT having anti-PD effects. Zervas and Fink (14) had all 3 patients respond. Serby et al. (28) noted improvement in all three patients. Fall et al. (29) reported benefits in 14 of 15 PD patients, with 8 of these sustaining their improvement for 3 months or longer. Pridmore and Pollard (30) treated 14 PD patients and had follow-up data on 12, of whom 9 sustained their improvement for 10 weeks to 35 months. Wengel et al. (31) reported improvement in two of four PD patients. Aarsland et al. (20) in a report on maintenance ECT had one PD patient without depression respond. A later study by Fall et al. (19) included improvement in all four nondepressed PD patients.

Since 1957 there have been 13 reports of ECT in nondepressed patients with PD with a clinically significant response in 55 of 76 patients (72%). The duration of improvement ranged from days to years. The modal duration of improvement has been about 3–4 weeks. Ongoing maintenance ECT typically given every 2 to 4 weeks has been effective in maintaining improvement for many patients, sometimes for a number of years (14,17,18,20,28,31). At present there are no robust clinical or biological predictors of response or duration of response. In one study, cerebrospinal fluid (CSF) levels of the norepinephrine metabolite 3 methoxy-4 hydroxy-phenylglycol (MHPG) were significantly lower in the group of patients with the longest lasting motor improvement (29).

Drug-induced parkinsonism (DIP) is highly responsive to ECT. Although DIP has become uncommon since the introduction of atypical antipsychotic agents, reports have found ECT to be uniformly effective in the treatment of DIP (32). These reports add credibility to the potential utility of ECT in PD. ECT has been tried in a number of Parkinson-plus patients with much more limited success. One of five progressive supranuclear palsy patients responded (33). Of five patients with multiple system atrophy, one had substantial improvement, two had minimal improvements, and two had no change in neurological status (34–36).

IV. MECHANISMS OF ACTION

ECT induces a plethora of neurotransmitter and receptor changes in the brain (37). Effects on serotonergic and noradrenergic systems are felt to be most relevant for the treatment of depression. Dopaminergic effects are posited to improve PD (38). In animal studies of chronic electroconvulsive shock (ECS), striatal dopamine levels as measured by brain dialysis increase substantially (39,40) as do frontal lobe levels of homovanillic acid (HVA) (41). Also of great interest is ECS causing an upregulation of dopamine D-1 receptors (42) and post-ECS increased responsiveness to a D-1 agonist (43). A body of work also has found ECS to potentiate many dopamine-mediated behaviors (44).

Human studies have also found ECT to have dopaminergic effects. Post-ECT increases in CSF HVA suggest overall increased dopamine metabolism (45). Studies have also found ECT to increase dopamine-mediated neuroendocrine function utilizing growth hormone and prolactin responses to apomorphine (46). The dopamine transporter is not affected by ECT as shown in a human study using beta-CIT to image the transporter with single photon emission computed tomography (SPECT) (19).

V. PRACTICAL MATTERS AND CONCLUSIONS

Patients with PD are particularly vulnerable to complications from ECT, most notably post-ECT delirium. This was described in 15 of 35 patients in four separate reports (14,16,29,31). In some instances the delirium lasted up to 2 weeks. This occurs if too many ECT are administered in too short a time period. The usual schedule of three ECT per week for depression should be reduced to two times per week for patients with PD. An additional complication can be the emergence of dyskinesias with ECT. This is assumed to be a manifestation of ECT's dopaminergic effects. Lowering the doses of levodopa and dopamine agonists by 25–33% has been found to be a practical means of circumventing the emergence of dyskinesias and delirium (47). In fact, many patients who have significant motor improvement with ECT can remain on a reduced medication regimen.

The optimal electrode placement for treating PD is unknown. Right (nondominant) unilateral and bifrontal electrode placements are widely used alternatives to the traditional bilateral frontotemporal placement. These alternatives are associated with less acute confusion and amnesia and are recommended initially. If improvement is not observed after four treatments, electrode placement should be switched to the bilateral frontotemporal position.

In conclusion, ECT can be an extremely useful treatment in PD both for severe depression which has not responded to medication or requires rapid intervention and for the motor disturbances that define PD. The model candidate for ECT who is not depressed is someone that has been treated with levodopa and dopamine agonists for 5 or more years and no longer has a satisfactory response and has dyskinesias or other treatment complications. Some very advanced patients who were bedridden and being tube-fed have regained considerable ability. Some patients may gain years of improvement in their quality of life with periodic maintenance ECT. With proper patient selection and attention to medication dosing and frequency of administration, ECT can be a highly effective adjunctive treatment for depression and motor dysfunction in PD.

REFERENCES

1. American Psychiatric Association Task Force on ECT. The Practice of ECT: Recommendations for Treatment, Training, and Privileging. Washington, DC: American Psychiatric Press, 1990.
2. American Psychiatric Association Task Force on ECT. The Practice of ECT: Recommendations for Treatment, Training, and Privileging. 2d ed. Washington, DC: American Psychiatric Press, 2001.
3. Meduna LJ. Über experimentelle Campher-epilepsie. Arch Psychiatry Nerv 1934; 102:333–339.
4. Sackeim HA, Prudic J, Devenand DP, Kiersky JE, Fitzsimons L, Moody BJ, McElhiney MC, Coleman EA, Settembrino JM. Effects of stimulus intensity and electrode placement on the efficacy and cognitive effects of electroconvulsive therapy. N Engl J Med 1993; 328:839–846.
5. Cummings JL. Depression and Parkinson's disease: a review. Am J Psychiatry 1992; 149:443–454.
6. Slaughter JR, Slaughter KA, Nichols SE, Martens MP. Prevalence, clinical manifestations, etiology, and treatment of depression in Parkinson's disease. J Neuropsychiatry Clin Neurosci 2001; 13: 187–196.
7. Hillen ME, Sage JI. Nonmotor fluctuations in patients with Parkinson's disease. Neurology 1996; 47:1180–1183.
8. Vazquez A, Jimenez-Jimenez FJ, Garcia-Ruiz P, Garcia-Urra D. 'Panic attacks' in Parkinson's disease. Acta Neurol Scand 1993; 87:14–18.
9. Maycux R, Stern Y, Williams JB, Cote L, Frantz A, Dyrenfurth I. Clinical and biochemical features of depression in Parkinson's disease. Am J Psychiatry 1986; 143:756–759.
10. Witjas T, Kaphan E, Azulay JP, Blin O, Ceccaldi M, Pouget J, Poncet M, Ali Cherif A. Nonmotor fluctuations in Parkinson's disease: frequent and disabling. Neurology 2002; 59:408–413.
11. Kalinowsky LB. Die Electrokrampfbehandlung in ihrer Beziehung zur Neurologie. Monatsschr Psychiatr Neurol 1949; 177:268–279.
12. Faber R, Trimble MR. Electroconvulsive therapy in Parkinson's disease and other movement disorders. Mov Disord 1991; 6:293–303.
13. Birkett DP. ECT in parkinsonism with affective disorder. Br J Psychiatry 1988; 152:712.
14. Zervas IM, Fink M. ECT for refractory Parkinson's disease. Convuls Ther 1991; 7:222–223.
15. Friedman J, Gordon N. Electroconvulsive therapy in Parkinson's disease: a report on five cases. Convuls Ther 1992; 8:204–210.
16. Oh JJ, Rummans TA, O'Connor MK, Ahlskog JE. Cognitive impairment after ECT in patients with Parkinson's disease and psychiatric illness. Am J Psychiatry 1992; 149:271.
17. Kramer BA. A naturalistic review of maintenance ECT at a university setting. J ECT 1999; 15:262–269.
18. Fall PA, Granerus AK. Maintenance ECT in Parkinson's disease. J Neural Transm 1999; 106:737–741.
19. Fall PA, Ekberg S, Granerus AK, Granerus G. ECT in Parkinson's disease-dopamine transporter visualized by (123I)-beta-CIT SPECT. J Neural Transm 2000; 107:997–1008.
20. Aarsland D, Larsen JP, Waage O, Langeveld JH. Maintenance electroconvulsive therapy for Parkinson's disease. Convuls Ther 1997; 13:274–277.
21. Young RC, Alexopoulos GS, Shamoian CA. Dissociation of motor response from mood and cognition in a parkinsonian patient treated with ECT. Biol Psychiatry 1983; 20:566–569.
22. Anderson K, Balldin J, Gottpries CG, Granerus CG, Modigh K, Svennerholm L, Wallin A. A double-blind evaluation of electroconvulsive therapy in Parkinson's disease with 'on-off' phenomena. Acta Neurol Scand 1987; 76:191–199.
23. Fromm GH. Observations on the effects of electroshock treatment on patients with parkinsonism. Bull Tulane Univ Med Faculty 1959; 18:71–73.
24. Ward C, Stern GM, Pratt RTC, McKenna P. Electroconvulsive therapy in parkinsonian patients with the "on-off" syndrome. J Neural Transm 1980; 49:133–135.
25. Balldin J, Eden S, Granerus AK, Modigh K, Svanborg A, Walinder J, Wallin L. Electroconvulsive therapy in Parkinson's syndrome with "on-off" phenomenon. J Neural Transm 1980; 47:11–21.

26. Balldin J, Granerus AK, Lindstedt G, Modigh K, Wanlinder J. Predictors for improvement after electroconvulsive therapy in parkinsonian patients with on-off symptoms. J Neural Transm 1981; 52:199–211.

27. Berger M, de Soto DA. The use of ECT for parkinson symptoms in a nondepressed patient. Psychosomatics 1990; 31:465–466.

28. Serby M, Moros D, Rowan J, Carlin L, Yahr M. Maintenance ECT as adjunctive treatment to dopaminergic drugs in Parkinson's disease. Biol Psych 1994; 35:654.

29. Fall PA, Ekman R, Granerus AK, Thorell LH, Walinder J. ECT in Parkinson's disease. Changes in motor symptoms, monoamine metabolites and neuropeptides. J Neural Transm Park Dis Dement Sect 1995; 10:129–140.

30. Pridmore S, Pollard C. Electroconvulsive therapy in Parkinson's disease: 30 month follow up. J Neurol Neurosurg Psychiatry 1996; 60:693.

31. Wengel SP, Burke WJ, Pfeiffer RF, Roccaforte WH, Paige SR. Maintenance electroconvulsive therapy for intractable Parkinson's disease. Am J Geriatr Psychiatry 1998; 6:263–269.

32. Faber R. Electroconvulsive therapy in Parkinson's disease. Koller WC, Paulson G. Therapy of Parkinson's Disease. 2nd ed. Marcel Dekker, 1995:533–537.

33. Barclay CL, Duff J, Sandor P, Lang AE. Limited usefulness of electroconvulsive therapy in progressive supranuclear palsy. Neurology 1996; 46:1284–1286.

34. Ruxin RJ, Ruedrich S. Case report and review: ECT in combined multiple system atrophy and major depression. Convuls Ther 1994; 10:298–300.

35. Hooten WM, Melin G, Richardson JW. Response of the parkinsonian symptoms of multiple system atrophy to ECT. Am J Psychiatry 1998; 155:1628.

36. Roane DM, Rogers JD, Helew L, Zarate J. Electroconvulsive therapy for elderly patients with multiple system atrophy: a case series. Am J Geriatr Psychiatry 2000; 8:171–174.

37. Kapur S, Mann JJ. Antidepressant action and the neurobiological effects of ECT: human studies. Coffey CE, ed. The Clinical Science of Electroconvulsive Therapy. Washington, DC: American Psychiatric Press, 1993:235–250.

38. Fochtmann L. A mechanism for the efficacy of ECT in Parkinson's disease. Convuls Ther 1988; 4:321–327.

39. Nomikos GG, Zis AP, Damsma G, Fibiger HC. Electroconvulsive shock produces large increases in interstitial concentrations of dopamine in the rat striatum: an in-vivo microdialysis study. Neuropsychopharmacology 1991; 4:65–69.

40. Yoshida K, Higuchi H, Kamata M, Yoshimoto M, Shimizu T, Hishikawa Y. Dopamine releasing response in rat striatum to single and repeated electroconvulsive shock treatment. Prog Neuro-Psychopharmacol Biol Psychiatry 1997; 21:707–715.

41. Yoshida K, Higuchi H, Kamata M, Yoshimoto M, Shimizu T, Hishikawa Y. Single and repeated electroconvulsive shocks activate dopaminergic and 5-hydroxytrptaminergic neurotransmission in the frontal cortex of rats. Prog Neuro-Psychopharmacol Biol Psychiatry 1998; 22:435–444.

42. Fochtmann LJ, Cruciani R, Aiso M, Potter WZ. Chronic electroconvulsive shock increases D-1 receptor binding in rat substantia nigra. Eur J Pharmacol 1989; 167:305–306.

43. Sharp T, Kingston J, Grahame-Smith DG. Repeated ECS enhances dopamine D-1 but not D-2 agonist-induced behavioral responses in rats. Psychopharmacology 1990; 100:110–114.

44. Nutt DJ, Glue P. The neurobiology of ECT: animal studies. In: Coffey CE, ed. The Clinical Science of Electroconvulsive Therapy. Washington, DC: American Psychiatric Press, 1993:213–234.

45. Rudorfer MV, Risby ED, Hsiao JK, Linnoila M, Potter WZ. ECT alters human monoamines in a different manner from that of antidepressant drugs. Psychopharm Bull 1988; 24:396–399.

46. Kamil R, Joffe RT. Neuroendocrine testing in electroconvulsive therapy. Psychiatr Clin North Am 1991:961–970.

47. Faber R. More on ECT and delirium in Parkinson's disease. J Neuropsychiatry Clin Neurosci 1992; 4:232.

27

Functional Radiosurgery in Movement Disorders

Susan M. Baser

*Drexel University School of Medicine and Allegheny General Hospital,
Pittsburgh, Pennsylvania, U.S.A.*

I. OVERVIEW OF STEREOTACTIC RADIOSURGERY

Stereotactic radiosurgery is a method of delivering high doses of ionizing radiation to small, well-defined intracranial targets. This technique differs from conventional radiotherapy, which involves exposing large areas of intracranial tissue to relatively broad fields of radiation over a number of sessions. This technology delivers highly focused convergent beams in a single session so that only the desired target is radiated, sparing adjacent structures. With major technological advances, the general role for radiosurgery as both an adjuvant and alternative to conventional neurosurgery has greatly expanded.

Five main methods of this technology exist: gamma-ray radiosurgery (gamma knife), linear-accelerator radiosurgery (LINAC), proton-beam radiosurgery, helium-ion radiosurgery, and neutron-beam radiosurgery (charged particles) (1,2).

1. Gamma knife: The energy source used in the gamma knife is gamma rays. In this technique, 201 separate cobalt-60 sources are arranged in a steel shell; beams intersect on a desired target.
2. Linear accelerator: X-rays consisting of photons with an average energy of 2 MeV are the energy source utilized in linear accelerator technology. Adapted for stereotactic use is a single beam of x-rays, rotated to produce multiple intersecting beams.
3. Charged particles: Three different energy sources used include protons, neutrons, or helium ions. Three to five fixed beams of charged particles have minimal scatter as they pass through tissue, depositing ionizing energy at a precise depth.

The gamma knife and linear accelerator systems are similar in concept; both use multiple photon radiation arcs that intersect at a stereotactically determined target, allowing higher doses of radiation delivery with sparing of surrounding normal tissues. The differences between the two relate to how the energy is produced (i.e., through decaying cobalt or from x-rays) and the number of energy sources used (i.e., multiple energy sources in the gamma knife versus one in the linear accelerator system). LINAC differs from the gamma knife in the way the radiation beams are delivered. In LINAC, the radiation beams are emitted by a single source, which rotates slowly around the patient's head.

Charged-particle beams are fundamentally different in that they take advantage of the Bragg peak phenomenon, i.e., the deposition of energy at a specific depth with minimal scatter. Typically three to five fixed beams are used, similar to the beam arrangement in conventional radiotherapy.

Prior to performing the radiosurgical procedure is a process of localizing the target, which can be performed with one or more of the following techniques: cerebral angiography, computed tomography (CT), and magnetic resonance imaging (MRI).

A. Fractionated Stereotactic Radiotherapy

When stereotactic radiation therapy is delivered over a course of days rather than in a single session, the technique is referred to as fractionated stereotactic radiotherapy. Fractionation of radiation over several sessions is desirable because the tolerability of the brain to irradiation increases with the number of sessions. The most common applications of stereotactic radiosurgery include treatment of intracranial metastases, arteriovenous malformations (AVMs) (3), acoustic neuromas (4), and other tumors such as meningiomas, gliomas, or pituitary adenomas (5–7).

B. Functional Neuroradiosurgery

Stereotactic radiosurgery has been investigated as a treatment of functional disorders, such as trigeminal neuralgia, epileptic seizures, and chronic pain. More recently, functional neuroradiosurgery is being used as a treatment for movement disorders such as Parkinson's disease (PD) and essential tremor (ET).

Using MRI for target localization, a noninvasive stereotactic lesion is made in the area of the ventral intermediate (VIM) nucleus of the thalamus or the internal segment of the globus pallidus (GPi). This approach has been proposed for patients who are high surgical risks for an invasive procedure such as deep brain stimulation (DBS), pallidotomy, or thalamotomy.

II. THE GAMMA KNIFE

A. History and Development of the Gamma Knife

The basic concept of radiosurgery developed more than 50 years ago. In 1946 Wilson first proposed the clincial use of charged-particle beams because of their unique characteristics (8). Leksell and Larsson developed a radiosurgical tool as a method for cerebral lesion generation without opening the skin and skull. Using a cyclotron, they used a cross-fired proton beam in initial experiments in animals and in the first treatments of human patients. Leksell addressed the theoretical and many practical aspects of stereotactic radiosurgery in 1951 (9). The prototype irradiation tool developed was called a gamma knife (10).

Clinical application of the gamma knife rapidly developed over the next several decades. Tumors, including skull base lesions, were treated using this new technology. Leksell performed the first such treatment, radiating a vestibular schwannoma in

1969 (11). Stereotactic treatment of AVMs began in 1963 and was based on a stereotactic guidance device and angiograms (12).

B. The Gamma Knife and Functional Radiosurgery

Functional applications for gamma knife radiosurgery have expanded over the past two decades. Uses of gamma knife technology include lesion generation for PD (ventrolateral thalamotomy), pain (medial thalamotomy), affective disorders (anterior capsulotomy and cingulotomy), trigeminal neuralgia, and epilepsy (13–17).

The Leksell gamma knife delivers a single high dose of ionizing radiation. The radiation unit of the gamma knife contains 201 cobalt-60 sources secured within a hemispheric or circular array. Each beam channel has a source bushing assembly, a tungsten alloy precollimator, and a primary collimator. Secondary collimation is achieved via one of the four helmets containing 201 channels of different sizes. The radiation beams are collimated and converge precisely to the common focal point at the center of the radiation unit. Since each individual gamma ray is of relatively weak intensity, the normal brain tissue surrounding the abnormality is protected. Only at the point where the beams converge is the radiation at its most powerful and tissues destroyed. The Leksell gamma knife is provided with four helmets with collimators of different sizes: 4, 8, 14, and 18 mm. Helmets may be used individually for a single spherical lesion, such as a 4 mm for a functional target.

For stereotactic radiosurgery, MRI, CT scanning, and/or angiography are used in conjunction with special computer-assisted instruments to produce three-dimensional views of the lesion and the surrounding brain structures. Using these images, the physician can precisely locate the target and focus the gamma radiation beams emitted by the gamma knife.

As a lesion generator the gamma knife has proved to be a reliable tool. Single session doses from 50 to 200 Gy can cause tissue necrosis within 6 months, depending on target volume (18,19). Smaller volumes require more radiation. There exists a therapeutic range in which nerve or brain parenchyma can be affected without requiring total parenchymal injury. This range differs with brain location, target volume, and desired response time.

C. Gamma Knife Thalamotomy for Tremor

Since the early 1960s, the VIM nucleus of the thalamus has been regarded as the most satisfactory target for the surgical control of tremor. Regardless of etiology or pathophysiology, patients with most types of tremor have some benefit from VIM thalamotomy (20,21).

D. Radiofrequency Lesioning Versus Thalamic Stimulation Versus Gamma Knife Radiosurgery

Several papers reported complication rates higher than 1–2% for radiofrequency lesioning procedures (21,22). Tasker (23), in an extensive literature review of radiofrequency thalamotomy for tremor, described a 0–5% mortality rate, permanent hemiparesis in up to 6.3% of patients, permanent dysphasia in up to 3%, permanent dysarthria in up to 25%, and permanent gait disturbances in up to 6%. The benefits of radiofrequency thalamotomy also tend to lessen over time. Long-term follow-up for up to 10 years indicates that about half of patients may return to their preoperative tremor level (24). Although thalamotomy and DBS electrode implantation are performed under local anesthesia, there is a subgroup of patients who have conditions that predispose them to higher risks from invasive procedures. These patients include those with advanced respiratory or cardiac disease. Radiosurgical thalamotomy is an attractive option for these patients (25). In radiosurgical thalamotomy, such as gamma knife thalamotomy, imaging definition alone is used for lesion placement. Because of the absence of electrophysiological information and the inability to confirm the target site intraoperatively, most surgeons consider radiosurgical thalamotomy only for patients with medical disorders that preclude invasive procedures. The typical delay of 1–4 months for clinical results is another disadvantage (26). Niranjan et al. (27) compared the results of surgical approaches for the management of intractable tremor in 39 patients undergoing neurosurgical procedures. Procedures evaluated included stereotactic radiofrequency thalamotomy, gamma knife thalamotomy, and thalamic stimulation. Gamma knife radiosurgery was performed in elderly patients with concurrent medical problems. The three procedures had similar results with good relief of tremor. The authors concluded that all three stereotactic procedures for tremor control are safe and effective, but each procedure has specific advantages and disadvantages that are important for patient selection.

E. Type of Tremor and Gamma Knife Radiosurgery

In a review of ET surgery, only five studies with more than 10 patients were found (28). Radiosurgical lesions for ET or MS tremor (with more than 6 months follow-up) provided effective reduction in tremor in 100% of a series of 11 patients. Although objective assessment of tremor showed major improvement in 8 out of 11 patients, overall functional outcome was considered as excellent by 9 (82%) patients and good by 2 (18%) patients (29). In a study of eight patients undergoing gamma knife thalamotomy for ET, five patients were reported tremor-free, two were "nearly" tremor-free, and one had failed (30).

MRI after gamma knife thalamotomy typically shows a ring-enhancing lesion of 4 mm in diameter on T1-weighted, contrast-enhanced images (Fig. 1). The T2-weighted images

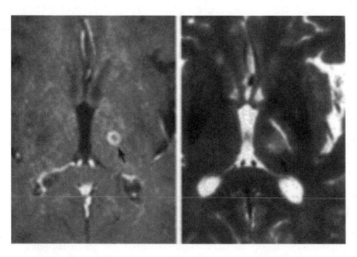

Figure 1 Contrast-enhanced axial MRI 4 months after gamma knife thalamotomy. T1-weighted MRI (left) shows a 4–5 mm enhancing lesion (arrow); T2-weighted MRI (right) shows a hyperintense area at the target site (arrow). (From Ref. 31).

demonstrate a hyperintense signal involving a relatively larger area with some hyper-intensity outlining the internal capsule. T2-weighted signal change probably represents increased water content and is unlikely to represent necrosis; its presence even in the internal capsule does not produce a neurological deficit. Serial scans show that this perilesional effect decreases over time. The T1 change represents necrosis and is limited to a 4–5 mm area. It matches the position and shape of the 50% isodose line used for targeting.

Improvement in gamma knife technology has improved control of lesion size and results. Early reports from the 1980s that involved an 8 mm collimator were associated with higher irradiation volumes and adverse effects. The 4 mm collimator of the gamma knife can be used in different ways. Traditionally, surgeons use the 50% isodose line as the marginal radiation dose. However, one can create a smaller volume by using the 80% isodose line with a 4 mm collimator. A very small target volume can be accurately irradiated with the gamma knife (32).

Higher doses of radiation appear to be associated with a higher rate of complication. The dose administered to the thalamotomy patients in a series reviewed by Okun and colleagues was 200 Gy (33). Patients now selected for gamma knife thalamotomy typically receive smaller doses in the range of 130–140 Gy (32,34).

The size of the radiation-generated lesion is dependent on dose as well as collimator size. In a recent study, Kondziolka et al. performed a baboon thalamotomy with a dose of 100 Gy and were able to achieve an area of necrosis 6 mm in diameter at 6 months (35). With careful patient selection, appropriate targeting, and dose selection, the complication rate has remained low. Bilateral radiosurgical thalamotomy is not recommended.

In summary, gamma knife thalamotomy can be an effective treatment for disabling tremor in selected patients for whom radiofrequency techniques or DBS may not be appropriate.

F. Gamma Knife Pallidotomy and Parkinson's Disease

The use of radiosurgical lesions in the pallidum is controversial. Control of lesion size and damage to nearby visual pathways remains a major concern. Despite these concerns, Young et al. (36) reported results for gamma knife pallidotomy with improvements in 18 of 28 PD patients with bradykinesia, 12 of 14 with dyskinesias, 18 of 28 with rigidity, and 0 of 3 with akinesia. One patient did experience a complete left homonymous hemianopsia after a right gamma knife pallidotomy.

Other published reports are less encouraging. One patient lesioned with gamma knife pallidotomy suffered a permanent contralateral homonymous hemianopsia and transient contralateral hemiparesis with some improvement in contralateral parkinsonian symptoms (37). Another report of four patients showed that only one patient changed significantly, with resolution of dyskinesia on the side contralateral to the lesion (38).

REFERENCES

1. Phillips MH, Stelzer KJ, Griffin TW, et al. Stereotactic radiosurgery: a review and comparison of methods. J Clin Oncol 1994; 12:1085–1089.
2. Luxton G, Petrovich Z, Jozsef G, et al. Stereotactic radiosurgery: principles and comparison of treatment methods. Neurosurgery 1993; 32:241–259.
3. Kirkeby OJ, Bakke S, Tveraa K, Hirschberg H. Fractionated stereotactic radiation therapy for intracranial arteriovenous malformation. Stereotact Funct Neurosurg 1996; 66:10–14.
4. Andrews DW, Silverman CL, Glass J, et al. Preservation of cranial nerve function after treatment of acoustic neurinomas with fractionated stereotactic radiotherapy. Stereotact Funct Neurosurg 1995; 64:165–182.

5. Song DY, Williams JA. Fractionated stereotactic radiosurgery for treatment of acoustic neuromas. Stereotact Funct Neurosurg 1999; 73:45–49.
6. Meijer OW, Wolbers JG, Baayen JC, et al. Fractionated stereotactic radiation therapy and single high-dose radiosurgery for acoustic neuroma: early results of a prospective clinical trial. Int J Radiat Oncol Biol Phys 2000; 46:45–49.
7. Ryu SI, Chang SD, Kim DH, et al. Image-guided hypo-fractionated stereotactic radiosurgery to spinal lesions. Neurosurgery 2001; 49:838–846.
8. Wilson RR. Radiological use of fast protons. Radiology 1946; 47:487–491.
9. Leksell L. The stereotaxic method and radiosurgery of the brain. Acta Chir Scand 1951; 102:316–319.
10. Larsson B, Leksell L, Rexed B, et al: The high energy proton beam as a neurosurgical tool. Nature 1958; 182:1222–1223.
11. Leksell L. A note on the treatment of acoustic tumors. Acto Chir Scand 1969; 137:763–765.
12. Kjellberg RN, Hanamura T, Davis KR, Lyons SL, Adams RD. Bragg-peak proton-beam therapy for arteriovenous malformations of the brain. N Engl J Med 1983; 309:269–274.
13. Leksell L. Stereotactic radiosurgery. J Neurol Neurosurg Psych 1983; 46:797–803.
14. Lindquist C, Kihlstrom L, Hellstrand E. Functional neurosurgery—a future for the gamma knife? Stereotact Funct Neurosurg 1991; 57:72–81.
15. Barcia Salorio JL, Roldan T, Hernandez G, et al. Radiosurgical treatment of epilepsy. Appl Neurophysiol 1985; 48:400–403.
16. Leksell L, Backlund EO. Stereotactic gammacapsulotomy. In: Hitchchock ER, Ballantine HT, Meyerson BA, eds. Modern Concepts in Psychiatric Surgery. New York: Elsevier, 1979:213–216.
17. Steiner L, Forster D, Leksell L, et al. Gammathalamatomy in intractable pain. Acta Neurochir 1980; 52:173–184.
18. Kondziolka D, Linskey ME, Lunsford LD. Animal models in radiosurgery. In: Alexander E, Loeffler J, Lunsford LD, eds. Stereotactic Radiosurgery. New York: McGraw-Hill, 1993:51–64.
19. Kondziolka D, Lunsford LD, Claassen D, et al. Radiobiology of radiosurgery: Part I. The normal rat brain model. Neurosurgery 1992; 31:271–279.
20. Goldman MS, Kelly PJ. Symptomatic and functional outcome of stereotactic ventralis lateralis thalamotomy for intention tremor. J Neurosurgery 1992; 77:223–229.
21. Jankovic J, Cardoso F, Grossman RG, Hamilton WJ. Outcome after stereotactic thalamotomy for parkinsonian, essential and other types of tremor. Neurosurgery 1995; 37:680–687.
22. Pahwa R, Lyons KE, Wilkinson SB, et al. Comparison of thalamotomy to deep brain stimulation of the thalamus in essential tremor. Mov Disord 2001; 16:140–143.
23. Tasker RR. Thalamotomy for Parkinson's disease and other types of tremor, II: the outcome of thalamotomy for tremor. In: Gildenberg PL, Tasker RR, eds. Textbook of Stereotactic and Functional Neurosurgery. New York: McGraw-Hill, 1998:1179–1198.
24. Broggi G, Giorgi C, Servello D. Stereotactic neurosurgery in the treatment of tremor. Acta Neurochir 1987; 39(suppl):73–76.
25. Kondziolka D. Functional radiosurgery. Neurosurgery 1999; 44:12–20.
26. Duma CM, Jacques D, Kopyov OV. Gamma knife radiosurgery for thalamotomy in parkinsonian tremor: a five year experience. J Neurosurg 1998; 88:1044–1049.
27. Niranjan A, Jawahar A, Kondziolka D, Lunsford LD. A comparison of surgical approaches for the management of tremor: radiofrequency thalamotomy, gamma knife thalamotomy and thalamic stimulation. Stereotact Funct Neurosurg 1999; 72(2–4):178–184.
28. Speelman JD, Schuurman PR, de Bie RMA, Bosch DA. Thalamic surgery and tremor. Mov Disord 1998; 13:103–106.
29. Niranjan A, Kondziolka D, Baser S, Heyman R, Lunsford LD. Functional outcomes after gamma knife thalamotomy for essential tremor and MS-related tremor. Neurology 2000; 55:443–446.
30. Young RF, Shumway–Cook A, Vermeulen SS, et al. Gamma knife radiosurgery as a lesioning technique in movement disorder surgery. J Neurosurg 1998; 89:183–193.
31. Niranjan A, Kondziolka D, Baser S, Heyman R, Lunsford LD. Functional outcomes after gamma knife thalamotomy for essential tremor and MS-related tremor. Neurology 2000; 55:443–446.
32. Kondziolka D. Gamma knife thalamotomy for disabling tremor. Arch Neurol 2002; 59(10):1660; author reply 1662–1664.
33. Okun MS, Stover NP, Subramanian T, et al. Complications of gamma knife surgery for Parkinson disease. Arch Neurol 2001; 58:1995–2002.
34. Niranjan A, Kondziolka D, Baser S, Heyman R, Lunsford LD. Functional outcomes after gamma knife thalamotomy for essential tremor and MS-related tremor. Neurology 2000; 55:443–446.
35. Kondziolka D, Conce M, Niranjan A, Maesawa S, Fellows W. Histology of the 100 Gy thalomotomy in the baboon. Radiosurgery 2002; 4:279–284.

36. Young RF, Shumway-Cook A, Vermeulen SS, Grimm P, Blasko J, Posewitz A, Burkhart WA, Goiney RC. Gamma knife radiosurgery as a lesioning technique in movement disorder surgery. J Neurosurg 1998; 89(2):183–193.
37. Bonnen JG, Iacono RP, Lulu B, Mohamed AS, Gonzalez A, Schoonenberg T. Gamma knife pallidotomy: case report. Acta Neurochir (Wien) 1997; 139(5):442–445.
38. Friedman JH, Epstein M, Sanes JN, Lieberman P, Cullen K, Lindquist C, Daamen M. Gamma knife pallidotomy in advanced Parkinson's disease. Ann Neurol 1996; 39(4):535–538.

28

Transcranial Magnetic Stimulation

Laura S. Boylan and Seth L. Pullman

Columbia-Presbyterian Medical Center and New York University, New York, New York, U.S.A.

I. INTRODUCTION

Transcranial magnetic stimulation (TMS), introduced just over 15 years ago (1), has become a key method of studying the normal conductivity and excitability of the corticospinal system, as well as the pathophysiology of cortical modulation circuitry in Parkinson's disease (PD). TMS is applied using a quick (100 μs) electrical discharge from a series of capacitors through a wire coil. The coil is embedded in a nonconductive plastic or rubber material and fashioned into a figure eight, butterfly, round, or cap shape and held over the part of the brain under study. The high-intensity electric current passes through the wires and induces a magnetic field, which in turn induces electrical current in the underlying cerebral cortex. Unlike transcranial electrical stimulation, TMS is relatively painless, with only a brief acoustic click, occasionally some mild scalp/facial muscle activation, and a momentary sense of disorientation with maximal TMS stimulation and virtually no sensation at low stimulation intensities. Also, unlike transcranial electrical stimulation, which directly affects cortical long tracts, the induced electrical field with TMS preferentially excites neural elements oriented parallel to the surface of the brain, i.e., primarily interneurons (2–4).

TMS devices are now available for delivering single or paired TMS pulses as well as repetitive trains of stimulation (rTMS). rTMS has become a powerful tool for studying human brain function by transient inhibition or stimulation of different brain areas in awake and behaving subjects (5). Effects of rTMS on cortical excitability and inhibition have been found to outlast transiently (at least for several minutes) the stimulation itself (6–8), raising the possibility of therapeutic applications of rTMS. Clinical trials aimed at determining therapeutic effects of rTMS have been conducted primarily in depression, but PD, epilepsy, obsessive-compulsive disorders, and schizophrenia also have been

---

Portions of this chapter are adapted from Ref. (53 and 71) with permission from Elsevier Science.

studied in small numbers of subjects (for a recent and thorough review, see Ref. 9). In this chapter, basic TMS and rTMS measures, their clinical significance in PD, and investigations of rTMS intervention in PD as a potential therapeutic approach are discussed.

II. SINGLE-PULSE TMS

A. MEP Amplitude, Latency, and Threshold

The motor-evoked potential (MEP) latency and amplitude are thought to measure most directly the integrity of pathways and related membrane excitability characteristics of the upper motor neuron. The central motor conduction time (10) is obtained by a single high-intensity TMS over the primary motor cortex and is derived by subtracting MEP peripheral latencies at the levels of the cervical and lumbosacral proximal roots from the total TMS conduction time. While the central motor conduction time is of importance in helping to determine the presence of upper motor neuron conduction abnormalities, it is of limited value in idiopathic PD where long tract integrity is known to be normal. MEP amplitudes and latencies are influenced by multiple factors, including configuration and placement of the TMS coil, stimulus intensity, presence of conditioning pulses, and muscle facilitation. A suprasegmental modulation of MEPs by these influences can be inferred in several ways such as by demonstration of relatively unchanged F wave and other spinal responses under the same stimulus conditions (11).

Peri-stimulus time histograms obtained using single-fiber electromyography (EMG) recordings after cortical stimulation reveal several peaks. The first of these peaks, referred to as the D wave, represents the direct activation of the upper motor neuron. Subsequent peaks, termed I waves, are thought to result from indirect excitation of upper motor neurons via cortical interneurons. Interpeak intervals corresponding to synaptic transmission support this interpretation (2–4,12).

By convention, motor threshold is defined as the lowest stimulus intensity that evokes MEPs of $50 \mu V$ in amplitude in 5 of 10 trials (13). Stimulus intensity is expressed as a percentage of the TMS device's maximum output. MEP amplitude is usually measured peak-to-peak, increases with stimulus intensity, and plateaus at approximately 80% of the peripherally induced M wave (6).

B. Recruitment and Facilitation

Motor thresholds are lowered and MEP amplitudes increased by muscle activation (see Fig. 1). Facilitation by muscle activation is also associated with decreased latencies (14). Mechanisms for this facilitation may include an increased number and greater synchronization of descending impulses from the motor cortex as well as reafferent facilitation at the segmental level (15).

Recruitment is measured by plotting a stimulus-response curve of stimulus intensity versus MEP amplitude. The slope of this curve is normally increased by facilitation as well as by maneuvers that enlarge cortical representation of muscles (16). Temporal summation can also be shown with stimuli delivered repeatedly. Immediately following trains at low (1 Hz) and high (10 Hz) stimulus frequencies, decreases and increases, respectively, of single-pulse MEP amplitudes have been demonstrated (6,7). These latter phenomena bear some resemblance to long-term depression and facilitation.

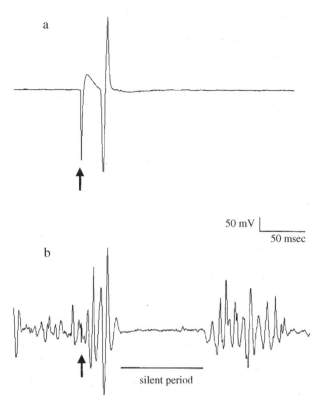

50 mV

50 msec

silent period

Figure 1 MEPs evoked from relaxed (a) and facilitated (b) first dorsal interosseus (FDI) in the same subject. Motor-evoked potential (MEP) amplitudes are equivalent, but in (a) stimulus intensity was 76% machine output and in (b) stimulus intensity was 40% machine output. Note the silent period following the MEP in (b). Arrows indicate stimuli onset.

C. Silent Period

The electromyographic silent period is a temporary suppression of EMG activity brought on during active muscle contraction and can be induced with many forms of peripheral or central stimuli. The cortical silent period may occur for up to 300 ms after a single TMS (see Fig. 1). It typically follows an MEP, but a silent period may also be induced by central stimulation that is subthreshold to produce an MEP (17). Though the origin of the initial segments of the silent period induced by TMS are controversial, the latter part of the cortical silent period is considered to be modulated by central mechanisms (12,18–21).

III. PAIRED-PULSE TMS

Measures of MEPs using paired pulses time-locked at precise interstimulus intervals (ISIs) can demonstrate changes in cortical excitability, specifically intracortical inhibition and facilitation. The first pulse, or conditioning stimulus, is generally just subthreshold compared to the second or test pulse in studies using short ISIs between 1 and 15 ms. At ISIs up to 6 ms, an inhibition of the test MEP amplitude is normally found, while facilitation of MEP amplitudes may occur at ISIs between 6 and 15 ms (22) (see Fig. 2).

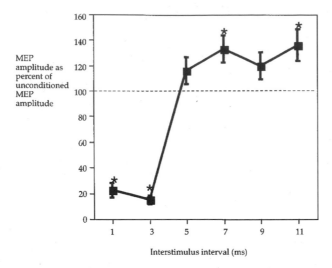

Figure 2 Paired pulse curve. Test pulses are preceded by subthreshold conditioning stimuli by 1 ± 11 ms. Interstimulus intervals of 1 ± 3 ms are associated with decreased motor-evoked potential (MEP) amplitude as compared with test pulse alone (intracortical inhibition), while interstimulus intervals of 7 ± 11 ms are associated with increased MEP amplitude (intracortical facilitation).

Paired-pulse TMS at longer ISIs (100–250 ms) using suprathreshold stimuli for both conditioning and test pulses (23) has been used to investigate longer-term effects. Cortical inhibitory mechanisms underlying short- and long-interval ISIs appear to be distinct (24).

IV. CORTICAL STIMULATION IN PARKINSON'S DISEASE

Normal central motor conduction time has been found in PD, consistent with the absence of direct involvement of the corticospinal tract (25,26). Increased central motor conduction time has been demonstrated in atypical parkinsonian syndromes in comparison to idiopathic PD, a finding with potential diagnostic utility (27). Enhanced resting MEP amplitudes have been reported (26,28), as has diminished facilitation of MEP size with either muscle activation or increased stimulus intensity (29), though it is difficult to obtain a true resting state in PD without motor activity.

A consistent finding in PD is an abnormally short silent period that is thought to be due to reduced intracortical inhibition (23,26,30,31). One report presented in abstract form suggests that the presence of this shortened silent period might distinguish PD from essential tremor early in the illness (32) and thus be a useful marker of PD, although there have been no follow-up reports. Of particular interest is the fact that dopaminergic therapy and anticholinergic agents lengthen the abnormally short silent period in patients with PD. Furthermore, the silent period appears to be shorter and more dopa responsive contralateral to a patient's most affected limbs (31).

Investigators have found decreased intracortical inhibition as measured in short- and long-interval paired-pulse paradigms (30,33,34). In one study these abnormalities were reversed with acute infusion of apomorphine (35). Another study found that intracortical inhibition was normalized and clinical improvement maintained during 12 months of chronic treatment with levodopa, but not with pergolide (36).

Different functional surgical treatments, e.g., deep brain stimulation (DBS) or lesioning of subcortical nuclei, have been shown to be associated with distinct changes in short- and long-interval intercortical inhibition and the silent period, suggesting that there is a difference in the modulation of motor cortical excitability by these interventions (37–40). Intracortical inhibition was examined in a study on patients with typical and atypical parkinsonian syndromes including vascular parkinsonism and the various multiple system atrophy (MSA) syndromes (41). Abnormalities in intracortical inhibition were found in all patient subgroups except those with predominantly cerebellar MSA. The decrease in intracortical inhibition was partially reversed by levodopa treatment in patients with vascular parkinsonism and MSA in the absence of clinical improvement.

V. CLINICAL STUDIES IN PARKINSON'S DISEASE

The therapeutic potential of TMS for PD has been considered a painless and potentially safe alternative to electrical stimulation of the brain, due in part to early clinical work showing that electroshock therapy had some lasting motoric benefit in severe parkinsonism (42,43). Electrophysiological (44) and some metabolic imaging (45) studies suggest that in patients with PD, motor and premotor areas of the cortex including the supplementary motor area (SMA) are both tonically underactivated and inadequately reactive to meet the needs of normal movements. Abnormal cortical inhibition in PD is thought to be due to reduced excitation from thalamocortical projections (46).

The potential of rTMS to enhance cortical excitability is supported by an increase in MEP amplitudes with rTMS (6), by persistent focal metabolic activation on positron emission tomography (PET) following rTMS (47), and by facilitation of picture naming following high-frequency rTMS (20Hz) to Wernicke's area (48). Persistent focal activation to the dorsolateral prefrontal cortex is thought to underlie the clinical trial data suggesting therapeutic efficacy of rTMS in major depression (49).

Open studies have found some significant clinical improvement in patients with PD lasting up to 3 months following rTMS (50,51). Many of these studies, however, suffer from the lack of undetectably different sham stimulation. One controlled study used a problematic sham technique in which the TMS coil was held completely off the head and therefore quite recognizable by the subjects. In this study, clinical benefit including decreased Hoehn and Yahr staging and improvement on the Schwab and England Activities of Daily Living scale was found in all eight of the patients who received rTMS and in none of the seven subjects who received sham treatment (52). Even when the coil is placed on the head, subjects may be able to discern sham or active TMS due to local skin and muscle stimulation. This issue is particularly salient in crossover studies where the same subject receives both sham and active stimulation (53). Such investigations form the basis of many of the acute challenge studies in PD (53–56) and in writer's cramp (57). One study specifically looking into the effective blinding and truly inactive stimulation found that some "sham" conditions did stimulate underlying brain (58).

Improvement in motor performance as tested *during* stimulation to the motor cortex was found among patients with PD and not among controls (59), but these results were not reproduced in a larger replicative study (60). In both studies stimulation was delivered at 90% of motor threshold over the primary motor cortex during performance of the Grooved Pegboard Task. In the latter study, stimuli delivered at these parameters grossly disrupted task performance with induction of twitches.

Improvement *following* rTMS was found in a controlled study demonstrating improvements in speed and smoothness as measured by kinematic analysis of a ballistic pointing task (54), though it is unclear if these changes would be clinically significant. Another study by this group used the Unified Parkinson's Disease Rating Scale (UPDRS) and found overall improvement following 5 Hz stimulation to the motor cortex with active but not sham stimulation (55). An issue with this study is that examiners were not blind to the treatment condition. Another report compared the effect of various rTMS frequencies delivered to the motor cortex on patients with PD but found no change in UPDRS, a timed walking task, or reaction time at 1, 5, 10, and 20 Hz (61).

Applying rTMS over the SMA interferes with the execution of complex movements and motor sequences (62). TMS stimulation can be administered at stimulation intensities up to 150% motor threshold of the primary motor cortex and not directly induce MEPs. In a blinded sham-controlled study, Boylan et al. applied high-intensity rTMS over the SMA without noticeable motor responses to determine if delivery of higher stimulation might yield effects of greater magnitude (53). No changes were found in the UPDRS scores or performance of timed motor tasks, but there was subclinical worsening of computer-analyzed spiral drawings, a method of objectively quantifying and rating complex movements (63), and reaction time 30–45 minutes following active but not sham stimulation.

Sommer et al. used the novel technique of cortical stimulation with rTMS repetitive trains of paired pulse stimuli (56). They found increased tapping speed among PD patients but not among healthy controls following all active stimulation including single- and paired-pulse stimulation trains. They demonstrated differential effects of paired-pulse stimuli given at inhibitory and facilitatory intervals on MEP size, but these did not correlate with motor responses to rTMS. Three subjects with tapping speed improvements immediately following rTMS were retested 30 minutes following stimulation, and no persistent benefit was found. Finally, in a protocol designed to assess the antidepressant effects of rTMS in PD patients with depression, rTMS was given daily over a 10-day period. Depression, but not parkinsonian motor symptoms (assessed by UPDRS), modestly improved for up to 2 weeks following the end of treatment in this open study (64).

VI. CONCLUSION

Although our understanding of the effects of rTMS in PD is improving, the precise mechanisms by which TMS affects cortical excitability and the resulting clinical significance remain unclear. In general, it has been suggested that low-frequency rTMS is inhibitory, while higher frequencies have facilitatory effects (6,54). However, the relationship of stimulus frequency to physiological effect remains to be determined, and, overall, disruption or deterioration rather than improvement of behavioral processes has been demonstrated.

Disturbance of ongoing cognitive and motor tasks can be found during high-frequency (15–20 Hz) rTMS (62,65,66), and facilitation of finger tapping has been demonstrated with low-frequency (1 Hz) rTMS in healthy subjects (8) as well as among PD patients (56). On the other hand, Tergau et al. found no change in movements among PD subjects assessed by global clinical rating scales following stimulation using four sets of frequencies over the entire testing range from 1 to 20 Hz (61). The effects of TMS administered at any frequency, even when applied to the same brain region, will likely differ between and among healthy subjects and those with different diseases

(56,57,66–68). Also, enhanced function will not necessarily be associated with increased cortical excitability just as dysfunction does not always represent cortical inhibition. For example, improvements in writing among patients with focal brachial dystonia were associated with enhanced intracortical inhibition on TMS paired-pulse studies (57), supporting the concept that reduced intracortical inhibition is likely involved in the pathophysiology of focal dystonia. On the other hand, alterations in intracortical inhibition were not correlated with improvement in tapping frequency following TMS in PD (56). In another study in healthy subjects, rTMS increased motor threshold and suppressed input-output curves for 30 minutes but had no effect on basic motor behavior (69).

The correlation between the effects rTMS, cortical excitability, and lasting changes in motor behavior remains elusive. There are many reasons for this, including difficulty in standardizing the administration of rTMS, determining the most appropriate brain areas to stimulate, the intensity and frequency of application, and the problems in developing a meaningful sham stimulation for truly blinded and perhaps more objective studies. Furthermore, even focally applied TMS affects both local and distant parts of the brain functionally connected through complex networks (70). While the use of noninvasive brain stimulation is still an attractive option for the treatment of PD, data from trials thus far do not support robust, lasting, or clinically beneficial effects with rTMS.

REFERENCES

1. Barker AT, Jalinous R, Freeston IL. Non-invasive magnetic stimulation of human cortex. Lancet 1985; 1:1106–1107.
2. Amassian VE, Cracco RQ, Maccabee PJ. Focal stimulation of human cerebral cortex with the magnetic coil: a comparison with electrical stimulation. Electroencephalogr Clin Neurophysiol 1989; 74:401–416.
3. Amassian VE, Quirk GJ, Stewart M. A comparison of corticospinal activation by magnetic coil and electrical stimulation of monkey motor cortex. Electroencephalogr Clin Neurophysiol 1990; 77:390–401.
4. Day BL, Dressler D, Maertens de Noordhout A, Marsden CD, Nakashima K, Rothwell JC, Thompson PD. Electric and magnetic stimulation of human motor cortex: surface EMG and single motor unit responses. J Physiol 1989; 412:449–473.
5. Hallett M. Transcranial magnetic stimulation and the human brain. Nature 2000; 406:147–150.
6. Pascual-Leone A, Valls-Sole J, Wassermann EM, Hallett M. Responses to rapid-rate transcranial magnetic stimulation of the human motor cortex. Brain 1994; 117:847–858.
7. Chen R, Classen J, Gerloff C, Celnik P, Wassermann EM, Hallett M, Cohen LG. Depression of motor cortex excitability by low-frequency transcranial magnetic stimulation. Neurology 1997; 48:1398–1403.
8. Wassermann EM, Grafman J, Berry C, Hollnagel C, Wild K, Clark K, Hallett M. Use and safety of a new repetitive transcranial magnetic stimulator. Electroencephalogr Clin Neurophysiol 1996; 101:412–417.
9. Wassermann EM, Lisanby SH. Therapeutic application of repetitive transcranial magnetic stimulation: a review. Clin Neurophysiol 2001; 112:1367–1377.
10. Eisen AA, Shtybel W. Clinical experience with transcranial magnetic stimulation. Muscle Nerve 1990; 13:995–1011.
11. Sohn YH, Kaelin-Lang A, Jung HY, Hallett M. Effect of levetiracetam on human corticospinal excitability. Neurology 2001; 57:858–863.
12. Berardelli A, Inghilleri M, Cruccu G, Manfredi M. Descending volley after electrical and magnetic transcranial stimulation in man. Neurosci Lett 1990; 112:54–58.
13. Rothwell JC, Hallett M, Berardelli A, Eisen A, Rossini P, Paulus W. Magnetic stimulation: motor evoked potentials. The International Federation of Clinical Neurophysiology. Electroencephalogr Clin Neurophysiol Suppl 1999; 52:97–103.
14. Hess CW, Mills KR, Murray NM. Responses in small hand muscles from magnetic stimulation of the human brain. J Physiol 1987; 388:397–419.

15. Rossini PM, Barker AT, Berardelli A, Caramia MD, Caruso G, Cracco RQ, Dimitrijevic MR, Hallett M, Katayama Y, Lucking CH, et al. Non-invasive electrical and magnetic stimulation of the brain, spinal cord and roots: basic principles and procedures for routine clinical application. Report of an IFCN committee. Electroencephalogr Clin Neurophysiol 1994; 91:79–92.
16. Ridding MC, Inzelberg R, Rothwell JC. Changes in excitability of motor cortical circuitry in patients with Parkinson's disease. Ann Neurol 1995; 37:181–188.
17. Rossini PM, Caramia MD, Iani C, Desiato MT, Sciarretta G, Bernardi G. Magnetic transcranial stimulation in healthy humans: influence on the behavior of upper limb motor units. Brain Res 1995; 676:314–324.
18. Uncini A, Treviso M, Di Muzio A, Simone P, Pullman S. Physiological basis of voluntary activity inhibition induced by transcranial cortical stimulation. Electroencephalogr Clin Neurophysiol 1993; 89:211–220.
19. Brasil-Neto JP, Cammarota A, Valls-Sole J, Pascual-Leone A, Hallett M, Cohen LG. Role of intracortical mechanisms in the late part of the silent period to transcranial stimulation of the human motor cortex. Acta Neurol Scand 1995; 92:383–386.
20. Hallett M. Transcranial magnetic stimulation. Negative effects. Adv Neurol 1995; 67:107–113.
21. Chen R, Lozano AM, Ashby P. Mechanism of the silent period following transcranial magnetic stimulation. Evidence from epidural recordings. Exp Brain Res 1999; 128:539–542.
22. Kujirai T, Caramia MD, Rothwell JC, Day BL, Thompson PD, Ferbert A, Wroe S, Asselman P, Marsden CD. Corticocortical inhibition in human motor cortex. J Physiol 1993; 471:501–519.
23. Berardelli A, Inghilleri M, Priori A, Marchetti P, Curra A, Rona S, Manfredi M. Inhibitory cortical phenomena studied with the technique of transcranial stimulation. Electroencephalogr Clin Neurophysiol Suppl 1996; 46:343–349.
24. Sanger TD, Garg RR, Chen R. Interactions between two different inhibitory systems in the human motor cortex. J Physiol 2001; 530:307–317.
25. Dick JP, Cowan JM, Day BL, Berardelli A, Kachi T, Rothwell JC, Marsden CD. The corticomoto-neurone connection is normal in Parkinson's disease. Nature 1984; 310:407–409.
26. Cantello R, Gianelli M, Bettucci D, Civardi C, De Angelis MS, Mutani R. Parkinson's disease rigidity: magnetic motor evoked potentials in a small hand muscle. Neurology 1991; 41:1449–1456.
27. Abbruzzese G, Marchese R, Trompetto C. Sensory and motor evoked potentials in multiple system atrophy: a comparative study with Parkinson's disease. Mov Disord 1997; 12:315–321.
28. Eisen A, Siejka S, Schulzer M, Calne D. Age-dependent decline in motor evoked potential (MEP) amplitude: with a comment on changes in Parkinson's disease. Electroencephalogr Clin Neurophysiol 1991; 81:209–215.
29. Valls-Sole J, Pascual-Leone A, Brasil-Neto JP, Cammarota A, McShane L, Hallett M. Abnormal facilitation of the response to transcranial magnetic stimulation in patients with Parkinson's disease. Neurology 1994; 44:735–741.
30. Berardelli A, Rona S, Inghilleri M, Manfredi M. Cortical inhibition in Parkinson's disease. A study with paired magnetic stimulation. Brain 1996; 119:71–77.
31. Priori A, Berardelli A, Inghilleri M, Accornero N, Manfredi M. Motor cortical inhibition and the dopaminergic system. Pharmacological changes in the silent period after transcranial brain stimulation in normal subjects, patients with Parkinson's disease and drug-induced parkinsonism. Brain 1994; 117:317–323.
32. Pardal AM, Gatto EM, Reisin RC, Pardal MMF. Cortical silent period in patients with de novo Parkinson's disease and essential tremor. Neurology 1999; 52:A167.
33. Ridding MC, Rothwell JC. Stimulus/response curves as a method of measuring motor cortical excitability in man. Electroencephalogr Clin Neurophysiol 1997; 105:340–344.
34. Valzania F, Strafella AP, Quatrale R, Santangelo M, Tropeani A, Lucchi D, Tassinari CA, De Grandis D. Motor evoked responses to paired cortical magnetic stimulation in Parkinson's disease. Electroencephalogr Clin Neurophysiol 1997; 105:37–43.
35. Pierantozzi M, Palmieri MG, Marciani MG, Bernardi G, Giacomini P, Stanzione P. Effect of apomorphine on cortical inhibition in Parkinson's disease patients: a transcranial magnetic stimulation study. Exp Brain Res 2001; 141:52–62.
36. Strafella AP, Valzania F, Nassetti SA, Tropeani A, Bisulli A, Santangelo M, Tassinari CA. Effects of chronic levodopa and pergolide treatment on cortical excitability in patients with Parkinson's disease: a transcranial magnetic stimulation study. Clin Neurophysiol 2000; 111:1198–1202.
37. Young MS, Triggs WJ, Bowers D, Greer M, Friedman WA. Stereotactic pallidotomy lengthens the transcranial magnetic cortical stimulation silent period in Parkinson's disease. Neurology 1997; 49:1278–1283.

38. Chen R, Garg RR, Lozano AM, Lang AE. Effects of internal globus pallidus stimulation on motor cortex excitability. Neurology 2001; 56:716–723.

39. Gironell A, Kulisevsky J, Sedano BP, Molet J. Effects of internal globus pallidus stimulation on motor cortex excitability. Neurology 2002; 58:669–670.

40. Cunic D, Roshan L, Khan FI, Lozano AM, Lang AE, Chen R. Effects of subthalamic nucleus stimulation on motor cortex excitability in Parkinson's disease. Neurology 2002; 58:1665–1672.

41. Marchese R, Trompetto C, Buccolieri A, Abbruzzese G. Abnormalities of motor cortical excitability are not correlated with clinical features in atypical parkinsonism. Mov Disord 2000; 15: 1210–1214.

42. Levy LA, Savit JM, Hodes M. Parkinsonism: improvement by electroconvulsive therapy. Arch Phys Med Rehabil 1983; 64:432–433.

43. Friedman J, Gordon N. Electroconvulsive therapy in Parkinson's disease: a report on five cases. Convuls Ther 1992; 8:204–210.

44. Cunnington R, Iansek R, Johnson KA, Bradshaw JL. Movement-related potentials in Parkinson's disease. Motor imagery and movement preparation. Brain 1997; 120:1339–1353.

45. Eidelberg D, Moeller JR, Dhawan V, Spetsieris P, Takikawa S, Ishikawa T, Chaly T, Robeson W, Margouleff D, Przedborski S, et al. The metabolic topography of parkinsonism. J Cereb Blood Flow Metab 1994; 14:783–801.

46. DeLong MR. Primate models of movement disorders of basal ganglia origin. Trends Neurosci 1990; 13:281–5.

47. Siebner HR, Peller M, Willoch F, Minoshima S, Boecker H, Auer C, Drzezga A, Conrad B, Bartenstein P. Lasting cortical activation after repetitive TMS of the motor cortex: a glucose metabolic study. Neurology 2000; 54:956–963.

48. Mottaghy FM, Hungs M, Brugmann M, Sparing R, Boroojerdi B, Foltys H, Huber W, Topper R. Facilitation of picture naming after repetitive transcranial magnetic stimulation. Neurology 1999; 53:1806–1812.

49. George MS, Lisanby SH, Sackeim HA. Transcranial magnetic stimulation: applications in neuropsychiatry. Arch Gen Psychiatry 1999; 56:300–311.

50. Pascual-Leone A, Alonso MD, Pascual-Leone Pascual A, Catala MD. Lasting beneficial effect of radip-rate transcranial magnetic stimulation on slowness in Parkinson's disease. Neurology 1995; 45(suppl):A315.

51. Mally J, Stone TW. Improvement in Parkinsonian symptoms after repetitive transcranial magnetic stimulation. J Neurol Sci 1999; 162:179–184.

52. Shimamoto H, Morimitsu H, Sugita S, Nakahara K, Shigemori M. Therapeutic effect of repetitive transcranial magnetic stimulation in Parkinson's disease. Rinsho Shinkeigaku 1999; 39:1264–1267.

53. Boylan LS, Pullman SL, Lisanby SH, Spicknall KE, Sackeim HA. Repetitive transcranial magnetic stimulation to SMA worsens complex movements in Parkinson's disease. Clin Neurophysiol 2001; 112:259–264.

54. Siebner HR, Mentschel C, Auer C, Conrad B. Repetitive transcranial magnetic stimulation has a beneficial effect on bradykinesia in Parkinson's disease. Neuroreport 1999; 10:589–594.

55. Siebner HR, Rossmeier C, Mentschel C, Peinemann A, Conrad B. Short-term motor improvement after sub-threshold 5-Hz repetitive transcranial magnetic stimulation of the primary motor hand area in Parkinson's disease. J Neurol Sci 2000; 178:91–94.

56. Sommer M, Kamm T, Tergau F, Ulm G, Paulus W. Repetitive paired-pulse transcranial magnetic stimulation affects corticospinal excitability and finger tapping in Parkinson's disease. Clin Neurophysiol 2002; 113:944–950.

57. Siebner HR, Tormos JM, Ceballos-Baumann AO, Auer C, Catala MD, Conrad B, Pascual-Leone A. Low-frequency repetitive transcranial magnetic stimulation of the motor cortex in writer's cramp. Neurology 1999; 52:529–537.

58. Loo CK, Taylor JL, Gandevia SC, McDarmont BN, Mitchell PB, Sachdev PS. Transcranial magnetic stimulation (TMS) in controlled treatment studies: are some "sham" forms active?. Biol Psychiatry 2000; 47:325–313.

59. Pascual-Leone A, Valls-Sole J, Brasil-Neto JP, Cammarota A, Grafman J, Hallett M. Akinesia in Parkinson's disease. II. Effects of subthreshold repetitive transcranial motor cortex stimulation. Neurology 1994; 44:892–898.

60. Ghabra MB, Hallett M, Wassermann EM. Simultaneous repetitive transcranial magnetic stimulation does not speed fine movement in PD. Neurology 1999; 52:768–770.

61. Tergau F, Wassermann EM, Paulus W, Ziemann U. Lack of clinical improvement in patients with Parkinson's disease after low and high frequency repetitive transcranial magnetic stimulation. Electroencephalogr Clin Neurophysiol Suppl 1999; 51:281–288.

62. Gerloff C, Corwell B, Chen R, Hallett M, Cohen LG. Stimulation over the human supplementary motor area interferes with the organization of future elements in complex motor sequences. Brain 1997; 120:1587–1602.
63. Pullman SL. Spiral analysis: a new technique for measuring tremor with a digitizing tablet. Mov Disord 1998; 13:85–89.
64. Potrebic A, Dragasevic N, Svetel M. Kostic VS. [Effect of slow repetitive transcranial magnetic stimulation on depression in patients with Parkinson disease]. Srp Arh Celok Lek 2001; 129:1–4.
65. Mottaghy FM, Krause BJ, Kemna LJ, Topper R, Tellmann L, Beu M, Pascual-Leone A, Muller-Gartner HW. Modulation of the neuronal circuitry subserving working memory in healthy human subjects by repetitive transcranial magnetic stimulation. Neurosci Lett 2000; 280:167–170.
66. Pascual-Leonc A, Gates JR, Dhuna A. Induction of speech arrest and counting errors with rapid-rate transcranial magnetic stimulation. Neurology 1991; 41:697–702.
67. Cunnington R, Iansek R, Thickbroom GW, Laing BA, Mastaglia FL, Bradshaw JL, Phillips JG. Effects of magnetic stimulation over supplementary motor area on movement in Parkinson's disease. Brain 1996; 119:815–822.
68. Maeda F, Keenan JP, Tormos JM, Topka H, Pascual-Leone A. Interindividual variability of the modulatory effects of repetitive transcranial magnetic stimulation on cortical excitability. Exp Brain Res 2000; 133:425–430.
69. Muellbacher W, Ziemann U, Boroojerdi B, Hallett M. Effects of low-frequency transcranial magnetic stimulation on motor excitability and basic motor behavior. Clin Neurophysiol 2000; 111:1002–1007.
70. Paus T, Jech R, Thompson CJ, Comeau R, Peters T, Evans AC. Transcranial magnetic stimulation during positron emission tomography: a new method for studying connectivity of the human cerebral cortex. J Neurosci 1997; 17:3178–3184.
71. Boylan LS, Sackeim HA. Magnetoelectric brain stimulation in the assessment of brain physiology and pathophysiology. Clin Neurophysiol 2000; 111:504–512.

29

Autonomic Nervous System Disturbances

Amos D. Korczyn and Tanya Gurevich

*Tel Aviv Sourasky Medical Center, Sackler School of Medicine,
Tel Aviv University, Ramat-Aviv, Israel*

I. INTRODUCTION

The parkinsonian syndromes are a group of disorders with clinical, pathological, and genetic heterogeneity. Although considered to be predominantly motor disorders, other manifestations frequently coexist which, at times, may play a prominent role. More attention is being given to nonmotor aspects of Parkinson's disease (PD), including cognitive, affective, and sensory disturbances. Autonomic nervous system (ANS) disturbances, although much less prominent in PD than in multiple system atrophy (MSA), may still adversely affect the quality of life of PD patients. Patients with PD often complain of difficulties in micturition and gastrointestinal function and may also have defective cardiovascular control and temperature regulation as well as salivary drooling (1–4). Seborrhea, a classic feature of parkinsonism, is frequently considered a vegetative symptom, although the pathogenesis is obscure (5,6).

PD primarily affects the brain, but autonomic symptoms may be ascribed not only to faulty central regulation (7–9), but also to changes in the peripheral autonomic system. There is some evidence of changes in the autonomic ganglia and in the adrenal glands in PD (10,11). Evidence supporting a peripheral contribution to the autonomic dysfunction in PD is the finding of cardiac sympathetic denervation seen during scintigraphy with [123I]-metaiodobenzylguanidine (MIBG), which enables the quantification of postganglionic sympathetic cardiac innervation (12). Positron emission tomography (PET) scanning with 6-[18F]-fluorodopa, which enables visualization of sympathetic innervation to the heart, was also found to be reduced in PD (13). Thus, dysautonomia in PD can be related to both central and peripheral components.

It is important to differentiate manifestations that are an integral part of the clinical spectrum of PD from those that are iatrogenic. Autonomic manifestations in patients with PD are rarely specific. Changes in various functions, such as those of the gastrointestinal tract, are common in old age and have similar characteristics in normal aging and in parkinsonian patients, but data on their respective frequencies are not easily available (14). A formidable question in a particular patient is whether constipation, for example, is a manifestation of age, disease, therapy, or any combination of these factors. Another problem that may occur, particularly in the diagnosis of patients in whom the autonomic problems predominate, is whether the disturbances indicate MSA rather than PD. These questions require detailed understanding of not only the pathophysiology but also relevant pharmacological issues.

MSA has been distinguished from PD based on clinical, pathological, and imaging data (15–18). In many cases of MSA the autonomic symptoms are responsible for the main disability of the patient. In other cases it may be clinically more difficult, or even impossible, to decide whether the patient suffers from PD or from MSA. However, the treatment of the autonomic dysfunction is basically identical in PD and in MSA.

II. GASTROINTESTINAL FUNCTION

Various disturbances of gastrointestinal function occur in patients with PD. Sialorrhea, a common manifestation of PD, most often results from a reduction of automatic swallowing and should therefore be regarded as a manifestation of hypokinesia rather than a purely autonomic dysfunction. This symptom responds satisfactorily to treatment with levodopa and dopaminomimetic drugs. Some patients with prominent sialorrhea may derive benefit from high dosages of a peripherally acting anticholinergic drug (such as propantheline, 15–45 mg/d in divided doses), which acts on the salivary glands to reduce its activity. When these agents are employed in this high concentration, decreased salivation may be achieved, while central anticholinergic toxicity is avoided because of its poor penetration through the blood-brain barrier. Transdermal scopolamine (Scopoderm) is also helpful in the reduction of sialorrhea and rarely causes central anticholinergic side effects (19). The use of antimuscarinic drugs may further impair swallowing by increasing the viscosity of the saliva. The difficulties in swallowing saliva may also be relieved by drugs that liquefy the saliva. Bromhexine, a mucolytic agent, given in a dose of 8 mg three times daily may be helpful. A novel approach is the use of botulinum toxin injections into the parotid glands (20–22).

The pathophysiology of swallowing disturbances in PD is incompletely understood. The relevance of this problem is underscored by the fact that patients may aspirate food, leading to pneumonia. Recurrent pneumonia should alert the neurologist to the possibility of swallowing difficulties. The abnormality is partially responsive to levodopa (10), presumably because it involves the striated muscles of the oropharynx. Smooth muscle dysfunction in the esophagus may additionally be manifested as gastroesophageal reflux that is poorly responsive to medication. Some patients may require a feeding gastrostomy to prevent malnutrition and reflux aspiration pneumonia (23,24).

Probably the most common gastrointestinal manifestation of PD is constipation, and this frequently predates the diagnosis or the motor manifestations of the disease (10,25). Constipation was described by James Parkinson (26). Abbott et al. (27) showed that infrequent bowel movements were associated with an elevated risk of future PD. A more detailed analysis of the underlying mechanisms responsible for the constipation and its characteristics is needed. It is important to look systematically for Lewy bodies in mesenteric ganglia (10), since these peripheral structures may provide confirmatory tissue diagnosis of PD. The most severe gastrointestinal complication of PD is intestinal pseudo-obstruction, with the development of paralytic or adynamic ileus. Patients may have to undergo emergency explorative laparotomy and sigmoidostomy for the treatment of the ileus.

Patients with PD are not immune to other disorders. Therefore, patients suffering from constipation should undergo the usual investigations, particularly if a change occurs in the pattern of gastrointestinal functions (e.g., the development of subileus or ileus), if the constipation alternates with diarrhea, or if it is accompanied by iron-deficiency anemia. The constipation may be exacerbated by antiparkinsonian drugs, particularly antimuscarinics and amantadine. The constipation in PD will frequently respond to various dietary and drug manipulations, including high-fiber diet and mild laxatives, but may eventually lead to dependence on enemas. Macrogol 3350/electrolyte produced a marked improvement in constipation in patients with PD and MSA (28).

Stimulation of cholinergic receptors in the gastrointestinal tract should be efficacious in patients in whom neurogenic hypoactivity is responsible for the constipation. This can be achieved by the use of direct stimulants (such as bethanechol) or by using inhibitors of cholinesterase, which enhance the action of endogenous acetylcholine. Unfortunately, clinical experience shows that oral neostigmine or bethanechol are not helpful in the treatment of this condition. Even the intravenous administration of these agents, while undoubtedly stimulating intestinal motility, does not usually result in fecal evacuation. Since the desired action of the drug in constipated patients is on the colon, another approach is the use of a cholinergic agent given by enema. The dose required is 20–50 mg of bethanechol (dissolved in a small amount of saline), usually administered two or three times weekly.

Weight loss frequently accompanies PD, although it is relatively mild (29). Several factors may contribute to this phenomenon, including swallowing impairment (30), anorexia, or nausea caused by dopaminergic therapy. Another contributing factor could be bradykinesia. One cause of anorexia that must be considered in a patient with PD is depression. In such cases antidepressants may counteract the affective changes and increase the appetite. Many antidepressants are known to increase weight. In our study (31), patients with PD treated with the dopaminergic drug lisuride gained weight. This observation is consistent with animal data (32). Weight gain was also seen in parkinsonian patients after unilateral pallidotomy, with high correlation between weight gain and improvement in off motor scores. It was suggested that this phenomenon is related to the changes in the cardinal manifestations of PD (33).

The weight of parkinsonian patients is important for proper drug management. It was shown that body weight influences the pharmacokinetics of levodopa in PD patients, and thus lighter patients receive a greater relative dose of the drug per kilogram of body weight and are more predisposed to drug-induced peak-dose dyskinesias (34). If weight loss is a problem, a high-calorie diet should be recommended (35). In addition, domperidone can be efficacious. Domperidone is a quaternary dopamine receptor–blocking drug that can affect the chemoreceptor trigger zone in the medulla oblongata and thus counteracts nausea and vomiting. Other antidopaminergics cross the blood-brain barrier and may enhance the parkinsonism and are therefore contraindicated in PD.

III. CARDIOVASCULAR SYSTEM

Livedo reticularis, or cutis marmorata, frequently occurs among patients treated with amantadine and for unknown reasons is particularly common in women. The mechanism underlying this phenomenon is unclear but may be related to venular dilation. Although this phenomenon is innocuous, it is important to recognize as a drug effect.

Edema of the legs is another common feature in advanced PD. It is almost always absent or less conspicuous upon awakening and develops during the day. In patients with predominantly unilateral disease, the affected limb is more edematous than the contralateral limb. In such cases, leg edema is probably due to a loss of the propelling forces on venous flow by muscular activity, particularly in advanced stages of PD. Dopaminergic drugs are frequently helpful since they affect hypokinesia, but several studies have recently shown that dopamine agonists may cause leg edema (36–39). Amantadine may also increase edema, particularly if high dosages are being used.

Cardiac arrhythmias are rare in patients with PD. These have been reported as side effects of levodopa therapy, but the use of peripheral decarboxylase inhibitors markedly reduced the frequency of this adverse event.

The most disabling and dangerous cardiovascular manifestation of autonomic failure is dysregulation of blood pressure. This is manifested mainly as orthostatic hypotension (OH), frequently accompanied by recumbent hypertension. Occasionally patients complain of dizziness and actually fall, but the relationship to blood pressure may not be immediately obvious. Hypotension in PD is more common following meals (40), although patients may not be aware of the association with food intake. Conversely, lack of energy or tiredness may be a reflection of hypotension rather than an off state. Although postprandial hypotension may be frequent in PD patients, OH is rare in the early, untreated stages of PD. It usually appears in response to dopaminergic treatment. Occurrence of OH in the early stages of the disease, with or without other prominent autonomic disturbances such as urinary incontinence and impotence, suggests that the patient may not be suffering from PD but from MSA.

It must be realized that OH may not necessarily occur as a full-blown condition. This is because the symptoms result from decreased perfusion of the brain, which may occur when venous return to the heart, and thus cardiac output, are reduced, even while peripheral vasoconstriction prevents the blood pressure from falling significantly. Patients may complain of vague symptoms such as weakness, dizziness, or blurred vision, and if these occur in the upright posture, blood pressure monitoring is required. However, these patients can be treated as OH even if blood pressure fall cannot be documented.

In a study with PET scanning after injection of the radioactive tracer 6-[^{18}F]-fluorodopa for visualization of sympathetic innervation, the derived radioactivity was reduced in the myocardium and in the thyroid and renal cortex of patients with PD. It was therefore suggested that OH reflects sympathetic neurocirculatory failure resulting from generalized sympathetic denervation (13).

Drugs may constitute an important factor contributing to OH in patients with PD (41). Several antiparkinsonian agents, including levodopa, may cause or exacerbate OH. The peripheral conversion of levodopa to dopamine may also contribute to hypotension. Dopamine may stimulate presynaptic receptors in noradrenergic sympathetic terminals, which act by negative feedback to reduce noradrenaline release. This latter component is eliminated by the coadministration of decarboxylase inhibitors (9).

The monoamine oxidase type B (MAO-B) inhibitor selegiline may also cause OH due to its amphetamine- and tyramine-like effects (42). Rasagiline mesylate is a new potent, selective, non-reversible MAO-B inhibitor that is not metabolized to amphetamine or methamphetamine and has no tyramine-potentiating effect. It is currently being evaluated as an adjunct therapy to levodopa in PD. In clinical trials at doses of up to 5 mg per day, the incidence of side effects was not distinguishable from those reported by placebo-treated patients. At doses of 10 mg per day it caused hypertension and postural hypotension in two out of five patients when given with levodopa (43).

Activation of dopamine receptors located on sympathetic terminals inhibits norepinephrine release. This action may be abolished by coadministration of the D_2 receptor antagonist domperidone. Amitriptyline and other tricyclic antidepressants may also cause OH.

PD and MSA patients with autonomic disturbances are also prone to supine hypertension that may possibly be ascribed to dysregulation of blood pressure. It was hypothesized that nocturnal hypertension is a risk factor in the development of cerebrovascular disease in patients who are affected by autonomic failure (40). All drugs used to treat OH may cause, or exacerbate, recumbent hypertension. The dangers of supine hypertension make the treatment of OH more complicated. Therefore treatment of any patient with OH requires close monitoring of nocturnal blood pressure.

A practical approach to the management of OH in PD is to reduce as much as possible the dose of levodopa and dopamine agonists or block their peripheral effect by employing domperidone. The dose of domperidone to be used is 10 mg three times daily, 30 minutes before giving antiparkinsonian medications (44,45).

A comprehensive approach to OH treatment includes nonpharmacological measures, such as good hydration, diet with salt supplementation, and the use of high elastic hose. Symptomatic patients with OH who are not responsive to nonpharmacological measures and domperidone treatment must receive medications to control their OH. The standard and commonly used medications are fludrocortisone and the α-receptor agonist midodrine. In a multinational, multi-center, dose-ranging study, 300 mg of twice-daily L-threo-DOPS seemed to offer effective control of symptomatic neurogenic hypotension and was well tolerated by the patients (46). A subset of MSA patients have postural hypotension that may be associated with normocytic normochromic anemia. A therapeutic trial with recombinant erythropoietin may be worthwhile in MSA patients with autonomic failure and anemia (47). The antidiuretic V_2 receptor–specific vasopressin analogue desmopressin increases the intravascular volume and may be a useful alternative to, or may supplement, other forms of treatments in some patients. Given in the dose of 2–4 μg intramuscularly at 8p.m. it reduced nocturnal polyuria, diminished overnight weight loss, and reduced the postural blood pressure fall, especially in the morning, but raised supine blood pressure (48). Desmopressin may also be given intranasally (49). The synthetic somatostatin analogue octreotide has also been proposed for the treatment of both postprandial and orthostatic hypotension. It mainly mediates splanchnic venoconstriction, which explains its beneficial effect, which is more significant in postprandial hypotension. In different studies it was used in the dose of 25 μg subcutaneously or 0.4–0.5 μg/kg subcutaneously (50,51). The combination of midodrine and octreotide was shown to be more potent than either drug alone (52). Use of these drugs, especially midodrine and fludrocortisone, for OH is limited because of the frequent appearance of supine hypertension in response to treatment.

Hydralazine and enalapril, given at night, are other antihypertensive agents that were found to be beneficial in the treatment of nocturnal hypertension in patients with OH, but the dose should be individualized and used with caution (53,54). Shannon et al. (55) found that patients with autonomic failure are particularly susceptible to the hypotensive effect of transdermal nitroglycerin.

IV. BLADDER DYSFUNCTION

Urination disturbances (urgency, frequency, nocturia, and incontinence) may appear in PD at a significantly higher frequency than in controls (56–58). It is difficult to dissociate these from other age-related changes, and they seem to be particularly common among men. If these problems cannot be explained by prostate hypertrophy, the contribution of drug-induced changes must be considered.

Micturition difficulties in PD are thought to be frequently due to detrusor hyper-reflexia, influenced by the basal ganglia (59). However, dysfunction of the striated urethral sphincter and pelvic musculature can also be seen in PD, with the main abnormality consisting of delayed relaxation at the time of initiation of voluntary voiding (60). Urinary incontinence was reported to result from bromocriptine (61,62,63) and urinary frequency with pramipexole (64) and pergolide (65). It has not been reported with ropinirole (38). The suggested mechanism was related to that reported for levodopa, which decreases detrusor tone, possibly through a central action (66).

Levodopa, and the D_1/D_2 receptor agonist apomorphine were reported to reduce bladder hyperactivity and to improve continence in parkinsonian patients (66–68). These data were confirmed in animal studies. These findings suggest that concurrent activation of D_1 and D_2 receptors, rather than selective stimulation of D_2 receptors alone, might be beneficial for treating urinary symptoms caused by detrusor hyperreflexia in PD (69).

Antimuscarinic drugs used for the treatment of PD can cause urinary retention, although this is usually seen only with high doses. These agents include not only antiparkinsonian drugs but also tricyclic antidepressants and other medications. Whether or not an anatomical obstruction can be demonstrated in the bladder outlet, treatment with α_1-adrenergic blockers (phenoxybenzamine, prazosin, terazosin, alfuzosin and others), 5α-reductase inhibitors (finasteride), or a combination can be offered (70,71). These should be used cautiously since they may exacerbate preexisting OH or unmask it as a new manifestation. Bethanechol chloride is commonly used to stimulate bladder contractions, but physicians should be careful when prescribing it for elderly patients with cardiovascular problems because it may induce bradycardia or hypotension.

For the treatment of urinary urgency, frequency, and incontinence, anticholinergic agents such as oxybutynin, flavoxate, tolterodine, and propantheline are effective (72,73). Tricyclic agents, particularly imipramine, may also be beneficial, as they are in nocturnal enuresis (74). Nocturia may be treated with desmopressin (intranasal, 10–40 µg, or oral, 0.1 mg, at bedtime) (75–77).

V. SEXUAL DYSFUNCTION

Sexual problems have been reported to occur in PD, particularly among males. The most frequent complaints are erectile dysfunction and premature ejaculation. The prevalence of erectile dysfunction in men with PD may be as high as 60%, almost double the frequency among age-matched nonparkinsonian male subjects (78,79). Sildenafil citrate (50 mg) was shown to be efficacious in the treatment of erectile dysfunction in parkinsonism due to either PD or MSA. It may unmask or exacerbate hypotension in MSA (80), although in patients with PD it seems to be safe and effective.

VI. MEDICATIONS AND AUTONOMIC FAILURE

Patients with autonomic failure may have unusual or exaggerated responses to some medications. For example, patients with MSA are prone to the malignant neuroleptic syndrome due to an imbalance of neurotransmitters and receptors in the central ANS (81). Neuroleptic malignant syndrome can be triggered by a reduction of dopaminergic medications, stress to the body, and heating by a variety of factors. Neuroleptic malignant syndrome was also described in patients with PD after withdrawal or alteration of dopaminergic therapy (82). Menstruation and changes of sodium serum concentration rarely precipitate neuroleptic malignant syndrome in PD patients (83).

Autonomic failure is associated with impaired baroreflex buffering and extreme sensitivity to changes in vascular tone (84,85) or volume status (86). Some hemodynamic "stressors" that would be considered trivial in healthy subjects can cause dramatic changes in blood pressure in those with autonomic failure (87). Food intake, environmental heat, and exercise acutely decrease blood pressure in patients with autonomic failure. In contrast, drinking water elicits a potent and acute pressor effect, which can improve symptoms of OH (88). Loss of autonomic function makes patients extremely volume-sensitive and also causes fluctuations in the volume status (86).

Loss of buffering capacity of the baroreflex may additionally enhance the vascular sensitivity and risk of adverse effects from vasoactive medications (89). It was suggested that even moderate changes in baroreflex function may have a substantial effect on the sensitivity to vasoactive medications. It was shown that patients with MSA were particularly sensitive to phenylephrine and nitroprusside and that they may have increased risk of side effects from over-the-counter medications, such as phenylpropanolamine or ephedra alkaloids (89–91). However, the response to a pressor agent cannot be predicted by autonomic function testing or plasma catecholamines. Empiric testing with a sequence of medications, based on the risk of side effects in the individual patient, is a useful approach (85).

VII. CONCLUSIONS

Patients with PD manifest impaired ANS activity and reactions. The pattern of impairment, with prominent gastrointestinal manifestations, is different from the abnormalities observed in progressive autonomic failure. Understanding of the pathogenesis and pathophysiology of autonomic dysfunction is still unsatisfactory.

Clinical autonomic dysfunction is rarely a problem in the initial stages of PD (with the notable exception of constipation). Instead, the existence of definite and conspicuous autonomic manifestations at onset should be an important indication that the underlying disease producing the extrapyramidal features is not PD, but another parkinsonian syndrome, such as MSA.

REFERENCES

1. Appenzeller O, Goss JE. Autonomic deficits in Parkinson's syndrome. Arch Neurol 1971; 24:50–57.
2. Rajput AH, Rozdisky B. Dysautonomia in parkinsonism: a clinicopathological study. J Neurol Neurosurg Psychiatry 1976; 11:1092–1100.
3. Tanner CM, Goetz CG, Klawans HL. Autonomic nervous system disorders. Koller WC, ed. Handbook of Parkinson's Disease. New York: Marcel Dekker, 1987:145–170.
4. Korczyn AD. Autonomic nervous system disturbances in Parkinson's disease. Adv Neurol 1990; 53:463–468.
5. Martignoni E, Godi L, Pacchetti C, Martignoni, E, Godi L, Pacchetti C, Berardesca E, Vignoli GP, Albani G, Mancini F, Nappi G. Is seborrhea a sign of autonomic impairment in Parkinson's disease. J Neural Transm 1997; 104(11–12):1295–1304.
6. Fischer M, Gemende I, Marsch W, Fischer P. Skin function and skin disorders in Parkinson's disease. J Neural Transm 2001; 108(2):205–213.
7. Aminoff MJ, Wilcox CS. Assessment of autonomic function in patients with a parkinsonian syndrome. Br Med J 1971; 4:80–84.
8. Gross M, Bannister R, Godwin-Austen R. Orthostatic hypotension in Parkinson's disease. Lancet 1972; 1:174–176.
9. Sachs C, Berglund B, Kaijser L. Autonomic cardiovascular responses in parkinsonism: effect of levodopa with dopa-decarboxylase inhibition. Acta Neurol Scand 1985; 71:37–42.
10. Korczyn AD. Autonomic nervous dysfunction in Parkinson's disease. Calne DB, Comi G, Crippa D, Horowski R, Trabucci M, eds. Parkinsonism and Aging. New York: Raven Press, 1989:211–220.
11. Jellinger KA. Post mortem studies in Parkinson's disease—is it possible to detect brain areas for specific symptoms? J Neural Transm 1999; 56:1–29.
12. Braune S, Reinhardt M, Schnitzer R, Riedel A, Lucking CH. Cardiac uptake of [^{123}I]MIBG separates Parkinson's disease from multiple system atrophy. Neurology 2000; 54:1877–1878.
13. Goldstein DS, Holmes CS, Dendi R, Bruce SR, Li ST. Orthostatic hypotension from sympathetic denervation in Parkinson's disease. Neurology 2002; 58:1247–1255.
14. Catz A, Korczyn AD. Aging and the autonomic nervous system. Vinken PJ, Bruyn GW, eds. Handbook of Clinical Neurology: The Autonomic Nervous System, Part I. New York: Elsevier, 1999:I:225–243.
15. Lantos PL. The definition of multiple system atrophy: a review of recent developments. J Neuropathol Exp Neurol 1998; 57:1099–1111.
16. Davie C, Wenning G, Barker G, Tofts P, Kendall B, Quinn N, McDonald W, Marsden C, Miller D. Differentiation of multiple system atrophy from idiopathic Parkinson's disease using proton magnetic resonance spectroscopy. Ann Neurol 1995; 37:204–210.
17. Eidelberg D, Takikawa S, Moeller JR, Dhawan V, Redington K, Chaly T, Robertson W, Dahl J, Margouleff D, Fazzini E, Przedborski S, Fahn S. Striatal hypometabolism distinguishes striatonigral degeneration from Parkinson's disease. Ann Neurol 1993; 33:518–527.
18. Kraft E, Trenkwalder C, Auer DP. T2*-weighted MRI differentiates multiple system atrophy from Parkinson's disease. Neurology 2002; 59:1265–1267.
19. Talmi YP, Finkelstein Y, Zohar Y. Reduction of salivary flow with transdermal scopolamine: a four-year experience. Otolaryngol Head Neck Surg 1990; 103:613–618.
20. Jost WH. Treatment of drooling in Parkinson's disease with botulinum toxin. Mov Disord 1999; 14:1057.
21. O'Sullivan JD, Bhatia KP, Lees AJ. Botulinum toxin A as treatment for drooling saliva in PD. Neurology 2000; 55:606–607.
22. Pal PK, Calne DB, Calne S, Tsui JKC. Botulinum toxin A as treatment for drooling saliva in PD. Neurology 2000; 54:244–247.
23. Lieberman AN, Horowitz L, Redmond P, Pachter L. Dysphagia in Parkinson's disease. Am J Gastroenterol 1980; 74:157–160.
24. Buchholz DW. Dysphagia associated with neurological disorders. Acta Otorhinolaryngol Belg 1994; 48:143–155.
25. Eadie MJ, Tyrer JH. Alimentary disorder in parkinsonism. Aust Ann Med 1965; 14:13–22.
26. Parkinson J. An Essay on the Shaking Palsy. London: Sherwood, Neely and Jones, 1817:7.
27. Abbott RD, Petrovitch H, White LR, Masaki KH. Frequency of bowel movements and the future risk of Parkinson's disease. Neurology 2001; 57:456–462.
28. Eichhorn TE, Oertel WH. Macrogol 3350/electrolyte improves constipation in Parkinson's disease and multiple system atrophy. Mov Disord. 2001; 16:1176–1177.

29. Durrieu G, LLau ME, Rascol O, Senard JM. Parkinson's disease and weight loss: a study with anthropometric and nutritional assessment. Clin Auton Res. 1992; 2:153–157.
30. Nozaki S, Saito T, Matsumura T, Miyai I, Kang J. Relationship between weight loss and dysphagia in patients with Parkinson's disease. Rinsho Shinkeigaku 1999; 39:1010–1014.
31. Rabey JM, Treves T, Streifler M, Korczyn AD. Comparison of efficacy of lisuride hydrogen maleate with increased doses of levodopa in parkinsonian patients. Adv Neurol. 1987; 45:569–572.
32. Horowski R, Wachtel H. Direct dopaminergic action of lisuride hydrogen maleate, an ergot derivative, in mice. Eur J Pharmacol 1976; 36:373–383.
33. Ondo WG, Ben-Aire L, Jankovic J, Lai E. Weight gain following unilateral pallidotomy in Parkinson's disease. Acta Neurol Scand 2000; 101:79–84.
34. Zappia M, Crescibene L, Arabia G, Nicoletti G. Body weight influences pharmacokinetics of levodopa in Parkinson's disease. Clin Neuropharmacol 2002; 25:79–82.
35. Kempster PA, Wahlqvist ML. Dietary factors in the management of Parkinson's disease. Nutr Rev 1994; 52:51–58.
36. Blackard WG. Edema—an infrequently recognized complication of bromocriptine and other ergot dopaminergic drugs. Am J Med 1993; 94:445.
37. Inzelberg R, Nisipeanu P, Rabey JM, Orlov E, Catz T, Kippervasser S, Schechtman E, Korczyn AD. Double-blind comparison of cabergoline and bromocriptine in Parkinson's disease patients with motor fluctuations. Neurology 1996; 47:785–788.
38. Schrag AE, Brooks DJ, Brunt E, Fuell D, Korczyn AD, Poewe A, Quinn W, Rascol O, Stocchi F. The safety of ropinirole, a selective nonergoline dopamine agonist, in patients with Parkinson's disease. Clin Neuropharmacol 1998; 21:169–175.
39. Tan EK, Ondo W. Clinical characteristics of pramipexole-induced peripheral edema. Arch Neurol 2000; 57:729–732.
40. Plaschke M, Trenkwalder P, Dahlheim H, Lechner C, Trenkwalder C. Twenty-four-hour blood pressure profile and blood pressure responses to head-up tilt tests in Parkinson's disease and multiple system atrophy. Hypertension 1998; 16:1433–1441.
41. Korczyn AD, Rubenstein AE. Autonomic nervous system complications of therapy. Silverstein A, ed. Neurological Complications of Therapy. New York: Futura, 1982:405–418.
42. Churchyard A, Mathias CJ, Lees AJ. Selegiline-induced postural hypotension in Parkinson's disease: a longitudinal study on the effects of drug withdrawal. Mov Disord 1999; 14:246 251.
43. Rabey JM, Sagi I, Huberman M, Melamed E, Korczyn AD, Giladi N, Inzelberg R, Djaldetti R, Klein C, Berecz G. Rasagiline Study Group. Rasagiline mesylate, a new MAO-B inhibitor for the treatment of Parkinson's disease: a double-blind study as adjunctive therapy to levodopa. Clin Neuropharmacol 2000; 23:324–330.
44. Montastruc JL, Chamontin B, Senard JM, Rascol O. Domperidone in the management of orthostatic hypotension. Clin Neuropharmacol 1985; 8:191–192.
45. Lang AE. Acute orthostatic hypotension when starting dopamine agonist therapy in Parkinson disease: the role of domperidone therapy. Arch Neurol 2001; 58:835.
46. Mathias CJ, Senard JM, Braune S, Watson L. L-Threo-dihydroxyphenylserine (L-threo-DOPS; droxidopa) the management of neurogenic orthostatic hypotension: a multi-national, multi-center, dose-ranging study in multiple system atrophy and pure autonomic failure. Clin Auton Res. 2001; 11:235–242.
47. Winkler AS, Marsden J, Parton M, Watkins PJ, Chaudhuri KR. Erythropoietin deficiency and anaemia in multiple system atrophy. Mov Disord. 2001; 16:233–239.
48. Mathias CJ, Fosbraey P, da Costa DF, Thornley A, Bannister R. The effect of desmopressin on nocturnal polyuria, overnight weight loss, and morning postural hypotension in patients with autonomic failure. Br Med J 1986; 293:353–354.
49. Riley DE. Orthostatic hypotension in multiple system atrophy. Curr Treat Options Neurol 2000; 2:225–230.
50. Armstrong E, Mathias CJ. The effects of the somatostatin analogue, octreotide, on postural hypotension, before and after food ingestion, in primary autonomic failure. Clin Auton Res. 1991; 1:135–140.
51. Lamarre-Cliche M, Cusson J. Octreotide for orthostatic hypotension. Can J Clin Pharmacol 1999; 6:213–215.
52. Hoeldtke RD, Horvath GG, Bryner KD, Hobbs GR. Treatment of orthostatic hypotension with midodrine and octreotide. J Clin Endocrinol Metab 1998; 83:339–343.
53. Fealey RD, Robertson D. Management of orthostatic hypotension. Low PA, ed. Clinical Autonomic Disorders. Philadelphia: Lippincott Raven, 1997:763–775.
54. Slavachevsky I, Rachmani R, Levi Z, Brosh D, Lidar M, Ravid M. Effect of enalapril and nifedipine on orthostatic hypotension in older hypertensive patients. J Am Geriatr Soc 2000; 48:807–810.

55. Shannon J, Jordan J, Costa F, Robertson RM, Biaggioni I. The hypertension of autonomic failure and its treatment. Hypertension 1997; 30:1062–1067.
56. De Marinis M, Argenta G, Mele D, Carbone A, Baffigo G, Agnoli A. Evaluation of vesico-urethral and sweating function in disorders presenting with parkinsonism. Clin Auton Res. 1993; 3:125–130.
57. Sakakibara R, Hattori T, Uchiyama T, Yamanishi T. Videourodynamic and sphincter motor unit potential analyse in Parkinson's disease and multiple system atrophy. J Neurol Neurosurg Psychiatry 2001; 71:600–606.
58. Siddiqui MF, Rast S, Lynn MJ, Auchus AP, Pfeiffer RF. Autonomic dysfunction in Parkinson's disease: a comprehensive symptom survey. Parkinsonism Relat Disord. 2002; 8:277–284.
59. Fitzmaurice H, Fowler CJ, Rickards D, Kirby RS. Micturition disturbance in Parkinson's disease. Br J Urol 1985; 57:652–656.
60. Singer C. Urinary dysfunction in Parkinson's disease. Clin Neurosci 1998; 5:78–86.
61. Gopinathan G, Calne DB. Incontinence of urine with long-term bromocriptine therapy. Ann Neurol 1980; 8:204.
62. Sandyk R, Gillman MA. Urinary incontinence in patient on long-term bromocriptine. Lancet 1983; 2:1260–1261.
63. Caine M. Bromocriptine and urinary incontinence. Lancet 1984; 1:228.
64. Dooley M, Markham A. Pramipexole. A review of its use in the management of early and advanced Parkinson's disease. Drugs Aging 1998; 12:495–514.
65. Uchiyama T, Sakakibara R, Hattori T. Effect of pergolide on micturition disturbance in Parkinson disease with wearing-off phenomenon (abstr). V-PD-18. The 5th International Conference on Progress in Alzheimer's and Parkinson's Disease, Kyoto, Japan 2001:110..
66. Benson GS, Raezer DM, Anderson JR, Saunders CD, Corriere JN. Effect of levodopa on urinary bladder. Urology 1976; 7:24–28.
67. Aranda B, Cramer P, Adba MA. Effect of apomorphine on the bladder of parkinsonian patients. J Urol 1992; 98:25–29.
68. Sakakibara R, Hattori T, Uchiyama T, Yamanishi T. Urodynamic evaluation in Parkinson's disease before and after l-dopa treatment (abstr). IV-ICS-36. The 9th International Catecholamine Symposium, Kyoto, Japan, 2001:81..
69. Yoshimura N, Mizuta E, Yoshida O, Kuno S. Therapeutic effects of dopamine D1/D2 receptor agonists on detrusor hyperreflexia in 1-methyl-4-phenyl-1–2,3,6-tetrahydropyridine-lesioned parkinsonian cynomolgus monkeys. J Pharmacol Exp Ther 1998; 286:228–233.
70. Nickel JC. Long-term implications of medical therapy on benign prostatic hyperplasia end points. Urology 1998; 51:50–57.
71. McVary KT. Medical therapy for benign prostatic hyperplasia progression. Curr Urol Rep 2002; 3:269–275.
72. Atala A, Amin M. Current concepts in the treatment of genitourinary tract disorders in the older individual. Drugs Aging 1991; 1:176–193.
73. Garely AD, Burrows LJ. Current pharmacotherapeutic strategies for overactive bladder. Expert Opin Pharmacother 2002; 3:287–233.
74. Korczyn AD, Kish I. The mechanism of imipramine in enuresis nocturna. Clin Exp Pharmacol Physiol. 1979; 6:31–35.
75. Partinen M. Sleep disorder related to Parkinson's disease. J Neurol 1997; 244:3–6.
76. Suchowersky O, Furtado S, Rohs G. Beneficial effect of intranasal desmopressin for nocturnal polyuria in Parkinson's disease. Mov Disord. 1995; 10:337–340.
77. Kuo HC. Efficacy of desmopressin in treatment of refractory nocturia in patients older than 65 years. Urology 2002; 59:485–489.
78. Singer C, Weiner WJ, Sanchez-Ramos J, Ackerman M. Sexual function in patients with Parkinson's disease. J Neurol Neurosurg Psychiatry 1991; 54:942.
79. Bronner G, Royter V, Korczyn AD, Giladi N. Sexuality and Parkinson's disease. Bedard M, Agid Y, Chouinard S, Fahn S, Korczyn AD, Lesperance P, eds. Mental and Behavioral Dysfunction in Movement Disorders. Totowa, NJ: Humana Press, 2003:517–526.
80. Hussain IF, Brady CM, Swinn MJ, Mathias CJ, Fowler CJ. Treatment of erectile dysfunction with sildenafil citrate (Viagra) in parkinsonism due to Parkinson's disease or multiple system atrophy with observations on orthostatic hypotension. J Neurol Neurosurg Psychiatry 2001; 71:371–374.
81. Kumagai R, Harada T, Kurokawa K, Okazaki, M, Egi N, Shimote K, Nakamura S. A case of impending neuroleptic malignant syndrome associated with Shy-Drager syndrome. No To Shinkei 1998; 50:745–749.
82. Keyser DL, Rodnitzky RL. Neuroleptic malignant syndrome in Parkinson's disease after withdrawal or alteration of dopaminergic therapy. Arch Intern Med 1991; 151:794–796.

83. Cao L, Katz RH. Acute hypernatremia and neuroleptic malignant syndrome in Parkinson disease. Am J Med Sci 1999; 318:67–68.
84. Robertson D, Hollister AS, Carey EL, Tung CS, Goldberg MR, Robertson RM. Increased vascular beta$_2$-adrenoreceptor responsiveness in autonomic dysfunction. J Am Coll Cardiol 1984; 3:850–856.
85. Jordan J, Shannon JR, Biaggioni I, Norman R, Black BK, Robertson D. Contrasting actions of pressor agents in severe autonomic failure. Am J Med 1998; 105:116–124.
86. Wilcox CS, Puritz R, Lightman SL, Bannister R, Aminoff MJ. Plasma volume regulation in patients with progressive autonomic failure during changes in salt intake or posture. J Lab Clin Med 1984; 104:331–339.
87. Shannon JR, Jordan J, Robertson RM. Blood pressure in autonomic failure: drinks, meals, and other ordeals. Clin Sci 1998; 94:5.
88. Jordan J, Shannon JR, Black BK, Ali, Y, Farley M, Costa F, Diedrich A, Robertson RM, Biaggioni I, Robertson D. The pressor response to water drinking in humans: a sympathetic reflex? Circulation 2000; 101:504–509.
89. Jordan J, Tank J, Shannon JR, Diedrich A, Lipp A, Schroder C, Arnold G, Sharma AM, Baggioni I, Robertson D, Luft FC. Baroreflex buffering and susceptibility to vasoactive drugs. Circulation 2002; 105:1459–1464.
90. Kernan WN, Viscoli CM, Brass LM, Broderick JP, Brott T, Feldman E, Morgenstern LB, Wilterdink JL, Horwitz RI. Phenylpropanolamine and the risk of hemorrhagic stroke. N Engl J Med 2000; 343:1826–1832.
91. Haller CA, Benowitz NL. Adverse cardiovascular and central nervous system events associated with dietary supplements containing ephedra alkaloids. N Engl J Med 2000; 343:1833–1838.

30
Sleep Problems

Pradeep K. Sahota

University of Missouri Health Care, Columbia, Missouri, U.S.A.

Kapil D. Sethi

Medical College of Georgia, Augusta, Georgia, U.S.A.

Sleep problems, while reported even in the original description by James Parkinson (1) and subsequently by Charcot (2), are now better defined with the recent emergence of and progress in the field of sleep medicine. There are multiple reasons for sleep problems in patients with Parkinson's disease (PD). Neuronal substrates of sleep may be affected in PD patients. Sleep is best understood in terms of its structural, neuronal, and neurochemical substrates. Several neurotransmitter systems are involved in sleep-wake functioning, including serotonin (dorsal raphe nuclei), norepinephrine (locus ceruleus), acetylcholine (pedunculopontine nucleus), and dopamine (striatonigral system, ventral tegmentum, and mesocorticolimbic system). In PD, neuronal loss occurs in the substantia nigra, locus ceruleus, and possibly in the dorsal raphe nuclei and pedunculopontine nucleus. This alteration in neuronal substrates may form the basis for sleep disturbances in patients with PD.

Sleep is also affected by physical state. Timing of sleep, along with physical and mental relaxation, in the setting of good sleep hygiene contributes to sleep onset and quality of sleep. Pain, discomfort, and physical disability have negative effects on sleep. Patients with PD are more prone to sleep problems due to limitation of movements and dyskinesias. Cognitive problems such as sun downing and visual hallucinations also contribute to sleep problems. Patients with PD may also suffer from depression and other problems that may affect sleep.

There are age-related changes in sleep that include advanced sleep phase syndrome, decreased quality of nocturnal sleep with increased arousals and awakenings, and daytime naps, which may affect patients with PD. Sleep disorders such as periodic limb movements in sleep (PLMS) and sleep apnea also increase in incidence with age. Patients with PD are also reported to develop some unique sleep disorders, such as rapid eye movement (REM) behavior disorder (RBD), which are not as common in age-matched healthy controls.

Patients with PD may be on several medications with the potential to cause sleep problems. The effect of newer therapeutic modalities including pallidotomies and subthalamic nucleus (STN) deep brain stimulation (DBS) in sleep on patients with PD is not well defined.

Sleep can also affect the clinical features of PD, which can have direct implications on the functioning ability of patients. Therefore, patients with PD can develop sleep problems with multifactorial etiologies.

I. SPECTRUM OF SLEEP PROBLEMS IN PD

While the exact incidence of sleep disturbances in PD is not known, sleep complaints have been reported in 60–90% of patients (3). These include light, fragmented sleep with an increased number of arousals and awakenings and PD-specific problems affecting sleep, including nocturnal immobility, tremor, eye-blinking, dyskinesia, periodic and aperiodic limb movements, restless leg syndrome (RLS), fragmentary myoclonus, and respiratory dysfunction. Depression, hallucinations/psychosis, and RBD with violent behavior can also cause sleep disturbances.

A recent report compared three groups—PD patients, their spouses, and healthy controls (153 PD patient and spouse pairs, 103 healthy controls) (4). Measurements included Zung self-rating depression scale and self-rating of sleep disturbance. In the PD patient group, 25% of the men and 41% of the women reported sleep problems, and these were best predicted by depression scores. Thus depression seems to play a role in sleep disturbance in patients with PD. Another study compared 90 nondepressed PD patients with 71 age-matched controls and reported more severe disturbance of sleep maintenance in patients with PD due to nocturia, pain, stiffness, and problems turning in bed (5). Daytime sleepiness was similar in both groups.

A 20-item questionnaire was used to compare 1575 PD patients with 2504 controls (6). PD patients had increased complaints of sleep-wake disturbance, frequent awakenings at night, early morning awakening, daytime sleepiness, use of sleeping pills, parasomnias, RLS, and nocturnal myoclonus, with RLS and nocturnal myoclonus increasing significantly with the worsening of PD symptoms. A larger (48 items) interview-based study of 97 untreated, nondepressed, non-demented PD patients and age- and sex-matched controls was conducted with interviews at study entry and at the initiation of levodopa therapy. There were no significant differences in sleep disruption scores or individual complaints between the two groups at study entry (7). However, increased sleep disruption scores and increased sleep complaints [significant only for excessive daytime sleepiness (EDS)] were reported in 17 patients with PD progression, suggesting that there is an increase in sleep complaints with PD progression unrelated to depression or dementia. These studies suggest that sleep problems do occur in patients with PD and may be related to both PD symptoms and other concomitant issues such as depression and may have a tendency to worsen with the progression of PD.

II. SLEEP AND COGNITIVE/MOOD PROBLEMS IN PD

Cognitive problems in PD may be accompanied by or contribute to sleep problems. There is an increased incidence of depression in patients with PD. In a retrospective survey of

339 PD patients, the prevalence of depression was 47% (8). Depression can contribute to sleep disturbances such as insomnia—specifically early morning insomnia. As mentioned earlier (4), sleep problems in a group of PD patients were best predicted by patients' depression scores. In addition to depression, visual hallucinations may occur in approximately one third of patients with PD who are on treatment. In a study of 214 consecutive patients with PD, 55 had visual hallucinations (9). Dementia, age, duration of disease, history of depression, and history of a sleep disorder were strongly associated with hallucinations.

Kline et al. compared 29 PD patients with visual hallucinations to 58 age- and disease duration–matched PD patients without visual hallucinations (10). There was a higher frequency of sleep disturbance (disorder of initiating or maintaining sleep) and dementia in patients with visual hallucinations (22 vs. 7 in the nonhallucination group). These patients were also more frequently on selegiline, more often developed wearing off and freezing phenomenon, and had lower Mini-Mental Status Examination (MMSE) scores. A study (11) of 10 nondepressed, nondemented PD patients on only dopaminergic medication carbidopa/levodopa and a dopamine agonist) was reported. Five of these patients had visual hallucinations and 5 did not. The PD patients with visual hallucinations had decreased sleep efficiency, decreased total sleep time, and decreased REM proportion. Both groups also had decreased K-complexes, decreased spindle formation, and motor activity in REM sleep consistent with RBD. Thus, cognitive and affective disturbances can also contribute to or are associated with sleep problems.

III. REM SLEEP BEHAVIOR DISORDER (RBD) IN PD

RBD was described by Schenk and colleagues (12,13) and is characterized by vigorous and injurious behavior in REM sleep that usually represents attempted dream enactment of vivid, action-filled, violent dreams. Normally, there is significant loss of muscle tone during REM sleep, with the exception of the respiratory, extraocular, and middle ear muscles. Thus, while dreaming occurs in REM sleep, it is not accompanied by dream enactment. In RBD, however, this loss of muscle tone does not occur and dream enactment may result. While Schenk and colleagues first described this disorder, increased chin electromyography (EMG) activity had been reported earlier in a study of 33 patients with PD who were recorded for 2–3 consecutive nights (14). These patients were either on no treatment or withdrawn from treatment 15 days prior to the study. They were reported to have repetitive blinking at the beginning of the night, persistence of EMG activity of chin muscles during paradoxical sleep, occurrence of rapid eye movements during slow-wave sleep and before onset of paradoxical sleep, and presence of alpha rhythm during paradoxical sleep. It was further noted that this association between blinking and persistence of activity of chin muscles during paradoxical sleep had hitherto not been encountered. A decrease in paradoxical sleep was suggested to be due to the possible involvement of the locus ceruleus.

Schenk et al. studied 29 patients over the age of 50 with RBD and reported that 11 of 29 patients developed PD with a mean interval of 3.7 years after the diagnosis of RBD and a mean interval of 12.7 years after the onset of RBD symptoms (15). They suggested the pedunculopontine nucleus as a likely site of pathology in combined RBD-PD patients.

In a study of 93 patients with RBD, neurological disorders were present in 57% of patients (16). Of these, 86% had PD, dementia without parkinsonism, or multiple system atrophy. In patients with PD, RBD preceded the onset of PD symptoms in 52% of patients. Clonazepam was effective for most patients with RBD, although it did not decrease the REM-related chin EMG activity.

IV. PERIODIC LEG MOVEMENTS IN SLEEP (PLMS) IN PD

Periodic leg movements in sleep (PLMS) occur in up to one third of patients with PD (17). Fragmentary myoclonus with irregular myoclonic twitches and jerks of extremities may occur in non-REM sleep. However, it does not seem that the incidence of PLMS is significantly higher in patients with PD as compared to age-matched controls.

V. RESPIRATORY PROBLEMS DURING SLEEP IN PD

There does not seem to be an increase in the incidence of sleep apnea in patients with PD when compared to age-matched controls. However, there may be an increase in central sleep apnea and obstructive sleep apnea in patients with PD with accompanying autonomic dysfunction (18). These findings were reported in only two patients who had autonomic dysfunction along with features of parkinsonism.

VI. EFFECT OF MEDICAL TREATMENT OF PD ON SLEEP

Dopaminergic medications are known to affect sleep, and this effect may be dose-dependent. Low dosages may be sedating and induce sleep (19,20), whereas high dosages may prolong sleep latency and cause sleep disruption (21). The appropriate dosage of dopaminergic medication at bedtime may help ameliorate PD symptoms resulting from wearing off or on-off phenomenon and reduce the nocturnal akinesia and rigidity, thereby improving sleep. It is critical to find a balance in the dosages of these medicines. A high dose may predispose the patient to dyskinesias that may adversely affect sleep. One study reported on 158 PD patients who were on a stable dose of carbidopa/levodopa and were switched to controlled-release carbidopa/levodopa (L-CR). While there was no significant change in dyskinesias, the patients on L-CR had fewer sleep interruptions per night and there was a decrease in the number of patients with sleep disturbances (45). A double-blind, placebo-controlled trial of 11 PD patients found significant improvement in sleep after nocturnal dosing of levodopa (22). A study that compared the nocturnal sleep pattern in six patients with PD treated with bromocriptine and then with levodopa found no difference between the two groups (23).

Dopaminergic medications may cause side effects that lead to sleep disturbance. Klawans et al. reported levodopa-induced myoclonus in PD patients on long-term levodopa therapy consisting of single unilateral or bilateral abrupt jerks of the extremities occurring most frequently during sleep (24).

Dopaminergic medications were recently reported to cause "sleep attacks" in nine patients on pramipexole and one patient on ropinirole, causing them to fall asleep while driving and leading to accidents (25). Of these, five patients experienced no warning before the attack. The attacks ceased when these medications were discontinued. EDS was reported in a patient on levodopa and ropinirole, and the symptoms disappeared when the treatment was changed to ropinirole monotherapy (47).

Six patients with PD reported sudden onset of sleep when a dopaminergic medication was added to levodopa therapy (26). The patients were evaluated by a sleep diary, the

Epworth Sleepiness Scale (ESS), polysomnography (PSG), multiple sleep latency test (MSLT), standard vigilance test, and driving simulation. They noted a disrupted sleep-wake pattern with the tendency toward decreased sleep efficiency, slow-wave sleep, and REM sleep. The patients had increased ESS scores and abnormal results on the MSLT or the vigilance test in five cases. The authors concluded that sudden onset of sleep in PD patients in this setting may be a phenomenon of daytime sleepiness.

The issue of sleep attacks in PD patients is not without criticism. It is suggested that EDS is common in PD and is likely to be related to both the disease process and drug therapy (27). A detailed sleep history should be a regular part of the clinical evaluation of PD patients.

Selegiline is unique among antiparkinsonian medications in that it may have an alerting effect and thus the potential to cause difficulty initiating sleep in patients with PD. However, there are reports that while it has an alerting effect it may not cause insomnia (28).

VII. EFFECT OF SURGICAL TREATMENT OF PD ON SLEEP

STN DBS is an effective treatment for patients with PD. A recent study reported 10 insomniac patients with PD who had undergone bilateral STN DBS (48). The patients were studied with stimulation on and stimulation off during the night. STN stimulation reduced nighttime akinesia by 60% and completely suppressed axial and early morning dystonia. However, it did not alleviate PLMS (3 patients) or RBD (5 patients). Total sleep time increased by 47%, and the time spent awake after initial sleep onset decreased by 51 minutes.

Another study reviewed 11 consecutive patients with advanced PD who had STN-DBS. Both subjective (sleep interview and Pittsburgh Sleep Quality Index Questionnaire) and objective (polysomnography) evaluations were performed (49). Of the 8 patients who rated their sleep quality as unsatisfactory, 7 reported marked improvement after surgery. There was an increase in the longest period of uninterrupted sleep and a decrease in the arousal index. There was also an increase in nocturnal mobility after surgery but no change in RBD. It was concluded that STN-DBS is associated with subjective improvement in sleep quality that may be secondary to increased mobility and a decrease in sleep fragmentation.

VIII. POLYSOMNOGRAPHIC SLEEP EVALUATION IN PD

Multiple PSG studies have reviewed sleep patterns in patients with PD. Kales et al. reported increased sleep onset latency and frequent awakenings with increased time in the wake state after sleep onset (29). There was an increase in stage 1 sleep and a decrease in stages 3 and 4 and REM sleep. Patients with rigidity had less REM sleep, and reports of prominent alpha waves during REM sleep have been suggested (14). Another study suggested that the increase in sleep-onset latency and the number of awakenings are proportional to the severity of PD symptoms (30). A decrease in sleep spindles during slow-wave sleep (SWS) was also reported (30). In a study of 10 PD patients compared with 5 age-matched controls, PD patients had increased sleep-onset latency and decreases in stage 3, 4 and REM sleep. Low levels of serotonin and dopamine were thought to be the neurochemical substrate of these findings (31). Decreased total REM sleep and decreased sleep efficiency in PD patients with visual hallucinations was reported (11).

The severity of PD appears to be an important factor. In a sleep laboratory study of 26 patients with untreated mild to moderate PD for less than 5 years, sleep architecture and respiration did not differ significantly from age-matched controls (32). A study comparing 12 PD patients with 12 controls and 10 patients with Huntington's disease reported that PD patients have fragmented sleep with increased arousals and awakenings, decreased sleep period time, decreased SWS, decreased REM sleep, increased stage 1, and decreased sleep spindle density (33). Another study compared 12 PD patients with 12 normal controls and 2 patients with parkinsonian features with autonomic dysfunction. PD patients had more frequent awakenings, increased waking through the night, and a significant decrease in REM sleep (18). They did not have sleep apnea but did have increased respiratory rate during the awake state and during REM sleep. Central and obstructive apneas were reported in the 2 patients who had autonomic dysfunction.

IX. ACTIGRAPHIC STUDIES IN PATIENTS WITH PD

Actigraphic monitoring of wrist movements in a continuous fashion offers the advantage of relatively cheap, in-home extended recording. In a study of 89 PD patients and 83 age-matched controls for 6 successive nights, PD patients had increased nocturnal activity, indicating more disturbed sleep (21). The mean duration of nocturnal immobility was similar in the two groups. Daily levodopa dosage or use of dopamine agonists (rather than disease severity) were the best predictors of nocturnal activity. The authors suggested that in mild to moderate PD, levodopa or dopamine agonists can cause sleep disruption by their effect on sleep regulation.

X. EFFECT OF SLEEP ON PD

Diurnal fluctuation of PD symptoms has been reported, with motor symptoms typically less severe in the morning than in the afternoon (34). In addition, circadian fluctuation of contrast sensitivity (a nonmotor variable) has also been reported in PD patients (35). Most movement disorders improve during sleep but do not disappear entirely (36,37). In a study of four patients with PD, brief episodes of tremor were reported in sleep in association with cursory arousals or body movement at any stage of sleep and without body movement or arousal in REM sleep (46). Another study of five patients with PD of longer than 5 years duration noted that tremor disappears with relaxation and during sleep and reappears with awakening. The study further reported that tremor does recur during sleep in an unpredictable fashion with electrographic features of different sleep stages (38). Tremor was also reported to occasionally reappear during sleep. Dyskinesias occurred most commonly after an awakening and to a lesser extent after a shift to the light sleep stages, but rarely during REM sleep (39).

Sleep may provide an improvement in symptoms that could last for 1–3 hours after awakening. PD patients often function best in the mornings (40). An interview based study of 162 consecutive patients examined disability upon awakening. Thirty-three percent of the PD patients reported experiencing sleep benefit. These patients tended to have earlier disease onset, longer disease duration, higher daily dosages of levodopa, longer duration of levodopa treatment, and less cognitive and physical disability (41). In a questionnaire-based study of 312 consecutive PD patients, sleep benefit was noted in 55% of patients, with 33% reporting that awakening was their best time of the day (42). Because of the sleep benefit, 21% were able to skip or delay their first dose of antiparkinsonian medication.

Patients who reported sleep benefit in this study were older, more often men, and had PD for a longer period. However, no differences were noted in the hours of sleep or sleep latency when compared with patients without sleep benefit. Another study compared 10 PD patients with sleep benefit to 10 PD patients without sleep benefit and noted small but significant motor improvement in patients with sleep benefit (43). Sleep benefit was more pronounced in patients with a higher frequency of arousals and awakenings and more disrupted REM sleep. Levodopa levels were undetectable in the morning.

Sleep may provide some benefit to PD patients. The exact mechanism of sleep benefit is unknown. It is known that individuals may have short-duration or long-duration response to levodopa that does not correspond to levodopa levels. Individuals who show benefit may possibly have more long-duration levodopa response. Restoration of the endogenous store of dopamine is another suggested explanation. There may also be a slowing of the inner clocks and a subjective change in perception such that patients may not perceive that they were doing as poorly as they did (43).

XI. SLEEP EVALUATION IN PD

Sleep disturbances are common in PD patients and need to be carefully evaluated to optimize PD therapy and treat the sleep disorder. A restful sleep may indeed provide some benefit to PD patients. A complete history of change in PD symptoms during sleep-wake hours is needed. This should include a history of motor as well as cognitive/behavioral features, including sundowning and the presence of hallucinations. Selective appearance of abnormal movements (painful dystonias or dyskinesias, extremity movements) and abnormal behaviors (nocturnal vocalizations, nightmares, nocturia, dream enactment, etc.) should be recorded. A history of urinary problems should also be obtained. A complete sleep diary reflecting hours of sleep, timing and dosage of medications (anti-parkinsonian and other) can be useful. Apart from the patient, the caregiver can provide useful information regarding sleep problems. Various sleepiness scales including the ESS and the Parkinson's Disease Sleep Scale may be useful (27). Finally, evaluation in a sleep disorders clinic may help diagnose the sleep disorder and provide help in the management of these patients. Polysomnographic studies may be needed in selective patients with respiratory problems or abnormal behaviors during the night. In-home actigraphic studies provide some information but do not have a defined clinical role in the evaluation of sleep disorders in PD.

XII. MANAGEMENT OF SLEEP PROBLEMS IN PD

Appropriate treatment of PD with an evaluation of both daytime and nighttime symptoms is important. Dopaminergic therapy may be reduced if nocturnal dyskinesias are present. An increase in the nighttime dosage may be necessary if increased rigidity or nocturnal immobility are disturbing sleep. Controlled release levodopa preparations provide added benefit in some patients. In patients with early morning worsening of symptoms, a slow-release preparation at night may be beneficial.

Good sleep hygiene with regular sleep-wake hours and regular mealtimes is helpful. Daytime activity, avoidance of long daytime naps, and bright lights early in the evening to prevent advance in sleep phase may be helpful.

The recognition and treatment of other related disorders is important. Depression is usually treated with serotonin reuptake inhibitors. There is a report of treatment of depression with fluoxetine in four PD patients resulting in a worsening of PD (44). One should be aware of this potential worsening of symptoms with treatment. Tricyclic antidepressants are used as they may benefit nocturnal sleep.

Visual hallucinations and psychosis need to be treated appropriately. Quetiapine and clozapine are the preferred drugs. The need for hematological monitoring in patients on clozapine makes it less likely to be the initial treatment of choice. RBD can be effectively treated with clonazepam in a majority of patients.

Patients treated with dopamine agonists need to be aware of the possibility of sudden somnolence while engaged in activities of daily living. If EDS does occur, wake-promoting medications such as modafinil can be useful. Modafinil seems to be effective for the management of EDS in patients with PD (50–52). In a case report, a dose of 400 mg/day was helpful in treating EDS in a patient with levodopa-responsive PD, with the ESS improving from 13 to 8 after 2 weeks of treatment (50). In a study of 10 consecutive patients with PD with EDS, a 4-week open-label trial of modafinil resulted in significant improvement, with the ESS improving from a mean of 14 to 6 (53). Headache, generalized paresthesias, and hallucinations were the reported adverse effects. The usual starting dose is 100–200 mg in the morning and it is increased gradually with most patients with EDS responding to 200–400 mg/day. In a stereological study on the neuroprotective action of acute modafinil treatment on 1-methyl-4-phenyl-1,2,3,6-tetrahydropyridine (MPTP)–induced nigral lesions in the male black mouse, co-administration of modafinil restored to normal the decreased number of tyrosine hydroxylase (TH) immunoreactive neurons and the non-TH-immunoreactive neurons (54). This suggests a potential neuroprotective role for modafinil in the substantia nigra for dopaminergic neurons and the non-dopaminergic nerve cell population affected by MPTP lesions. A similar neuroprotective role for modafinil in the MPTP-treated common marmoset has been suggested (55). Modafinil therefore holds promise as both a wake-promoting agent and a neuroprotective agent.

In summary, sleep disturbances are common in patients with PD. The relationship between sleep and PD still needs to be defined. It is important that a complete sleep history be part of the evaluation of PD patients. This will help tailor their antiparkinsonian medication to the sleep-wake changes and help treat underlying sleep disorders to improve quality of sleep and in turn quality of life. Larger prospective studies with longitudinal follow-up are needed to provide more information regarding the presence and evolution of sleep disorders in PD.

REFERENCES

1. Parkinson J. An Essay on the Shaking Palsy. London: Whittingham and Rowland, 1817.
2. Charcot JM. Lectures on the Diseases of the Nervous System. London: The New Sydenham Society, 1877.
3. Trenkwalder C. Sleep dysfunction in Parkinson's disease. Clin Neurosci 1998; 5(2):107–114.
4. Smith MC, Ellgring H, Oertel WH. Sleep disturbances in Parkinson's disease patients and spouses. J Am Geriatr Soc 1997; 45(2):194–199.
5. van Hilten JJ, Waggeman M, van der Velde EA, et al. Sleep, excessive daytime sleepiness and fatigue in Parkinson's disease. J Neural Transm 1993; 5(3):235–244.
6. Horiguchi J, Inami Y, Nishimatsu O, et al. Sleep wake complaints in Parkinson's disease (Japanese). Rinsho Shinkeigaku Clin Neurol 1990; 30(2):214–216.
7. Carter J, Carroll VS, Lannon MC, et al. Sleep disruption in untreated Parkinson's disease. Neurology 1990; 40 (suppl 1):220.
8. Dooneief G, Mirabello E, Bell K, et al. An estimate of the incidence of depression in idiopathic Parkinson's disease. Arch Neurol 1992; 49:305–307.

9. Sanchez-Ramos JR, Ortoll R, Paulson GW. Visual hallucinations associated with Parkinson disease. Arch Neurol 1996; 53:1265–1268.

10. Kline C, Kompf D, Pulkowski U, et al. A study of visual hallucinations in patients with Parkinson's disease. J Neurol 1997; 244:371–377.

11. Comella CL, Tanner CM, Ristanovic RK. Polysomnographic sleep measures in Parkinson's disease patients with treatment-induced hallucinations. Ann Neurol 1993; 34(5):710–714.

12. Schenk CH, Bundlie SR, Ettinger MG, et al. Chronic behavioral disorders of human REM sleep: a new category of insomnia. Sleep 1986; 9:293–308.

13. Schenk CH, Bundlie SR, Patterson AL, et al. Rapid eye movement sleep behavior disorder: a treatable parasomnia affecting older adults. JAMA 1987; 257:1786–1789.

14. Mouret J. Differences in sleep in patients with Parkinson's disease. Electroencephalogr Clin Neurophysiol 1975; 38(6):653–657.

15. Schenk CH, Bundlie SR, Mahowald MW. Delayed emergence of a parkinsonian disorder in 38% of 29 older men initially diagnosed with idiopathic rapid eye movement sleep behavior disorder. Neurology 1996; 46:388–393.

16. Olson EJ, Boeve BF, Silber MH. Rapid eye movement sleep behavior disorder: demographic, clinical and laboratory findings in 93 cases. Brain 2000; 123:331–339.

17. Aldrich MS. Parkinsonism. In: Kryger MH, Roth T, Dement WCPrinciples and Practice of Sleep Medicine. 3rd ed. Philadelphia: WB Saunders Company, 2000:1051–1057.

18. Apps MC, Sheaff PC, Ingram DA, et al. Respiration and sleep in Parkinson's disease. J Neurol Neurosurg Psychiatry 1985; 48:1240–1245.

19. Askenasy JJM, Yahr MD. Suppression of REM rebound by pergolide. J Neurol Trans 1984; 59:151–159.

20. Askenasy JJM, Yahr MD. Parkinsonian tremor loses its alternating aspect during non-REM sleep and is inhibited by REM sleep. J Neurol Neurosurg Psychiatry 1990; 52:749–753.

21. van Hilten B, Hoff JI, Middlekoop AM, et al. Sleep disruption in Parkinson's disease—assessment by continuous activity monitoring. Arch Neurol 1994; 51:922–928.

22. Leeman AL, O'Neil CJ, Nicholson PW, et al. Parkinson's disease in the elderly: response to and optimal spacing of night time dosing with levodopa. Br J Clin Pharmacol 1987; 24(5):637–643.

23. Vardi J, Glaubman H, Rabey J, et al. EEG sleep patterns in parkinsonian patients treated with bromocryptine and L-dopa: a comparative study. J Neural Transm 1979; 45(4):307–316.

24. Klawans HL, Goetz C, Bergen D. Levodopa-induced myoclonus. Arch Neurol 1975; 32:331–334.

25. Frucht S, Rogers JD, Greene PE, et al. Falling asleep at the wheel: motor vehicle mishaps in persons taking pramipexole and ropinirole. Neurology 1999; 52(9):1908–1910.

26. Moller JC, Stiasny K, Hargutt V, et al. Evaluation of sleep and driving performance with Parkinson's disease reporting sudden onset of sleep under dopaminergic medication: a pilot study. Mov Disord 2002; 17(3):474–481.

27. Chaudhuri KR, Pal S, Brefel-Courbon C. 'Sleep attacks' or 'unintended sleep episodes' occur with dopamine agonists: is this a class effect? Drug Safety 2002; 25(7):473–483.

28. Lavie P, Wajsbort J, Youdim MB. Deprenyl does not cause insomnia in parkinsonian patients. Commun Psychopharm 1980; 4(4):303–307.

29. Kales A, Ansel R, Markham C, et al. Sleep in patients with Parkinson's disease and normal subsets prior to and following levodopa administration. Clin Pharmacol Ther 1971; 12:397–406.

30. Freidman A. Sleep patterns in Parkinson's disease. Acta Med Pol 1980; 21:193–199.

31. Friedman A. Sleep pattern in parkinsonism. Preliminary communications (polish). Neurol Neurochir Pol 1977; 11(3):289–293.

32. Ferini-Strambi L, Franceschi M, Pinto P, et al. Respiration and heart rate variability during sleep in untreated Parkinson patients. Gerontology 1992; 38:92–98.

33. Emser W, Brenner M, Stober T, et al. Changes in nocturnal sleep in Huntington's and Parkinson's disease. J Neurol 1988; 235(3):177–179.

34. Yamamura Y, Sobue I, Ando K, et al. Paralysis agitans of early onset with marked diurnal fluctuation of symptoms. Neurology 1973; 23(3):239–244.

35. Struck LK, Rodnitzky RL, Dobson JK. Circadian fluctuations of contrast sensitivity in Parkinson's disease. Neurology 1990; 40:467–470.

36. Autret A, Lucas B, Henry F, et al. The influence of sleep on abnormal waking movements (French). Neurophys Clin 1994; 24(3):218–226.

37. Dyken ME, Rodnitzky RL. Periodic, aperiodic, and rhythmic motor disorders of sleep. Neurology 1992; 42(suppl 6):68–74.

38. April RS. Observations on parkinsonian tremor in all night sleep. Neurology 1966; 16:720–724.

39. Fish DR, Sawyers D, Allen PJ. The effect of sleep on the dyskinetic movements of Parkinson's disease, Gilles de la Tourette syndrome, Huntington's disease, and torsion dystonia. Arch Neurol 1991; 48(2):210–214.
40. Clark EC, Feinstein B. The on-off effect in Parkinson's disease treated with levodopa with remarks concerning the effect of sleep. Adv Exp Med Biol 1977; 90:175–182.
41. Currie LJ, Bennett JP jr, Harrison MB, et al. Clinical correlates of sleep benefit in Parkinson's disease. Neurology 1997; 48(4):1115–1117.
42. Morello M, Hughes A, Colosimo C, et al. Sleep benefit in Parkinson's disease. Mov Disord 1997; 12(4):506–508.
43. Hogl BE, Gomez-Arevalo G, Garcia S, et al. A clinical, pharmacologic, and polysomnographic study of sleep benefit in Parkinson's disease. Neurology 1998; 50(5):1332–1339.
44. Steur ENHJ. Increase of Parkinson disability after fluoxetine medication. Neurology 1993; 43:211–213.
45. Pahwa R, Busenbark K, Huber SJ, et al. Clinical experience with controlled-release carbidopa/ levodopa in Parkinson's disease. Neurology 1993; 43:677–681.
46. Stern M, Roffwarg H, Duvoisin R. The parkinsonian tremor in sleep. J Nerv Ment Dis 1968; 147:202–210.
47. Schafer D, Greulich W. Effect of parkinsonian medication on sleep. J Neurol 2000; 247(suppl 4): 24–27.
48. Arnulf I, Bejjani BP, Garma L, et al. Improvement of sleep architecture with subthalamic nucleus stimulation. Neurology 2000; 55:1732–1734.
49. Iranzo A, Valldeoriola F, Santamaria J, et al. Sleep symptoms and polysomnographic architecture in advanced Parkinson's disease after chronic bilateral subthalamic stimulation. J Neurol Neurosurg Psychiatry 2002; 72:661–664.
50. Rabinstein A, Shulman LM, Weiner WJ. Modafinil for the treatment of excessive daytime sleepiness in Parkinson's disease: a case report. Parkinsonism Relat Disord 2001; 7(4):287–288.
51. Happe S, Pirker W, Sauter C, et al. Successful treatment of excessive daytime sleepiness in Parkinson's disease with modafinil. J Neurol 2001; 248(7):632–634.
52. Hauser RA, Wahba MN, Zesiewicz TA, et al. Modafinil treatment of pramipexole-associated somnolence. Mov Disord 2001; 15(6):1269–1271.
53. Nieves AV, Lang AE. Treatment of excessive daytime sleepiness in patients with Parkinson's disease with modafinil. Clin Neuropharmacol 2002; 25(2):111–114.
54. Aguirre JA, Cintra A, Hillion J, et al. A stereological study on the neuroprotective actions of acute modafinil treatment on 1-methyl-4-phenyl-1,2,3,6-tetrahydropyridine-induced nigral lesions of the male black mouse. Neurosci Lett 1999; 275(3):215–218.
55. Jenner P, Zeng BY, Smith LA, et al. Antiparkinsonian and neuroprotective effects of modafinil in the MPTP-treated common marmoset. Exp Brain Res 2000; 133(2):178–188.

31

Psychosis and Dementia

Hubert H. Fernandez*

*Memorial Hospital of Rhode Island and Brown University School of Medicine,
Providence, Rhode Island, U.S.A.*

Leslie Shinobu

*Massachusetts General Hospital and Harvard Medical School,
Boston, Massachusetts, U.S.A.*

I. PSYCHOSIS

A. Introduction

Psychotic symptoms rarely occur in untreated Parkinson's disease (PD) (1,2) or in PD patients with a concomitant psychiatric illness such as schizophrenia (3). Much more commonly, psychotic symptoms occur as a complication of PD drug therapy (4–6), in which all anti-PD drugs have been implicated (7–9). It is the single most important factor precipitating nursing home placement (10–12). Psychotic symptoms in PD can be subdivided into three general categories: hallucinations, psychosis, and delirium.

Abnormal dream phenomena precede psychosis in some patients and include vivid dreams, nightmares, and night terrors (13,14). These can occur in more than 30% of PD patients and are perceived as risk factors for more serious forms of psychosis (15,16).

Hallucinations are usually visual, nonthreatening, and associated with preserved insight but can also be perceived as very real. They occur in 20–40% of treated PD patients (17,18). Auditory hallucinations are less common, usually associated with visual hallucinations (18,19), and are unlike the persecutory auditory hallucinations that characterize schizophrenia.

Current affiliation: McKnight Brain Institute at University of Florida, Gainesville, Florida, U.S.A.

Delusions, affecting about 8% of treated PD patients (4–6), usually carry a paranoid theme, such as suspicions of spousal infidelity, people stealing money, intruders living in the house, or nurses planning harmful plots. Thought broadcasting, ideas of reference, loosened associations, and "negative" symptoms, all common in schizophrenia, are less likely to be experienced by the PD patient with drug-induced psychosis.

In delirium, the patient's sensorium is clouded. It may start as nocturnal confusion or "sundowning," but when left untreated can carry over to daytime behaviors. This toxic mental state can be accompanied by agitation or aggression and often represents the trigger for nursing home placement.

B. Pathophysiology and Risk Factors

The exact pathophysiological basis of drug-induced psychosis has not been established. Excessive stimulation of dopamine receptors in the mesolimbic/mesocortical pathways is the most popular hypothesis. An increase in the number of striatal dopamine receptors has been shown in postmortem brains of PD patients with psychosis (20). This is thought to be due to denervation hypersensitivity resulting from the loss of presynaptic dopaminergic neurons. However, with long-term treatment, downregulation of these receptors often occurs, resulting in desensitization.

A process akin to the kindling effect described in epilepsy may explain this discrepancy (21). In this theory, two populations of dopamine-sensitive neurons exist. With chronic dopaminergic stimulation, dopamine-inhibited neurons in the striatum (responsible for motor control) exhibit downregulation, while dopamine-facilitated neurons in the limbic system become hypersensitive, resulting in psychosis.

Postsynaptic serotonergic hypersensitivity due to the partial loss of serotonergic projections may also contribute to the genesis of psychosis (22,23). Postmortem brains of PD patients with psychosis have shown a significant reduction of serotonin content in the brainstem (24). Levodopa challenges in laboratory animals have shown increased cortical and striatal levels of 5-hydroxyindoleacetic acid (the main metabolite of serotonin) and decreased levels of serotonin, suggesting increased serotonin turnover (25). Odansetron has been reported to alleviate psychosis due to its antiserotonergic properties (26). Similarly, the efficacy of atypical antipsychotic drugs have been attributed in part to their relative high affinity for 5-HT2 compared to D2 receptors.

Genetic variation analysis in PD patients with hallucinations did not reveal increased representations of the dopamine receptor gene DRD1 or DRD3, as reported in Alzheimer's disease (AD) patients with psychosis. Also, no association was found between PD patients with hallucinations and apolipoprotein E4 (27).

Reported risk factors for drug-induced psychosis include presence of dementia, advancing age, history and increased severity of depression, presence of sleep disorders, and longer disease duration (17,28). The type, duration, and dose of anti-PD drug therapy were not found to be associated with increased risk for psychosis.

C. General Treatment

As in any geriatric patient, urinary and pulmonary infections, metabolic and endocrine derangements, cerebral hypoperfusion states, and even social stress such as a change in environment are common precipitating factors for delirium and psychosis in PD. A search for these correctable causes is required, and resolution of the underlying medical illness may be all that is necessary to reverse psychosis (28–31). Another easily ignored etiology is the addition of medications with central nervous system (CNS) effects such as narcotics, hypnotics, antidepressants, anxiolytics, and virtually any other drug that crosses the blood-brain barrier, including anti-PD medications. If psychotic symptoms persist, anti-PD medications are slowly reduced, then discontinued. When a PD patient is on multiple medications, the following sequence of discontinuation of anti-PD medications is recommended: anticholinergic agents, selegiline, amantadine, dopamine agonists, catechol-*O*-methyltransferase (COMT) inhibitors, and, finally, levodopa (9,14). If psychosis improves, the patient is then maintained on the lowest possible dose of anti-PD medications. However, withdrawal of anti-PD drugs usually worsens parkinsonism and may not be tolerated. The use of an atypical antipsychotic agent is then recommended.

D. Specific Treatments

1. Clozapine

Clozapine is a dibenzodiazepine derivative. It does not cause catalepsy in rodents or parkinsonism in humans even at high doses (32). The first report on clozapine in PD included four patients and reported that clozapine was well tolerated and effective against psychosis (33). The next report concerned a single patient with chronic schizophrenia who developed PD while on neuroleptics (3). He did well on a combination of clozapine and anti-PD medication for 14 years and his autopsy confirmed PD (34).Over the next several years a large number of open-label reports were published describing clozapine as a successful antipsychotic that does not worsen motor function (see Table 1). The lone negative report was also the first double-blind, placebo-controlled trial (35). It used a small number of subjects at a single site and reported worsened parkinsonism and poor drug tolerance. However, this trial was undermined by the lack of experience with clozapine in the PD population at that time. The authors treated the patients as if they were young

Table 1 Summary of Double-Blind and Selected Larger Open-Label Reports with Clozapine for the Treatment of Psychosis in PD

Study (Ref.)	Design	No. of patients	Dosage[a] (mg/d)	No. in which psychosis improved	No. in which PD worsened
Wolters et al. (35)	Double-blind	6	75–250	3	3
Parkinson Study Group (36)	Double-blind	60	24.7	Improved mean BPRS	0
French Clozapine Study (37)	Double-blind	60	36	Improved mean CGIS, PANSS	7
Ostergard and Dupont (38)	Open-label	16	12.5	14	0
Kahn et al. (39)	Open-label	11	56	8	0
Factor et al. (40)	Open-label	19	35	Improved mean BPRS	1
Rabey et al. (41)	Open-label	27	42	Not documented	0
Ruggieri et al. (42)	Open-label	36	10.6	Improved mean BPRS	0

[a]Dosage given as mean or range.
BPRS = Brief Psychiatric Rating Scale; CGIS = Clinical Global Impression Scale; PANSS = Positive and Negative Symptom Scale.

schizophrenia patients, beginning with clozapine 25 mg/d and increasing by 25 mg each day. This resulted in severe sedation, partly manifested as worsened parkinsonism.

The cumulative experience of all open-label reports on clozapine in parkinsonism involves over 400 patients. The usual dose in schizophrenia is 300–900 mg/d. PD patients with psychosis required an average of 25 mg/d given as a single bedtime dose, with some patients requiring only 6.25 mg/d (29). Many patients had complete resolution of psychosis in one day, and most improved significantly in a week or two. A meta-analysis of all large clozapine reports on psychosis in PD showed an 85% improvement rate with acceptable tolerance (29,43). Most importantly, clozapine did not worsen motor symptoms and in some reports, it actually improved tremor (44–49).

It was not until 1999 that two well-designed, placebo-controlled, double-blind trials were published (36,37), making clozapine the gold standard atypical antipsychotic for the treatment of psychosis in PD. In the U.S. trial 60 subjects were enrolled at six sites and treated with clozapine, starting at 6.25 mg/d and increasing to a ceiling dose of 50 mg/d. Motor function was rated using the Unified Parkinson's Disease Rating Scale (UPDRS). Clozapine, at a mean dose of 25 mg/d, improved psychosis, as measured on each of four different neuropsychiatric scales. The overall motor function improved slightly but tremor improved significantly. Only one subject suffered a decline in white blood cell (WBC) count requiring termination, which was reversed within one week after discontinuing clozapine (36). The French study also involved 60 subjects using a very similar protocol. The results were less detailed than the U.S. study but almost identical (37).

Several cases of reversible WBC count decline have been reported (4,36,42,50). Since the agranulocytosis complication is not dose related (51,52), occurrence of this problem is assumed to be similar to age-matched schizophrenia patients. The U.S. Food and Drug Administration (FDA) mandates a weekly WBC monitoring for 6 months and bi-monthly thereafter for any patient on clozapine. Pharmacists will only dispense the week's supply pending a satisfactory WBC count.

Due to the differences in patient population and dosage used, clozapine side effects in PD do not mirror that in schizophrenia. No cases of myocarditis have been formally reported in PD patients. Hyperglycemia has been reported in PD patients on clozapine, but it appears to be less common than in schizophrenia (53). Clozapine-induced seizures, being a dose-related problem, have not yet been reported in PD. The potential anticholinergic side effects have not been a major problem in PD (36), and increased salivation, rather than dry mouth was observed at doses of 100 mg/d or more. A task force that considered all well-designed peer-reviewed reports on clozapine in PD concluded that "low-dose clozapine is efficacious in the short-term improvement of psychosis in PD with acceptable risk with specialized monitoring, but there is insufficient evidence on its long-term efficacy" (54).

In a long-term efficacy and safety study, a retrospective analysis of 39 parkinsonian patients on clozapine for a mean duration of 60 months showed 85% with continued partial/good response and 13% with complete resolution of psychosis (55). Thirty-three percent were eventually admitted to nursing homes while 28% died over a span of 5 years, a significantly improved mortality rate compared to previous 2-year mortality rate reports approaching 100% among PD nursing home residents with psychosis (56).

2. Risperidone

The second atypical antipsychotic drug released in the United States was found to be less atypical than clozapine (57,58). Risperidone induced dose-related problems typical of

Table 2 Summary of Reports with Risperidone for the Treatment of Psychosis in PD

Study (Ref.)	No. of patients	Dosage[a] (mg/d)	No in which psychosis improved	No in which PD worsened
Meco et al. (60)	6	0.67	6	0
Ford et al. (61)	6	1.5	6	6
Rich et al. (62)	6	0.5–4	4	5
Meco et al. (63)	10	0.73	9	3
Workman et al. (64)	9	1.9	9	0
Leopold (65)	39	1.1	33	6
Mohr et al. (66)	17	1.1	16	1

[a]Dosage given as mean or range.

conventional neuroleptics such as prolactin elevation and acute dystonic reactions (57,58). All reports but one (59) concerning risperidone in PD have been open-label (see Table 2). The first report was an open-label study in which all six patients' psychoses improved without an initial decline in motor function on a mean dose of 0.67 mg/d (60). Two retrospective reports involving six patients each (61,62) described 11 of the 12 patients as suffering significant motor worsening. The mean risperidone dose in one report was 1.5 mg/d, and doses in the other ranged from 0.5 to 4.0 mg/d. Further studies showed mixed results. Workman et al. (64) reported no worsening of parkinsonism in a prospective study of nine patients but did not formally measure parkinsonism. In a prospective study using the standard instruments for measuring PD, Leopold reported worsening of parkinsonism in only 6 of 39 patients and improved psychosis in 33 (65). Mohr et al. described a marked benefit of risperidone in 16 PD patients and only one with worsened parkinsonism, yet described other adverse effects such as hypokinesia and drooling (66). Why these side effects from a drug that does not induce sialorrhea were not ascribed to worsening parkinsonism has been challenged (67). Even more perplexing is the only double-blind study reported (59). In a trial comparing low-dose clozapine to low-dose risperidone in 12 subjects, 2 clozapine and one risperidone subject dropped out. Parkinsonism worsened in one clozapine and 3 risperidone patients. Although the mean UPDRS score improved in the clozapine group and worsened in the risperidone group, this was not statistically significant. On the contrary, the study showed a statistically significant benefit of risperidone but not clozapine for psychosis. This article perhaps best illustrates the dangers of overinterpreting a small, albeit double-blind, study.

One paper casting doubt on the atypicality of risperidone compared the development of various extrapyramidal symptoms on young neuroleptic-naïve patients with primary psychoses receiving either risperidone (mean dose 3.2 mg/d) or haloperidol (mean dose 3.7 mg/d) (68). There were no differences in the incidence of parkinsonism (59% vs. 52%) or akathisia (50% vs. 39%). Another study found that in subjects with schizophrenia under the age of 65, risperidone induced more prolactin elevation than higher haloperidol doses (69).

It is unclear why the results of risperidone studies in PD vary so much. It is likely that the conflicting results reflect the open-label aspects of the studies, the variable sophistication of the authors' ability to recognize and assess parkinsonism, the speed of titration, and the duration of the observations.

3. Olanzapine

Olanzapine is a thiobenzodiazepine of similar chemical structure to clozapine. It offered more promise than risperidone for being atypical (70,71). It either did not elevate prolactin or did so only transiently in humans. In animal models, only very high doses induced catalepsy or blocked amphetamine-induced stereotypy (58), but it has been reported to induce acute dystonic reactions and tardive dyskinesia.

As with risperidone, the first publication of olanzapine in PD was positive (72). Psychosis in 15 nondemented PD patients was prospectively evaluated. The UPDRS motor score was unchanged and the Brief Psychiatric Rating Scale (BPRS) improved significantly. The mean dosage required was 6.5 mg/d, not much lower than that used in schizophrenia. This was in contrast to clozapine, which required less than one-tenth of the dose in PD psychosis as compared to schizophrenia. Shortly thereafter, Jimenez-Jimenez et al. (73) and Friedman and Goldstein (74) published the first of several negative reports. Jimenez-Jimenez et al. (73) reported two patients having motor worsening on 5 mg/d of olanzapine, while Friedman and Goldstein (74) reported motor worsening in 10 of 19 psychotic patients with akinetic-rigid syndromes. Psychosis improved in 12 patients. Friedman et al. then attempted to slowly switch PD patients on clozapine to olanzapine, with poor results due to worsened parkinsonism (75). In each of the Friedman et al. studies, one subject required hospitalization for motor worsening. Five other publications describe further open-label experience with olanzapine (76–80), but only four specifically measured motor changes. A meta-analysis of these studies show motor worsening in about 40% of subjects (see Table 3).

A 12-week open-label comparison between nine consecutive PD patients treated with olanzapine, followed by nine consecutive PD patients treated with clozapine, reported that three olanzapine-treated patients dropped out due to severe gait deterioration (83). The six remaining subjects suffered a significant decline in mean PD motor scores. In contrast, all nine clozapine-treated patients had an improvement in mean motor scores. Only two

Table 3 Summary of Reports with Olanzapine for the Treatment of Psychosis in PD

Study (Ref.)	No. of patients	Dosage[a] (mg/d)	No. in which psychosis improved	No. experiencing motor worsening
Wolters et al. (72)	15	6.5	15	0
Jimenez et al. (73)	2	5	1	2
Friedman and Goldstein (74)	19	N/A	7	10
Friedman et al. (75)	12	4.4	12	7
Molho and Factor (76)	12	6.3	9	10
Weiner et al. (78)	21	5	13	9
Churchyard and Iansek (77)	22	7.5	17	N/A
Graham et al. (79)	5	5	5	3
Stover and Juncos (80)	22	N/A	12	8
Goetz et al. (81)	7	11.2	N/A	6
Aarsland et al. (82)	21	4.5	16	0
Gimenez-Roldan et al. (83)	9	4.7	6	9

[a]Dosage given as mean or range.
N/A = data not available.

olanzapine studies reported no patients with worsened motor function (72,82). The first positive study used only nondemented subjects (72). The other open-label trial involved 21 PD patients on olanzapine for drug-induced psychosis (82).

A single-site, double-blind trial comparing olanzapine to low-dose clozapine for psychosis in PD enrolled only 15 subjects before the safety monitoring committee aborted the study due to worsened motor function in six of seven olanzapine-treated subjects (81). No worsening occurred in the clozapine group. The mean olanzapine dose was 11.2 mg/d.

In a double-blind, placebo-controlled trial, olanzapine was tested in non-psychotic PD patients with levodopa-induced dyskinesias (84), based on similar reports using clozapine (85,86). Every patient suffered intolerable motor effects. The task force for evidence-based review of the treatment of psychosis in PD concluded "there is insufficient evidence to demonstrate efficacy of olanzapine and at low conventional doses it carries an unacceptable risk of motor deterioration" (54).

4. Quetiapine

Quetiapine is a dibenzothiazepine with the closest pharmacological resemblance to clozapine but without the risk of agranulocytosis. It is a strong 5-HT2 receptor antagonist and a moderate D2 receptor antagonist, does not block apomorphine-induced stereotypy, and does not alter prolactin levels (58). It has not been cited as a cause of any acute dystonic reaction among previously neuroleptic-naïve individuals. Quetiapine has not been subject to any double-blind trials. Several open-label studies involving over 200 PD patients have been reported (see Table 4).

The first description of quetiapine in parkinsonism was a letter (88), followed by a retrospective report involving two patients (87). Juncos et al. then reported that quetiapine improved psychosis in 15 of 15 parkinsonian subjects without worsening motor function (89). The same authors also reported the results of a one-year open-label study of quetiapine in psychotic parkinsonian patients (90). Eighty percent of the patients had improved psychosis. None experienced motor worsening. Further reports involved larger

Table 4 Summary of Reports with Quetiapine for the Treatment of Psychosis in PD

Study (Ref.)	No. of patients	Dosage[a] (mg/d)	No. in which psychosis improved	No. in which PD worsened[c]
Parsa and Bastani (87)	2	200–400	2	1
Evatt et al. (88)	10	50	10	0
Juncos et al. (89)	15	70	15	0
Juncos et al. (90)	40	25–800	40	8
Samanta and Stacy (91)	10	37.5	6	7
Fernandez et al. (92)	15	62.5	12	4
Targum and Abbott (93)	10	107	7	0
Reddy et al. (94)	43	54	32	5
Dewey and O'Suilleabhain (95)	75	86	40	0
Fernandez et al. (96)[b]	106	60.8	87	34

[a]Dosage given as mean or range.
[b]11 patients had Lewy body dementia, 2 had progressive supranuclear palsy, and 1 had dementia pugilistica.
[c]Motor worsening in all reports was described as minor.

numbers of subjects and included two crossover studies in which patients on clozapine were converted to quetiapine (92,97). Eighty percent of PD patients on clozapine were able to switch over to quetiapine without worsening motor function when a slow titration with a long overlap was instituted (92). Menza et al. reported three cases of PD or dementia with Lewy bodies (DLB) patients with psychosis switched successfully from clozapine at a mean dose of 34 mg/d to quetiapine 12.5–150 mg/d (98).

Reddy et al. reported a review on 43 consecutive quetiapine-treated PD patients for a mean duration of 9.7 months (94). Eighty-one percent had improved psychosis. Five patients (13%) experienced mild worsening of motor symptoms, but none were sufficient to stop the drug. Only demented patients had motor worsening on quetiapine. A chart review of 61 patients on quetiapine for psychosis showed that 40 (66%) had a good response psychiatrically. Nine patients switched to clozapine because of the lack of efficacy of quetiapine at a mean dose of 139 mg/d. Deterioration of motor function on quetiapine or clozapine was not observed. Two separate reports described PD patients whose parkinsonism worsened with olanzapine at 2.5 mg daily within 3 days but did well on quetiapine 25 mg and 37.5 mg at bedtime without motor impairment (99,100). Ten PD patients were given quetiapine at a mean dose of 37.5 mg/d. Six patients felt their hallucinations improved, one was unchanged, and 2 were worse. Although motor function declined mildly in 7, the drug was well tolerated in 9 of 10 patients (91). A prospective open-label study of 11 PD patients had 9 complete the first 12 weeks of the protocol. Of these, 2 stopped due to poor efficacy and 2 for other medical problems. There was no motor decline during the first 12 weeks and a slow decline thereafter, consistent with disease progression (93).

Fernandez et al. reported 106 parkinsonian patients treated at a single PD center with quetiapine (96). Seventy-eight out of 106 (74%) remained on quetiapine for a mean duration of 15 months at an average dose of 60 mg/d. Eighty-seven (82%) patients had partial or complete resolution of their psychosis, while 19 (18%) patients had no improvement on quetiapine. Motor worsening was noted in 34 (32%) patients but was typically not sufficient to warrant quetiapine discontinuation. Demented subjects had a 12-fold increased risk of nonresponse to quetiapine. Similar to Reddy et al.'s report, patients who developed motor worsening tended to be more demented.

With the lack of double-blind trials, the task force on evidence-based review of PD treatment concluded that "there is insufficient evidence to support the efficacy and safety of quetiapine and that its use for psychosis in PD should be considered investigational" (54). Nonetheless, available reports involving over 200 patients strongly suggest that quetiapine appears to be well tolerated and effective. However, despite the lack of head-to-head trials, quetiapine appears to be slightly less effective than clozapine against psychosis. Unlike clozapine, it does not improve tremor and may induce mild motor worsening. Unlike olanzapine and risperidone, there was no significant motor worsening on quetiapine. The majority of motor decline, especially in long-term trials, was mild or could be attributed to PD progression.

5. Ziprasidone

Ziprasidone is the latest atypical antipsychotic drug with a higher affinity for serotonin 5-HT2 than dopamine D2 receptors. There has been no report on its use in the PD population. With the historically lower dose requirement of antipsychotic drugs in PD compared to schizophrenia patients, the inability to cut ziprasidone in half as it comes in a capsule makes it a difficult and perhaps riskier drug to initiate in PD. A review of all available data on ziprasidone use in schizophrenia concluded that its extrapyramidal profile is "better than risperidone, the same as olanzapine but not quite as good as quetiapine or clozapine" (101).

6. Odansetron

Odansetron is an expensive antiemetic and a selective 5HT-3 receptor antagonist. Zoldan et al. reported two open-label trials of odansetron with a total of 40 PD patients with improvement of psychosis. Only one patient developed a headache and 7 patients had constipation (26,102). However, these positive findings were not reproduced by others (103).

7. Cholinesterase inhibitors

With the improvement of psychosis in DLB patients given cholinesterase inhibitors for dementia, this class of drug might be an alternative to antipsychotic agents in PD (104–108). Small open-label trials in PD show cholinesterase inhibitors improved not only dementia but hallucinations as well (109,110). Blinded studies on the use of cholinesterase inhibitors and head-to-head trials comparing them with atypical antipsychotics will be important in determining the best approach to psychosis in PD.

8. Electroconvulsive Therapy

Electroconvulsive therapy (ECT) has been reported to be beneficial in depressed PD patients with psychosis, and it may improve motor symptoms as well (111–114). However, experience with ECT for PD psychosis is limited. It may require a period of hospitalization, may cause significant confusion, and its efficacy can be short-lived. Thus, it should only be considered when drug manipulations have failed.

II. DEMENTIA

A. Introduction

Dementia is a syndrome defined as a progressive deterioration of cognition leading to impaired functional ability. The current working criteria for identifying primary degenerative dementias consist of: (a) impairment of memory, (b) impairment in at least one other cognitive domain, (c) a degree of impairment sufficient to interfere with work or usual activity, (d) without evidence of delirium, or (e) other major psychiatric problems (115).

In PD, dementia may be the single most important factor limiting the treatment for bradykinesia, rigidity, and tremor (116). PD patients with concomitant dementia are particularly prone to the development of dopamine-induced confusion, agitation, and visual misperceptions. These phenomena may be benign cognitive changes and can progress to include hallucinations, delusions, and even delirium.

In the early stages of cognitive decline, behavioral interventions designed to reinforce organizational strategies or enhance procedural learning may transiently benefit some PD patients. Efforts to test pharmacological strategies that may compensate for the loss of the neurotransmitters most likely to be determinants of the clinical features of dementia in PD have been extremely limited. Thus, the sequelae of dementia are now the most important contributors in late-stage PD to caregiver stress (117,118), poor quality of life (119), early nursing home placement (11,120), morbidity, and mortality (121,122).

B. Prevalence and Risk Factors

If one applies the Diagnostic and Statistical Manual of Mental Disorders (DSM) criteria for dementia to PD patients, approximately one-third of patients will meet the requirements. Apaydin et al. (123) identified 17 studies by 13 groups, published between 1984 and 2001, which reported the frequency and prevalence of dementia in PD. In clinic-hospital cohorts the frequency ranged from 6 to 29%; prevalence figures in community-based studies were between 12 and 41% (123).

The yearly incidence of dementia appearing in an initially nondemented PD cohort ranges from 2.7 to 9.5 per year (123). The relative risk for the development of dementia in PD, compared with controls, was reported as 1.7 in a New York–based cohort (121) and 5.9 in a Norwegian cohort (118). On average, PD appears to raise the risk of having dementia about threefold (123). Moreover, the cumulative risk of developing dementia for individuals with PD is substantial, and by 85 years the incidence of dementia in PD has been estimated to be more than 65% (124).

Environmental risk factors for PD (exposure to pesticides, well water, rural living) or for AD (head injury, smoking, hypertension, diabetes mellitus) are not predictors for the development of dementia in PD (125). In one study, current smoking was significantly associated with incident dementia (OR 4.5; 95% CI; $p = 0.02$) (125), despite the reported inverse association between smoking and development of PD.

The apolipoprotein E gene (APO-E4), clearly over-represented in the AD population, has not consistently been shown to occur with increased frequency in PD (19,121, 126–128). There is a single report that the presence of an APO-E4 allele is increased in cases with combined PD and AD pathologies (OR 2.5; 95% CI) (129). A report of a 12-fold increased relative risk of developing PD with a combined α-synuclein/APOE-E4 genotype has not yet been confirmed in a second population (130).

There is reasonable consensus that the overall risk of developing global cognitive impairment in PD increases with age (118,121,122,131–139) and with the severity of akinesia/rigidity (121,137,140). One study suggested that the important factor is the combination of these two features, rather than their separate effects (141). In the past, the presence of atypical features for PD (early freezing, prominent autonomic dysfunction, symmetrical disease presentation, poor balance, and limited response to levodopa) has been deemed significant (117,137), but it is more likely that these are signs of a different parkinsonian disorder. The following have not consistently been shown to be risk factors: age of onset of motor symptoms, longer duration of illness, gender, low level of formal education, depressive symptoms, psychosis precipitated by levodopa, and a family history of dementia (118,121,139,142).

C. Neurobiology of Dementia in PD

The pathology of PD affects function primarily in the striatum (caudate and putamen) and secondarily in the frontal cortex (143). Cell loss in the following areas contributes to cognitive decline in PD: the substantia nigra pars compacta (SNpc), nucleus basalis of Meynert, locus ceruleus, and limbic cortex. Cell loss in the SNpc shows a consistent gradient in PD—lateral to medial, dorsal to ventral—which results in a much greater loss of dopamine and dopamine transporter sites in the putamen than in the caudate (144–146). Reliable correlations have been demonstrated between clinical (motor) stage and dopamine metabolism in the putamen, but not the caudate nucleus (147). Conversely, metabolism in the caudate, but not the putamen, correlates with impairment in a cognitive task (verbal delayed recall) (148). This so-called functional division of the striatum is, perhaps, the main reason for the predominance of motor, and relative paucity of cognitive, symptoms due to loss of dopamine in uncomplicated PD.

Levodopa and dopamine agonists improve at least some aspects of attention and mild cognitive impairment (MCI) in the elderly (149). Comprehensive studies have not been carried out, but it is clear that these drugs can either improve or impair cognitive performance in PD, depending on the nature of the task, the basal level of dopaminergic function in underlying cortico-striatal circuitry, the dose of drug given, and the pattern of coexistent pathology (148,150–152). Regardless, there is no doubt that the benefit of dopaminergic therapy for cognitive dysfunction in PD is considerably less impressive than for motor symptoms (152).

Cholinergic networks mediate aspects of memory and attention in animal and human studies and are at least as damaged in PD as in patients with AD (153). In autopsy series, striking cell loss is found in the nucleus basalis of Meynert. Choline acetyltransferase (ChAT) activity has consistently been reported to be decreased to about 40–60% of control values in frontal, temporal, and hippocampal cortex accompanied by a decrease in acetylcholinesterase (AChE) activity (129,145,154–156). In cases of PD with dementia, ChAT activity is even lower, with lower residual levels in the neocortex compared to the hippocampus (157). Cognitive impairment correlated significantly with both prefrontal ChAT activity ($r = -0.52$; $p = 0.005$) and the density of D1 dopamine receptors in the caudate nucleus ($r = -0.40$; $p = 0.037$) (129). Nicotinic cholinergic receptor binding in the putamen is also decreased in PD (158). However, muscarinic cholinergic receptors have been reported to be relatively spared in PD with dementia, compared to AD (154). Therefore, from a theoretical point of view, there is a strong rationale for testing cholinesterase inhibitors in PD (159).

The noradrenergic system plays a major role in attentional control and depressed mood, both of which influence cognition, as well as the late-stage gait difficulties of PD related to postural instability, frequent falls, and freezing (160,161). These symptoms tend to be improved only marginally by levodopa or dopamine agonists. In older individuals with PD, with or without dementia, loss of cells in the locus ceruleus leads to low levels of norepinephrine in the neocortical and hippocampal projection fields (160,161). Norepinephrine metabolism in the locus ceruleus is subnormal only in PD with dementia and has been reported to be 13% of the value in control brains, and 26% of control values in the hypothalamus. Bradyphrenia, a subjective feeling of slowness and poor thinking, correlates with the severity of bradykinesia in the off state (162,163). However, the cognitive deficits are not necessarily improved by dopamine, and the phenomenon has been suggested to be related to noradrenergic dysfunction (116).

Finally, cell loss from the raphe nuclei leads to deficiency in the almost ubiquitous serotonin projection systems that help regulate mood. Some form of depression is experienced by at least 40% of patients with PD at some point in their clinical course (8). Mood fluctuators and patients with clinically apparent mood changes during their motor on and off states may be more likely to have dementia (164).

D. Cognitive Dysfunction in PD

Despite the many methodological difficulties that have hampered progress in the field, disturbances of frontal executive function remain consistently among the earliest and most robust cognitive manifestations of PD (143,165,166). Patients with PD who do not meet DSM criteria for dementia still tend to be impaired in concept formation, sequence planning, shifting and maintaining sets, and temporal ordering. Other studies cite specific cognitive deficits in visuospatial function, memory capacity, and linguistic abilities. In PD, problems in these areas of cognition are likely the result of dysfunction in either the maintenance of attention and/or a decrease in working memory (140,143,148,165,167,168). Patients (and more often their caregivers) often report that they are having problems with decision making, planning, and completion of goal-directed behaviors.

The relationship between early cognitive deficits and the later development of dementia remains unclear. For individuals in whom cognition is relatively spared early on, with a good motor response to levodopa, cognitive changes may proceed in at least three ways: they may continue to remain relatively unscathed throughout their clinical course with isolated or small groups of deficits that do not impair activities of daily living; they may begin to develop increasing behavioral, mood, and cognitive difficulties with a predominance of frontal lobe dysfunction; or they may develop more severe and global cognitive deficits. There is some support for progression from frontal lobe dysfunction to more widespread cognitive deficits (135). Typically, there is a long history consistent with idiopathic PD, followed by the late superimposition of fairly rapidly progressive cognitive and motor difficulties.

If early in the clinical course of parkinsonism cognitive difficulties are already noted, concomitant AD with PD or one of the parkinson-plus syndromes, fronto-temporal dementia with parkinsonism, progressive supranuclear palsy (PSP), or DLB, should be considered. The neuropathological features and clinical criteria for diagnosis of these disorders are reviewed elsewhere (169).

1. Dementia in PD Versus AD

The core symptoms of early AD also involve memory and language tasks such as impairment in immediate and delayed recall, naming, and category fluency. Although PD patients do not do as well on these tasks, the reasons for poor performance in PD are different. For example, normal controls tend to spontaneously use semantic organizational strategies at the time of learning and subsequent recall remains intact. Individuals with AD do not use these strategies and have a failure of encoding because of medial temporal lobe–hippocampal damage. Patients with AD have low immediate free recall rates and show an equivalent impairment in delayed recall and recognition. Delayed recall of word lists correlates best with early AD. PD groups also spontaneously use fewer organizational strategies during encoding and do worse than age-matched controls on immediate free recall, but their scores improve disproportionately for delayed recognition or cued recall (170). In a novel experimental design, patients with PD benefited significantly and progressively from three graded levels of cueing on the California Verbal Learning Test (171).

In general, individuals with PD show little cognitive decline over a period of one year (112,140). In contrast, patients with AD invariably change over the same time period. However, once dementia in PD becomes manifest, the time course of deterioration in PD dementia is usually faster than for AD (122,137,172). Patients with PD dementia, matched by age and disease duration to nondemented PD, had decreased survival (122). However, the presence of dementia per se does not add to the magnitude of the risk of death (120,173).

2. Dementia in PD Versus DLB

Although recent discussion has focused on whether PD, DLB, and PD dementia represent distinct nosological entities or whether they represent a spectrum of a single Lewy body disease, the clinical syndrome of DLB is different from PD. DLB is primarily a dementing syndrome. Its core clinical features include parkinsonism (92.4%), day-to-day cognitive fluctuations (89.1%), and visual hallucinations (77%) (174). These core features are found at presentation, early in the course. Exquisite sensitivity to the extrapyramidal side effects of neuroleptics is common. Compared to idiopathic PD, cognitive impairments, psychiatric manifestations, and myoclonus are more common in DLB, whereas there is more tremor and a better response to levodopa administration in PD; bradykinesia and rigidity are equally represented in both conditions (173).

The temporal relationship between the onset of parkinsonism and the development of the neuropsychiatric features of the disease has been used to distinguish DLB from PD with dementia. Patients who have "motor-only" symptoms for at least 12 months before the development of fluctuating cognition and hallucinations were grouped as having PD with dementia instead of DLB (169).

E. General Treatment

General approaches to treating dementia in PD follow the same principles applied to other geriatric populations and other dementing illnesses (175). Similar to psychosis, any sudden change in cognition or behavior is typically due to a medical cause. Infections, metabolic and endocrine derangements, hypoperfusion states, and social stress are common precipitating factors for worsened mental status. Substance abuse, including reliance on over-the-counter preparations containing antihistamines, may be underappreciated, especially in individuals who are living alone.

Medications with CNS effects such as narcotics, sedative hypnotics, antidepressants, anxiolytics, and antihistamines should be avoided or used sparingly. It is less appreciated that many other commonly prescribed medications, including antiemetics, antispasmodics for the bladder, H_2 receptor antagonists, antiarrhythmic agents, antihypertensive agents, and nonsteroidal anti-inflammatory agents, may also cause cognitive impairment (176). Any of these medications, even if previously well tolerated by the PD patient, can be expected to lower the threshold for cognitive decline as the disease progresses.

F. Specific Treatments

1. Cholinesterase Inhibitors

Four members of this class of compounds are currently FDA approved for the treatment of mild to moderate AD. Tacrine, donepezil, rivastigmine, and galantamine are all inhibitors of AChE enzymes and, in theory, help repair brain cholinergic deficits by increasing the amount of acetylcholine available for binding in the synaptic cleft to cholinergic receptors.

The pharmacokinetic properties and in vivo ability to modulate cholinergic networks of each of these compounds are quite different (see Table 5). Tacrine and rivastigmine also inhibit a second enzyme, butyryl cholinesterase, whose activity seems to be upregulated in AD brains in parallel with senile plaque formation. Galantamine has additional properties as an allosteric modulator of presynaptic nicotinic cholinergic receptors.

Donepezil and rivastigmine have shown comparable efficacy in maintaining Alzheimer's Disease Assessment Scale—cognitive portion (ADAS-cog) scores above baseline in double-blind controlled studies in AD (177,178). Brain metabolism by

Table 5 FDA-Approved Cholinesterase Inhibitors for the Treatment of Alzheimer's Disease

	Tacrine	Donepezil	Rivastigmine	Galantamine
Year approved	1993	1995	2000	2001
Chemical class	Acridine	Piperidine	Carbamate	Phenanthrene alkaloid
Cholinesterase inhibition	Non-competitive reversible	Non-competitive reversible	Non-competitive reversible; most potent	Competitive reversible; least potent
Butyryl cholinesterase	+	Negligible	+	Negligible
Nicotinic acetylcholine receptor inhibition	–	–	–	Allosteric modulation
Metabolism	Hepatic CYP450	Hepatic CYP450	Renal	Hepatic renal
Plasma $T_{1/2}$	2–4 h	~70 hrs	~1 h; enzyme dissociation time 8 h	~6 h
Dosing	qid	qd	bid	bid
Initial dose	5 mg	2.5 mg	1.5 mg	4 mg
Maximum dose	160 mg	10 mg	12 mg	32 mg
Warning label	Hepatotoxicity	–	–	–
Drug interactions	+	+	None known	+

fluoro-deoxyglucose positron emission tomography (FDG-PET) has been shown to increase in tandem with clinical benefit (179). In observational studies, long-term use of cholinesterase inhibitors translated into a 2-year delay in admission to nursing homes (180,181).

For all the cholinesterase inhibitors, the most common side effects are gastrointestinal distress (nausea, diarrhea, vomiting), fatigue, insomnia, and muscle cramps (182). Rivastigmine tends to be associated, additionally, with weight loss and dizziness. Documented hypersensitivity has rarely occurred with this class of compounds. Theoretical concerns about worsening seizures, asthma, conduction abnormalities, chronic obstructive pulmonary disease, and peptic ulcer disease seem not to have materialized as significant adverse events in the thousands of individuals with AD who have now been exposed to these drugs (183).

Use of the first cholinesterase inhibitor, tacrine, in the AD population was accompanied by anecdotal evidence of worsened parkinsonism (184), reports of fulminant hepatotoxicity resulting in the addition of a warning label, and only a modest clinical benefit. A small open-label trial of tacrine, in seven PD patients with psychosis reported five patients with complete resolution and two patients with partial improvement of hallucinations. The mean Mini-Mental State Examination (MMSE) score improved by 7.1 points, and the UPDRS scores improved dramatically (185).

It was not until recently that, encouraged by slow confirmation of the more benign side-effect profiles of the remaining three cholinesterase inhibitors and reports of perhaps even better efficacy in treating the cognitive and neuropsychiatric concomitants of

DLB (104–108,186–192), investigators began to reconsider their potential for treating dementia in PD.

An open-label study included 11 patients (average age 75 years) with PD dementia, treated for 26 weeks with either tacrine (7 patients) or donepezil (4 patients). For the combined group, scores for the ADAS-cog improved by 3.2 points ($p < 0.012$). No change in motor function as assessed by the Short Parkinson Evaluation Scale (SPES) was noted (193). Behavioral symptoms were not mentioned.

In an open-label trial of 12 PD patients with drug-induced psychosis (109), rivastigmine was initiated at 1.5 mg bid and increased every 2 weeks until either the maximum of 6 mg bid or the highest tolerated dose was achieved. The drug was well tolerated. Three withdrew: one due to death from unrelated sepsis, one because the caretaker became ill and the third from nausea. The MMSE improved from 20.8 to 25.4, while the UPDRS motor scale did not change, and the mean Neuropsychiatric Inventory (NPI) score improved on the subscales measuring hallucinations and sleep disturbance but not delusions. Caregiver distress also improved. Repeat measurements after a 3-week withdrawal showed a comparable decline. No worsening of tremor or parkinsonism was noted.

An open-label pilot study of rivastigmine in 19 patients with severe PD-associated dementia was reported (194). They were evaluated at baseline, after 26 weeks of treatment, and following an 8-week washout period. The average dose, from weeks 12 though 26 of treatment, was approximately 7.5 mg/day. Significant changes in total ADAS-cog and the attention subscore of the MMSE (both $p < 0.004$) were reported, but the actual scores were not given. The comment was made that "enhancement of tremor was the only extrapyramidal symptom worsened in some patients."

A double-blind, placebo-controlled, crossover study of 14 individuals with PD and cognitive impairment assigned to either donepezil (5 or 10 mg/d) or placebo during two sequential periods lasting 10 weeks each was reported (159). Patient characteristics at baseline included: a history of cognitive decline beginning one year or more after the onset of parkinsonism. The average duration of PD was 10.8 ± 5.2 years, the mean age was 71.0 ± 3.9 years, and average levodopa dose was 485 ± 256 mg/d. The average MMSE score at study entry was 20.8 ± 3.4, with all patients showing evidence of decline in memory and at least one other category of cognitive function. Significant effects of donepezil compared with placebo for MMSE (2.1 ± 2.7 vs. 0.3 ± 3.2, $p = 0.013$) and a clinicians interview-based impression of change combined with a caregiver input score (CIBIC) (3.3 ± 0.9 vs. 4.1 ± 0.8) were noted. Motor UPDRS subscores did not worsen during donepezil treatment. Three patients had improved scores on delusions, two on hallucinations, one on agiation, six on depression, and five on apathy. None of these improvements were statistically significant due to the low scores on these items at baseline and the small number of subjects involved.

In addition, two small case series targeting individuals with PD and dementia with psychosis were reported. The first involved six individuals treated with donepezil up to 10 mg/day for 6 weeks without obvious deterioration of parkinsonian symptoms (110); the second employed rivastigmine (195). Neither study noted obvious deterioration of parkinsonian symptoms or paradoxical worsening of behavior. Currently, there are no published data on the use of galantamine in PD.

In summary, although there is a strong biochemical rationale for the use of cholinesterase inhibitors in the treatment of dementia in PD, there are currently insufficient data on either the safety or the efficacy of donepezil, rivastigmine, or galantamine in this patient population. Until clinical trial data are available, clinicians should use caution when prescribing these agents (see Table 6).

A single trial using nicotinic patches did not show any benefit in either AD or PD (200). Other possible approaches to improving cholinergic function in the brain, such as dietary supplementation with cholinergic precursors (lecithin) or administration of cholinergic receptor agonists (bethanechol, milameline, tasaclidine), have not been found to be useful in AD and at this point are unlikely to be tried in patients with PD dementia.

2. Other Strategies

Few other pharmacological strategies for treating dementia in PD have been reported. The results of two attempts to compensate for noradrenergic deficits in PD have been reported. The first study employed L-threo-3,4-dihydroxyphenylserine (L-DOPS) in individuals with late-stage PD. A moderate improvement in gait freezing, bradyphrenia, and depression was observed (201). The benefit has not been reproduced. The second trial consisted of nine PD patients treated with naphtoxazine (SDZ-NVI-085), a selective noradrenergic alpha1-agonist (202). This compound appeared to improve subject performance on two classic tests of frontal lobe function: the Stroop and Odd-Man-Out tests.

Estrogen replacement therapy (ERT) may be a reasonable protective strategy for the development of dementia in women who have PD (142,203). The effect of ERT on the risk of development of dementia was investigated in 87 women with PD without dementia, 80 women with PD with dementia, and 989 nondemented healthy women. ERT did not affect the risk of PD, but appeared to be protective for the development of dementia arising within the setting of PD (OR 0.22; 95% CI, 0.05–1.0) (142). Another large survey of all PD nursing home residents in five U.S. states comparing women residents on ERT versus those who were not found PD residents on estrogen to be less cognitively impaired (203).

The concept that anti-inflammatory agents may be beneficial in the treatment of dementia is based on epidemiological studies showing a lower than expected prevalence or delayed onset of dementia in patient populations exposed to anti-inflammatory drugs. One study using a transgenic mouse model of AD reported that administration of ibuprofen suppressed senile plaque-associated inflammation and reduced amyloid accumulation (204). There are activated microglia in the substantia nigra in PD and in the cerebral cortex in DLB, even in the absence of coexisting AD pathology (205).

Table 6   Extrapyramidal and Behavioral Side-Effects of Cholinesterase Inhibitors

Drug	Disease/study type	Side effects	Ref.
Tacrine	AD/case report	Bradykinesia, rigidity	(184)
Donepezil	PD/open-label ($n=8$)	Worsened parkinsonism (2 out of 8)	(197)
Donepezil	AD/case report	Bradykinesia, rigidity	(196)
Donepezil	PSP/randomized trial ($n=21$)	Worsened UPDRS-ADL	(198)
Rivastigmine	PD/case report	Rigidity, bradykinesia anxiety, irritability	(199)

AD = Alzheimer's disease; PD = Parkinson's disease; PSP = Progressive supranuclear palsy; UPDRS-ADL = Unified Parkinson's Disease Rating Scale—Activities of Daily Living.

REFERENCES

1. Regis E. Precis de Psychiatrie. Paris: Gaston Doiz, 1906.
2. Jacson JA, Free GBM, Pike HV. The psychiatric manifestations in paralysis agitans. Arch Neurol Psychiatry 1923; 10:680–684.
3. Friedman JH, Max, J, Swift R. Idiopathic Parkinson's disease in a chronic schizophrenic patient. Long-term treatment with clozapine and L-Dopa. Clin Neuropharmacol 1987; 10:470–475.
4. Greene P, Cote'L, Fahn S. Treatment of drug-induced psychosis in Parkinson's disease with clozapine. Adv Neurol 1993; 60:703–706.
5. Melamed E, Achiron A, Shapira A, Davidovicz S. Persistent and progressive parkinsonism after discontinuation of chronic neuroleptic therapy: an additional tardive syndrome? Clin Neuropharmacol 1991; 14:273–278.
6. Klawans HL. Levodopa-induced psychosis. Psychiatr Am 1978; 8:447–471.
7. Fischer P, Danielczyk W, Simanyi M, Streifer MB. Dopaminergic psychosis in advanced Parkinson's disease. In: Striefler MB, Korczyn AD, Melamed E, Youdim MBH, eds. Advances in Neurology. Vol. 53. Parkinsons Disease: Anatomy, Pathology and Therapy. New York: Raven Press, 1990:391–397.
8. Cummings JL. Behavioral complications of drug treatment of Parkinson's disease. J Am Geriatr Soc 1991; 39:708–716.
9. Fernandez HH, Friedman JH. The role of atypical antipsychotics in the treatment of movement disorders. CNS Drugs 1999; 11(6):467–483.
10. Goetz CG, Stebbins GT. Risk factors for nursing home placement in advanced Parkinson's disease. Neurology 1993; 43:2227–2229.
11. Aarsland D, Larsen JP, Tandberg E, Laake K. Predictors of nursing home placement in Parkinson's disease: a population based prospective study. J Am Geriatr Soc 2000; 48:938–942.
12. Liu K, Manton KG. The characteristics and utilization pattern of an admission cohort of nursing home patients. Gerontologist 1983; 23:92–98.
13. Mendis T, Barclay CL, Mohr E. Drug-induced psychosis in Parkinson's disease: a review of management. CNS Drugs 1996; 5:166–174.
14. Friedman JH, Fernandez HH. The non-motor problems of Parkinson's disease. Neurologist 2000; 6:18–27.
15. Nausieda PA, Weiner WJ, Kaplan LR, et al. Sleep disruption in the course of chronic levodopa therapy: an early feature of levodopa psychosis. Clin Neuropharmacol 1982; 5:183–194.
16. Comella CL, Tanner CM, Ristanovic RK. Polysomnographic sleep measures in Parkinson's disease patients with treatment-induced hallucinations. Ann Neurol 1993; 34:710–714.
17. Sanchez-Ramos JR, Ortoll R, Paulson GW. Visual hallucinations associated with Parkinson's disease. Arch Neurol 1996; 53:1265–1268.
18. Fenelon G, Mahieux F, Huon R, Ziegler M. Hallucinations in Parkinson's disease : prevalence, phenomenology and risk factors. Brain 2000; 123:733–745.
19. Inzelberg R, Kiervasse S, Korczyn AD. Auditory hallucinations in Parkinson's disease. J Neurol Neurosurg Psychiatry 1998; 64:533–535.
20. Rinne UK. Brain neurotransmitter receptors in Parkinson's disease. In: Marsden CS, Fahn S, eds. Movement Disorders. Boston: Butterworth Scientific, 1982:59–74.
21. Moskovitz C, Moses H, Klawans HL. Levodopa-induced psychosis: a kindling phenomenon. Am J Psychiatry 1978; 135:669–675.
22. Nausieda P, Tanner C, Klawans H. Serotonergically active agents in levodopa-induced psychiatric toxic reactions. Adv Neurol 1983; 37:23–32.
23. van der Mast RC, Fekkes D. Serotonin and amino acids: patterns in delirium pathophysiology? Semin Clin Neuropsychiatry 2000; 5:125–131.
24. Birkmayer W, Riederer P. Responsibility of extrastriatal areas for the appearance of psychosis: biochemical and post-mortem findings. J Neural Transm 1975; 37:175–182.
25. Melamed E, Zoldan J, Friedberg G, et al. Is hallucinosis in Parkinson's disease due to central serotonergic hyperactivity? Mov Disord 1993; 8:406–407.
26. Zoldan J Friedberg G, Goldberg-Stern H, et al. Odansetron for hallucinosis in advanced Parkinson's disease. Lancet 1993; 341:562–563.
27. Goetz CG, Burke PF, Leurgans S, et al. Genetic variation analysis in Parkinson disease patients with and without hallucinations. Arch Neurol 2001; 58:209–213.
28. Aarsland D, Larsen JP, Cummings JL, Laake K. Prevalence and clinical correlates of psychotic symptoms in Parkinson's disease. A community-based study. Arch Neurol 1999; 56:595–601.

29. Factor SA, Friedman JH. The emerging role of clozapine in the treatment of movement disorders. Mov Disord 1997; 12(4):483–496.

30. Factor SA, Molho ES, Podskalny GD, Brown D. Parkinson's disease: drug-induced psychiatric states. Adv Neurol 1995; 65:115–138.

31. Friedman JH. The management of levodopa psychoses. Clin Neuropharmacol 1991; 14:283–295.

32. Meltzer HY, Matsubara S, Lee JC. Classification of typical and atypical antipsychotic drugs on the basis of D-1, D-2 and serotonin 2 pK values. J Pharmacol Exp Ther 1989; 251: 238–246.

33. Scholz E, Dichgans J. Treatment of drug-induced exogenous psychosis in parkinsonism with clozapine and fluperlapine. Eur Arch Psychiatr Neurol Sci 1985; 235:60–64.

34. Friedman JH, Fernandez HH. Autopsy follow-up of a patient with schizophrenia and presumed idiopathic Parkinson's disease. Clin Neuropharmacol 2001; 24:12.

35. Wolters ECH, Hurwitz TA, Mak E, et al. Clozapine in the treatment of parkinsonian patients with dopaminomimetic psychosis. Neurology 1990; 40:832–834.

36. Parkinson Study Group. Low dose clozapine for the treatment of drug-induced psychosis in Parkinson's disease. N Engl J Med 1999; 340:757–763.

37. The French Clozapine Study Group. Clozapine in drug-induced psychosis in Parkinson's disease. Lancet 1999; 353:2041–2042.

38. Ostergaard K, Dupont E. Clozapine treatment of drug-induced psychotic symptoms in late stages of Parkinson's disease. Act Neurol Scand 1988; 78:349–350.

39. Kahn N, Freeman A, Juncos JL, Manning D, Watts RL. Clozapine is beneficial for psychosis in Parkinson's disease. Mov Disord 1992; 41:1699–1700.

40. Factor SA, Brown D, Molho ES, Podskalny GD. Clozapine: a two-year open trial in Parkinson's disease patients with psychosis. Neurology 1994; 44:544–546.

41. Rabey JM, Treves TA, Neufeld MY, Orlov E, Korczyn AD. Low-dose clozapine in the treatment of levodopa-induced mental disturbances in Parkinson's disease. Neurology 1995; 45:432–434.

42. Ruggieri S, De Pandis MF, Bonamartini A, et al. Low dose of clozapine in the treatment of dopaminergic psychosis in Parkinson's disease. Clin Neuropharmacol 1997; 20:204–209.

43. Friedman JH, Factor SA. Atypical antipsychotics in the treatment of drug-induced psychosis in Parkinson's disease. Mov Disord 2000; 151:201–211.

44. Pakkenberg H, Pakkenberg B. Clozapine in the treatment of tremor. Acta Neurol Scand 1986; 73:295–297.

45. Fischer P, Danielczyk W, Simanyi M, Streifler MB. Dopaminergic psychosis in advanced Parkinson's disease. In: Streifler MB, Korczyn AD, Melamed E, Youdim MBH, eds. Advances in Neurology. Vol. 53. Parkinson's Disease: Anatomy, Pathology and Therapy. New York: Raven Press 1990:391–397.

46. Friedman JH, Lannon MC. Clozapine-responsive tremor in Parkinson's disease. Mov Disord 1990; 5:225–229.

47. Friedman JH, Lannon MC. Benztropine versus clozapine for the treatment of tremor in Parkinson's disease. Neurology 1997; 4(48):1077–1081.

48. Jansen ENH. Clozapine in the treatment of tremor in Parkinson's disease. Acta Neurol Scand 1994; 89:262–265.

49. Bonnucelli U, Ceravolo R, Salvetti S, et al. Clozapine in Parkinson's disease tremor: effects of acute and chronic administration. Neurology 1997; 49:1587–1590.

50. Rui-Silva M, Magalhaes M, Viseu M, Bastos Lima A. Clozapine in the treatment of psychosis in parkinsonism. J Neurol 1995; 242(suppl 2):138.

51. Alvir JMA, Lieberman JA, Safferman AZ. Clozapine induced agranulocytosis. Incidence and risk factors in the United State. N Engl J Med 1993; 329:162–167.

52. Honigfeld G, Arellano F, Sethi J, et al. Reducing clozapine-related morbidity and mortality: 5 years of experience with clozapine national registry. J Clin Psychiatry 1998; 59(suppl 3):3–7.

53. Fernandez HH, Friedman JH, Factor SA, Molho ES, Coskun DJ, Lansang MC. New onset diabetes among parkinsonian patients on long-term clozapine use. Presented at the 7th International Congress on Parkinson's Disease and Movement Disorders, Miami, FL, Nov 10–14, 2002.

54. Goetz CG, Koller WC, Poewe W et al. Management of Parkinson's disease: an evidence based review. Mov Disord 2002; 17(suppl 4):S120–S127.

55. Fernandez HH, Donnelly EM, Friedman JH. Long-term outcome of clozapine use for psychosis among parkinsonian patients. Presented at the 7th International Congress on Parkinson's Disease and Movement Disorders, Miami, FL Nov 10–14, 2002.

56. Goetz CG, Stebbins G. Mortality and hallucinations in nursing home patients with advanced Parkinson's disease. Neurology 1995; 45:669–671.

57. Grant S, Fiton A. Risperidone: a review of its pharmacology and therapeutic potential in the treatment of schizophrenia. Drugs 1994; 43:456–460.
58. Arndt J, Skarsfeld T. Do novel antipsychotics have similar pharmacological characteristics? A review of the evidence. Neuropsychopharmacology 1998; 18:63–101.
59. Ellis T, Cudkowicz ME, Sexton PM, Growdon JH. Clozapine and risperidone treatment of psychosis in Parkinson's disease. J Neuropsychiatry J Clin Neurosci 2000; 12:364–369.
60. Meco G, Allesandri A, Bonifati V, Guistini P. Risperidone for hallucinations in levodopa treated Parkinson's disease patients. Lancet 1994; 343:1370–1371.
61. Ford B, Lynch T, Greene P. Risperidone in Parkinson's disease. Lancet 1994; 344:681.
62. Rich SS, Friedman JH, Ott BR. Risperidone versus clozapine in the treatment of psychosis in six patients with Parkinson's disease and other akinetic-rigid syndromes. J Clin Psychiatry 1995; 56:556–559.
63. Meco G, Alessandri A, Guistini P, Bonifati V. Risperidone in levodopa-induced psychosis in advanced Parkinson's disease: an open label long term study. Mov Disord 1997; 12:610–612.
64. Workman RJ Jr., Orengo CA, Bakey AA, et al. The use of risperidone for psychosis and agitation in demented patients with Parkinson's disease. J Neuropsychiatry Clin Neurosci 1997; 9:594–597.
65. Leopold NA. Risperidone treatment of drug related psychosis in patients with parkinsonism. Mov Disord 2000; 15:301–304.
66. Mohr E, Mendis TF, Hildebrand K, DeDeyn PP. Risperidone in the treatment of dopamine induced psychosis is Parkinson's disease: an open pilot trial. Mov Disord 2000; 15:1230–1237.
67. Factor SA, Molho ES, Friedman JH. Risperidone and Parkinson's disease. Mov Disord 2002; 17:221–222.
68. Rosebush PI, Mazurek MF. Neurologic side effects in neuroleptic-naïve patients treated with haloperidol or risperidone. Neurology 1999; 52:782–785.
69. David SR, Taylor CC, Kinon BJ, Breier A. The effects of olanzapine, risperidone and haloperidol on plasma prolactin levels in patients with schizophrenia. Clin Ther 2000; 22:1085–1096.
70. Moore NA, Tye NC, Axton MS, et al. The behavioral pharmacology of olanzapine a novel atypical antipsychotic agent. J Pharmacol Exp Ther 1992; 262:545–551.
71. Moore NA, Coligaro DO, Wong DT, et al. The pharmacology of olanzapine and other new antipsychotic agents. Curr Opin Invest Drug 1993; 2:281–293.
72. Wolters EC, Jansen EN, Tuynman-Qua HG, Bergmens PL. Olanzapine in the treatment of dopaminomimetic psychosis in patients with Parkinson's disease. Neurology 1996; 47: 1085–1087.
73. Jimenez-Jimenez FJ, Talon-Barranco A, Orti-Pareja M, et al. Olanzapine can worsen parkinsonism. Neurology 1998; 50:1183–1184.
74. Friedman JH, Goldstein SM. Olanzapine in the treatment of dopaminomimetic psychosis in patients with Parkinson's disease. Neurology 1998; 50:1195–1196.
75. Friedman JH, Goldstein SM, Jacques C. Substituting clozapine for olanzapine in psychiatrically stable Parkinson's disease patients: results of an open-label pilot trial. Clin Neuropharmacol 1998; 21:285–288.
76. Molho ES, Factor SA. Worsening of motor features of Parkinson's disease with olanzapine. Mov Dis 1999; 14:1014–1016.
77. Churchyard A, Iansek R. Olanzapine as treatment of the neuropsychiatric complications of Parkinson's disease: an open-label study. Mov Dis 1998; 13(suppl 2):188.
78. Weiner WJ, Minagar A, Shulman L. Olanzapine for the treatment of hallucinations/delusions in Parkinson's disease. Mov Dis 1998; 13(suppl 2):62–79.
79. Graham JM, Sussman JP, Ford KS, Sagar HJ. Olanzapine in the treatment of hallucinosis in Parkinson's disease: a cautionary note. J Neurol Neurosurg Psychiatry 1998; 65:774–777.
80. Stover NP, Juncos JL. Olanzapine treatment of parkinsonian patients with psychosis. Neurology 1999; 52(suppl 2):A215.
81. Goetz CG, Blasucci LM, Leurgans S, Pappert EJ. Olanzapine and clozapine: Comparative effects on motor function in hallucinating PD patients. Neurology 2000; 55:789–794.
82. Aarsland D, Larsen J, Lim NG, Tandberg E. Olanzapine for psychosis in patients with Parkinson's disease with and without dementia. J Neuropsychiatry Clin Neurosci 1999; 11:392–394.
83. Gimenez-Roldan S, Mateo D, Navarro E, Gines MM. Efficacy and Safety of Clozapine and Olanzapine: an open label trial comparing two groups of Parkinson's disease patients with dopaminergic-induced psychosis. Parkinsonism Relat Disord 2001; 7:121–127.
84. Manson AJ, Schrag A, Lees AJ. Low-dose olanzapine for levodopa induced dyskinesias. Neurology 2000; 55:795–799.

85. Bennett JP Jr., Landow ER, Schuh LA, et al. Suppression of dyskinesia in advanced Parkinson's disease II: increasing daily clozapine doses suppress dyskinesias and improve motor symptoms. Neurology 1993; 43:1551–1555.

86. Bennett JP Jr., Landon ER, Dietrich S, Schuh LA. Suppression of dyskinesias in advanced Parkinson's disease: moderate daily clozapine doses provide long-term dyskinesia reduction. Mov Disord 1994; 9:409–414.

87. Parsa MA, Bastani B. Quetiapine (Seroquel) in the treatment of psychosis in patients with Parkinson's disease. J Neuropsychiatry Clin Neurosci 1998; 10:216–219.

88. Evatt ML, Lewart D, Juncos JL. "Seroquel" treatment of psychosis in parkinsonism. Mov Disord 1996; 11:595.

89. Juncos JL, Arvantis L, Swertzer D, et al. Quetiapine improves psychotic symptoms associated with Parkinson's disease. Neurol 1999; 52(suppl 2):A262.

90. Juncos JL, Evatt ML, Jewart D. Long term effect of quetiapine fumarate in parkinsonism complicated by psychosis. Neurology 1998; 50:A70–A71.

91. Samanta J, Stacy M. Quetiapine in the treatment of hallucinations in advanced Parkinson's disease. Mov Disord 1998; 13(suppl 2):274.

92. Fernandez HH, Lannon MC, Friedman JH, Abbot BP. Clozapine replacement by quetiapine for the treatment of drug induced psychosis in Parkinson's disease. Mov Disord 2000; 15:579–581.

93. Targum SD, Abbott JL. Efficacy of quetiapine in Parkinson's patients with psychosis. J Clin Psychopharmacol 2000; 20:54–60.

94. Reddy S, Factor SA, Molho ES, Feustel PJ. The effect of quetiapine on psychosis and motor function in patients with and without dementia. Mov Disord 2002; 17:676–681.

95. Dewey RB, O'Suilleabhain. Treatment of drug induced psychosis with quetiapine and clozapine in Parkinson's disease. Neurology 2000; 55:1753–1754.

96. Fernandez HH, Trieschmann ME, Burke MA, Jacques C, Friedman JH. Long-term outcome of quetiapine use for psychosis among parkinsonian patients. Mov Disord 2003; 18:510–514.

97. Fernandez HH, Friedman JH, Jacques C, Rosenfeld M. Quetiapine for the treatment of drug induced psychosis in Parkinson's disease. Mov Disord 1999; 14:484–487.

98. Menza MM, Palermo B, Mark M. Quetiapine as an alternative to clozapine in the treatment of dopamimetic psychosis in patients with Parkinson's disease. Ann Clin Psychiatry 1999; 11: 141–144.

99. Fernandez HH. Quetiapine for L-dopa-induced psychosis in PD. Neurology 2000; 55:899.

100. Weiner WJ, Minagar A, Shulman LM. Quetiapine for l-dopa-induced psychosis in PD. Neurology 2000; 54(7):1538.

101. Weiden PJ, Iqbal N, Mendelowitz AJ, Tandon R, Zimbroff DL, Ross R. Best Clinical practice with ziprasidone: update after one year of experience. J Psychiatr Pract 2002; 8:81–98.

102. Zoldan Y, Friedberg G, Livneh M, Melamed E. Psychosis in advanced Parkinson's disease: treatment with odansetron, a 5HT3 receptor antagonist. Neurology 1995; 45:1305–1308.

103. Eichhorn TE, Brunt E, Oertel WH. Odansetron treatment of L-dopa-induced psychosis. Neurology 1996; 47:1608–1609.

104. McKeith IG, Grace JB, Walker Z, et al. Rivastigmine in the treatment of dementia with Lewy bodies. Preliminary findings from an open trial. Int J Geriatric Psych 2000; 15:387–392.

105. McKeith I, Del Ser T, Spano P-F, Emre M, Wesnes K, Anand R, Cicin-Sain A, Ferrara R, Spiegel R. Efficacy of rivastigmine in dementia with Lewy bodies: a randomized, double-blind, placebo-controlled international study. Lancet 2000; 356:2031–2036.

106. Maclean LE, Collins CC, Byrne EJ. Dementia with Lewy bodies treated with rivastigmine: effects on cognition, neuropsychiatric symptomism and sleep. Int Psychogeriatr 2001; 13:277–288.

107. Grace J, Daniel S, Stevens T, Shankar KK, Walker Z, Byrne EJ, Butler S, Wilkinson D, Woolford J, Waite J, McKeith IG. Long-term use of rivastigmine in patients with dementia with Lewy bodies: an open-label trial. Int Psychogeriatr 2001; 13:199–205.

108. Rojas-Fernandez CH. Successful use of donepezil for the treatment of dementia with Lewy bodies. Ann Pharmacother 2001; 35:202–205.

109. Reading PJ, Luce Ak, McKeith IG. Rivastigmine in the treatment of parkinsonian psychosis and cognitive impairment: preliminary findings from an open trial. Mov Disord 2001; 16:1171–1174.

110. Bergman J, Lerner V. Successful use of donepezil for the treatment of psychotic symptoms in patients with Parkinson's disease. Clin Neuropharmacol 2002; 25:107–110.

111. Hurwitz TA, Calne DB, Waterman K. Treatment of dopaminomimetic psychosis in Parkinson's disease with electroconvulsive therapy. Can J Neurol Sci 1988; 15:32–34.

112. Douyen R, Serby M, Klutcho B, et al. ECT and Parkinson's disease revisited: a naturalistic study. Am J Psychiatry 1989; 146:1451–1455.

113. Balldin J, Eden S, Grerus AK, et al. Electroconvulsive therapy in Parkinson's syndrome with 'on-off' phenomenon. J Neural Transm 1980; 47:11–21.
114. Andersen K, Balldin J, Gottfires CG, et al. A double-blind evaluation of electroconvulsive therapy in Parkinson's disease with on-off phenomena. Acta Neurol Scand 1987; 76:191–199.
115. American Psychiatric Association. Diagnostic and Statistical Manual of Mental Disorders. Rev. 3rd ed. Washington, DC: American Psychiatric Press, 1987.
116. Mayeux R. A current analysis of behavioral problems in patients with idiopathic Parkinson's disease. Mov Disord 1989; 4:26–37.
117. Aarsland D, Tandberg E, Larsen JP, et al. Frequency of dementia in Parkinson's disease. Arch Neurol 1996; 53:538–542.
118. Aarsland D, Andersen K, Larsen JP, Lolk A, Nielsen H, Kragh-Sorensen P. Risk of dementia in Parkinson's disease: a community-based, prospective study. Neurology 2001; 56(6):730–736.
119. Schrag A, Ben-Shlomo Y, Quinn N. How common are complications of Parkinson's disease? J Neurol 2002; 249(4):419–423.
120. Fernandez HH, Lapane KL. Predictors of mortality among nursing home residents with a diagnosis of Parkinson's disease. Med Sci Monit 2002; 8(4):241–246.
121. Marder K, Tang MX, Cote L, Stern Y, Mayeux R. The frequency and associated risk factors for dementia in patients with Parkinson's disease. Arch Neurol 1995; 52:695–701.
122. Biggins CA, Boyd JL, Harrop FM, Madeley P, Mindham RH, Randall JI, Spokes EG. A controlled, longitudinal study of dementia in Parkinson's disease. J Neurol Neurosurg Psychiatry 1992; 55:566–571.
123. Apaydin H, Ahlskog JE, Parisi JE, Boeve BF, Dickson DW. Parkinson disease neuropathology: later-developing dementia and loss of the levodopa response. Arch Neurol 2002; 59(1): 102–112.
124. Mayeux R, Chen J, Mirabello E, et al. An estimate of the incidence of dementia in idiopathic Parkinson's disease. Neurology 1990; 40:1513–1517.
125. Levy G, Tang MX, Cote LJ, Louis ED, Alfaro B, Mejia H, Stern Y, Marder K. Do risk factors for Alzheimer's disease predict dementia in Parkinson's disease? An exploratory study. Mov Disord 2002; 17(2):250–257.
126. Ecrola J, Launes J, Hellstron O, Tienari PJ. Apolipoprotein E (APOE), PARKIN and catechol-O-methyltransferase (COMT) genes and susceptibility to sporadic Parkinson's disease in Finland. Neurosci Lett 2002, 330.296–298.
127. Parsian A, Racette B, Goldsmith LJ, Perlmutter JS. Parkinson's disease and apolipoprotein E: possible association with dementia but not age at onset. Genomics 2002; 79:458–461.
128. Zareparsi S, Camicioli R, Sexton G, Bird T, Swanson P, Kaye J, Nutt J, Payami H. Age at onset of Parkinson disease and apolipoprotein E genotypes. Am J Med Genet 2002; 105:156–161.
129. Mattila PM, Roytta M, Lonnberg P, Marjamaki P, Helenius H, Rinne JO. Choline acetyltransferase activity and striatal dopamine receptors in Parkinson's disease in relation to cognitive impairment. Acta Neuropathol (Berl) 2001; 102(2):160–166.
130. Kahn N, Graham E, Dixon P, et al. Parkinsons Disease is not associated with combined alphasynuclein/apolipoprotein E susceptibility genotype. Ann Neurol 2001; 49:665–668.
131. Elizan TS, Sroka H, Maker H, Smith H, Yahr MD. Dementia in idiopathic Parkinson's disease. Variables associated with its occurrence in 203 patients. J Neural Transm 1986; 65:285–302.
132. Ebmeier KP, Calder SA, Crawford JR, Stewart L, Besson JA, Mutch WJ. Clinical features predicting dementia in idiopathic Parkinson's disease: a follow-up study. Neurology 1990; 40:1222–1224.
133. Stern Y, Marder K, Tang MX, Mayeux R. Antecedent clinical features associated with dementia in Parkinson's disease. Neurology 1993; 43:1690–1692.
134. Caparros-Lefebre D, Pecheux N, Petit V, Duhamel A, Petit H. Which factors predict cognitive decline in Parkinson's disease? J Neurol Neurosurgery and Psychiatry 1995; 58:51–55.
135. Mindham RH, The place of dementia in Parkinson's disease: a methodologic saga. Adv Neurol 1999; 80:403–408.
136. Graham JM, Sagar HJ. A data-driven approach to the study of heterogeneity in idiopathic Parkinson's disease: identification of three distinct subtypes. Mov Disord 1999; 14:10–20.
137. Poewe WH, Wenning GK. The natural history of Parkinson's disease. Ann Neurol 1998; 44(suppl 1):S1–S9.
138. Giladi N, Treves TA, Paleacu D, Shabtai H, Orlov Y, Kandinov B, Simon ES, Korczyn AD. Risk factors for dementia, depression and psychosis in long-standing Parkinson's disease. J Neural Transm 2000; 107(1):59–71.

139. Hughes TA, Ross HF, Musa S, Bhattacherjee S, Nathan RN, Mindham RH, Spokes EG. A 10-year study of the incidence of and factors predicting dementia in Parkinson's disease. Neurology 2000; 54:1596–1602.
140. Growdon JH, Corkin S, Rosen TJ. Distinctive aspects of cognitive dysfunction in Parkinson's disease. Adv Neurol 1990; 53:365–376.
141. Levy G, Schupf N, Tang MX, Cote LJ, Louis ED, Mejia H, Stern Y, Marder K. Combined effect of age and severity on the risk of dementia in Parkinson's disease. Ann Neurol 2002; 51(6): 722–729.
142. Marder K, Tang MX, Alfaro B, Mejia H, Cote L, Jacobs D, Stern Y, Sano M, Mayeux R. Postmenopausal estrogen use and Parkinson's disease with and without dementia. Neurology 1998; 50(4):1141–1143.
143. Savage CR. Neuropsychology of subcortical dementias. In neuropsychiatry of the basal ganglia. Psychiatri Clin North Am. 1997; 20(4):911–931.
144. Kish SJ, Shannak K, Hornykiewicz O. Uneven pattern of dopamine loss in the striatum of patients with idiopathic Parkinson's disease. N Engl J Med 1988; 334:345–348.
145. Rinne JO, Lonnberg P, Marjamaki P, Rinne UK. Brain muscarinic receptor subtypes are differently affected in Alzheimer's disease and Parkinson's disease. Brain Res 1989; 483:402–406.
146. Murray AM, Weihmueller FB, Marshall JF, Hurtig HI, Gottlieb GL, Joyce JN. Damage to dopamine systems differs between Parkinson's disease and Alzheimer's disease with parkinsonism. Ann Neurol 1995; 37:300–312.
147. Holthoff-Detto VA, Kessler J, Herholz K, et al. functional effects of striatal dysfunction in Parkinson disease. Arch Neurol 1997; 54:145.
148. Owen AM, Sahakian BJ, Hodges JR, Summers BA, Polkey CE, Robbins TW. Dopamine-dependent frontostriatal planning deficits in early Parkinson's disease. Neuropsychology 1995; 9:126–140.
149. Nagaraja D, Jayashree S. Randomized study of the dopamine receptor agonist piribedil in the treatment of mild cognitive impairment. Am J Psychiatry 2001; 158(9):1517–1519.
150. Gotham AM, Grown RG, Marsden CD. "Frontal" cognitive function in patients with Parkinson's disease "on" and "off" levodopa. Brain 1988; 111:299–321.
151. Huber SJ, Shulman HG, Paulson GW, et al. Dose-dependent memory impairment in Parkinson's disease. Neurology 1989; 39:438–440.
152. Growdon JH, Kieburtz K, McDermott MP, Panisset M, Friedman JH. Levodopa improves motor function without impairing cognition in mild non-demented Parkinson's disease patients. Parkinson Study Group. Neurology 1998; 50:1327–1331.
153. Tiraboschi P, Hansen LA, Alford M, et al. Cholinergic dysfunction in diseases with Lewy bodies. Neurology 2000; 54:407–411.
154. Perry EK, McKeith I, Thompson P, Marshall E, Kerwin J, Jabeen S, Edwardson JA, Ince P, Blessed G, Irving D, Perry RH. Topography, extent, and clinical relevance of neurochemical deficits in dementia of Lewy body type, Parkinson's disease, and Alzheimer's disease. Ann NY Acad Sci 1991; 640:197–202.
155. Perry EK, Irving D, Kerwin JM, McKeith IG, Thompson P, Collerton D, Fairbairn AF, Ince PG, Morris CM, Cheng AV, Perry RH. Cholinergic transmitter and neurotrophic activities in Lewy body dementia: similarity to Parkinson's and distinction from Alzheimer disease. Alz Dis Assoc Disord 1993; 7:69–79.
156. Ruberg M, Ploska A, Javoy-Agid F, Agid Y. Muscarinic binding and choline acetyltransferase activity in parkinsonian subjects with reference to dementia. Brain Res 1982; 232: 129–139.
157. Kuhl DE, Minoshima S, Fessler JA, Frey KA, Foster NL, Ficaro EP, Wieland DM, Koeppe RA. In vivo mapping of cholinergic terminals in normal aging, Alzheimer's disease, and Parkinson's disease. Ann Neurol 1996; 40:399–410.
158. Martin-Ruiz C, Lawrence S, Piggot M, Kuryatov A, Lindstrom J, Gotti C, Cookson MR, Perry RH, Jaros E, Perry EK, Court JA. Nicotinic receptors in the putamen of patients with dementia with Lewy bodies and Parkinson's disease: relation to changes in alpha-synuclein expression. Neurosci Lett 2002; 25:134–138.
159. Aarsland D, Laake K, Larsen JP, Janvin C. Donepezil for cognitive impairment in Parkinson's disease: a randomized controlled study. J Neurol Neurosurg Psychiatry 2002; 72(6):708–712.
160. Scatton V, Javoy-Agid F, Roquier L, et al. Reduction of cortical dopamine, noradrenaline, serotonin and their metabolites in Parkinson's disease. Brain Res 1983; 275:321–328.
161. Jellinger K. Neuropathological substrates of Alzheimer's disease and Parkinson's disease. J Neural Trans 1987; 24(suppl):109–129.

162. Mortimer JA, Pirozzolo FJ, Hansch EC, Webster DD. Relationship of motor symptoms to intellectual deficits in Parkinson disease. Neurology 1982; 32:133–137.

163. Berger H, van Es N, van Spaendonck K, Teunisse JP, Horstink M, van't Hof M, Cools A. Relationship between memory strategies and motor symptoms in Parkinson's disease. J Clin Exp Neuropsych 1999; 21:677–684.

164. Racette BA, Harlein MJ, Hershey T, Mink JW, Perlmutter JS, Black KJ. Clinical features and comorbidity of mood fluctuations in Parkinson's disease. J Neuropsychiatry Clin Neurosci 2002; 14:438–442.

165. Saint-Cyr JA, Taylor AE, Nicholson K. Behavior and the basal ganglia. In: Weiner WJ, Lang AE, eds. Behavioral Neurology of Movement Disorders. New York: Raven Press, 1995:1–28.

166. Cahn-Weiner DA, Grace J, Ott BR, Fernandez HH, Friedman JH. Cognitive and behavioral features discriminate between Alzheimer's and Parkinson's disease. Neuropsychiatry Neuropsychol Behav Neurol 2002; 15(2):79–87.

167. Brown RG, Marsden CD. Neuropsychology and cognitive function in Parkinson's disease: an overview. In: Marsden CD, Fahn S, eds. Movement Disorders. New York & London: Butterworth's, 1987:99–123.

168. Tamaru F, Yanagisawa N. Shifting ability in Parkinson's disease: does shifting ability really deteriorate? Adv Neurol 1990; 53:317–320.

169. Litvan I, MacIntyre A, Goetz CG, et al. Accuracy of the clinical diagnoses of Lewy Body disease, Parkinson's disease, and dementia with Lewy bodies. Arch Neurol 1998; 55:969–978.

170. Heindel WC, Salmon DP, Butters N. Pictorial priming and cued recall in Alzheimer's and Huntington's disease. Brain Cogn 1990; 13:282–295.

171. Korczyn AD. Dementia in Parkinson's disease. J Neurol 2001; 248(suppl 3):III 1–4.

172. Jellinger KA, Seppi K, Wenning GK, Poewe W. Impact of coexistent Alzheimer pathology on the natural history of Parkinson's disease. J Neural Transm 2002; 109(3):329–339.

173. Louis ED, Klatka LA, Liu Y, Fahn S. Comparison of extrapyramidal features of 31 pathologically confirmed cases of diffuse lewy body disease and 34 pathologically confirmed cases of Parkinson's disease. Neurology 1997; 48:376–380.

174. McKeith IG, Galasko D, Kosaka K, et al. for the Consortium on Dementia with Lewy Bodies. Consensus guidelines for the clinical and pathologic diagnosis of dementia with Lewy bodies (DLB): report of the consortium on DLB international workshop. Neurology 1996; 47: 1113–1124.

175. Doody RS, Stevens JC, Beck C, et al. Practice parameter: management of dementia (an evidence-based review). Report of the Quality Standards Subcommittee of the American Academy of Neurology. Neurology 2001; 56:1145–1166.

176. AHCPR Clinical Practice Guidelines, No. 19. Publication #97–0702. USHHS. Washington, DC, November 1996.

177. Rogers SL, Friedhoff LT. Long-term efficacy and safety of donepezil in the treatment of Alzheimer's disease: an interim analysis of the results of a US multicenter open label extension study. Eur Neuropsychopharmacol 1998; 8:67–75.

178. Farlow M, Anand R, Messina J Jr., et al. A 52-week study of the efficacy of rivastigmine in patients with mild to moderately severe Alzheimer's disease. Eur Neurol 2000; 44:236–241.

179. Potkin SG, Anand R, Fleming K, Alva G, Keator D, Carreon D, Messina J, Wu JC, Hartman R, Fallon JH. Brain metabolic and clinical effects of rivastigmine in Alzheimer's disease. Int J Neuropsychopharmacol 2001; 4:223–230.

180. Lopez OL, Becker JT, Wisniewski S, Saxton J, Kaufer DI, DeKosky ST. Cholinesterase inhibitor treatment alters the natural history of Alzheimer's disease. J Neurol Neurosurg Psychiatry 2002; 72:310–314.

181. Winblad B, Engedal K, Soininen H, Verhey F, Waldemar G, Wimo A, Wetterholm AL, Zhang R, Haglund A, Subbiah P. Donepezil Nordic Study Group. A 1-year, randomized, placebo-controlled study of donepezil in patients with mild to moderate AD. Neurology 2001; 57(3):489–495.

182. Physicians Desk Reference. 56th Ed. Medical Economics Company, Inc., Montvale, NJ 2002.

183. Dunn NR, Pearce GL, Shakir SA. Adverse effects associated with the use of donepezil in general practice in England. J Psychopharmacol 2000; 14:406–408.

184. Ott BR, Lannon MC. Exacerbation of parkinsonism by tacrine. Clin Neuropharmacol 1992; 15:322–325.

185. Hutchison M, Fazzini E. Cholinesterase inhibition in Parkinson's disease. J Neurol Neurosurg Psychiatry 1996; 61:324–325.

186. Geizer M, Ancill RJ. Combination of risperidone and donepezil in Lewy body dementia. Can J Psychiatry 1998; 43:421–422.

187. Kaufer DI, Catt KE, Lopez OL, DeKosky ST. Dementia with Lewy bodies: response of delirium-like features to donepezil (lett). Neurology 1998; 51:1512.
188. Shea C, MacKnight C, Rockwood K. Donepezil for treatment of dementia with Lewy bodies: a case series of nine patients. Int Psychogeriatr 1998; 10:229–238.
189. Aarsland D, Bronnick K, Karlsen K. Donepezil for dementia with Lewy bodies: a case study. Int J Geriatr Psychiatry 1999; 14:69–72.
190. Lanctot KL, Herrmann N. Donepezil for behavioural disorders associated with Lewy bodies: a case series. Int J Geriatr Psychiatry 2000; 15:338–345.
191. Samuel W, Caliguri M, Galasko D, et al. 2000 Better cognitive and psychopathologic response to donepezil in patients prospectively diagnosed as dementia with Lewy bodies: a preliminary study. Int J Geriatric Psych 15, 794–802.
192. Skjerve A, Nygaard HA. Improvement in sundowning in dementia with Lewy bodies after treatment with donepezil. Int J Geriatric Psychiatry 2000; 15:1147–1151.
193. Werber EA, Rabey JM. The beneficial effect of cholinesterase inhibitors on patients suffering from Parkinson's disease and dementia. J Neural Transm 2001; 108(11):1319–1325.
194. Korczyn AD. Treating the cholinergic deficit in dementia: a therapeutic strategy with disease-modifying potential pp 260–262. In: Understanding Changes in Cholinergic Function: Implications for Treating Dementia [Academic Highlights].
195. Bullock R, Cameron A. Rivastigmine for the treatment of dementia and visual hallucinations associated with Parkinson's disease: a case series. Curr Med Res Opin 2002; 18:258–264.
196. Bourke D, Bruckenbrod RWS. Possible association between donepezil and worsening Parkinson's disease. Ann Pharmacother 1998; 32:610–611.
197. Fabbrini G, Barbanti P, Aurilia C, et al. Donepezil in the treatment of hallucinations and delusions in Parkinson's disease. Neurol Sci 2002; 41–43.
198. Litvan I, Philipps M, Pharr VL, Hallet M, Grafman J, Salazar A. Randomized placebo-controlled trial of donepezil in patients with progressive supranuclear palsy. Neurology 2001; 57:467–473.
199. Richard IH, Justus AW, Greig NH, Marshall F, Kurlan R. Worsening of motor function and mood in a patient with Parkinson's disease after pharmacologic challenge with oral rivastigmine. Clin Neuropharmacol 2002; 25:296–299.
200. Maelicke A. Allosteric modulation of nicotinic receptors as a treatment strategy for Alzheimer's disease. Dement Geriatr Cogn Disord 2000; 11(S):P11–P18.
201. Narabayashi H, Yokochi F, Ogawa T, Igakura T. Analysis of l-threo-3,4-dihydroxyphenylserine effect on motor and psychological symptoms in Parkinson's disease. No To Shinkei 1991; 43(3): 263–268.
202. Bedard MA, el Massioui F, Malapani C, Dubois B, Pillon B, Renault B, Agid Y. Attentional deficits in Parkinson's disease: partial reversibility with naphtoxazine (SDZ NVI-085), a selective noradrenergic alpha 1 agonist. Clin Neuropharmacol 1998; 21:108–117.
203. Fernandez HH, Lapane KL for the SAGE (Systematic Assessment of Geriatric Drug Use via Epidemiology) Study Group. Estrogen use among nursing home residents with a diagnosis of Parkinson's disease. Mov Disord 2000; 15:1119–1124.
204. Lim GP, Yang F, Chu T, et al. Ibuprofen suppresses plaque pathology and inflammation in a mouse model of Alzheimer's disease. J Neurosci 2000; 20:5709–5714.
205. McKenzie JE, Edwards RJ, Gentleman SM, Ince PG, Perry RH, Royston MC, Roberts GW. A quantitative comparison of plaque types in Alzheimer's disease and senile dementia of the Lewy body type. Acta Neuropathol (Berl) 1996; 91(5):526–529.

32
Anxiety and Depression

Alexander I. Tröster

*University of North Carolina School of Medicine,
Chapel Hill, North Carolina, U.S.A.*

Elizabeth A. Letsch

*University of Washington School of Medicine,
Seattle, Washington, U.S.A.*

I. INTRODUCTION

Anxiety and depression are among the most common neurobehavioral symptoms of Parkinson's disease (PD), yet often go unrecognized in clinical practice (1). Shulman et al. (1) observed that anxiety and depression detected by symptom inventories was undetected by neurologists in more than half the cases. Furthermore, in comparison to the proportion of parkinsonians with depressive symptoms, relatively few are prescribed antidepressants (2). The importance of diagnosing and treating anxiety and depression cannot be overstated, given that mental health symptoms in general (3), and depression in particular, profoundly impact the parkinsonian's quality of life (4–6). Early and successful treatment of depression is imperative because this condition is associated with depression in the caregiver (7) and diminishes the caregiver's quality of life (8). Depression exacerbates cognitive impairment (9–14), increases the risk of dementia (15,16), and is associated with excess functional disability (17–19) and more rapid disease progression (20). Indeed, depression may be a risk factor for PD and one of the earliest signs of the disease, preceding motor symptoms by several years (21–24). This chapter reviews depression and anxiety disorders in PD. Each section examines incidence and prevalence, phenomenology and diagnostic issues, potential causes, and treatment.

II. DEPRESSION

A. Incidence and Prevalence

Estimates of the incidence of depression in PD range from 4 to 75%, while prevalence estimates range from 7 to 90%. Commonly accepted prevalence estimates are 30–50%, with half of the depressed patients having major depression and the other half having minor depression or dysthymia (25). Community-based and case register studies (26–28), however, suggest that major depression may be less common than minor depression (with a prevalence of only about 3–8%). These large variations in prevalence estimates likely reflect differences in diagnostic criteria, case ascertainment and sampling methods, and whether cases include persons with only major depression or other affective disturbances, such as dysthymia, as well. It is commonly believed that community-based studies yield lower prevalence estimates than do studies conducted in hospitals and research centers and that studies employing depression symptom inventories or rating scales report higher prevalence rates than do studies using structured diagnostic interviews and strict diagnostic criteria (29). A recent meta-analysis (30), however, contradicts the latter belief. That meta-analysis found that the average prevalence of depression among studies using Diagnostic and Statistical Manual (DSM) criteria (10 studies, 1179 PD patients) was about 42%. By comparison, studies using depression rating scales or symptom inventories (21 studies, 1556 patients) showed a prevalence of about 37%, and studies using clinical diagnoses (chart review or structured interviews) (13 studies, 3176 patients) yielded an average depression prevalence of about 24%. This suggests that more rigorous diagnostic methods might actually yield higher prevalence estimates of depression in PD, a finding that would parallel that of dementia in PD (31).

B. Phenomenology of Depression in Parkinson's Disease

Depression in PD is thought to differ from idiopathic major depression in that the parkinsonian with depression is less likely to report self-reproach, feelings of failure, and guilt. Although less likely to suffer hallucinations or delusions (32,33), the parkinsonian with depression is more likely to experience comorbid anxiety (34–36). Even though suicidal ideation is common among depressed parkinsonians (37), completed suicide is not (38,39). Myslobodsky and colleagues (38), examining 1991–1996 mortality data from the National Center of Health Statistics (U.S.) database, found that among 144,364 decedents with a primary diagnosis of PD, 122 (0.08%) died by suicide. Although studies of depressed parkinsonians reveal that these patients experience dysphoria, sadness, irritability, pessimism, and anhedonia (40), this does not imply that the depressed parkinsonian will spontaneously complain of such symptoms at clinic visits. Indeed, Okun and Watts (41) cautioned that depressed PD patients may spontaneously complain only of fatigue and diminished energy and that such complaints should trigger a detailed interview about stressors and other possible symptoms of depression. This recommendation is consonant with the observation that depression in PD often occurs in the context of other nonmotor symptoms such as sleep disturbance, fatigue, anxiety, and sensory symptoms and that the presence of any nonmotor symptom should cue investigation of other nonmotor symptoms (42).

C. Diagnosis of Depression in Parkinson's Disease

In the Diagnostic and Statistical Manual of Mental Disorders (DSM-IV-TR) (43) entities that require consideration include depressive disorders (major depressive disorder, dysthymic disorder), other mood disorders (e.g., mood disorder due to a general medical condition, substance-induced mood disorder), and adjustment disorders (e.g., with depressed mood, with anxiety, or with mixed anxiety and depressed mood). Some of the

Table 1 Diagnostic Criteria for Major Depressive Disorder vs. Dysthymia

Major Depressive Disorder

    Major depressive episode requires at least a 2-week presence, generally almost daily, of at least five symptoms such as depressed mood or anhedonia (one or both of these two must be present), weight and/or appetite changes, sleep disturbance,[a] anergia and/or fatigue,[a] recurring thoughts of death or suicide, cognitive deficit in concentration or decision making, excessive self-reproach or guilt, and psychomotor agitation or retardation.[a]

    Symptoms are of clinical significance (inferred from role impairment and/or distress) and not due to psychosis, substance use, a medical condition, bereavement, or part of a mixed episode.

Dysthymia

    Depressed mood for more days than not, for at least 2 years, with no symptom-free period longer than 2 months, no major depression in the initial 2-year period, and no prior manic or mixed episode.

    While depressed, the person suffers from two or more of: anergia, appetite disturbance, sleep disturbance, hopelessness, difficulty with concentration and/or decision-making, low self-esteem.

    The symptoms are of clinical severity (cause marked distress or impede social or work roles).

    Symptoms are not better explained by psychotic disorder, substance use, or medical condition.

[a]Psychomotor retardation, early morning awakening, and anergia have empirically been shown to occur with similar frequency in PD without depression and PD with depression, and it is recommended that these symptoms are given less weight in the diagnosis of depression in PD. *Source*: Adapted from Ref. 43.

more important features of these diagnostic entities are presented in Tables 1 through 3. It is also important to differentiate these mood disorders from apathy and emotionalism.

    While the DSM is helpful in providing guidelines for the reliable and valid differentiation of conditions associated with depression, the practical application of these guidelines and criteria in PD occasionally faces difficulties. Depression in the context of PD is typically diagnosed under the rubric of mood disorders due to a general medical condition (44), which permits specification whether the mood disorder involves a major depressive episode, depressive features (when criteria for a major depressive episode are not met), or manic features. Meeting the diagnostic criterion that history, physical examination, and/or laboratory tests provide evidence that the mood disorder is a direct physiological

Table 2 Mood Disorder Due to Parkinson's Disease

Prominent and persistent mood disturbance evidenced by depressed mood or anhedonia and/or elevated or irritable mood that produces clinically remarkable distress or role impairment.

History, physical examination, or laboratory findings confirm that the mood disorder is a physiological consequence of Parkinson's disease.

The type (with depressive features, with major depressive-like episode, with manic features, or mixed features) is specified. To qualify for diagnosis of "with major depressive-like episode," the criteria for major depressive episode (see Table 1) must be met (except excluding a medical cause of the mood disturbance).

Source: Adapted from Ref. 43.

Table 3 Diagnostic Criteria for Adjustment Disorders

Emotional or behavioral symptom onset within 3 months in response to an identifiable stressor. Symptoms cause marked distress (excessive given the circumstances) and/or role impairment.

Symptoms are not better explained by another mental disorder or bereavement and are not simply an exacerbation of a preexisting mental disorder.

Symptoms resolve within 6 months of cessation of the stressor or its consequences (unless due to a chronic or protracted stressor such as a medical condition, which is of particular relevance in the case of Parkinson's disease).

The type (with depressed mood, with anxiety, with mixed anxiety and depressed mood, with conduct disturbance, with mixed emotional and conduct disturbance, or unspecified) is indicated.

Source: Adapted from Ref. 43.

consequence of PD may prove elusive in practice, and perhaps is more often assumed than conclusively demonstrated. One reason for this is that biological and nonbiological markers for idiopathic depression and for depression in PD overlap (40,45). For example, although functional neuroimaging findings support the contention that mood alterations and depression in PD are accompanied by physiological (metabolic) brain changes (46,47) and that response to antidepressants is associated with changes in regional cerebral metabolism (46), the cerebral metabolic abnormalities associated with depression overlap in PD and idiopathic depression (48). Similarly, nonsuppression of cortisol secretion after administration of dexamethasone (dexamethasone suppression test or DST) is seen in PD with depression and idiopathic depression (49), though some studies have failed to find nonsuppression rates in PD with depression that are comparable to those in idiopathic depression (50).

Determining whether depression in PD represents a feature of an adjustment reaction according to DSM criteria is also not straightforward. It has been suggested that depression is rarely merely a reaction to PD (51), but it is not clear that any empirical study has documented the prevalence of adjustment reactions using DSM criteria. One difficulty with the use of DSM criteria for adjustment reactions in PD is that the adjustment reaction must be deemed to be of clinical severity, as might be inferred from excessive distress or interference with occupational or social functioning. In practice, it may be difficult to determine whether: (a) the mood disturbance rather than physical and/or cognitive disability associated with PD leads to occupational and social functional changes; or (b) the mood disturbance is a reaction to, rather than a cause of, occupational and social functioning changes.

One issue in the diagnosis of depression in PD concerns potential symptom overlap between depression and PD (52,53). Patients with both PD and idiopathic depression may demonstrate psychomotor retardation, anergia, stooped posture, diminished facial animation and conversational prosody, cognitive alterations, and sleep disturbance, raising the possibility that depression is overdiagnosed in PD because symptoms of PD are mistaken for those of depression. Similarly, autonomic symptoms (e.g., dry mouth, decreased libido, impotence) associated with PD may lead to an erroneous diagnosis of depression or anxiety (54), though most investigators have found autonomic symptoms more generally to have adequate specificity for depression in PD (34,55,56). Several studies have fruitfully detailed those symptoms likely to overlap in PD and depression and those more likely to be manifestations of depression. Specifically, early morning awakening, anergia, and psychomotor retardation overlap significantly in PD with and without depression (56,57) and, thus, should be excluded from consideration when diagnosing depression in PD.

Given that some symptoms of depression and PD overlap, there is concern that self-report inventories (many of which quantify the presence and/or severity also of overlapping symptoms) might overdiagnose depression. Several studies have sought to identify and compare different measures' sensitivity and specificity and to propose potential alterations in cutoff scores used to diagnose depression in PD. In this regard, one might emphasize that the use of cutoff scores for diagnostic purposes suffers psychometric limitations, regardless of the instrument employed. Typically, the cutting scores are not corrected for base rates of the condition in question, are derived from small samples, and are not corrected for demographics that might be associated with the condition in question. Scores within one standard error of measurement of the cutting score may be difficult to interpret, particularly if the instrument has less than optimal test-retest reliability. Self-report inventories and rating scales are better used for screening, and the diagnosis of depression in the individual patient is best achieved by using self-report inventories in conjunction with detailed psychological or psychiatric diagnostic interviews (58). Table 4 lists some of the more commonly employed depression self-report and rating instruments and some preliminary, empirically determined, recommended cutoff scores for use in PD.

1. Apathy and Emotionalism

Apathy involves an absence or lack of feeling, concern, emotion, motivation, and interest (59). It may be mistaken for depression in PD, with which it frequently coexists, as well as for PD itself, given overlapping signs and symptoms such as absence of facial animation, reduced socialization, and reduced interest in hobbies (60). Among 50 patients, Starkstein et al. (61) found that 12% were clinically apathetic [defined by a score on an abbreviated version of Marin's apathy scale (62)], 26% were only depressed, while 30% of the PD patients had both depression and apathy. Levy et al. (63), using the Neuropsychiatric Inventory, found that 5% of 40 PD patients had apathy, 28% had depression, and 28% had apathy and depression. Although reliable morphometric correlates of apathy have not been identified in PD (64), a consistent finding is that, among cognitive impairments, executive dysfunction in particular is more pronounced in those with than without apathy, and in those with higher than lower levels of apathy (61,64,65). This strongly suggests that frontal systems are implicated in the apathy of PD. Clinically, assessment of apathy in PD is readily achieved with the Apathy Scale (62), the Neuropsychiatric Inventory (66), or the Frontal Systems Behavior Scale (formerly called the Frontal Lobe Personality Scale) (67).

Depression also needs to be differentiated from emotionalism, meaning excessive and heightened sentimentality that is inappropriate, involuntary, and unmotivated (68). Madeley and colleagues (69) found that about 40% of patients with PD reported excessive tearfulness and 11% more widespread emotionalism.

D. Etiology of Depression in Parkinson's Disease

The debate whether depression is intrinsic to PD or a reaction to it is unlikely to be resolved. Supporting evidence for both viewpoints is readily mustered, and it may be more productive to elucidate more precisely the interactions among biological and environmental factors that lead to and maintain depression (70).

Table 4   Self-Report and Rating Scales Used to Detect Depression in Parkinson's Disease

Scale (Ref.)	Example of study of scale in Parkinson's disease	PD sample size; [depressed/not depressed]; and criteria	Number of items; maximum score; traditional cutoff [a]	Recommended cutoff to distinguish depressed vs. non-depressed PD (sensitivity/specificity)	Recommended screening cutoff for PD (sensitivity/specificity)	Recommended diagnostic cutoff for PD (sensitivity/specificity)
Beck Depression Inventory (181). *Note:* Updated version of this scale available (182)	Leentjens et al. (58)	N = 53; [12 depressed, 41 not depressed]; DSM-IV "depressive disorder"	21 items; maximum = 63 10 = mild 12 = moderate 30 = severe	13/14 (0.67/0.88)	8/9 (0.92/0.59)	16/17 (0.42/0.98)
Hamilton Rating Scale for Depression (17-item) (183)	Leentjens et al. (184)	N = 63; [16 depressed, 47 not depressed]; DSM-IV "depressive disorder"	17 items; maximum = 50 8 = mild 14 = moderate 19 = severe 23 = very severe	13/14 (0.88/0.89)	11/12 (0.94/0.75)	16/17 (0.75/0.98)
	Naarding et al. (185)	N = 85; [20 depressed, 65 not depressed]; DSM-IV "major depression"		12/13 (0.80/0.92)	9/10 (0.95/0.98)	15/16 (0.99/0.93)
Montgomery-Åsberg Depression Rating Scale (186)	Leentjens et al. (184)	N = 63; [16 depressed, 47 not depressed]; DSM-IV "depressive disorder"	10 items; maximum = 60 15 = mild 25 = moderate 31 = severe 44 = very severe	14/15 (0.88/0.89)	14/15 (0.88/0.89)	17/18 (0.63/0.94)

Scale	Study	Sample					Scoring
			—	—	—	—	
			—	—	—	—	
			—	—	—	—	
Geriatric Depression Scale (30-item) (187); (15-item)(188)	Meara et al. (2)	N = 132; [84 depressed, 48 not depressed]; GDS-15; traditional cutoff					30-item form; maximum = 30; 9/10 = mild; 15 item-form; maximum = 15; 4/5 = cutoff
Hospital Anxiety and Depression Scale (189)	Marinus et al. (190)	N = 177; [38 possible depressed, HADS 8–10; 30 probable depressed, HADS ≥ 11; 109 not depressed]					14 items; maximum = 21 (7 depression, 7 anxiety) 8 = mild 11 = moderate 15 = severe
Zung Self Rating Depression Scale (191)	Kuopio et al. (6)	N = 228; [55 possible depressed, Zung 38–44; 66 probable depressed, Zung ≥ 45]					20 items; maximum = 80 50 = mild 60 = moderate 70 = severe
Neuropsychiatric Inventory (66)	Levy et al. (63)	N = 40; [22 depressed, 18 not depressed]; symptom presence per NPI					—
	Åarsland et al. (8)	N = 139; [53 depressed, 86 not depressed]; Symptom presence per NPI					—

aTraditional cutoffs from test manuals or per Task Force for the Handbook of Psychiatric Measures (166).

1. Neurochemical and Neuroanatomical Correlates of Depression

Possible dopaminergic mechanisms underlying depression in PD traditionally have been minimized because levodopa seems to have a limited effect on depression (52). The observation that chronic levodopa treatment has minimal impact on depression, however, does not exclude a dopaminergic role in depression because levodopa principally affects the nigrostriatal system rather than the mesolimbic system, which is involved in emotional regulation. Infusion of methylphenidate, which primarily activates the mesolimbic system, does indeed lead to a lesser euphoric response in depressed than non-depressed patients with PD (71), suggesting a dopaminergic role in PD mood changes. Furthermore, newer dopamine agonists, such as pramipexole, that have a higher affinity for postsynaptic D_3 receptors may have more notable antidepressant effects (72).

Other findings pointing toward a dopaminergic role in depression in PD include Torack and Morris's (73) observation of more pronounced degeneration of ventral tegmental dopaminergic neurons in PD with mood disturbance and dementia than without. This ventral tegmental area send afferents to orbital and prefrontal cortical regions that have been shown to be hypometabolic by functional neuroimaging in parkinsonians with depression (46,74) or dysphoria (47). Although strong evidence of a dopaminergic role in depression remains elusive (75), it may be that dopamine plays different roles in what Burn (52) has termed phasic versus tonic mood changes in PD and/or that dopaminergic mechanisms influence the expression, if not presence, of depressive symptoms.

Fluctuations in mood accompanying motor fluctuations (76,77) are widely described, and such nonmotor fluctuations may be even more disconcerting to patients than the motor fluctuations (78). Unlike tonic depression, phasic depression in PD may bear a reasonable relationship to dopaminergic mechanisms. The findings of Cantello et al. (71) might be considered as supportive of a role of dopaminergic mechanisms in phasic rather than tonic mood disturbance. Dose-related mood elevations and anxiety reductions observed in a placebo-controlled study of the effects of levodopa infusion in parkinsonians with motor fluctuations (79,80) might similarly be interpreted as supporting a dopaminergic role in phasic depression or dysphoria, particularly since this effect of levodopa is attenuated in early PD (81), when dopaminergic depletion is less pronounced. The hypothesis that there is a stronger relationship between dopaminergic mechanisms and phasic rather than tonic depression is, however, clouded by at least two findings. First, nonfluctuating (tonic) clinical depression is much more likely to occur in parkinsonians with mood and motor fluctuations as opposed to those with only motor fluctuations (82), meaning that there is an association between tonic and phasic mood disturbance. Second, while it is typically the case that dysphoria or depression, in some instances co-occurring with anxiety, accompany the motor off state and elevated mood accompanies the on or mobile state, this relationship probably is not linear (83).

Noradrenergic abnormalities have also been only weakly linked to depression, and the strongest evidence, perhaps, is that depression in PD responds to tricyclic antidepressants (84). Other supportive evidence includes the findings that locus ceruleus cell loss relates to atypical depression in PD (85), though more general depression in PD may not relate to such abnormalities (86), and that cerebrospinal fluid (CSF) level of 3-methoxy-4-hydroxyphenyl-glycol (MHPG), a metabolite of norepinephrine, is associated with depression in PD (87).

Stronger evidence implicates serotonergic mechanisms in the depression of PD. However, orbitofrontal targets of dopaminergic pathways project back to the serotonergic dorsal raphe nuclei, and thus, some serotonergic abnormalities may be secondary to dopaminergic changes. Reductions in the metabolite of serotonin, 5-hydroxyindoleacetic acid (5-HIAA), in CSF have been associated with depression PD in some (88,89) but not all studies (90), and lower 5-HIAA levels are observed in major depression than in dysthymia in PD (88). Greater loss of serotonergic dorsal raphe neurons has been observed in depressed than nondepressed patients with PD (86). Recent functional neuroimaging studies suggest that depression in PD may be related to both loss of serotonergic output and diminished cortical responsiveness to serotonin (91). Specifically, using ^{11}C-WAY 100635 positron emission tomography (PET), Doder and colleagues (92) found significant reductions in presynaptic 5-HT$_{1A}$ binding in the midbrain raphe in both depressed and nondepressed PD patients, but reduced cortical postsynaptic 5-HT$_{1A}$ binding in only depressed parkinsonians. Murai et al. (93) found that single photon emission computed tomography (SPECT) –measured [^{123}I] β-CIT binding ratios were reduced in the dorsal midbrain of depressed PD patients, and this was interpreted as reflective of regional serotonin transporter abnormalities. Structural alterations in the midline brainstem indicative of raphe abnormalities have been demonstrated by both magnetic resonance imaging (MRI) and transcranial sonography in depressed PD patients (94).

There may be a genetic susceptibility to serotonergic abnormalities and depression in PD. The serotonin transporter is of importance in determining serotonergic tone, and a polymorphism in the promoter of the transporter gene (5-HTTLPR) is of particular interest. The long allele (l) of the transporter gene is more efficiently transcribed than the short allele (s), which has a 44-base-pair deletion, and thus, the long allele is associated with greater transporter production, and hence serotonin uptake. The s-s and s-l genotypes of 5-HTTLPR have been associated with anxiety, especially in elderly (95), and more recently, the short allele has been linked to depression and anxiety in PD (96,97)

2. Treatment-Induced (Iatrogenic) Depression

Levodopa treatment has been associated with depression, perhaps related to levodopa's effect on the metabolism of serotonin (98), although this is not suspected to be a frequent cause of depression. Huber et al. (99) found that patients with PD and depression had been taking levodopa for a longer time and in higher doses than those without depression.

Mood-altering effects of surgical therapies such as deep brain stimulation (DBS), have also been described. Although depressive symptoms have been reported to improve soon after DBS (100–102), it has been noted that depression and suicide attempts can occur in the context of DBS (103–105). Although depression may be attributable to stimulation of the substantia nigra instead of the subthalamic nucleus (106), it may be that a subgroup of persons with a history of significant depression pre-operatively may be at increased risk for depression after surgery or that alterations in medication in association with DBS are related to depression. Further research is needed to disentangle the mechanisms underlying depression observed in conjunction with DBS.

E. Treatment of Depression in Parkinson's Disease

1. Pharmacotherapy

Very few well-designed, randomized, blinded, placebo-controlled studies of antidepressant efficacy in PD have been undertaken. Klaassen et al.'s review (107) showed that in 12 trials, positive outcomes were observed for selegiline (10 mg/day), desipramine

(100 mg/day), imipramine (30–75 mg/day in patients older than 55 years, 50–100 mg in patients younger than 55 years), nortriptyline (100 mg/day), and bupropion (maximum 450 mg). An evidence-based review of treatment of PD (108) shows that little progress has been made in evaluating antidepressants in PD since the review by Klaassen et al. (107). This evidence-based review classified studies into three classes: Class I studies that are randomized, controlled trials; Class II studies that involve controlled clinical or observational trials; and Class III studies that are non-controlled and case studies. The studies were scored for methodological adequacy and based on the strength and quality of evidence. Conclusions were offered about efficacy and safety of various treatments (Table 5). This table makes it evident that when only methodologically rigorous studies are considered, there is insufficient empirical evidence to support the efficacy and/or safety of virtually any class of antidepressant treatment specifically in PD.

Given the limited empirical guidance available in the selection of antidepressants in PD, selection of an agent will often rest on the side effect profile (72), though consideration need also be given to age-related factors, medical comorbidity, pharmacokinetics and pharmacodynamics of the agent, previous response (if applicable), drug interactions, cost, and compliance issues (41).

Though many pharmacological agents might potentially be considered for treating depression in PD (109), a survey of Parkinson Study Group investigators revealed that selective serotonin reuptake inhibitors (SSRIs) and tricyclics are, respectively, the first and second most frequent first-line therapies for depression selected by these clinicians (110). The most typical side effects of tricyclics in PD include anticholinergic effects (e.g., confusion, urinary retention) and antiadrenergic effects such as hypotension (111). However, the sedating properties of tricyclics may make them a reasonable choice in the parkinsonian with agitated depression, and tricyclics' anticholinergic properties may alleviate tremor.

Concerns have been expressed about the possibility that SSRIs such as fluvoxamine (112), fluoxetine (113), sertraline (114), and paroxetine (115) may exacerbate parkinsonian symptoms and that citalopram (116) or fluvoxamine (117) may be associated with new onset parkinsonism. Other studies, in contrast, have found SSRIs to be well tolerated without exacerbation of motor symptoms (118,119), and indeed, some studies have found an improvement in bradykinesia (120).

Several other agents have received scant attention in the empirical literature about depression treatment in PD. Selegiline was thought to have antidepressant properties (107). However, Klaassen's review (107) found positive support for its antidepressant effect in only one of five studies. The use of selegiline with antidepressants is rarely associated with serotonergic syndrome, which occured in fewer than 0.3% of more than 4000 patients treated with selegiline and an antidepressant (121). It has been proposed that venlafaxine, inhibiting reuptake of both serotonin and norepinephrine, may be helpful in the PD patient with hypotension, but that it needs to be used cautiously in the agitated depressed patient given the drug's activating properties (41). Mirtazapine is a presynaptic adrenergic (α_2) antagonist as well as an antagonist of serotonergic ($5HT_{1,2, and 3}$) receptors that also increases norepinephrin release. While it may reduce insomnia, nausea, and anxiety in comparison to other antidepressants (41), a recent case study invites caution given a possible association with rapid eye movement (REM) sleep behavior disorder in parkinsonism (122). While its mechanism of action remains poorly understood, preliminary support exists for bupropion's effectiveness in treating PD depression (123,124). Nefazodone and trazodone may also be effective (41), although empirical support remains to be

Table 5 Summary of Evidence-Based Recommendations Concerning Antidepressants in Parkinson's Disease

Class of antidepressants	Agent	Number of studies per class[a]			Adjudicated efficacy	Adjudicated safety
		I	II	III		
Tricyclics Imipramine Class	Nortriptyline	1	0	0	Likely efficacious Insufficient evidence	Insufficient evidence
MAO Inhibitors	Moclobemide	0	0	0	Insufficient evidence	Insufficient evidence
	Selegiline	0	1	0		
	Moclobemide and selegiline	1	0	0		Combined treatment with MAO inhibitor and either tricyclic or SSRI involves unacceptable risk
Serotonin reuptake Inhibitors	Paroxetine	0	0	2	Insufficient evidence	Insufficient evidence
Electroconvulsive therapy		0	0	1	Insufficient evidence	Insufficient evidence

[a]Class I: controlled, randomized study; Class II: controlled study; Class III: uncontrolled study or case report.
Source: Adapted from Ref. 108.

gathered. Reboxetine, a norepinephrine reuptake inhibitor (not approved for use in the United States), may be effective in treating depression in PD, though at least transient side effects seem common (125).

2. Electroconvulsive Therapy

While Tom and Cummings (109) indicated that electroconvulsive therapy (ECT) is appropriate for use in suicidal patients with PD, Rabinstein and Shulman (72) propose that this is rarely appropriate in PD because suicidal ideation and intractable depression are rare in PD. When used, ECT may improve motor symptoms of PD (126,127). The antidepressant effect and safety of ECT in PD, although receiving preliminary support (126,128), remains to be investigated in a randomized, controlled, clinical trial.

3. Psychotherapy

No controlled trials of psychotherapy have been undertaken to evaluate its efficacy in treating depression in PD. One study suggests that brief psychotherapy (consisting of five 2-hour sessions of cognitive restructuring, relaxation, coping skills training, and role playing) will benefit PD patients (129).

4. Repetitive Transcranial Magnetic Stimulation

Repetitive transcranial magnetic stimulation (rTMS) may provide relief from depression under experimental conditions, and in PD it produces transient alterations in motor function and mood (130). Only one uncontrolled study of rTMS has been undertaken in a small number of depressed PD patients (131). Among 10 patients with major depression or dysthymia, bilateral prefrontal slow rTMS was found to decrease (improve) Hamilton Depression Rating Scale and Beck Depression Inventory scores immediately after the 10-day treatment and up to 2 and 3 weeks after treatment. It is unclear whether caseness changed (i.e, whether patients no longer met diagnostic criteria for depression or dysthymia).

III. ANXIETY DISORDERS

Although anxiety disorders have received less attention than depressive disorders and are thus less recognized in patients with PD, anxiety disorders also contribute substantially to morbidity and caregiver burden (132) and have been associated with cognitive dysfunction (133,134). Anxiety disorders including generalized anxiety, panic, social phobia, and obsessive-compulsive disorder occur in up to 40% of patients with PD (135,136). Recognition of a specific anxiety disorder in patients with PD and a depressive disorder is difficult (36) because anxiety and depressive disorders have symptoms in common (35). Yet, as many as 75% of patients with PD and depression have a concomitant anxiety disorder (137).

A. Phenomenology of Anxiety Disorders in Parkinson's Disease

Anxiety disorders in patients with PD are phenomenologically indistinct from anxiety disorders in other populations (138,139). Although the DSM (43) excludes diagnosis of an anxiety disorder if it is due to the physiological effects of a medical condition, treatment is warranted if the anxiety results in significant patient distress or impairment (140).

1. Generalized Anxiety Disorder

Generalized anxiety may be present in nearly one fifth of patient's with PD and is not related to motor disability or treatment with levodopa (138). It is characterized by excessive anxiety and worry about multiple issues or events and is difficult for the patient to control. To meet DSM-IV-TR diagnostic criteria, patients must experience this worry and three additional symptoms of anxiety (i.e., restlessness, easily fatigued, concentration difficulty, irritability, muscle tension, disturbed sleep) for at least 6 months with significant distress or functional impairment. The focus of the worry cannot be limited to features of other psychiatric disorders.

2. Panic

In persons with PD treated with levodopa, up to 24% have been found to have recurrent panic attacks (139). Idiopathic panic attacks are circumscribed events reaching their greatest severity within 10 minutes of the onset with at least four of the following symptoms: heart palpitations, sweating, trembling, perceived shortness of breath, choking feeling, chest pain or discomfort, nausea or abdominal distress, dizziness or lightheadedness including feeling unsteady or faint, derealization or depersonalization, fear of losing control or going crazy, fear of dying, paresthesias, and chills or hot flashes (43). However, panic states in PD may be protracted, lasting for several hours, and 90% predictably occur during the off state (139). Agoraphobia, anxiety regarding and/or avoidance of places or situations in which retreat or assistance may not be easily attained, may also be present. A diagnosis of panic disorder includes recurrent panic attacks and at least one month of concern about having another attack or a change in behavior related to the attacks. Although symptoms of panic frequently occur in PD as isolated symptoms, the diagnosis in patients with PD should not be overlooked because patients may self-medicate with levodopa or a sedative in order to seek relief (141).

3. Phobias

Phobic disorders are characterized by a marked and recognizably unreasonable or irrational specific fear with an immediate anxiety response upon exposure to the feared stimulus or avoidance that results in significant distress or functional impairment for the patient (43). Although patients with PD may justifiably manifest some specific concerns or fears (e.g., fear of falling, fear of being judged in social situations), patients with a specific phobia recognize its excessive and extreme nature. Social phobia, the marked and excessive fear of a social situation in which unfamiliar people are present, or when scrutiny by others, humiliation, and embarrassment are feared, is the most common phobia in persons with PD (138), although other phobias may also develop. Stein and colleagues (138) found that nearly 20% of their subjects met diagnostic criteria for social phobia and an additional 20% experienced significant disabling social anxiety specifically related to their symptoms of PD. Although fears focused primarily on symptoms associated with a medical condition is an exclusionary condition for diagnosis of a phobia, treatment of the anxiety is warranted whenever it contributes to patient distress or impairment (140).

4. Obsessive-Compulsive Disorder

Obsessive-compulsive (OC) disorder has been linked to dysfunction of the basal ganglia, and thus, OC symptoms are found in patients with medical disorders affecting that brain region (e.g., Tourette's syndrome, blepharospasm) (142). OC disorder is characterized by recurrent obsessions (i.e., persistent ideas, thoughts, or images that the patient perceives as intrusive or unusual) or compulsions (i.e., repetitive behaviors in which the patient engages to reduce or prevent anxiety) that are time consuming for the patient and result in distress or interfere with daily functioning (43). The content of common obsessions includes thoughts about becoming contaminated, doubts regarding activities (e.g., leaving a door unlocked), aggressive impulses, and sexual images. Common compulsions include hand washing, ordering of objects, praying, counting, and checking. Although patients with PD may meet diagnostic criteria for OC disorder, it is more likely that they will experience OC symptoms (138,143). OC symptoms tend to appear late in the course of PD (143), and left-sided motor dysfunction was found to be a reliable predictor of the overall severity of OC symptoms (144).

B. Etiology of Anxiety in Parkinson's Disease

Although the psychological impact of PD and its effects on multiple domains of quality of life cannot be ignored, this is an incomplete explanation of the genesis of anxiety in patients with PD. If anxiety in patients with PD were simply or primarily a psychological response to disability, then patients whose dominant hand was affected would be expected to have more anxiety (145). Two studies, however, have shown that anxiety was associated with mainly left-sided symptoms (146,147). A common pathophysiological process, pharmacological effects, and surgical effects are etiological factors.

Anxiety may be related to the neurochemical changes of PD. Abnormalities of norepinephrine, serotonin, dopamine, and γ-aminobutyric acid (GABA), implicated in the pathogenesis of anxiety (148–151), have been demonstrated in patients with PD (152). The exact mechanism, however, remains unproven. Dopaminergic deficits may contribute to anxiety through the disinhibition of the locus ceruleus (138,153) or interaction with norepinephrine and serotonin deficiencies (154,155). Because of the pathophysiological changes in PD, patients may also be more sensitive to the effects of a functional polymorphism in the human serotonin transporter gene that influences synaptic serotonin physiology (96).

Symptoms of anxiety and panic have also been attributed to levodopa therapy (139), especially when occurring in patients not predisposed before the onset of PD (156). Evidence to support this etiology includes the high prevalence of anxiety in patients with levodopa-induced motor fluctuations, especially in the off state (82,147,157). Also, patients with prior symptomatology have reported worsening of their anxiety syndromes upon initiation of levodopa (158). This remains somewhat controversial, however, because some studies have found that levodopa dose did not differ between anxious and nonanxious patients (138) and did not significantly correlate with anxiety levels (36). Pergolide and selegiline (in combination with levodopa) have also been associated with a significant incidence of anxiety (159,160) though one study found no relationship between either drug and anxiety level (36). Bilateral subthalamic stimulation may increase or decrease preexisting anxiety symptoms (105,161). Pallidotomy (132,162,163) and globus pallidus or thalamus stimulation (164) may result in decreased levels of anxiety, unrelated to change in motor symptoms.

C. Evaluation of Anxiety Disorders in Parkinson's Disease

1. Cautions in Evaluating Anxiety Disorders

Brief self-report measures of anxiety are commonly used to screen for symptoms of anxiety, although a thorough psychiatric interview is usually necessary for diagnostic specificity. Sensory and somatic symptoms commonly experienced by patients with PD may overlap with the symptoms of anxiety. These need to be evaluated carefully because misdiagnosis may lead to subsequent mismanagement (165). Autonomic dysfunction and related symptoms (e.g., flushing, dizziness, changes in heart rate) may occur independent of an anxiety disorder. Akathisia, inner restlessness relieved by movement, may be misinterpreted as a sign of anxiety when the patient notes an inability to sit still. Another phenomenon occurring in PD and associated with anxiety is internal tremor.

2. Instruments

Multiple brief and long symptom inventories for assessing anxiety symptoms and specific anxiety disorders exist [e.g., Handbook of Psychiatric Measures (166)]. Though several measures are considered the gold standard for brief assessment and monitoring of change across time, validity for their use in PD has rarely been established. The majority of these instruments need to be interpreted with caution given the overlap of symptoms of anxiety and PD, and the consequent possible overestimation of anxiety in PD (167). The Beck Anxiety Inventory (BAI) (168) is a 21-item self-report questionnaire that takes approximately 5 minutes to complete. It has high internal consistency and test-retest correlation and discriminates anxious diagnostic groups (panic disorder, generalized anxiety disorder, etc.) from nonanxious psychiatric groups and nonpatient groups (169). Despite overlap between anxiety and depression symptoms, this inventory discriminated between anxiety and depression more accurately than other self-report measures of anxiety including the State-Trait Anxiety Inventory (STAI) (168,170) in non-PD patients. Higginson and colleagues (167), however, found that in PD the BAI and Profile of Mood States (POMS) yielded scores associated with clinically significant anxiety more frequently than did clinical interview. Elimination of items loading on the neurophysiological and autonomic factors is not advised, however, given that this method probably leads to egregious underestimation of anxiety in PD (167).

The Yale-Brown Obsessive Compulsive Scale (171) measures the severity of obsessive-compulsive symptoms through a clinically administered semi-structured interview (20–30 min administration time) or self-report questionnaire (10–15 min completion time) (172). Neither method, however, specifically assesses the presence of the DSM-IV-TR diagnostic criteria. The two methods are adequately correlated (172), and each has moderate internal consistency and high test-retest correlation (171,172). A separate associated self-report questionnaire assesses the content of the obsessions and compulsions (171).

The Social Phobia and Anxiety Inventory (SPAI) (173) is a 45-item self-report questionnaire requiring 20–30 minutes that assists in the diagnosis of social phobia (174). With excellent internal consistency and good test-retest reliability (173), the SPAI facilitates discrimination among persons with social phobia, agoraphobia, other anxiety disorders, and nonpatients.

D. Treatment of Anxiety Disorders in Parkinson's Disease

There is no clinical trial evidence regarding the treatment of anxiety in patients with PD (135). Optimal treatments have not been established, but some guidelines have been proposed (175).

1. Pharmacological Interventions

If anxiety appears related to dopamimetic medication, dose modification or addition or substitution of a different medication may be considered with a goal of reducing off time. Long-term use of benzodiazepines can lead to the development of tolerance and need for increasing doses to evoke the same response. Elderly patients are more sensitive to benzodiazepines and thus, at greater risk of oversedation, falls, and concomitant medical conditions. Also, benzodiazepines may increase parkinsonian symptoms (176).

Low-dose tricyclic antidepressants may be helpful in those patients not responding well to benzodiazepines (138). Buspirone may be chosen when reduction of the severity of levodopa-induced dyskinesias is also valued (177). Ludwig and colleagues (178) found that higher doses of buspirone (100 mg/day) increased parkinsonian symptoms, but when administered in conventional anxiolytic doses (10–40 mg/day) it was well tolerated. SSRIs may be beneficial in patients experiencing both depression and anxiety. Some suggest that individual susceptibility or sensitivity to SSRIs may exist (179).

2. Psychotherapy

Psychological interventions are often beneficial by helping patients learn strategies for managing their anxiety symptoms and coping skills for managing stressful situations. Interventions include both cognitive and behavioral approaches in combination with examination of the psychosocial effects of the disease. Treatment by psychologists or other mental health practitioners knowledgeable about the potential multifocal etiology of anxiety disorders in patients with PD and the psychosocial effects of chronic illness is crucial to ensure appropriate intervention. Controlled trials of such interventions remain to be conducted.

REFERENCES

1. Shulman LM, Taback RL, Rabinstein AA, Weiner WJ. Non-recognition of depression and other non-motor symptoms in Parkinson's disease. Park Rel Disord 2002; 8:193–197.
2. Meara J, Mitchelmore E, Hobson P. Use of the GDS-15 geriatric depression scale as a screening instrument for depressive symptomatology in patients with Parkinson's disease and their carers in the community. Age Ageing 1999; 28:35–38.
3. Chrischilles EA, Rubenstein LM, Voelker MD, Wallace RB, Rodnitzky RL. Linking clinical variables to health-related quality of life in Parkinson's disease. Park Rel Disord 2002; 8: 199–209.
4. Cubo E, Rojo A, Ramos S, Quintana S, Gonzalez M, Kompoliti K, Aguilar M. The importance of educational and psychological factors in Parkinson's disease quality of life. Eur J Neurol 2002; 9:589–593.
5. The Global Parkinson's Disease Survey Steering Committee. Factors impacting on quality of life in Parkinson's disease: results from an international survey. Mov Disord 2002; 17:60–67.
6. Kuopio AM, Marttila RJ, Helenius H, Toivonen M, Rinne UK. The quality of life in Parkinson's disease. Mov Disord 2002; 15:216–223.
7. Fernandez HH, Tabamo RE, David RR, Friedman JH. Predictors of depressive symptoms among spouse caregivers in Parkinson's disease. Mov Disord 2001; 16:1123–1125.
8. Aarsland D, Larsen JP, Karlsen K, Lim NG, Tandberg E. Mental symptoms in Parkinson's disease are important contributors to caregiver distress. Int J Geriatr Psychiatry 1999; 14:866–874.
9. Boller F, Marcie P, Starkstein S, Traykov L. Memory and depression in Parkinson's disease. Eur J Neurol 1998; 5:291–295.
10. Fields JA, Norman S, Straits-Tröster KA, Tröster AI. The impact of depression on memory in neurodegenerative disease. In: Tröster AI, ed. Memory in Neurodegenerative Disease: Biological, Cognitive, and Clinical Perspectives. New York: Cambridge University Press, 1998:314–337.
11. Kuzis G, Sabe L, Tiberti C, Leiguarda R, Starkstein SE. Cognitive functions in major depression and Parkinson disease. Arch Neurol 1997; 54:982–986.
12. Norman S, Tröster AI, Fields JA, Brooks R. Effects of depression and Parkinson's disease on cognitive functioning. J Neuropsychiatry Clin Neurosci 2002; 14:31–36.
13. Tröster AI, Stalp LD, Paolo AM, Fields JA, Koller WC. Neuropsychological impairment in Parkinson's disease with and without depression. Arch Neurol 1995; 52:1164–1169.
14. Tröster AI, Paolo AM, Lyons KE, Glatt SL, Hubble JP, Koller WC. The influence of depression on cognition in Parkinson's disease: a pattern of impairment distinguishable from Alzheimer's disease. Neurology 1995; 45:672–676.

15. Marder K, Tang MX, Cote L, Stern Y, Mayeux R. The frequency and associated risk factors for dementia in patients with Parkinson's disease. Arch Neurol 1995; 52:695–701.
16. Stern Y, Marder K, Tang MX, Mayeux R. Antecedent clinical features associated with dementia in Parkinson's disease. Neurology 1993; 43:1690–1692.
17. Cole SA, Woodard JL, Juncos JL, Kogos JL, Youngstrom EA, Watts RL. Depression and disability in Parkinson's disease. J Neuropsychiatry Clin Neurosci 1996; 8:20–25.
18. Gupta A, Bhatia S. Depression in Parkinson's disease. Clin Geronto 2000; 22:59–70.
19. Menza MA, Mark MH. Parkinson's disease and depression: the relationship to disability and personality. J Neuropsychiatry Clin Neurosci 1994; 6:165–169.
20. Starkstein SE, Mayberg HS, Leiguarda R, Preziosi TJ, Robinson RG. A prospective longitudinal study of depression, cognitive decline, and physical impairments in patients with Parkinson's disease. J Neurol Neurosurg Psychiatry 1992; 55:377–382.
21. Hubble JP, Cao T, Hassanein RE, Neuberger JS, Koller WC. Risk factors for Parkinson's disease. Neurology 1993; 43:1693–1697.
22. Schuurman AG, van den Akker M, Ensinck KT, Metsemakers JF, Knottnerus JA, Leentjens AF, Buntinx F. Increased risk of Parkinson's disease after depression: a retrospective cohort study. Neurology 2002; 58:1501–1504.
23. Shiba M, Bower JH, Maraganore DM, McDonnell SK, Peterson BJ, Ahlskog JE, Schaid DJ, Rocca WA. Anxiety disorders and depressive disorders preceding Parkinson's disease: a case-control study. Mov Disord 2000; 15:669–677.
24. Taylor AE, Saint-Cyr JA, Lang AE, Kenny FT. Parkinson's disease and depression A critical re-evaluation. Brain 1986; 109:279–292.
25. Davous P, Auquier P, Grignon S, Neukirch HC. A prospective study of depression in French patients with Parkinson's disease: The Depar Study. Eur J Neurol 1995; 2:455–461.
26. Hantz P, Caradoc-Davies G, Caradoc-Davies T, Weatherall M, Dixon G. Depression in Parkinson's disease. Am J Psychiatry 1994; 151:1010–1014.
27. Tandberg E, Larsen JP, Aarsland D, Cummings JL. The occurrence of depression in Parkinson's disease. A community-based study. Arch Neurol 1996; 53:175–179.
28. Nilsson FM, Kessing LV, Sorensen TM, Andersen PK, Bolwig TG. Major depressive disorder in Parkinson's disease: a register-based study. Acta Psychiatr Scand 2002; 106:202–211.
29. Edwards E, Kitt C, Oliver E, Finkelstein J, Wagster M, McDonald WM. Depression and Parkinson's disease: a new look at an old problem. Depress Anxiety 2002; 16.39–48.
30. Slaughter JR, Slaughter KA, Nichols D, Holmes SE, Martens MP. Prevalence, clinical manifestations, etiology, and treatment of depression in Parkinson's disease. J Neuropsychiatry Clin Neurosci 2001; 13:187–196.
31. Cummings JL. The dementias of Parkinson's disease: prevalence, characteristics, neurobiology, and comparison with dementia of the Alzheimer type. Eur Neurol 1988; 28(suppl 1):15–23.
32. Brown RG, MacCarthy B. Psychiatric morbidity in patients with Parkinson's disease. Psychol Med 1990; 20:77–87.
33. Brown RG, MacCarthy B, Gotham AM, Der GJ, Marsden CD. Depression and disability in Parkinson's disease: a follow-up of 132 cases. Psychol Med 1988; 18:49–55.
34. Gotham AM, Brown RG, Marsden CD. Depression in Parkinson's disease: a quantitative and qualitative analysis. J Neurol Neurosurg Psychiatry 1986; 49:381–389.
35. Henderson R, Kurlan R, Kersun JM, Como P. Preliminary examination of the comorbidity of anxiety and depression in Parkinson's disease. J Neuropsychiatry Clin Neurosci 1992; 4:257–264.
36. Menza MA, Robertson-Hoffman DE, Bonapace AS. Parkinson's disease and anxiety: comorbidity with depression. Biol Psychiatry 1993; 34:465–470.
37. Miyoshi K, Ueki A, Nagano O. Management of psychiatric symptoms of Parkinson's disease. Eur Neurol 1996; 36(suppl 1):49–48.
38. Myslobodsky M, Lalonde FM, Hicks L. Are patients with Parkinson's disease suicidal? J Geriatr Psychiatry Neurol 2001; 14:120–124.
39. Stenager EN, Wermuth L, Stenager E, Boldsen J. Suicide in patients with Parkinson's disease. An epidemiological study. Acta Psychiatr Scand 1994; 90:70–72.
40. Cummings JL. Depression and Parkinson's disease: a review. Am J Psychiatry 1992; 149:443–454.
41. Okun MS, Watts RL. Depression associated with Parkinson's disease: clinical features and treatment. Neurology 2002; 58(suppl 1):S63–S70.
42. Shulman LM, Taback RL, Bean J, Weiner WJ. Comorbidity of the nonmotor symptoms of Parkinson's disease. Mov Disord 2001; 16:507–510.
43. American Psychiatric Association. Diagnostic and Statistical Manual of Mental Disorders—Text Revision. Washington, DC: American Psychiatric Association, 2000.

44. Kremer J, Starkstein SE. Affective disorders in Parkinson's disease. Int Rev Psychiatry 2000; 12:290–297.
45. Leentjens AF, Lousberg R, Verhey FR. Markers for depression in Parkinson's disease. Acta Psychiatr Scand 2002; 106:196–201.
46. Mayberg HS, Brannan SK, Mahurin RK, Jerabek PA, Brickman JS, Tekell JL, Silva JA, McGinnis S, Glass TG, Martin CC, Fox PT. Cingulate function in depression: a potential predictor of treatment response. Neuroreport 1997; 8:1057–1061.
47. Mentis MJ, McIntosh AR, Perrine K, Dhawan V, Berlin B, Feigin A, Edwards C, Mattis P, Eidelberg D. Relationships among the metabolic patterns that correlate with mnemonic, visuospatial, and mood symptoms in Parkinson's disease. Am J Psychiatry 2002; 159:746–754.
48. Ring HA, Bench CJ, Trimble MR, Brooks DJ, Frackowiak RS, Dolan RJ. Depression in Parkinson's disease. A positron emission study. Br J Psychiatry 1994; 165:333–339.
49. Kostic VS, Covickovic-Sternic N, Beslac-Bumbasirevic L, Ocic G, Pavlovic D, Nikolic M. Dexamethasone suppression test in patients with Parkinson's disease. Mov Disord 1990; 5:23–26.
50. Frochtengarten ML, Villares JC, Maluf E, Carlini EA. Depressive symptoms and the dexamethasone suppression test in parkinsonian patients. Biol Psychiatry 1987; 22:386–389.
51. Cummings JL, Masterman DL. Depression in patients with Parkinson's disease. Int J Geriatr Psychiatry 1999; 14:711–718.
52. Burn DJ. Depression in Parkinson's disease. Eur J Neurol 2002; 9(suppl 3):44–54.
53. Poewe W, Luginger E. Depression in Parkinson's disease: impediments to recognition and treatment options. Neurology 1999; 52:S2–S6.
54. Berrios GE, Campbell C, Politynska BE. Autonomic failure, depression and anxiety in Parkinson's disease. Br J Psychiatry 1995; 166:789–792.
55. Levin BE, Llabre MM, Weiner WJ. Parkinson's disease and depression: psychometric properties of the Beck Depression Inventory. J Neurol Neurosurg Psychiatry 1988; 51:1401–1404.
56. Starkstein SE, Preziosi TJ, Forrester AW, Robinson RG. Specificity of affective and autonomic symptoms of depression in Parkinson's disease. J Neurol Neurosurg Psychiatry 1990; 53:869–873.
57. Hoogendijk WJ, Sommer IE, Tissingh G, Deeg DJ, Wolters EC. Depression in Parkinson's disease. The impact of symptom overlap on prevalence. Psychosomatics 1998; 39:416–421.
58. Leentjens AFG, Verhey FRJ, G-J Luijckx, Troost J. The validity of the Beck Depression Inventory as a screening and diagnostic instrument for depression in patients with Parkinson's disease. Mov Disord 2000; 15:1221–1224.
59. Marin RS. Apathy: a neuropsychiatric syndrome. J Neuropsychiatry Clin Neurosci 1991; 3:243–254.
60. Shulman LM. Apathy in patients with Parkinson's disease. Int Rev Psychiatry 2000; 12:298–306.
61. Starkstein SE, Mayberg HS, Preziosi TJ, Andrezejewski P, Leiguarda R, Robinson RG. Reliability, validity, and clinical correlates of apathy in Parkinson's disease. J Neuropsychiatry Clin Neurosci 1992; 4:134–139.
62. Marin RS. Differential diagnosis and classification of apathy. Am J Psychiatry 1990; 147:22–30.
63. Levy ML, Cummings JL, Fairbanks LA, Masterman D, Miller BL, Craig AH, Paulsen JS, Litvan I. Apathy is not depression. J Neuropsychiatry Clin Neurosci 1998; 10:314–319.
64. Isella V, Melzi P, Grimaldi M, Iurlaro S, Piolti R, Ferrarese C, Frattola L, Appollonio I. Clinical, neuropsychological, and morphometric correlates of apathy in Parkinson's disease. Mov Disord 2002; 17:366–371.
65. Pluck GC, Brown RG. Apathy in Parkinson's disease. J Neurol Neurosurg Psychiatry 2002; 73:636–642.
66. Cummings JL, Mega M, Gray K, Rosenberg-Thompson S, Carusi DA, Gombein J. The Neuropsychiatric Inventory: comprehensive assessment of psychopathology in dementia. Neurology 1994; 44:2308–2314.
67. Grace J, Malloy PF. Frontal Systems Behavior Scale Professional Manual. Lutz, FL: Psychological Assessment Resources, Inc., 2001.
68. Marsh L. Neuropsychiatric aspects of Parkinson's disease. Psychosomatics 2000; 41:15–23.
69. Madeley P, Biggins CA, Boyd JL, Mindham RHS, Spokes EGS. Emotionalism in Parkinson's disease. Irish J Psychol Med 1992; 9:24–25.
70. Brown R, Jahanshahi M. Depression in Parkinson's disease: a psychosocial viewpoint. Adv Neurol 1995; 65:61–84.
71. Cantello R, Aguggia M, Gilli M, Delsedime M, Chiardo Cutin I, Riccio A, Mutani R. Major depression in Parkinson's disease and the mood response to intravenous methylphenidate: possible role of the "hedonic" dopamine synapse. J Neurol Neurosurg Psychiatry 1989; 52:724–731.
72. Rabinstein AA, Shulman LM. Management of behavioral and psychiatric problems in Parkinson's disease. Park Rel Disord 2000; 7:41–50.

73. Torack RM, Morris JC. The association of ventral tegmental area histopathology with adult dementia. Arch Neurol 1988; 45:497–501.
74. Mayberg HS, Starkstein SE, Sadzot B, Preziosi T, Andrezejewski PL, Dannals RF, Wagner HN, Jr., Robinson RG. Selective hypometabolism in the inferior frontal lobe in depressed patients with Parkinson's disease. Ann Neurol 1990; 28:57–64.
75. Zesiewicz TA, Gold M, Chari G, Hauser RA. Current issues in depression in Parkinson's disease. Am J Geriatr Psychiatry 1999; 7:110–118.
76. Nutt JG. Motor fluctuations and dyskinesia in Parkinson's disease. Park Rel Disord 2001; 8: 101–108.
77. Raudino F. Non motor off in Parkinson's disease. Acta Neurol Scand 2001; 104:312–315.
78. Witjas T, Kaphan E, Azulay JP, Blin O, Ceccaldi M, Pouget J, Poncet M, Chérif AA. Nonmotor fluctuations in Parkinson's disease: frequent and disabling. Neurology 2002; 59:408–413.
79. Maricle RA, Nutt JG, Carter JH. Mood and anxiety fluctuation in Parkinson's disease associated with levodopa infusion: preliminary findings. Mov Disord 1995; 10:329–332.
80. Maricle RA, Nutt JG, Valentine RJ, Carter JH. Dose-response relationship of levodopa with mood and anxiety in fluctuating Parkinson's disease: a double-blind, placebo-controlled study. Neurology 1995; 45:1757–1760.
81. Maricle RA, Valentine RJ, Carter J, Nutt JG. Mood response to levodopa infusion in early Parkinson's disease. Neurology 1998; 50:1890–1892.
82. Racette BA, Hartlein JM, Hershey T, Mink JW, Perlmutter JS, Black KJ. Clinical features and comorbidity of mood fluctuations in Parkinson's disease. J Neuropsychiatry Clin Neurosci 2002; 14:438–442.
83. Richard IH, Justus AW, Kurlan R. Relationship between mood and motor fluctuations in Parkinson's disease. J Neuropsychiatry Clin Neurosci 2001; 13:35–41.
84. Tröster AI, Fields JA, Koller WC. Parkinson's disease and parkinsonism. In: Coffey CE, Cummings JL, eds. Textbook of Geriatric Neuropsychiatry. 2nd ed. Washington, DC: American Psychiatric Press, 2000:559–600.
85. V Chan-Palay, Asan E. Alterations in catecholamine neurons of the locus coeruleus in senile dementia of the Alzheimer type and in Parkinson's disease with and without dementia and depression. J Comp Neurol 1989; 287:373–392.
86. Paulus W, Jellinger K. The neuropathologic basis of different clinical subgroups of Parkinson's disease. J Neuropathol Exp Neurol 1991; 50:743–755.
87. Chia LG, Cheng LJ, Chuo LJ, Cheng FC, Cu JS. Studies of dementia, depression, electrophysiology and cerebrospinal fluid monoamine metabolites in patients with Parkinson's disease. J Neurol Sci 1995; 133:73–78.
88. Mayeux R, Stern Y, Cote L, Williams JB. Altered serotonin metabolism in depressed patients with parkinson's disease. Neurology 1984; 34:642–646.
89. Mayeux R, Stern Y, Sano M, Williams JB, Cote LJ. The relationship of serotonin to depression in Parkinson's disease. Mov Disord 1988; 3:237–244.
90. Kuhn W, Muller T, Gerlach M, Sofic E, Fuchs G, Heye N, Prautsch R, Przuntek H. Depression in Parkinson's disease: biogenic amines in CSF of "de novo" patients. J Neural Transm 1996; 103:1441–1445.
91. Brooks DJ, Doder M. Depression in Parkinson's disease. Curr Opin Neurol 2001; 14:465–470.
92. Doder M, Rabiner EA, Turjanski N, Lees AJ, Brooks DJ. Brain serotonin 1A receptors in Parkinson's disease with and without depression measured by positron emission tomography with 11C-WAY 100635. Mov Disord 2000; 15:213.
93. Murai T, Muller U, Werheid K, Sorger D, Reuter M, Becker T, von Cramon DY, Barthel H. In vivo evidence for differential association of striatal dopamine and midbrain serotonin systems with neuropsychiatric symptoms in Parkinson's disease. J Neuropsychiatry Clin Neurosci 2001; 13:222–228.
94. Berg D, Supprian T, Hofmann E, Zeiler B, Jager A, Lange KW, Reiners K, Becker T, Becker G. Depression in Parkinson's disease: brainstem midline alteration on transcranial sonography and magnetic resonance imaging. J Neurol 1999; 246:1186–1193.
95. Ricketts MH, Hamer RM, Sage JI, Manowitz P, Feng F, Menza MA. Association of a serotonin transporter gene promoter polymorphism with harm avoidance behaviour in an elderly population. Psychiatr Genet 1998; 8:41–44.
96. Menza MA, Palermo B, DiPaola R, Sage JI, Ricketts MH. Depression and anxiety in Parkinson's disease: possible effect of genetic variation in the serotonin transporter. J Geriatr Psychiatry Neurol 1999; 12:49–52.

97. Mössner R, Henneberg A, Schmitt A, Syagailo YV, Grassle M, Hennig T, Simantov R, Gerlach M, Riederer P, Lesch KP. Allelic variation of serotonin transporter expression is associated with depression in Parkinson's disease. Mol Psychiatry 2001; 6:350–352.

98. Andersen J, Aabro E, Gulmann N, Hjelmsted A, Pedersen HE. Anti-depressive treatment in Parkinson's disease. A controlled trial of the effect of nortriptyline in patients with Parkinson's disease treated with L-DOPA. Acta Neurol Scand 1980; 62:210–219.

99. Huber SJ, Paulson GW, Shuttleworth EC. Relationship of motor symptoms, intellectual impairment, and depression in Parkinson's disease. J Neurol Neurosurg Psychiatry 1988; 51:855–858.

100. Daniele A, Albanese A, Contarino MF, Zinzi P, Barbier A, Gasparini F, Romito LM, Bentivoglio AR, Scerrati M. Cognitive and behavioural effects of chronic stimulation of the subthalamic nucleus in patients with Parkinson's disease. J Neurol Neurosurg Psychiatry 2003; 74:175–182.

101. P Martínez-Martín, Valldeoriola F, Tolosa E, Pilleri M, Molinuevo JL, Rumià J, Ferrer E. Bilateral subthalamic nucleus stimulation and quality of life in advanced Parkinson's disease. Mov Disord 2002; 17:372–377.

102. Tröster AI, Fields JA. The role of neuropsychological evaluation in the neurosurgical treatment of movement disorders. In: Tarsy D, Vitek JL, Lozano AM, eds. Surgical Treatment of Parkinson's Disease and Other Movement Disorders. Totowa, NJ: Humana Press, 2003:213–240.

103. Berney A, Vingerhoets F, Perrin A, Guex P, Villemure J-G, Burkhard PR, Benkelfat C, Ghika J. Effect on mood of subthalamic DBS for Parkinson's disease: a consecutive series of 24 patients. Neurology 2002; 59:1427–1429.

104. Doshi PK, Chhaya N, Bhatt MH. Depression leading to attempted suicide after bilateral subthalamic nucleus stimulation for Parkinson's disease. Mov Disord 2002; 17:1084–1085.

105. Houeto JL, Mesnage V, Mallet L, Pillon B, Gargiulo M, Du Moncel ST, Bonnet AM, Pidoux B, Dormont D, Cornu P, Agid Y. Behavioural disorders, Parkinson's disease and subthalamic stimulation. J Neurol Neurosurg Psychiatry 2002; 72:701–707.

106. Bejjani BP, Damier P, Arnulf I, Thivard L, Bonnet AM, Dormont D, Cornu P, Pidoux B, Samson Y, Agid Y. Transient acute depression induced by high-frequency deep-brain stimulation. N Engl J Med 1999; 340:1476–1480.

107. Klaassen T, Verhey FR, Sneijders GH, Rozendaal N, de Vet HC, van Praag HM. Treatment of depression in Parkinson's disease: a meta-analysis. J Neuropsychiatry Clin Neurosci 1995; 7:281–286.

108. Movement Disorder Society Task Force. Management of Parkinson's disease: an evidence-based review. Mov Disord 2002; 17 (suppl 4):S1–S166.

109. Tom T, Cummings JL. Depression in Parkinson's disease. Pharmacological characteristics and treatment. Drugs Aging 1998; 12:55–74.

110. Richard IH, Kurlan R. The Parkinson Study Group. A survey of antidepressant drug use in Parkinson's disease. Neurology 1997; 49:1168–1170.

111. Valldeoriola F, Nobbe FA, Tolosa E. Treatment of behavioural disturbances in Parkinson's disease. J Neural Transm Suppl 1997; 51:175–204.

112. Leo RJ. Movement disorders associated with the serotonin selective reuptake inhibitors. J Clin Psychiatry 1996; 57:449–454.

113. Simons JA. Fluoxetine in Parkinson's disease. Mov Disord 1996; 11:581–582.

114. Richard IH, Maughn A, Kurlan R. Do serotonin reuptake inhibitor antidepressants worsen Parkinson's disease? A retrospective case series. Mov Disord 1999; 14:155–157.

115. Jiménez-Jiménez FJ, Tejeiro J, Martinez-Junquera G, Cabrera-Valdivia F, Alarcon J, Garcia-Albea E. Parkinsonism exacerbated by paroxetine. Neurology 1994; 44:2406.

116. Stadtland C, Erfurth A, Arolt V. De novo onset of Parkinson's disease after antidepressant treatment with citalopram. Pharmacopsychiatry 2000; 33:194–195.

117. Gonul AS, Aksu M. SSRI-induced parkinsonism may be an early sign of future Parkinson's disease. J Clin Psychiatry 1999; 60:410.

118. Dell'Agnello G, Ceravolo R, Nuti A, Bellini G, Piccinni A, D'Avino C, Dell'Osso L, Bonuccelli U. SSRIs do not worsen Parkinson's disease: evidence from an open-label, prospective study. Clin Neuropharmacol 2001; 24:221–227.

119. Wermuth L, Sorenson PS, Timm S, Christensen B, Utzon NP, Boas J, Dupont E, Hansen E, Magnussen I, Mikkelsen B, Worm-Petersen J, Lauritzen L, Bayer L, Bech P. Depression in idiopathic Parkinson's disease treated with citalopram: a placebo-controlled trial. Nord J Psychiatry 1998; 52:163–169.

120. Rampello L, Chiechio S, Raffaele R, Vecchio I, Nicoletti F. The SSRI, citalopram, improves bradykinesia in patients with Parkinson's disease treated with L-dopa. Clin Neuropharmacol 2002; 25:21–24.

121. Richard IH, Kurlan R, Tanner C, Factor S, Hubble J, Suchowersky O, Waters C. The Parkinson Study Group. Serotonin syndrome and the combined use of deprenyl and an antidepressant in Parkinson's disease. Neurology 1997; 48:1070–1077.
122. Onofrj M, Luciano AL, Thomas A, Iacono D, G D'Andreamatteo. Mirtazapine induces REM sleep behavior disorder (RBD) in parkinsonism. Neurology 2003; 60:113–115.
123. Flint AJ. Pharmacologic treatment of depression in late life. CMAJ 1997; 157:1061–1067.
124. Goetz CG, Tanner CM, Klawans HL. Bupropion in Parkinson's disease. Neurology 1984; 34: 1092–1094.
125. Lemke MR. Effect of reboxetine on depression in Parkinson's disease patients. J Clin Psychiatry 2002; 63:300–304.
126. Faber R, Trimble MR. Electroconvulsive therapy in Parkinson's disease and other movement disorders. Mov Disord 1991; 6:293–303.
127. Wengel SP, Burke WJ, Pfeiffer RF, Roccaforte WH, Paige SR. Maintenance electroconvulsive therapy for intractable Parkinson's disease. Am J Geriatr Psychiatry 1998; 6:263–269.
128. Mollentine C, Rummans T, Ahlskog JE, Harmsen WS, Suman VJ, O'Connor MK, Black JL, Pileggi T. Effectiveness of ECT in patients with parkinsonism. J Neuropsychiatry Clin Neurosci 1998; 10:187–193.
129. Ellring H, Seiler S, Perleth B, Frings W, Gasser T, Oertel W. Psychosocial aspects of Parkinson's disease. Neurology 1993; 43(suppl 6):S41–S44.
130. George MS, Wassermann EM, Post RM. Transcranial magnetic stimulation: a neuropsychiatric tool for the 21st century. J Neuropsychiatry Clin Neurosci 1996; 8:373–382.
131. Dragasevic N, Potrebic A, Damjanovic A, Stefanova E, Kostic VS. Therapeutic efficacy of bilateral prefrontal slow repetitive transcranial magnetic stimulation in depressed patients with Parkinson's disease: an open study. Mov Disord 2002; 17:528–532.
132. Marsh L, Solvasson B, Cahn DA, Shear PK, Teitelbaum J, Wasserstein P, Heit G, Silvergerg GD, Sullivan F. Psychiatric outcome after pallidotomy for Parkinson's disease. Biol Psychiatry 1997; 41:1075.
133. Marsh L, Vaughan C, Schretlen D, Brandt J, Mandir AS. Psychomotor aspects of mood disorders in Parkinson's disease. Biol Psychiatry 2000; 47:S165.
134. Ryder KA, Gontkovsky ST, McSwan KL, Scott JG, Bharucha KJ, Beatty WW. Cognitive function in Parkinson's disease: association with anxiety but not depression. Aging Neuropsychol Cogn 2002; 9:77–84.
135. Richard IH, Schiffer RB, Kurlan R. Anxiety and Parkinson's disease. J. Neuropsychiatry Clin Neurosci 1996; 8:383–392.
136. Starkstein SF, Robinson RG, Leiguardia R, Preziosi TJ. Anxiety and depression in Parkinson's disease. Behav Neurol 1993; 6:151–154.
137. Schiffer RB, Kurlan R, Rubin A, Boer S. Evidence for atypical depression in Parkinson's disease. Am J Psychiatry 1988; 145:1020–1022.
138. Stein MB, Heuser IJ, Juncos JL, Uhde TW. Anxiety disorders in patients with Parkinson's disease. Am J Psychiatry 1990; 147:217–220.
139. Vazquez A, Jimenez-Jimenez FJ, Garcia-Ruiz P, Garcia-Urra D. "Panic attacks" in Parkinson's disease. A long-term complication of levodopa therapy. Acta Neurol Scand 1993; 87:14–18.
140. Moutier CY, Stein MB. The history, epidemiology, and differential diagnosis of social anxiety disorder. J Clin Psychiatry 1999; 60(suppl 9):4–8.
141. Nausieda PA. Sinemet "abusers." Clin Neuropharmacol 1985; 8:318–327.
142. Müller N, Putz A, Kathmann N, Lehle R, Günther W, Straube A. Characteristics of obsessive-compulsive symptoms in Tourette's syndrome, obsessive-compulsive disorder, and Parkinson's disease. Psychiatry Res 1997; 70:105–114.
143. Alegret M, Junqué C, Valldeoriola F, Vendrell P, Marti MJ, Tolosa E. Obsessive-compulsive symptoms in Parkinson's disease. J Neurol Neurosurg Psychiatry 2001; 70:394–396.
144. Tomer R, Levin BE, Weiner WJ. Obsessive-compulsive symptoms and motor asymmetries in Parkinson's disease. Neuropsychiatry Neuropsychol Behav Neurol 1993; 6:26–30.
145. Walsh K, Bennett G. Parkinson's disease and anxiety. Postgrad Med J 2001; 77:89–93.
146. Fleminger S. Left-sided Parkinson's disease is associated with greater anxiety and depression. Psychol Med 1991; 21:629–638.
147. Siemers ER, Shekhar A, Quaid K, Dickson H. Anxiety and motor performance in Parkinson's disease. Mov Disord 1993; 8:501–506.
148. Gold PW, Goodwin FK, Chrousos GP. Clinical and biochemical manifestations of depression. Relation to the neurobiology of stress (1). N Engl J Med 1988; 319:348–353.

149. Heninger GR, Charney DS. Monoamine receptor systems and anxiety disorders. Psychiatr Clin North Am 1988; 11:309–326.
150. Nutt D, Lawson C. Panic attacks. A neurochemical overview of models and mechanisms. Br J Psychiatry 1992; 160:165–178.
151. Roy-Byrne PP, Uhde TW, Sack DA, Linnoila M, Post RM. Plasma HVA and anxiety in patients with panic disorder. Biol Psychiatry 1986; 21:849–853.
152. Mayeux R, Stern Y, Williams JB, Cote L, Frantz A, Dyrenfurth I. Clinical and biochemical features of depression in Parkinson's disease. Am J Psychiatry 1986; 143:756–759.
153. Lauterbach EC. The locus ceruleus and anxiety disorders in demented and nondemented familial parkinsonism. Am J Psychiatry 1993; 150:994.
154. Iruela LM, V Ibañez-Rojo, Palanca I, Caballero L. Anxiety disorders and Parkinson's disease. Am J Psychiatry 1992; 149:719–720.
155. Lauterbach EC, Duvoisin RC. Anxiety disorders in familial parkinsonism. Am J Psychiatry 1991; 148:274.
156. Celesia GG, Barr AN. Psychosis and other psychiatric manifestations of levodopa therapy. Arch Neurol 1970; 23:193–200.
157. Nissenbaum H, Quinn NP, Brown RG, Toone B, Gotham AM, Marsden CD. Mood swings associated with the 'on-off' phenomenon in Parkinson's disease. Psychol Med 1987; 17:899–904.
158. Rondot P, de Recondo J, Coignet A, Ziegler M. Mental disorders in Parkinson's disease after treatment with L-DOPA. Adv Neurol 1984; 40:259–269.
159. Lang AE, Quinn N, Brincat S, Marsden CD, Parkes JD. Pergolide in late-stage Parkinson disease. Ann Neurol 1982; 12:243–247.
160. Yahr MD, Mendoza MR, Moros D, Bergmann KJ. Treatment of Parkinson's disease in early and late phases. Use of pharmacological agents with special reference to deprenyl (selegiline). Acta Neurol Scand Suppl 1983; 95:95–102.
161. Dujardin K, Defebvre L, Krystkowiak P, Blond S, Destée A. Influence of chronic bilateral stimulation of the subthalamic nucleus on cognitive function in Parkinson's disease. J Neurol 2001; 248:603–611.
162. Masterman D, DeSalles A, Baloh RW, Frysinger R, Foti D, Behnke E, C Cabatan-Awang, Hoetzel A, Intemann PM, Fairbanks L, Bronstein JM. Motor, cognitive, and behavioral performance following unilateral ventroposterior pallidotomy for Parkinson disease. Arch Neurol 1998; 55:1201–1208.
163. Riordan HJ, Flashman LA, Roberts DW. Neurocognitive and psychosocial correlates of ventroposterolateral pallidotomy surgery in Parkinson's disease [electronic manuscript]. Neurosurg Focus 2:Manuscript 7, 1997.
164. Higginson CI, Fields JA, Tröster AI. Which symptoms of anxiety diminish after surgical interventions for Parkinson's disease. Neuropsychiatry Neuropsychol Behav Neurol 2001; 14:117–121.
165. Marsh L. Anxiety disorders in Parkinson's disease. Int Rev Psychiatry 2000; 12:307–318.
166. AJ Rush Jr., Pincus AH, First MB, Blacker D, Endicott J, Keith SJ, Philips KA, Ryan ND, GR Smith Jr., Tsuang MT, Widiger TA, Zarin DA. Handbook of Psychiatric Measures. Washington, DC: American Psychiatric Association, 2000.
167. Higginson CI, Fields JA, Koller WC, Tröster AI. Questionnaire assessment potentially overestimates anxiety in Parkinson's disease. J Clin Psychol Med Set 2001; 8:95–99.
168. Beck AT, Epstein N, Brown G, Steer RA. An inventory for measuring clinical anxiety: psychometric properties. J Consult Clin Psychol 1988; 56:893–897.
169. Creamer M, Foran J, Bell R. The Beck Anxiety Inventory in a non-clinical sample. Behav Res Ther 1995; 33:477–485.
170. Spielberger CD, Gorsuch RR, Luchene RE. State-Trait Anxiety Inventory. Palo Alto, CA: Consulting Psychologists Press, 1970.
171. Goodman WK, Price LH, Rasmussen SA, Mazure C, Fleischmann RL, Hill CL, Heninger GR, Charney DS. The Yale-Brown Obsessive Compulsive Scale. I. Development, use, and reliability. Arch Gen Psychiatry 1989; 46:1006–1011.
172. Steketee G, Frost R, Bogart K. The Yale-Brown Obsessive Compulsive Scale: interview versus self-report. Behav Res Ther 1996; 34:675–684.
173. Turner SM, Beidel DC, Dancu CV, Stanley MA. An empirically derived inventory to measure social fears and anxiety: the Social Phobia and Anxiety Inventory. Psychol Assessment 1989; 1:35–40.
174. Beidel DC, Turner SM, Cooley MR. Assessing reliable and clinically significant change in social phobia: validity of the social phobia and anxiety inventory. Behav Res Ther 1993; 31:331–337.
175. Lieberman A. Managing the neuropsychiatric symptoms of Parkinson's disease. Neurology 1998; 50(suppl 6):S33–S38.

176. Suranyi-Cadotte BE, Nestoros JN, Nair NP, Lal S, Gauthier S. Parkinsonism induced by high doses of diazepam. Biol Psychiatry 1985; 20:455–457.
177. Bonifati V, Fabrizio E, Vanacore N, Meco G. Buspirone in levodopa-induced dyskinesias. Clin Neuropharmacol 1994; 17:73–82.
178. Ludwig CL, Weinberger DR, Bruno G, Gillespie M, Bakker K, PA LeWitt, Chase TN. Buspirone, Parkinson's disease, and the locus ceruleus. Clin Neuropharmacol 1986; 9:373–378.
179. Montastruc JL, Fabre N, Blin O, Senard JM, Rascol O, Rascol A. Does fluoxetine aggravate Parkinson's disease? A pilot prospective study. Mov Disord 1995; 10:355–357.
180. Olanow CW, Koller WC. An algorithm (decision tree) for the management of Parkinson's disease: treatment guidelines. Neurology 1998; 50:S1–S57.
181. Beck AT, Ward CH, Mendelson M, Mock J, Erbaugh J. An inventory for measuring depression. Arch Gen Psychiatry 1961; 4:53–63.
182. Beck A, Steer RA, Brown GK. Beck Depression Inventory–II. San Antonio: The Psychological Corporation, 1996.
183. Hamilton M. A rating scale for depression. J Neurol Neurosurg Psychiatry 1960; 23:56–62.
184. Leentjens AF, Verhey FR, Lousberg R, Spitsbergen H, Wilmink FW. The validity of the Hamilton and Montgomery-Asberg depression rating scales as screening and diagnostic tools for depression in Parkinson's disease. Int J Geriatr Psychiatry 2000; 15:644–649.
185. Naarding P, Leentjens AF, F Van Kooten, Verhey FR. Disease-specific properties of the Hamilton Rating Scale for depression in patients with stroke, Alzheimer's dementia, and Parkinson's disease. J Neuropsychiatry Clin Neurosci 2002; 14:329–334.
186. Montgomery SA, Asberg M. A new depression scale designed to be sensitive to change. Br J Psychiatry 1979; 134:382–389.
187. Yesavage JA, Brink TL. Development and validation of a geriatric depression screening scale: a preliminary report. J Psychiatr Res 1983; 17:37–49.
188. Sheikh JI, Yesavage JA. Geriatric Depression Scale (GDS): recent evidence and development of a shorter version. Clin Gerontol 1986; 5:165–173.
189. Zigmond AS, Snaith RP. The Hospital Anxiety and Depression Scale. Acta Psychiatr Scand 1983; 67:361 370.
190. Marinus J, Leentjens AF, Visser M, Stiggelbout AM, Van Hilten JJ. Evaluation of the Hospital Anxiety and Depression Scale in patients with Parkinson's disease. Clin Neuropharmacol 2002; 25:318–324.
191. Zung WWK. A self-rating depression scale. Arch Gen Psychiatry 1965; 12:63–70,

33
Diet and Nutrition

Kathrynne E. Holden
Springfield, Missouri, U.S.A.

People with Parkinson's disease (PD) experience a broad spectrum of obstacles to nutritional health, both direct and indirect (1). These may result from PD, from medications used to treat PD, or the increasing infirmities, mental, emotional, and physical, that occur as the disease progresses. However, malnutrition, when properly understood, its risks assessed, and nutrition therapy provided, can often be prevented and is more successfully treated than many conditions that occur with PD. Both the physician and the dietitian play important roles in the nutritional well-being of the patient.

I. ETIOLOGIES OF MALNUTRITION IN PARKINSON'S DISEASE PATIENTS

Malnutrition may arise from a disorder of the autonomic nervous system (2,3), mental or emotional disturbances or medications used to treat PD, and other conditions (4,5,6) (Table 1). However, nutrition-related concerns are complex and often multifactorial, and the physician must be aware of the role of nutrition in the overall health of the individual with PD. Ideally, patients should be referred to a dietitian following diagnosis of PD. The dietitian will provide ongoing medical nutrition therapy as the disease progresses. This will include: (a) establishing a baseline nutritional status; (b) patient/family education regarding the adverse effects of PD on nutritional well-being; (c) individualized diet planning, evolving with disease progression; (d) notifying the physician of potential nutrition-related health concerns. Table 2 summarizes various disorders common in PD that can be related to nutrition.

Table 1 Etiologies of Malnutrition in Parkinson's Disease

Disorders occurring as a result of PD that impact nutritional health
   Slowed peristalsis of the gastrointestinal (GI) tract
   Cognitive impairment
   Depression
   Dysphagia
   Fatigue
   Physical impairment: loss of manual dexterity, tremor, rigidity, bradykinesia
   Impaired gait and balance, with decreased weight-bearing exercise
   Loss of olfaction, sense of taste, appetite
Medication side effects that directly or indirectly affect nutritional health
   Nausea/vomiting
   Constipation, fecal impaction
   Protein-levodopa interaction
   Appetite loss
   Dry mouth
Relation of B vitamins to levodopa and their relevance in PD
   Homocysteinemia/levodopa use
   Decreased stomach acids and intrinsic factor
   Changed eating habits, nutrient depletion
Unintentional weight loss

II. DISORDERS RELATED TO NUTRITION THAT COMMONLY OCCUR IN PD

A. Slowed Peristalsis of the Gastrointestinal Tract

1. Gastroparesis

Slowed peristalsis of the gastrointestinal tract (GI) tract (Table 2) is of concern for several reasons. When it affects the stomach it results in gastroparesis, (7–9) and can delay the passage of food into the small intestine, prevent or slow the absorption of medication, cause early satiety, so that the person is unwilling or unable to finish meals, or increase the likelihood of gastroesophageal reflux disease (GERD).

Table 2 Disorders Related to Nutrition That Commonly Occur in PD

Gastroesophageal reflux disease, Barrett's esophagus
Aspiration pneumonia
Unplanned weight loss
Sarcopenia (muscle wasting)
Bone thinning
Fractures
Fecal impaction, colorectal cancer
Motor fluctuations exacerbated by delayed stomach emptying, protein-levodopa interactions
Oral diseases, tooth loss
Homocysteinemia, B vitamin deficiencies
Other nutrient deficiencies

In the early stages of gastroparesis, a dietary approach is preferable to use of medications. Small meals are ideal, as they are less likely to slow gastric emptying. Also, patients who experience early satiety may be better able to consume a small portion of food than a large meal. Fat and soluble fibers can slow stomach emptying and should be used in moderation. This approach may provide better absorption of medications.

Levodopa should be taken 30 minutes prior to meals so that it can exit the stomach before food arrives. Delayed gastric emptying may affect medication uptake, especially when taken with meals, slowing drug release into the bloodstream. With gastroparesis, use of a liquid levodopa preparation, may be helpful (10).

GERD may over time increase risk for injury to the esophagus and lower esophageal sphincter, and increases the possibility of Barret's esophagus, a precancerous condition (11). GERD is of particular concern for those with PD when dysphagia is present, because impaired swallowing can lead to aspiration of refluxed stomach contents and aspiration pneumonia. Agents that raise stomach pH can interfere with the metabolism of some nutrients, including vitamin B_{12} and iron. When GERD is present, the avoidance of "trigger foods," such as alcohol, citrus, tomatoes, caffeine, and other acid foods, is helpful. Small meals may be helpful, as is consuming the last meal of the day about 4 hours prior to bedtime so that the stomach is empty before lying down.

2. Constipation

Slowed peristalsis of the colon with resultant constipation is common (2). Studies have shown that it may predate the diagnosis of PD by several years (12). Chronic constipation can raise the risk for fecal impaction (13) as well as for colorectal cancer (14–16).

Long-term laxative use, including herbal laxatives such as senna and cascara sagrada, may damage the colon. Sennosides also pose the possibility of cancer risk (17). Vigilance in the management of constipation, therefore, is preferred to laxative use. The physician should educate patients and caregivers concerning the signs of fecal impaction, advise annual screening for colorectal cancer, and encourage as much activity as the patient is able to perform.

The use of insoluble fiber, preferably from foods, has been shown to decrease colon transit time and improve stool bulk. Further, Astarloa, et al., in a small study of PD patients with motor fluctuations, found that a fiber-rich diet improves "on time" (18). Fiber-rich foods providing a minimum of 25 g of dietary fiber daily and at least six 8-ounce glasses of water or other fluids are an important part of constipation management. Use of probiotics such as yoghurt with live cultures and prebiotics, such as fructooligosaccharides (19,20), may be helpful. Use of laxative foods, such as prunes (21), kiwi (22), and sweet potatoes may be helpful, for constipation. The dietitian, using a food diary, should assess fiber and fluid intake and educate patients regarding appropriate food choices.

As PD advances, both physicians and dietitians should be aware that pelvic floor dysfunction can occur (23) and dietary measures may be insufficient to manage constipation. Although these remain protective and should always be continued, it may eventually be necessary for the physician to prescribe appropriate stool softeners and/or laxatives. Both the physician and dietitian should work together to manage constipation via lifestyle changes for as long as possible, keeping in mind that in later stages of PD, medical management may be necessary.

B. Cognitive Impairment

It is estimated that about 19% of patients sustain cognitive impairment while a further 27% suffer from dementia (24–27). All degrees of cognitive impairment can affect eating habits.

Table 3 Signs of Deficiencies of B Vitamins

B vitamin	Signs of deficiency
B_1 (thiamine)	Fatigue, insomnia, weakness, confusion, memory loss; uncoordinated movements, numbness, paralysis of the extremities, muscle fatigue; poor appetite, emaciation; personality change, irritability, depression; beriberi
B_2 (riboflavin)	Burning of tongue, lips, mouth, cracks at corners of mouth; burning, itching of eyes; vision loss, sensitivity to light; dermatitis, dryness, greasy scaling of skin; depression, hysteria, behavior changes
B_3 (niacin)	Weakness, loss of appetite, lethargy; dermatitis (scaly, dark pigmentation); swollen tongue; tremor; inflamed mucous membranes, disorientation, irritability, insomnia, memory loss, delirium, dementia; pellagra
B_6 (pyridoxine)	Depression; increased susceptibility to infections; dermatitis, anemia, inflammation of the nerves, nausea; lethargy; elevated serum homocysteine
B_{12} (cobalamin)	Anemia (pernicious or megaloblastic); fatigue, poor concentration; nerve damage including disorientation, numbness, tingling, dementia, moodiness, confusion, agitation, dimmed vision, delusions, hallucinations, dizziness; poor absorption of food; neuropathy; elevated serum homocysteine
Folic acid (folacin)	Anemia (macrocytic); impaired nutrient absorption, appetite loss, weight loss, weakness, apathy, sore tongue, headache, irritability, behavior change, depression; elevated serum homocysteine
B_7 (biotin)	Dermatitis, appetite loss, nausea, depression, alopecia (thinning of hair), dermatitis; anemia; tingling and numbness in the hands and feet, lethargy, muscle pain
Pantothenic acid	Fatigue, dermatitis, lack of coordination, staggering gait, muscle cramps; poor wound healing, appetite loss, rapid pulse, depression; burning sensation in the feet

Mild forgetfulness can affect shopping for, and preparation of, food. Patients may also forget to take medications, which affects manual dexterity and other physical abilities. Dementia can also influence the willingness to eat.

The person suffering from significant cognitive impairment is best aided by the presence of an able caregiver. It is necessary, therefore, to provide careful instruction to both patient and caregiver; the patient should be more likely to follow the caregiver's directions and the caregiver will be aware of the importance of meticulous supervision.

It is important to note that malnutrition itself may be the cause of, or a contributing factor to, cognitive impairment and dementia. Therefore, it is necessary to guard against nutrient deficiencies, particularly of the B vitamins B_1 (thiamine), B_2 (riboflavin), B_3 (niacin), B_6 (pyridoxine), and folate, all of which are implicated in cognitive impairment, memory loss, confusion, and dementia (Table 3).

C. Depression

In an examination of the neuropsychiatric symptoms of PD, Lieberman (27) states that approximately 40% of patients suffer from either endogenous or exogenous depression. Depression can range from sadness to major depression and may predate the diagnosis of PD by several years (28,29). Depression can impact nutritional repletion in several ways: Depression significantly affects functional ability in PD patients (30). It may also adversely affect the appetite and desire to eat (31). These symptoms then result in reduced food intake and nutritional deficiencies that can exacerbate existing depression, appetite loss and unwillingness to eat, creating a downward, self-promoting cycle to malnutrition.

It is important for the physician to determine the kind and degree of depression, whether it is best treated by counseling or medication (30), and whether dietary measures should be applied. Tests for deficiencies of B vitamins (Table 3) should be included (32,33) and repletion performed if needed.

Both lack of B vitamins and a limited intake of omega-3 fatty acids have been implicated in some forms of depression (34). The role of the dietitian is to regularly request a food record of at least 2–3 days and determine whether dietary intake of B vitamins and omega-3 fatty acids is adequate and whether supplements are being used or are indicated. Prophylactic measures may deter some instances of depression without use of medication.

D. Dysphagia

Dysphagia (8) can lead to choking, fear of choking, and inability to swallow, all of which impact energy and nutrient ingestion, as well as aspiration of food, liquids, saliva, or refluxed stomach contents (35,36), which may cause pneumonia. Tongue movement and bolus formation may be affected and jaw rigidity may make chewing difficult (37). The physician should question the patient and/or caregiver periodically as to whether any chewing or swallowing problems are present, and if so, should refer the patient to a speech pathologist for a swallowing evaluation and education regarding safe swallowing techniques. If the speech pathologist determines that a modified food consistency, such as thickened liquids or pureed foods, is needed, the individual should be referred to a dietitian for appropriate diet planning.

E. Fatigue

Fatigue can alter the individual's ability to shop for, prepare, and eat food. Complaints of exhaustion and sleepiness are common among patients (38) and can be either an effect of PD or a side effect of medications, particularly an additive effect from multiple medications; however, dietary causes should not be ruled out. Where there is decreased food intake, there may be a resulting drop in blood glucose, with attendant fatigue. Also, a prolonged reduction in caloric intake may result in deficiencies of B vitamins and iron, which can further worsen the condition (Table 3).

Reports of recent weight loss along with fatigue should be investigated. Tests for deficiencies of iron and B vitamins should be performed. Also, a dietitian, using a food diary, should determine the frequency and amount of food eaten and its adequacy, making appropriate recommendations. Often small, nourishing snacks between meals can prevent nutrition-related fatigue by ensuring a constant supply of blood glucose.

F. Physical Impairment

Disabilities increase as PD advances and include tremor, dyskinesia, rigidity, bradykinesia, and loss of manual dexterity, which all may affect the ability to manipulate eating utensils. Some individuals may require several hours to complete a meal and cannot ingest sufficient food to maintain weight or nutrient repletion. A referral to an occupational therapist for help with special plates, cups, and utensils is needed. A dietitian should provide recommendations for finger foods, nourishing drinks and shakes, and foods that are easy to scoop and do not need to be cut or speared with a fork.

G. Impaired Gait and Balance, Decreased Weight-Bearing Exercise

When impairment of gait and balance occurs, the individual is less likely to perform weight-bearing exercise. This results in muscle wasting and bone thinning (39), a combination that notably raises the risk for falls and subsequent fractures (40). If poor dietary habits are also present, this possibility is increased. The risk for bone thinning and fractures is increased in men as well as women, and prevention of these should be considered of the highest importance (41). Bone thinning usually takes place over an extended period of time. Dietary sources of calcium, magnesium, and vitamins D and K, adequate protein to maintain muscle mass, supplements as appropriate, and prevention of unplanned weight loss should be addressed. Additionally, physicians should regularly order fall risk assessment and fracture risk assessment (42,43), including a dual energy x-ray absorptiometry (DEXAscan), to determine baseline bone density, and consider use of such aids as hip protectors to help prevent fractures in case of falls (44). Prompt initiation of a diet sufficient in bone-strengthening nutrients, supplements as needed, protein, and as much weight-bearing and other exercise as the individual is capable of can bring about a long-term maintenance of both muscle mass and bone density. Regular nutrition risk assessment will guide nutrition therapy, and use of hip protectors if needed offers protection in case of falls.

H. Loss of Olfaction, Sense of Taste, Appetite

Loss of the sense of smell is common among patients with PD (45) and is thought in some cases to predate the diagnosis (46,47). Loss of smell is closely tied to the ability to taste, and therefore taste sensation is also impaired. Inability to experience smell and taste does not necessarily affect the willingness to eat; however, it can be a factor, particularly if other conditions, such as medication-induced appetite loss or depression, are present. Loss of appetite can seriously affect energy and nutrient intake.

The physician is well positioned to obtain an early determination of olfactory loss, as it may be incorporated into the diagnosis of PD, and can then also determine whether loss of taste is present and whether the appetite is affected. At this point, the patient should be referred to a dietitian for education with regard to the importance of diet. Individualized counseling on nutrient adequacy is important, including use of small, frequent meals and snacks, energy-dense foods, with multivitamins or canned supplements as appropriate.

I. Nausea/Vomiting

Many patients experience varying degrees of nausea, and sometimes vomiting, upon initiation of PD medications (48–57). Nausea can impact the desire for food and willingness to eat, while vomiting results in loss of nutrients and deranged electrolyte balance. Medications, such as carbidopa (Lodosyn) and domperidone (58), can be prescribed to allay nausea; however, dietary measures should be the first line of defense.

Initially the patient may take medications with meals. In the case of medications containing levodopa, especially the immediate-release form, this may interfere with levodopa absorption. However, in time most people adapt to the medications, so that within a few weeks they may be able to take the levodopa with a small low-protein snack, such as juice and crackers, and later on an empty stomach. Use of some form of ginger (as tea or crystallized) may allay mild nausea.

J. Protein-Levodopa Interaction

The large neutral amino acids, breakdown products of dietary proteins, compete with levodopa for absorption, both from the gut and at the blood-brain barrier. This becomes increasingly problematic as PD advances and motor fluctuations occur (59–61). In both immediate and controlled-release formulations, protein has been found to influence the response to the drugs (62,63). Additionally, some patients are more sensitive to protein than others, even in the early stages of PD. It is important, therefore, to instruct patients to take immediate release carbidopa/levodopa about 30 minutes prior to meals. The controlled-release form may be taken with meals; however, it requires a longer time before it takes effect.*

If motor fluctuations are not controlled by taking levodopa prior to meals, further adjustment may be necessary. It is important, however, to assure that patients' health and protein needs are met. Initially it was thought best for the patient experiencing problems to avoid protein during daytime hours, consuming the day's allotment of protein at the evening meal, to allow for best mobility (64) and/or to severely restrict protein intake. The amount of protein allotted ranged from 0.5 g/kg body weight (65) to 0.75–0.8 g/kg body weight per day (66). However, such menus are unnatural and disagreeable and can increase the likelihood of food avoidance and wasting. Additionally, patients may find they are unable to move at night, turn in bed or adjust the covers, or use the bathroom. Some patients avoid protein at the evening meal leading to protein-energy malnutrition.

Another approach is for the patient to eat meals that contain a high ratio of carbohydrate to protein—from 5:1 to 7:1 (67,68). The influx of glucose into the bloodstream creates an insulin release sufficient to remove some of the amino acids from the bloodstream, allowing the levodopa to reach and cross the blood-brain barrier unhindered. However, this requires careful diet planning. The patient and family members must be referred to a dietitian for individualized counseling and meal plans.

By far the simplest and often a very effective method for maintaining mobility and minimizing off time is for the dietitian to assess the patient's individual protein needs and divide the total grams of protein equally among three meals per day—morning, midday, and evening (67). This generally lowers the total amount of protein consumed, while still meeting the patient's dietary needs. Protein needs must be assessed carefully— elderly adults require 1–1.2 g of protein per kilogram body weight. Persons who have experienced unplanned weight loss, pressure ulcers, and/or muscle wasting may require additional protein. Also, patients with osteopenia or osteoporosis require extra protein (69).

K. Appetite Loss

There are many possible reasons for loss of appetite, including depression, medications, early satiety, nausea, loss of olfaction, and reduced sense of taste. When this occurs, it is important to determine the reason for the appetite loss. Early satiety may be due to gastroparesis, which might be treated by increasing gastric motility. Appetite loss due to depression may be best treated by counseling or an antidepressant. Nausea and loss of

---

*If the patient experiences increasing "off time," it may be preferable to take controlled-release preparations about 30 minutes before meals.

olfaction may also be related to appetite loss. If medications contribute, consider whether it is possible to reduce or eliminate one or more of the drugs.

L. Xerostomia (Dry Mouth)

Dry mouth is common among individuals with PD (70–72). It may be a side effect of medications, or due to mouth breathing [or occasionally, Sjogren's syndrome (72,73)]. Dry mouth may lead to candidiasis, periodontal disease, caries, and other oral diseases. People with PD may have greater difficulty with brushing and flossing, and also may have less success with dentures, and greater problems receiving dental care due to PD symptoms. Dental health is of special concern to dietitians, as mastication is of primary importance in maintaining nutritional health. Physicians and dietitians should inquire about dry mouth and oral health and recommend consultation with a dentist in order to prevent tooth loss and oral disease.

III. RELATIONSHIP OF B VITAMINS TO LEVODOPA AND THEIR RELEVANCE IN PD

The various B vitamins may play a role in the nutritional health of people with PD for several reasons: (a) homocysteinemia may occur with long-term use of levodopa; (b) aging is often accompanied by decreased production of stomach acids and intrinsic factor needed for metabolism of B_{12}; (c) changed eating habits may cause a depletion of nutrients and a gradual depletion can effect B vitamin deficiencies, the signs of which closely resemble symptoms of PD.

It is, therefore, important to understand the relationship of the B vitamins to medications and PD symptoms.

A. Homocysteinemia

Homocysteine is normally cleared from the bloodstream by the combined action of vitamins B_6, B_{12}, and folate. An elevation may indicate a deficiency of one or more of these vitamins. Muller et al. (73) found a relationship between long-term levodopa use and elevated serum homocysteine, while Duan et al. (74), using a mouse model, found that a folate-deficient diet led to elevated serum homocysteine and sensitized neurons to injury and death. Researchers have found an association between serum homocysteine and cognitive impairment/Alzheimer-type dementia (75,76), while Seshadri and colleagues state that plasma homocysteine is an independent risk factor for dementia (77). Because of the prevalence of cognitive impairment and dementia in PD, serum homocysteine should be regularly assessed.

B. Atrophic Gastritis

Many PD patients suffer from atrophic gastritis. The stomach secretes less of the acid needed to cleave B_{12} from dietary protein, resulting in megaloblastic anemia (78).

C. Reduced Intrinsic Factor

There may also be insufficient production of intrinsic factor, required for absorption of B_{12} in the ileum, with pernicious anemia ensuing (79).

D. Interpreting Laboratory Values for the Aged

Evidence exists that some elderly individuals with B_{12} levels in the low-normal range may nevertheless develop complications of deficiency (80,81).

E. Folate Masking

An excess of folate may mask B_{12} deficiency (82).

F. Signs of B Vitamin Deficiencies

Deficiencies of B vitamins may closely resemble symptoms of PD. While these symptoms are sometimes vague and often involve two or more of the B vitamins (83), it is worthwhile to examine them because patients' eating habits often change, leading to a narrowed range of nutrient intake (Table 3).

It is important for patients to receive comprehensive blood tests. Tests for cobalamine deficiency in cases of pernicious anemia are not always conclusive; tests for methyl malonate and serum homocysteine should also be conducted (84). Annual tests for macrocytic and pernicious anemias, serum homocysteine, and deficiencies of B_6, B_{12}, folate and other B vitamins will provide a better picture of nutritional status (73,74,76,85–89). Severe deficiencies, when discovered, may be best remedied by intramuscular injections of B vitamins.

The physician, therefore, should consider symptoms such as paresthesia, impaired gait, personality or behavior changes, sore or burning mouth or tongue, burning feet, dementia, and depression (89) and should rule out the possibility of B vitamin deficiencies by ordering comprehensive laboratory testing. The dietitian should periodically request a 3-day food-medication diary to determine whether the diet is adequate; if inadequate, the physician should be notified and laboratory testing ordered. A B-complex supplement or intramuscular injection may be needed to provide repletion.

IV. UNINTENTIONAL WEIGHT LOSS

Unplanned weight loss is very common in PD (90) and is of concern because it raises the risk for both morbidity and mortality (91). It is a significant factor in malnutrition, contributing to hospitalization, with longer length of stay and greater likelihood of home health care upon discharge (92). The weight loss may be slow and gradual, occurring over a period of years. Cornoni-Huntley et al. found that a loss of 10% of the maximum adult weight in 10 years increases the risk for mortality (93). Current instruments, however, are designed to detect weight loss occurring over a much shorter period of time, generally 1–6 months (94).

Experts are recommending intervention in older adults who have a body mass index below 24 (95), although Somes et al. conclude that annualized weight change is a better predictor of mortality than body mass index (96). Patients with PD are apt to lose weight, and early detection and intervention are needed (97). In order to help the patient arrest weight loss, and in some cases to regain weight, it is necessary to assess the etiology of the unintended weight loss (98). It may occur for a variety of reasons and may also be multifactorial (99). Treatment will depend on cause and requires a team approach, consisting of a physician, psychiatrist or psychologist, dietitian, speech–language pathologist, and occupational therapist.

A. Medication–Induced Weight Loss

Selegeline, amantadine, dopamine agonists, carbidopa/levodopa or levodopa/benserizide, and catechol–O–methyltransferase (COMT) inhibitors may induce side effects that adversely impact nutritional health (1,100). Nausea, dry mouth, metallic taste, loss of appetite, and anorexia may lead to an unwillingness to eat. Laboratory tests should be obtained, as zinc deficiency may contribute to loss of taste and appetite. Drowsiness and fatigue may lead to low blood glucose and nutrient deficiency due to low food intake. Cognitive impairment, dementia, hallucinations, agitation, and anxiety (101) may interfere with the ability or desire to eat. This may require counseling or medication adjustment. Laboratory tests for B vitamin deficiencies should be considered as these deficiencies can cause depression, behavior change, and cognitive impairment including dementia. Constipation may lead to fear of fecal impaction and unwillingness to eat.

B. PD Symptom–Induced Weight Loss

Caloric expenditure may be greater than intake. These conditions may require medication adjustments or a referral to an occupational therapist for specialized eating utensils, and to a dietitian for help with diet planning (102–104) (Table 3).

C. Depression–Induced Weight Loss

The depressed individual may refuse food (97) and may require counseling or medication. Alleviation of depression may restore enjoyment to mealtimes (Table 3).

D. Dysphagia–Induced

Choking or fear of choking can lead to unwillingness to eat.

REFERENCES

1. Markus HS, Tomkins AM, Stern GM. Increased prevalence of undernutrition in Parkinson's disease and its relationship to clinical disease parameters. J Neural Transm Park Dis Dement Sect 1993; 5:117–125.
2. Siddiqui MF, Rast S, Lynn MJ, Auchus AP, Pfeiffer RF. Autonomic dysfunction in Parkinson's disease: a comprehensive symptom survey. Parkinsonism Relat Disord 2002; 8(4):277–284.
3. Martignoni E, Pacchetti C, Godi L, Micieli G, Nappi G. Autonomic disorders in Parkinson's disease. J Neural Transm 1995; (suppl 45):11–19.
4. Hurtig HI. Problems with current pharmacologic treatment of Parkinson's disease. Exp Neurol 1997; 144(1):10–16.
5. Schafer D, Greulich W. Effects of parkinsonian medication on sleep. J Neurol 2000; 247(suppl 4):IV/24–27.
6. Okada K, Suyama N, Oguro H, Yamaguchi S, Kobayashi S. Medication-induced hallucination and cerebral blood flow in Parkinson's disease. J Neurol 1999; 246(5):365–368.
7. Pfeiffer RF. Gastrointestinal dysfunction in Parkinson's disease. Clin Neurosci 1998; 5(2):136–146.
8. Jost WH. Gastrointestinal motility problems in patients with Parkinson's disease. Effects of antiparkinsonian treatment and guidelines for management. Drugs Aging 1997; 10(4):249–258.
9. Hardoff R, Sula M, Tamir A, Soil A, Front A, Badarna S, Honigman S, Giladi N. Gastric emptying time and gastric motility in patients with Parkinson's disease. Mov Disord 2001; 16(6):1041–1047.
10. Kurth MC. Using liquid levodopa in the treatment of Parkinson's disease. A practical guide. Drugs Aging 1997; 10(5):332–340.
11. Duque JM, Betes MT, de la Riva S, Subtil JC, Munoz–Navas M. Barrett's esophagus. Rev Med Univ Navarra 1998; 42(3):145–155.
12. Abbott RD, Petrovitch H, White LR, Masaki KH, Tanner CM, Curb JD, Grandinetti A, Blanchette PL, Popper JS, Ross GW. Frequency of bowel movements and the future risk of Parkinson's disease. Neurology 2001; 14;57(3):456–462.

13. Bassotti G, Maggio D, Battaglia E, Giulietti O, Spinozzi F, Reboldi G, Serra AM, Emanuelli G, Chiarioni G. Manometric investigation of anorectal function in early and late stage Parkinson's disease. J Neurol Neurosurg Psychiatry 2000; 68(6):768–770.
14. Ghadirian P, Maisonneuve P, Perret C, Lacroix A, Boyle P. Epidemiology of sociodemographic characteristics, lifestyle, medical history, and colon cancer: a case–control study among French Canadians in Montreal. Cancer Detect Prev 1998; 22(5):396–404.
15. Shimotoyodome A, Meguro S, Hase T, Tokimitsu I, Sakata T. Decreased colonic mucus in rats with loperamide-induced constipation. Comp Biochem Physiol A Mol Integr Physiol 2000; 126(2):203–212.
16. Jacobs EJ, White E. Constipation, laxative use, and colon cancer among middle–aged adults. Epidemiology 1998; 9(4):385–391.
17. van Gorkom BA, Karrenbeld A, van der Sluis T, Zwart N, de Vries EG, Kleibeuker JH. Apoptosis induction by sennoside laxatives in man; escape from a protective mechanism during chronic sennoside use? J Pathol 2001; 194(4):493–499.
18. Astarloa R, Mena MA, Sanchez V, de la Vega L, de Yebenes JG. Clinical and pharmacokinetic effects of a diet rich in insoluble fiber on Parkinson disease. Clin Neuropharmacol 1992; 15(5):375–380.
19. Scheppach W, Luehrs H, Menzel T. Beneficial health effects of low-digestible carbohydrate consumption. Br J Nutr 2001; 85(suppl 1):S23–S30.
20. Cummings JH, Macfarlane GT, Englyst HN. Prebiotic digestion and fermentation. Am J Clin Nutr 2001; 73(2 suppl):415S–420S.
21. Stacewicz–Sapuntzakis M, Bowen PE, Hussain EA, Damayanti-Wood BI, Farnsworth NR. Chemical composition and potential health effects of prunes: a functional food? Crit Rev Food Sci Nutr 2001; 41(4):251–286.
22. Rush EC, Patel M, Plank LD, Ferguson LR. Kiwifruit promotes laxation in the elderly. Asia Pac J Clin Nutr 2002; 11(2):164–168.
23. Ashraf W, Wszolek ZK, Pfeiffer RF, Normand M, Maurer K, Srb F, Edwards LL, Quigley EM. Anorectal function in fluctuating (on–off) Parkinson's disease: evaluation by combined anorectal manometry and electromyography. Mov Disord 1995; 10(5):650–657.
24. Wang H, Wang Y, Wang D, Cui L, Tian S, Zhang Y. Cognitive impairment in Parkinson's disease revealed by event-related potential N270. J Neurol Sci 2002; 194(1):49–53.
25. Kulisevsky J, Pascual-Sedano B. Parkinson disease and cognition. Neurologia 1999; 14(suppl 1): 72–81.
26. Sawamoto N, Honda M, Hanakawa T, Fukuyama H, Shibasaki H. Cognitive slowing in Parkinson's disease: a behavioral evaluation independent of motor slowing. J Neurosci 2002; 22(12):5198–5203.
27. Lieberman A. Managing the neuropsychiatric symptoms of Parkinson's disease. Neurol 1998; 50(suppl 6):S33–S38.
28. Fukunishi I, Hosokawa K, Ozaki S. Depression antedating the onset of Parkinson's disease. Jpn J Psychiatry Neurol 1991; 45(1):7–11.
29. Schuurman AG, van den Akker M, Ensinck KT, Metsemakers JF, Knottnerus JA, Leentjens AF, Buntinx F. Increased risk of Parkinson's disease after depression: a retrospective cohort study. Neurology 2002; 58(10):1501–1504.
30. Liu CY, Wang SJ, Fuh JL, Lin CH, Yang YY, Liu HC. The correlation of depression with functional activity in Parkinson's disease. J Neurol 1997; 244(8):493–498.
31. Cote L. Depression: impact and management by the patient and family. Neurology 1999; 52(7 suppl 3):S7–S9.
32. Bottiglieri T, Laundy M, Crellin R, Toone BK, Carney MW, Reynolds EH. Homocysteine, folate, methylation, and monoamine metabolism in depression. J Neurol Neurosurg Psychiatry 2000; 69(2):228–232.
33. Gottfries CG. Late life depression. Eur Arch Psychiatry Clin Neurosci 2001; 251(suppl 2):II57–61.
34. Severus WE, Littman AB, Stoll AL. Omega-3 fatty acids, homocysteine, and the increased risk of cardiovascular mortality in major depressive disorder. Harv Rev Psychiatry 2001; 9(6): 280–293.
35. Nagaya M, Kachi T, Yamada T, Igata A. Videofluorographic study of swallowing in Parkinson's disease. Dysphagia 1998; 13:95–100.
36. Bassotti, G, Germani U, Pagliaricci S, Plesa A, Giulietti O, Mannarino E, Morelli A. Esophageal manometric abnormalities in Parkinson's disease. Dysphagia 1998; 13(1):28–31.
37. Leopold NA, Kagel MC. Prepharyngeal dysphagia in Parkinson's disease. Dysphagia 1996; 11(1):14–22.

38. Karlsen K, Larsen JP, Tandberg E, Jorgensen K. Fatigue in patients with Parkinson's disease. Mov Disord 1999; 14:237–241.
39. McIntosh GC, Holden KE. Risk for malnutrition and bone fracture in Parkinson's disease: a pilot study. J Nutr Elderly 1999; 18(3):21–31.
40. Lemmer J. Management of sarcopenia in the elderly. Nutrition M.D. 2002; 28(7).
41. Holden K. Reducing fracture risk in patients with Parkinson's disease. Nutrition M.D. 2001; 27(4).
42. Runge, M. Diagnosing fall risk in the elderly. Ther Umsch 2002; 59(7):351–358.
43. Stack E, Ashburn A. Fall events described by people with Parkinson's disease: implications for clinical interviewing and the research agenda. Physiother Res Int 1999; 4(3):190–200.
44. Conzelmann, M. Hip protectors offer a new method for reducing the risk of hip fractures. Ther Umsch 2002; 59(7):359–365.
45. Tissingh G, Berendse HW, Bergmans P, DeWaard R, Drukarch B, Stoof JC, Wolters EC. Loss of olfaction in de novo and treated Parkinson's disease: possible implications for early diagnosis. Mov Disord 2001; 16(1):41–46.
46. Doty RL. Olfaction. Annu Rev Psychol 2001; 52:423–452.
47. Daum RF, Sekinger B, Kobal G, Lang CJ. Olfactory testing with "sniffin' sticks" for clinical diagnosis of Parkinson disease. Nervenarzt 2000; 71(8):643–650.
48. Dooley M, Markham A. Pramipexole. A review of its use in the management of early and advanced Parkinson's disease. Drugs Aging 1998; 12(6):495–514.
49. Pogarell O, Gasser T, van Hilten JJ, Spieker S, Pollentier S, Meier D, Oertel WH. Pramipexole in patients with Parkinson's disease and marked drug resistant tremor: a randomised, double blind, placebo controlled multicentre study. J Neurol Neurosurg Psychiatry 2002; 72(6):713–720.
50. Brooks DJ, Abbott RJ, Lees AJ, Martignoni E, Philcox DV, Rascol O, Roos RA, Sagar HJ. A placebo-controlled evaluation of ropinirole, a novel D2 agonist, as sole dopaminergic therapy in Parkinson's disease. Clin Neuropharmacol 1998; 21(2):101–107.
51. Korczyn AD, Brooks DJ, Brunt ER, Poewe WH, Rascol O, Stocchi F. Ropinirole versus bromocriptine in the treatment of early Parkinson's disease: a 6-month interim report of a 3-year study. 053 Study Group. Mov Disord 1998; 13(1):46–51.
52. Najib J. Entacapone: a catechol-O-methyltransferase inhibitor for the adjunctive treatment of Parkinson's disease. Clin Ther 2001; 23(6):802–832.
53. Davis TL, Roznoski M, Burns RS. Effects of tolcapone in Parkinson's patients taking L-dihydroxyphenylalanine/carbidopa and selegiline. Mov Disord 1995; 10(3):349–351.
54. Block G, Liss C, Reines S, Irr J, Nibbelink D. Comparison of immediate-release and controlled release carbidopa/levodopa in Parkinson's disease. A multicenter 5-year study. The CR First Study Group. Eur Neurol 1997; 37(1):23–27.
55. Bayulkem K, Erisir K, Tuncel A, Bayulkem B. A study on the effect and tolerance of lisuride on Parkinson's disease. Adv Neurol 1996; 69:519–530.
56. Bosch MF, Ludin HP. Apomorphine as adjuvant treatment in idiopathic Parkinson syndrome. Schweiz Arch Neurol Psychiatr 1994; 145(5):8–13.
57. Vezina P, Mohr E, Grimes D. Deprenyl in Parkinson's disease: mechanisms, neuroprotective effect, indications and adverse effects. Can J Neurol Sci 1992; 19(1 suppl):142–146.
58. Soykan I, Sarosiek I, Shifflett J, Wooten GF, McCallum RW. Effect of chronic oral domperidone therapy on gastrointestinal symptoms and gastric emptying in patients with Parkinson's disease. Mov Disord 1997; 12(6):952–957.
59. Cotzias, GC, Vanwoert MH, Schiffer L. Aromatic amino acids and modification of parkinsonism. N Eng J Med 1967; 276:374.
60. Nutt JG, Woodward WR, Hammerstad JP, Carter JH, Anderson JL. The "on-off" phenomenon in Parkinson's disease. Relation to levodopa absorption and transport. N Engl J Med 1984; 310(8):483–488.
61. Nutt JG, Woodward WR, Carter JH, Trotman TL. Influence of fluctuations of plasma large neutral amino acids with normal diets on the clinical response to levodopa. J Neurol Neurosurg Psychiatry 1989; 52(4):481–487.
62. Garcia de Yebenes J, Mateo D, Pino MA, Cordero M, Pastor M, Chacon J, Morales B, Sanchez V, Mena MA, Gimenez Roldan S. The effect of controlled release of DOPA and carbidopa on clinical response and plasma pharmacokinetics of DOPA in parkinsonian patients. Neurologia 1997; 12(4):145–156.
63. Contin M, Riva R, Martinelli P, Albani F, Baruzzi A. Effect of meal timing on the kinetic–dynamic profile of levodopa/carbidopa controlled release [corrected] in parkinsonian patients. Eur J Clin Pharmacol 1998; 54(4):303–308. (Erratum in: Eur J Clin Pharmacol 1998; 54(7):577.)

64. Pincus JH, Barry K. Protein redistribution diet restores motor function in patients with dopa–resistant "off" periods. Neurology 1988; 38(3):481–483.
65. Mena I, Cotzias GC. Protein intake and treatment of Parkinson's disease with levodopa. N Engl J Med 1975; 23;292(4):181–184.
66. Vilming ST. Diet therapy in Parkinson disease. Tidsskr Nor Laegeforen 1995; 115(10):1244–1247.
67. Berry EM, Growdon JH, Wurtman JJ, Caballero B, Wurtman RJ. A balanced carbohydrate: protein diet in the management of Parkinson's disease. Neurology 1991; 41(8):1295–1297.
68. Holden, K. Levodopa effects. In: Parkinson's Disease: Guidelines for Medical Nutrition Therapy. Fort Collins, CO: Five Star Living Inc., 2000:LE.3–LE.4.
69. Sato Y, Kaji M, Tsuru T, Satoh K, Kondo I. Vitamin K deficiency and osteopenia in vitamin D–deficient elderly women with Parkinson's disease. Arch Phys Med Rehabil 2002; 83(1):86–91.
70. Clifford T, Finnerty J. The dental awareness and needs of a Parkinson's disease population. Gerodontology 1995; 12(12):99–103.
71. Hashimoto S, Sawada T, Inoue T, Yamamoto K, Iwata M. Cholinergic–drug induced sicca syndrome in Parkinson's disease: a case report and a review of the literature. Clin Neurol Neurosurg 1999; 101(4):268–270.
72. Nagao T, Takagi K, Hashida H, Masaki T, Sakuta M. A case of progressive systemic sclerosis and Sjögren's syndrome complicated by parkinsonism with special reference to the beneficial effect of corticosteroid. Rinsho Shinkeigaku 1991; 31(11):1238–1240.
73. Muller T, Woitalla D, Hauptmann B, Fowler B, Kuhn W. Decrease of methionine and S-adenosylmethionine and increase of homocysteine in treated patients with Parkinson's disease. Neurosci Lett 2001; 308(1):54–56.
74. Duan W, Ladenheim B, Cutler RG, Kruman II, Cadet JL, Mattson MP. Dietary folate deficiency and elevated homocysteine levels endanger dopaminergic neurons in models of Parkinson's disease. J Neurochem 2002; 80(1):101–110.
75. Miller JW, Green R, Mungas DM, Reed BR, Jagust WJ. Homocysteine, vitamin B_6, and vascular disease in AD patients. Neurology 2002; 58(10):1471–1475.
76. Selley ML, Close DR, Stern SE. The effect of increased concentrations of homocysteine on the concentration of (E)-4-hydroxy-2-nonenal in the plasma and cerebrospinal fluid of patients with Alzheimer's disease. Neurobiol Aging 2002; 23(3):383–388.
77. Seshadri S, Beiser A, Selhub J, Jacques PF, Rosenberg IH, D'Agostino RB, Wilson PW, Wolf PA. Plasma homocysteine as a risk factor for dementia and Alzheimer's disease. N Engl J Med 2002; 346(7):476–483.
78. Krasinski SD, Russell RM, Samloff M, Jacob RA, Dallal GE, McGandy RB, Hartz SC. Fundic atrophic gastritis in an elderly population. Effect on hemoglobin and several serum nutritional indicators. J Am Geriatr Soc 1986; 34:800–806.
79. Carmel R. Prevalence of undiagnosed pernicious anemia in the elderly. Arch Int Med 1996; 156:1097–1100.
80. Joosten E, van den Berg A, Riezler R, Naurath HJ, Lindenbaum J, Stabler SP, Allen RH. Metabolic evidence that deficiencies of vitamin B-12 (cobalamin), folate, and vitamin B-6 occur commonly in elderly people. Am J Clin Nutr 1993; 58:468–476.
81. Naurath HJ, Joosten E, Riezler R, Stabler SP, Allen RH, Lindenbaum J. Effects of vitamin B_{12}, folate, and vitamin B6 supplements in elderly people with normal serum vitamin concentrations. Lancet 1995; 346:85–89.
82. Allen LH, Casterline J. Vitamin B_{12} deficiency in elderly individuals: diagnosis and requirements [comment]. Am J Clin Nutr 1994; 60:12–14.
83. Somer E. The essential guide to vitamins and minerals. In: The Vitamins. New York: HarperCollins Publishers Inc., 1995:43–75.
84. Marcaud V. Pernicious anemia. Rev Prat 2001; 51(11):1211–1214.
85. Duthie SJ, Whalley LJ, Collins AR, Leaper S, Berger K, Deary IJ. Homocysteine, B vitamin status, and cognitive function in the elderly. Am J Clin Nutr 2002; 75(5):908–913.
86. Muller T. Non–dopaminergic drug treatment of Parkinson's disease. Expert Opin Pharmacother 2001; 2(4):557–572.
87. Kuhn W, Roebroek R, Blom H, van Oppenraaij D, Przuntek H, Kretschmer A, Buttner T, Woitalla D, Muller T. Elevated plasma levels of homocysteine in Parkinson's disease. Eur Neurol 1998; 40(4):225–227.
88. Yasui K, Kowa H, Nakaso K, Takeshima T, Nakashima K. Plasma homocysteine and MTHFR C677T genotype in levodopa-treated patients with PD. Neurology 2000; 55(3):437–440.
89. Healton EB, Savage DG, Brust JC, Garrett TJ, Lindenbaum J. Neurologic aspects of cobalamin deficiency. Med 1991; 70(4):229–245.

90. Beyer PL, Palarino MY, Michalek D, Busenbark K, Koller WC. Weight change and body composition in patients with Parkinson's disease. J Am Diet Assoc 1995; 95(9):979–983.
91. Reynolds MW, Fredman L, Langenberg P, Magaziner J. Weight, weight change, mortality in a random sample of older community-dwelling women. J Am Geriatr Soc 1999; 47(12):1409–1414.
92. Chima CS, Barco K, Dewitt ML, Maeda M, Teran JC, Mullen KD. Relationship of nutritional status to length of stay, hospital costs, and discharge status of patients hospitalized in the medicine service. J Am Diet Assoc 1997; 97(9):975–978.
93. Cornoni-Huntley JC, Harris TB, Everett DF, Albanes D, Micozzi MS, Miles TP, Feldman JJ. An overview of body weight of older persons, including the impact on mortality. The National Health and Nutrition Examination Survey I—Epidemiologic Follow-up Study. J Clin Epidemiol 1991; 44(8):743–753.
94. Holden, K. Unintentional weight loss. Parkinson's Disease: Guidelines for Medical Nutrition Therapy. Fort Collins, CO: Five Star Living Inc., 2000:WL.1–WL.6.
95. Beck AM, Ovesen L. At which body mass index and degree of weight loss should hospitalized elderly patients be considered at nutritional risk? Clin Nutr 1998; 17(5):195–198.
96. Somes GW, Kritchevsky SB, Shorr RI, Pahor M, Applegate WB. Body mass index, weight change, and death in older adults: the systolic hypertension in the elderly program. Am J Epidemiol 2002; 156(2):132–138.
97. Holden K. Unintended weight loss in Parkinson's disease. Nutr Clin Care 2001; 4(3):131–139.
98. Roberts SB. Regulation of energy intake in older adults: recent findings and implications. J Nutr Health Aging 2000; 4(3):170–171.
99. Fischer J, Johnson MA. Low body weight and weight loss in the aged. J Am Diet Assoc 1990; (12):1697–1706.
100. Pronsky ZM. Food-Medication Interactions. Pottstown, PA: Food-Medication Interactions, 2002.
101. Keller HH, Ostbye T. Do nutrition indicators predict death in elderly Canadians with cognitive impairment? Can J Public Health 2000; 91(3):220–224.
102. Louis ED, Marder K, Jurewicz EC, Watner D, Levy G, Mejia-Santana H. Body mass index in essential tremor. Arch Neurol 2002; 59(8):1273–1277.
103. Markus HS, Cox M, Tomkins AM. Raised resting energy expenditure in Parkinson's disease and its relationship to muscle rigidity. Clin Sci (Colch) 1992; 83(2):199–204.
104. Romagnoni F, Zuliani G, Bollini C, Leoci V, Soattin L, Dotto S, Rizzotti P, Valerio G, Lotto D, Fellin R. Disability is associated with malnutrition in institutionalized elderly people. Aging (Milano) 1999; 11(3):194–199.

34
Speech, Voice, and Swallowing Disorders

Lorraine Olson Ramig

University of Colorado-Boulder and National Center for Voice and Speech, Denver, Colorado, U.S.A.

Shimon Sapir

University of Haifa, Haifa, Israel, and National Center for Voice and Speech, Denver, Colorado, U.S.A.

Cynthia Fox

National Center for Voice and Speech, Denver, Colorado, U.S.A.

I. INTRODUCTION

As many as 50–90% of individuals with idiopathic Parkinson's disease (PD) will develop speech and voice disorders. The most common perceptual features of these disorders are reduced loudness (hypophonia), reduced prosodic pitch inflection (hypoprosodia or monotone speech), hoarse voice, and imprecise articulation (1–12). These disorders may be among the first signs of PD (13), with hypophonia and hoarseness typically preceding hypoprosodia and imprecise articulation (6,14,15). The voice and speech abnormalities associated with PD have been termed hypokinetic dysarthria (16). Hypokinetic dysarthria in individuals with PD typically results in reduced intelligibility, negatively affecting interpersonal communication and quality of life, including the ability to socialize, convey important medical information, interact with family members, and maintain employment (8,17).

Swallowing disorders (dysphagia) are also common in PD, occurring in as many as 95% of patients (18,19). Dysphagia symptoms in PD include difficulty with lingual motility, reduced initiation of swallow, difficulty with bolus formation, delayed pharyngeal response, and decreased pharyngeal contraction (18,20,21). These symptoms are often accompanied by weight loss and lack of enjoyment of eating. Aspiration pneumonia is not uncommon, especially in the later stages of the disease, and is sometimes the cause of death (22).

While neuropharmacological (23,24) and neurosurgical (25,26) approaches have been shown to be effective in improving many symptoms of PD, their impact on speech and swallowing remains unclear (27,28). Speech treatment of hypokinetic dysarthria has traditionally focused on rate, articulation, and prosody, with only modest and short-tem results (29,30). Swallowing treatment has focused on behavioral changes and diet modifications (21). A speech and voice treatment approach, the Lee Silverman Voice Treatment (LSVT®), has generated the first short-and long-term efficacy data (20,31,32) for successfully treating voice and speech disorders in this population.

II. SPEECH AND VOICE CHARACTERISTICS IN PARKINSON'S DISEASE

Disorders of laryngeal, respiratory, articulatory, and velopharyngeal function (33–36) have been documented in individuals with PD through perceptual, acoustic, aerodynamic, kinematic, videostroboscopic, electroglottographic, and electromyographic studies. The neural mechanisms underlying these voice and speech disorders are unclear (37–40). Traditionally, these abnormalities have been attributed to the primary physical characteristics of PD (rigidity, bradykinesia, and tremor), yet there is little evidence in support of these etiological factors. Alternative explanations for the speech and voice disorders have been proposed, in particular, deficits in internal cueing and sensory gating (15,41,42).

III. LARYNGEAL AND RESPIRATORY DISORDERS

Darley et al. (16) reported one of the first systematic descriptions of perceptual characteristics of speech and voice in individuals with PD (16,43,44). They identified reduced loudness, monopitch, monoloudness, reduced stress, breathy, hoarse voice quality, imprecise articulation, and short rushes of speech as classic features of speech and voice in these individuals. The vocal characteristics were further described by Logemann, et al. (6,45), who reported voice quality problems such as hoarseness, roughness, breathiness and tremor in 89% of 200 patients. These patients were nonmedicated (de novo) or off medication during the study, with most patients being diagnosed with PD and the rest with postencephalitic parkinsonism. Ho and colleagues (14) studied 200 individuals with PD and found that voice problems were first to occur, with other speech problems, prosody, articulation, and fluency, gradually appearing later and accompanying more severe motor signs of the disease. Sapir (15) studied the prevalence of voice, prosody, fluency, and articulation abnormalities in 42 individuals with PD who sought treatment for their speech problems. Eighty-six percent of the subjects had an abnormal voice, and these problems tended to occur early in the course of the disease. Later in the course of the disease, prosodic, fluency, and articulation abnormalities were reported to occur. These reports of voice problems occurring early in the course of PD are also consistent with the clinical reports by Aronson (13) and Stewart et al. (46).

Acoustic (speech signal) data have been used to describe speech and voice characteristics of individuals with PD and seem to parallel perceptual descriptions. Sound pressure level (SPL) has been measured in individuals with PD. Early studies (3,4,46–50) did not confirm a reduction in SPL consistent with perceptual reports of reduced loudness in these individuals. However, a report by Fox and Ramig (51) documented SPL that was 2–4 decibels (at 30 cm) lower across a number of speech tasks when comparing 29 individuals with PD and an age- and gender-matched control group. A 2–4 decibel change is equal to a 40% perceptual change in loudness (51). Ho et al. (52) found the voice intensity of individuals with PD to decay much faster than that observed in neurologically normal speakers during various speech tasks. They interpreted this fading speech as evidence for motor instability within the speech motor system, implicating specifically a deficit in the frontostriatal circuit. Prosodic pitch inflection in speech, measured acoustically as fundamental frequency variability, has been reported to be consistently lower in PD when compared to a healthy control group (3,4,47). These findings support the perceptual characteristics (43–45) of monopitch or monotonous speech typically observed in PD. A reduction in maximum fundamental frequency range has also been observed in the dysarthric speech of individuals with PD when compared to the normal speech of healthy speakers (3,47,53). Measures of short-term phonatory stability (e.g., jitter, shimmer, harmonics-to-noise ratio) are consistent with various perceptual characteristics of disordered voice quality (e.g., hoarse, breathy, harsh) (54,55). Long-term phonatory instability, reflecting vocal tremor in the range of 3–7 Hz during sustained vowel phonation, has been documented in PD (55–59).

Disordered laryngeal function has been documented through a number of video-endoscopic studies. Hansen, et al. (37) reported vocal fold bowing (lack of medial vocal fold closure) in 30 of 32 individuals with PD together with greater amplitude of vibration and laryngeal asymmetry. Smith and colleagues (60) made videostroboscopic observations of individuals with PD and reported that 12 of 21 patients had a form of glottal incompetence (bowing, anterior or posterior chink) on fiberoptic views. Perez et al. (61) observed laryngeal tremor in 55% of 29 individuals with PD. The primary site of tremor was vertical laryngeal motion; however, the most striking stroboscopic findings were abnormal phase closure and phase asymmetry.

Additional data to support laryngeal closure problems in individuals with PD come from analysis of the electroglottographic (EGG) signal. Uziel (11) reported EGG waveforms with reduced amplitude in individuals with PD relative to nondisordered speakers. Gerratt et al. (62) reported abnormally large speed quotient and poorly defined closing period in PD. These observations were consistent with slow vocal fold opening relative to the rate of closure and incomplete closure of the vocal folds.

Hirose and Joshita (63) studied data from the thyroarytenoid (TA) muscles in an individual with PD who had limited vocal fold movement. They observed no reduction in the number of motor unit discharges and no pathological discharge patterns (such as polyphasic or high-amplitude voltages). They reported loss of reciprocal suppression of the TA during inspiration and interpreted this as evidence of deterioration in the reciprocal adjustment of the antagonist muscles associated with rigidity. This finding is consistent with deficits in sensory gating characteristics of PD (64). Luschei et al. (65) studied single motor unit activity in the TA muscle in individuals with PD and suggested the firing rate of the TA motor units was decreased in male PD subjects. The authors report that these findings as well as past reports suggest that PD affects rate and variability in motor unit firing in the laryngeal musculature. Baker et al. (36) found that absolute TA amplitudes during a known loudness level task in individuals with PD were the lowest of three groups studied: young normal adults, normal aging adults, and adults with PD. Relative TA amplitudes were also decreased in both the aging and PD groups when compared to the young normal adults. The authors concluded that reduced levels of TA muscle activity may contribute to the reduced vocal loudness that is observed in PD and aging populations. The reduction in TA activity may also reflect sensory gating anomalies and is contrary to the notion of laryngeal muscle rigidity as the cause of hypophonia in PD.

A number of studies have documented disordered respiratory function in individuals with PD through various aerodynamic measurements. Reduced vital capacity has been reported (66–68) as well as a reduction in the total amount of air expended during maximum phonation tasks (69). Reduced intraoral air pressure during consonant/vowel productions has been reported (69–71) as well as abnormal airflow patterns (72,73). It has been suggested that the origin of these airflow abnormalities may be variations in airflow resistance. This may be caused by abnormal movements of the vocal folds and supralaryngeal area (73) or abnormal chest wall movements and respiratory muscle activation patterns (38,71,74).

IV. ARTICULATORY AND VELOPHARYNGEAL DISORDERS

Imprecise consonants have been observed in individuals with PD (6,45,66). Logemann et al. (6,45) reported articulation problems in 45% of 200 unmedicated patients. They suggested that inadequate narrowing of the vocal tract may underlie problems with stops /p/, /b/, affricates /sh/, /ch/, and fricatives /s/, /f/. Sapir et al. (15) reported abnormal articulation in 50% of 42 medicated patients with PD.

Disordered rate of speech has also been reported in some individuals with PD. While rapid rate or short rushes of speech have been reported in 6–13% of individuals with PD (3,4,75–77), Canter (48) reported slower than normal rates. Pallilalia or stuttering-like speech dysfluencies have been observed in a small percentage of individuals with PD (43,78).

Acoustic correlates of disordered articulation have been studied and include problems with timing of vocal onsets and offsets (voicing during normally voiceless closure intervals of voiceless stops) (11,39,79) and spirantization (presence of fricative-like, aperiodic noise during stop closures). In another study (80) dysarthric speakers with PD showed longer voice onset times (VOTs) than normal. Such abnormal VOTs may reflect a problem with movement initiation (80), which may be related to deficits in internal cueing, timing, and/or sensory gating (15,81).

Disordered articulatory movements have been documented in PD through kinematic analysis of jaw movements (80,82–89). It has been consistently reported that individuals with PD show a significant reduction in the size and peak velocity of jaw movements during speech when compared to healthy individuals with normal speech (80,86,90). On average, jaw movement of individuals with PD has been reported to be approximately half the size of the jaw movements observed in nondisordered subjects. The reduction in range of movement has been attributed to rigidity of the articulatory muscles (91,92); however, this may be related to a problem with sensorimotor perception and/or scaling of speech and nonspeech movements (14,41,42,81). In contrast to range of movements, durations of movements in individuals with PD have been reported to be similar to those of healthy individuals (80).

Electromyographic (EMG) studies of the lip and jaw muscles in individuals with and without PD have provided some evidence for increased levels of tonic resting and background activity (33–35,93,94) as well as for loss of reciprocity between agonist and antagonistic muscle groups (33,34,87,88,93). These findings are consistent with evidence for abnormal sensorimotor gating in the orofacial and limb systems, which are presumably related to basal ganglia dysfunction (95–97). Whether or not these abnormal sensorimotor findings are indicative of excess stiffness or rigidity in the speech musculature is not clear (98–100). Hunker et al. (89) studied lip muscle stiffness and labial speech movements and found evidence to suggest a positive correlation between muscle stiffness (quantified by applying known forces and observing the resultant displacements) and decrements in the range of lip movement. Connor and colleagues (99,100) found no evidence for excess stiffness or rigidity in jaw muscles during speech movements, but they did find some abnormalities during nonspeech visually guided movements. They concluded that motor impairment in PD may be task-dependent. Caligiuri (98) obtained measures of labial muscle rigidity and movement for 12 PD and 9 age-matched control subjects. Displacement amplitude, peak instantaneous velocity, and movement time were evaluated during repetitive syllable productions. The results showed that while mean displacement amplitudes and velocities were lower for the subjects with PD, than the normal control subjects, there was no statistical relationship between labial rigidity and the degree of movement abnormality. He concluded that while rigidity may play a part in overall disability, it does not sufficiently explain the labial articulatory difficulties associated with PD. He further indicated that these findings were in agreement with the literature on limb rigidity and movement aberrations in PD, suggesting that rigidity and bradykinesia probably represent independent pathophysiological phenomena.

While nasality and nasal emission have not been significant or consistent perceptual problems in the speech of individuals with PD, aerodynamic and kinematic studies suggest that velopharyngeal movements may be reduced in some of these individuals (40,87,101).

V. SENSORY OBSERVATIONS

While the speech and voice problems associated with PD are generally considered in relation to motor output problems, sensory problems in PD have been recognized for years (23,102,103). Sensorimotor deficits in the orofacial system (95–97,104) and abnormal auditory, temporal, and perceptual processing of voice and speech (41,42,81,105) have been documented in individuals with PD (96,97,106) and have been implicated as important etiological factors in hypokinetic dysarthria secondary to PD (107). Schneider and colleagues (96,97) have described marked sensorimotor deficits in the orofacial and limb systems of individuals with PD. They observed that individuals with PD, compared to neurologically normal age-matched controls, showed greater deficits in tests of sensory function and sensorimotor integration than in tests of motor function. Based on these findings they suggested that one aspect of PD might consist of complex deficits in the utilization of specific sensory inputs to organize and guide movements. They attributed these deficits to abnormal sensory gating or filtering associated with basal ganglia motor dysfunction. Caligiuiri and Abbs (95) have described abnormal orofacial reflexes in some, individuals with PD. Problems in sensory perception of effort have been identified as an important focus of successful speech and voice treatment for individuals with PD (108). Consistent with previous research (42), it has been observed that when individuals with PD are asked to produce "loud" speech (i.e., attempt large movements) they increased their otherwise underscaled "soft" speech to a level within normal limits. However, when they produce this "louder" speech that is perceived to be within normal limits to a listener, individuals with PD complain that they are talking "too loud." Furthermore, individuals with PD often report people around them "must need hearing aides," rather than recognize that their speech has become too soft. Thus, it appears that sensory kinesthesia problems may be a factor in the speech and voice disorder observed in PD. Sensory and perceptual deficits and their role in voice and speech abnormalities in PD have been discussed by Ho and colleagues (41,109). They compared voice loudness perception in individuals with PD and hypophonic dysarthria with that of neurologically normal speakers (42). They found that, unlike normal speakers, the PD patients overestimated the loudness of their speech during both reading and conversation. Ho et al. (42) interpreted these findings to suggest that either impaired speech production is driven by a basic perceptual fault or abnormal speech perception is a consequence of impaired mechanisms involved in the generation of soft speech. The latter explanation is related to the phenomenon of central inhibitory influences of the vocal motor system, via feed-forward mechanisms, on auditory cortical activity during self-produced vocalization. This phenomenon has been demonstrated both in humans and animals (110–112). Ho et al. (41) examined the ability of individuals with PD and the ability of neurologically normal individuals to adjust their voice volume in response to two types of implicit cues: background noise (BGN) and instantaneous auditory feedback (IAF). Control subjects demonstrated the Lombard effect by automatically speaking louder in the presence of BGN. They also decreased speech loudness in the presence of increasing levels of facilitative IAF. Subjects with PD demonstrated decreased overall speech loudness; they were less able than controls to appropriately increase loudness as BGN increased and to decrease volume as IAF increased. However, under explicit loudness instructions, the ability of subjects with PD to regulate loudness was similar to that of the normal controls, suggesting that individuals with PD have the capacity to speak with normal loudness, provided that they consciously attend to speaking loudly. The subjects with PD had overall speech loudness that was always lower than for control subjects, suggesting either a reduction of cortical motor input to the speech subsystems or abnormal perception of their own voice via motor-to-sensory inhibitory mechanisms.

Albin et al. (113) and Penny and Young (114) have suggested that basal ganglia excitatory circuits inadequately activate cortical motor centers and, as a result, motor-neuron pools are not provided with adequate facilitation, thus movements are small and slow. Berardelli et al. (115) has suggested that the defect in motor cortex activation is due to a perceptual failure to select the muscle commands to match external force and speed requirements. Demirci et al. (116) referred to this as a problem with kinesthesia and stated that when individuals with PD match their effort to their kinesthetic feedback, they constantly underscale their movement.

In summary, the neurophysiological mechanisms underlying hypokinetic dysarthria in PD are still poorly understood, especially as far as sensorium is concerned. Research on the role of sensory problems in speech and voice disorders in PD will likely further enhance our understanding of this relationship (96) and improve our ability to successfully treat these individuals.

VI. SWALLOWING DISORDERS

Swallowing disorders occur in upto 95% of individuals with PD (107) and may be among the first signs of the disease (21). Identification of swallowing disorders is extremely important in PD given the ramifications on nutrition and the ability to take oral medication appropriately. Silent aspiration may be observed and pneumonia is sometimes the cause of death in the later stages of PD (117).

Swallowing abnormalities have been reported in all stages of PD (117), and many individuals have more than one type of swallowing dysfunction (18). Disorders in both oral and pharyngeal stages of swallowing have been observed (18,117,118). Sharkawi et al. (20) found dysfunctions during the oral phase of swallowing, in individuals with PD, which included reduced tongue control and strength and reduced oral transit times. Others have reported a "rocking-like"motion of the tongue during the oral phase (21). This motion seemed to occur when the patients were unable to lower the posterior portion of the tongue to propel the bolus into the pharynx. Inability or delayed ability to trigger the swallowing reflex has also been observed in PD (21). These disorders may limit the ability of the individual with PD to control the food or liquid bolus while in the oral cavity. This may lead to choking, penetration, or aspiration of the food or liquid. Reduced nutritional intake, lack of enjoyment in eating, and difficulty taking medications also result from oral phase swallowing dysfunction. The specific neurophysiological mechanisms underlying such dysphagic abnormalities in PD are not clear. Sensory gating and internal cueing deficits, which have been implicated in hypokinetic dysarthria, may also be etiological factors in dysphagia during the oral phase.

Pharyngeal stage dysfunction includes residue in the valleculae due to reduced tongue base retraction. Sharkawi et al. (20) reported this to be the most common disorder in the pharyngeal stage of swallowing. Aspiration may occur in these patients as a result of the residue left in the pharynx after the swallow is complete (21). Leopold and Kagel (18) found several disorders of laryngeal movement during swallowing. These included slow closure, incomplete closure, absent closure, and slowed or delayed laryngeal excursion (18). Increased pharyngeal transit time has also been reported. Silent aspiration has been observed in the later stages of PD and can be a contributory cause of death (22). Dysfunction in the pharyngeal stage of swallowing may also lead to choking, penetration, aspiration, reduced nutritional intake or reduced ability to take medication orally. Again, sensory and internal cueing deficits may underlie these swallowing problems. It is unlikely that muscle rigidity is responsible for dysphagia, since swallowing dysfunction can occur when individuals with PD are optimally medicated for motor symptoms (117).

VII. IMPACT OF PARKINSON'S DISEASE TREATMENTS ON SPEECH AND SWALLOWING

Neuropharmacological and neurosurgical approaches for the treatment of PD have had positive effects on motor function. However, the impact of these treatments on speech, voice, and swallowing production is less compelling. While some studies have reported positive effects of levodopa on motor function (119–125), the magnitude and consistency of improvement in speech tends to be much less impressive (123,124). Studies have reported little variation in speech, voice, and respiratory characteristics at different points in the drug treatment cycle (27,71). Few systematic studies exist on the effect of various surgical treatments on speech and voice. Baker et al. (28) observed a limited effect of fetal dopamine transplant on speech. In addition, significant negative effects on speech, voice, and swallowing have been reported following bilateral thalamotomy (126) and pallidotomy (127). In a study by Schultz et al. (128) acoustic measures were analyzed following unilateral pallidotomy in six individuals with PD. At 3 months postsurgery all individuals demonstrated positive changes in at least one acoustic measure, but not all of the six patients consistently demonstrated those changes. It appears that at this time neuropharmacological and neurosurgical approaches alone do not improve speech and voice consistently and significantly. Therefore, behavioral speech treatment should be considered even for optimally medicated individuals and for those having neurosurgical procedures.

VIII. BEHAVIORAL SPEECH, VOICE, AND SWALLOWING TREATMENT FOR INDIVIDUALS WITH PARKINSON'S DISEASE

Although the incidence of speech and voice disorders in individuals with PD is extremely high, only 3–4% of these individuals receive speech treatment (7,12). One explanation for this discrepancy may be that carryover and long-term treatment outcomes have been disappointing (129–132). This challenge of carryover and long-term treatment outcomes has been observed consistently over a wide range of speech treatments that have been applied in PD (77). These approaches have included training in control of speech rate, prosody, loudness, articulation, and respiration (29). Treatment with instruments such as delayed auditory feedback (DAF), voice amplification devices, and pacing boards have also been of limited long-term success (30,49,77,133).

Carryover and long-term effects are two major challenges in the treatment of hypokinetic dysarthria associated with PD. In general, when dysarthric individuals with PD are in the treatment room and receiving direct stimulation, prodding, or feedback from the speech clinician or an instrument (external cue) (77,134,135), they often show dramatic improvement in their speech and voice production. However, maintaining these improvements (i.e. internalizing the cues to produce loud phonation and increase articulatory movements) is often difficult for these individuals. This consistent observation provides potential insight into the underlying basis for the problems in carryover experienced by most individuals with PD. One explanation for the inability of individuals with PD to maintain treatment gains may be their deficits in sensory gating and internal cueing (23,96,115). Recognition of these problems may improve treatment of motor speech output. Support for these ideas has come from the work of Ramig et al. (31,32), who have documented that training sensory perception of vocal effort appears to be a key element in successful speech treatment for individuals with PD. In addition, neuropsychological problems, such as deficits in implicit or procedural learning (136,137), may underlie the challenges that individuals with PD have in maintaining long-term treatment effects and in learning to automatize newly acquired speech habits.

IX. INTENSIVE VOICE TREATMENT FOR PARKINSON'S DISEASE

Ramig and colleagues (55) have developed an approach to the treatment of speech difficulties in individuals with PD. Unlike approaches that focused on rate or articulation, the LSVT focuses on the speech problem most often observed in individuals with PD, which is, disordered voice.

It is has been hypothesized by Ramig and colleagues that there are at least three features underlying the voice disorder in individuals with PD:

1. An overall amplitude scale down (23,113,114) to the speech mechanism (reduced amplitude of neural drive to the muscles of the speech mechanism), which may result in a "soft voice that is monotone."
2. A problem in sensory perception of effort (23,115), which prevents the individual with PD from accurately monitoring his or her vocal output.
3. Resultant difficulty in independently generating (internal cueing/scaling) the right amount of effort (116,138) to produce adequate loudness.

It is hypothesized that the combination of these factors underlies the speech and voice problems in individuals with PD and makes them particularly resistant to successful

PRE-TREATMENT

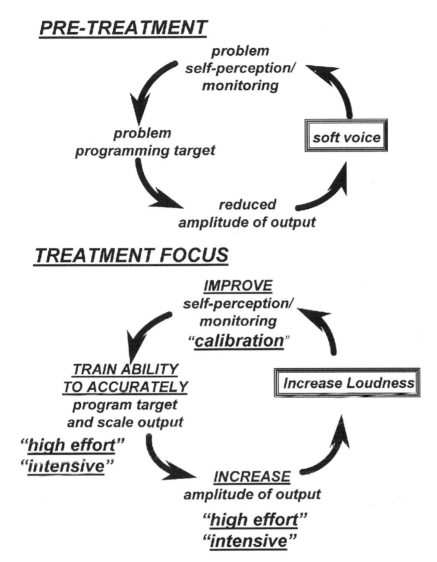

TREATMENT FOCUS

Figure 1 Hypothesized neural basis for the LSVT approach to treating individuals with Parkinson's disease. Pretreatment (top): the soft voice of the patient may be a result of reduced amplitude of output to the speech mechanism. The soft voice is maintained because patients have reduced self-perception/monitoring and fail to realize that the voice is too soft. Therefore, when they program output for another utterance, they downscale the output and continue to produce a soft voice. The LSVT focus (bottom) addresses the soft voice at three levels. High-effort, intensive treatment is designed to train increased amplitude of output to the respiratory phonatory system to generate increased loudness. Patients are then trained to improve self-perception/monitoring of effort so they understand the relationship between increased effort and successful communication. In this way, when they generate an utterance on their own they are able to carry over adequate effort and loudness for communication success outside the treatment room.

treatment. The LSVT has been designed to address these problems. The LSVT has five essential concepts:

1. Focus on voice (increase the amplitude of phonatory output).
2. Improve sensory perception of effort, i.e., "calibration."
3. Administer treatment in a high effort style.
4. Administer treatment intensively (4 times a week for 16 sessions in one month).
5. Quantify treatment-related changes.

Treatment techniques are designed to scale up amplitude to the respiratory and phonatory systems and train sensory perception of effort, internal cueing, and scaling of adequate output (Fig. 1). Administration of treatment four times a week for one month is consistent with principles of motor learning, skill acquisition (139,140), and muscle training (141). In addition, the LSVT is administered in a manner to maximize patient compliance by assigning treatment activities that make an immediate impact on daily functional communication. The rationale for the five concepts of the LSVT is shown in Fig. 2.

X. TREATMENT EFFECTIVENESS DATA FOR THE LSVT®

The LSVT was initially developed during the late 1980s, and initial Phase 1 studies (e.g., case studies, single subject designs, nonrandomized studies) were published (142,143). These studies documented the first evidence of successful treatment outcomes for individuals with PD and suggested that intensive treatment (four times a week for one month) focusing on increasing phonatory effort and self-monitoring of such effort could improve vocal communication in individuals with PD.

Based upon those findings, a number of Phase 2 experimental studies (e.g., randomized, blinded) were carried out. In one study 45 individuals with PD were randomly assigned to one of two forms of treatment: respiratory treatment or respiratory and voice treatment (LSVT). Short- (31) and long-term (32,144,145) outcome data have been reported from these studies. Significant pre- to posttreatment improvements were observed for more variables and were of greater magnitude for the subjects who received the voice and respiratory treatment (LSVT) than for the subjects who received the respiratory treatment alone. Only subjects who received the LSVT had a significant decrease in the impact of PD on their communication. Corresponding perceptual ratings by blinded raters (146) revealed only the male subjects who had the LSVT improved in ratings of breathiness and intonation. The acoustic findings were supported in studies at 1-year (32,147) and 2-year follow-up (145). Only those subjects in the LSVT group improved or maintained vocal SPL above pretreatment levels. In addition, perceptual reports by patients and family members supported the positive impact of treatment on functional daily communication.

In another study (148) 29 individuals with PD were studied over 6 months. Half the group received LSVT and half of the group served as an untreated control group. In addition, an age-matched, healthy, nontreated control group was studied over this time period. Only subjects who received the LSVT demonstrated significant increases in variables such as vocal SPL (related to loudness) and semitone standard deviation (related to intonation) at the 6 month follow-up.

An important aspect of this work was to evaluate the underlying speech mechanism changes accompanying treatment. A study by Smith et al. (60) documented increases in

Goal: Improved functional **oral communication** that "lasts"

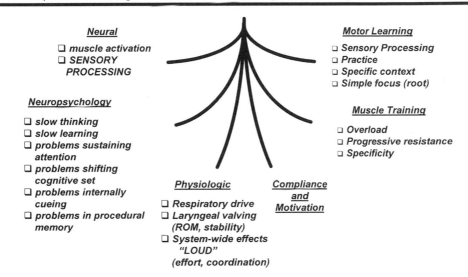

Figure 2 Rationale underlying the five essential concepts and techniques of the LSVT from neural, speech mechanism physiology, motor learning, muscle training, neuropsychological, and compliance perspectives. The neural bases are the reduction in muscle activation and self-monitoring and consequent problem in programming an output target with adequate amplitude. The physiological basis is the focus on respiratory drive and laryngeal valving to generate a maximally efficient vocal source. "LOUD" is used as the system trigger for improving effort and coordination across the speech mechanism. The LSVT is administered in a manner consistent with principles of motor learning in order to maximize treatment effectiveness. Emphasis on sensory processing, increased practice, practice within specific context, and and a simple, root focus (e.g., "LOUD") are key elements of treatment. The neuropsychological aspects of Parkinson disease—slow thinking, slow learning, problems sustaining attention, problems shifting cognitive set, problems internally cueing, and problems in procedural memory—are also taken into account with the LSVT. The LSVT is also administered in a way consistent with muscle training. Treatment technique overloads the muscles using progressive resistance in specific activities. The LSVT is designed to maximize patient compliance. From day 1 of treatment, activities are designed to maximize impact on daily functional communication.

vocal fold closure following treatment in individuals who received the LSVT but not in individuals who received only respiratory treatment. These data were collected outside of the treatment clinic by clinicians not directly involved in the study and therefore support generalization of treatment effects. There was no evidence of hyperfunctional laryngeal behaviors posttreatment in the patients with increased vocal intensity. In fact, Countryman et al. (126) reported a decrease in pretreatment hyperfunctional behavior (false fold overclosure, anterior-posterior hyperfunction, laryngeal elevation) following

LSVT. Consistent with these findings, Ramig and Dromey (149) reported increased subglottal air pressure and maximum flow declination rate accompanying increased vocal SPL following the LSVT. These findings were interpreted to reflect increased respiratory drive and improved vocal fold adduction.

To evaluate application of the LSVT to individuals with other neurological disorders or conditions, a number of case studies were reported. In one case study, the LSVT was applied to an individual with PD who had bilateral thalamotomies (126). In another study, the LSVT was applied to three individuals who had multiple system atrophy or progressive supranuclear palsy (150). While improvements were documented in speech and voice characteristics in these individuals following treatment, the magnitude was not as great as in the subjects with PD.

A finding of interest following the LSVT has been the apparent generalization of phonatory effort from a focus on voice to additional changes throughout the vocal tract. Not only does increased phonatory effort apparently improve vocal characteristics (loudness, pitch variability, vocal quality), it appears to trigger effort and coordination across the speech mechanism. The observation of apparently larger movements in the upper articulatory system following LSVT is consistent with the reports of Schulman (151) that as a speaker talks louder there are accompanying vocal tract and articulatory changes. Ramig et al. documented this observation in individuals with PD (152). Dromey (90) compared the effects of two treatment approaches, LSVT vs. exaggerated articulation during speech, and found the LSVT significantly more effective in improving speech articulation. These generalized effects have been shown to be long-lasting and treatment-specific (144,153). These findings, illustrated in Figure 3, may be useful in the attempt to improve efficiency and simplify speech treatment for individuals who may have multiple speech mechanism problems as well as cognitive limitations, as is common in motor speech disorders.

Positron emission tomography (PET) scan data (154) have demonstrated functional reorganization of speech-motor areas within the brain following the LSVT. Treatment-related changes were found in the right globus pallidus (GP) and in the supplementary motor area (SMA). In the GP, resting state regional cerebral blood flow (rCBF) was significantly reduced posttreatment when compared to pretreatment and significantly increased during sustained phonation when compared to rest. The authors concluded that the LSVT reduced baseline GP over-activity resembling the effect of pallidotomy. However, in addition, the LSVT increased GP activity during vocalization. These findings document the neural basis for behavioral changes following the LSVT.

The goal of the LSVT is to improve functional communication for at least 6–12 months without additional treatment. After the 16 sessions of individual treatment in one month, most patients are able to maintain speech and voice changes for at least 6 months and sometimes for up to 2 years (32,145) without additional speech treatment. Within the 16 initial sessions of treatment, patients are encouraged to establish a daily routine that they maintain on their own once treatment is over. All patients are encouraged to return for a reassessment at 6 months, at which time some patients may benefit from a few "tune-up" sessions. Details of the LSVT have been described in detail elsewhere (108).

Treatment data suggest that individuals with mild to moderate PD have the most positive treatment outcomes following the LSVT. Patients with co-occurring mild to moderate depression and dementia have succeeded in treatment as well (31). Because treatment focuses on voice, all patients must have a laryngeal examination before

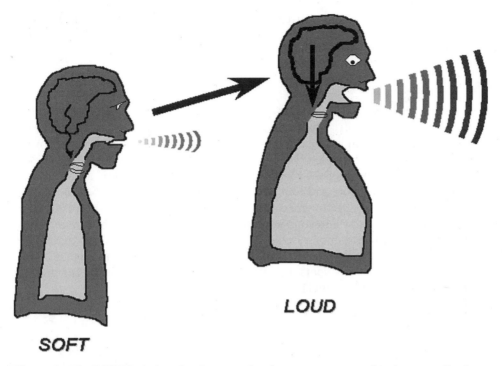

Figure 3 The LSVT is designed to improve the phonatory source and scale up amplitude across the speech mechanism with the global variable LOUD. Increases in loudness can trigger increases in respiratory volumes, vocal fold adduction, articulatory valving, and vocal tract opening. These factors may all contribute to improved speech intelligibility with the simple target of LOUD.

treatment to rule out any contraindications (e.g., vocal nodules, gastric reflux, laryngeal cancer). It is important to clarify that the goal of the LSVT is to maximize phonatory efficiency. It is never the goal to teach "tight or pressed" voice, but rather to improve vocal fold adduction for optimum loudness and quality without undue strain.

XI. SWALLOWING TREATMENT FOR INDIVIDUALS WITH PARKINSON'S DISEASE

Treatment of the swallowing disorders that occur in PD has not been extensively studied. Conventional treatment techniques have included oral motor exercises to improve muscle strength, range of motion and coordination, and behavioral modifications such as the Mendelsohn maneuver, effortful breath-hold, swallow/cough, chin positioning, double swallow, effortful swallow, and diet and liquid modifications (21,155). Effectiveness of these techniques varies and can be dependent upon patient motivation and cooperation, family support, and the timeliness of the referral for a swallowing evaluation. Sharkawi et al. (20) found that the LSVT reduced the swallowing motility disorders by 51%. Some temporal measures of swallowing were also reduced, as was the amount of residue. This is the first study to find positive changes in both voice and swallowing function following intensive voice therapy alone without a therapy focusing on swallowing. De Angelis et al. (156) documented improved voice, speech, and swallowing functions in individuals with PD participating in an intensive treatment with a schedule similar to that of the LSVT with a clinical goal of improved glottic closure. These studies support the utility of intensive voice treatment for the reduction of swallowing dysfunction.

XII. CONCLUSION

Speech, voice, and swallowing problems occur in the majority of individuals with PD and significantly hinder quality of life. While all aspects of speech production may be affected, disordered voice is one of the most common problems. Previous forms of treatment for the disorder of speech and voice in individuals with PD have had modest effectiveness. The LSVT, an intensive treatment program that addresses increased vocal effort and improved sensory perception of vocal effort and loudness, has been documented to be a successful approach in the short and long-term management of PD. The LSVT has been shown to produce favorable effects on swallowing dysfunction in individuals with PD, although these findings are based on preliminary efficacy data. Although the degenerative course of PD cannot be altered at this time, improving functions of oral communication and swallowing are important components in developing the highest levels of functioning and independence for these individuals.

ACKNOWLEDGMENT

This work was supported in part by NIH-NIDCD R01 DC01150, P60 DC00976, and OE-NIDRR 8133G40108.

REFERENCES

1. Scott S, Caird FI, Williams, BO. Communication in Parkinson's Disease. Rockville, MD: An Aspen Publication, 1985.
2. Atarashi J, Uchida E. A clinical study of parkinsonism. Recent Adv Res Nervous Syst 1959; 3:871–882.
3. Canter GJ. Speech characteristics of patients with Parkinson's disease: III. Articulation, diadochokinesis and overall speech adequacy. J Speech Hearing Disord 1965; 30:217–224.
4. Canter GJ. Speech characteristics of patients with Parkinson's disease: II Physiological support for speech. J Speech Hearing Disord 1965b; 30:44–49.
5. Hoberman SG. Speech techniques in aphasia and parkinsonism. J Mich State Med Soc 1958; 57:1720–1723.
6. Logemann J, Fisher H, Boshes B, Blonsky E. Frequency and concurrence of vocal tract dysfunctions in the speech of a large sample of Parkinson patients. J Speech Hearing Disord 1978; 43:47–57.
7. Mutch R, Strucwick A, Roy S, Downie A. Parkinson's disease: disability review and management. BMJ 1986; 293:675–677.
8. Oxtoby M. Parkinson's Disease Patients and Their Social Needs. London: Parkinson's Disease Society, 1982.
9. Selby G. Parkinson's disease. In: Vinken PJ, Bruyn GW, eds. Handbook of Clinical Neurology. Amsterdam: North Holland, 1968.
10. Streifler M, Hofman S. Disorders of verbal expression in parkinsonism. In: Hassler RG, Christ JF, eds. Advances in Neurology. New York: Raven Press, 1984.
11. Uziel A, Bohe M, Cadilhac J, Passouant P. Les troubles de la voix et de la parole dans les syndromes Parkinson'siens. Fol Phoniatr 1975; 27(3):166–176.
12. Hartelius L, Svensson P. Speech and swallowing symptoms associated with Parkinson's disease and multiple sclerosis: a survey. Fol Phoniatr Logoped 1994; 46:9–17.
13. Aronson AE. Clinical Voice Disorders. New York: Thieme-Stratton, 1990.
14. Ho AK, Iansek R, Marigliani C, Bradshaw JL, Gates S. Speech impairment in a large sample of patients with Parkinson's disease. Behav Neurol 1998; 11:131–137.

15. Sapir S, Ramig L, Hoyt P, O'Brien C, Hoehn M. Phonatory-respiratory effort (LSVT®) vs. respiratory effort treatment for hypokinetic dysarthria: comparing speech loudness and quality before and 12 months after treatment. Fol Phoniatr 2002; 54:296–303.

16. Darley FL, Aronson AE, Brown JR. Motor Speech Disorders. Philadelphia: W.B. Saunders, 1975.

17. King J, Ramig LO, Lemke J. Communication ability in Parkinson's disease in relation to employment satisfaction: a survey. Unpublished manuscript, 1996.

18. Leopold NA, Kagel MA. Laryngeal deglutition movement in Parkinson's disease. Neurology 1997; 48:373–375.

19. Croxson SC, Pye I. Dysphagia as the presenting symptom of Parkinson's disease. Geriatr Med 1988.

20. Sharkawi AE, Ramig LO, Logemann JA, Pauloski BR, Rademaker AW, et al. Swallowing and voice effects of Lee Silverman Voice Treatment (LSVT®): A pilot study. J Neurol Neurosurg Psychiatry 2002; 72:31–36.

21. Logemann JA. Evaluation and Treatment of Swallowing Disorders. Austin, TX: Pro-ed publisher, 1998.

22. Robbins J, Logemann JA, Kirshner H. Swallowing and speech production in Parkinson's disease. Ann Neurol 1986; 11:283–287.

23. Barbeau A, Sourkes TL, Murphy CF. Les catecholamines de la maladie de Parkinson's. In: Ajuriaguerra J, ed. Monoamines et Systeme Nerveux Central. Geneve: George, 1962.

24. Birkmayer W, Kiewicz GH. Oder l-Dioxyphenyalanin (l-dopa) Effekt beim Parkinson-syndrom des Menschen. Arch Psychiatr Nervenkr 1962; 203:560–574.

25. Svennilson E, et al. Treatment of parkinsonism by stereotactic thermolesions in the pallidal region. A clinical evaluation of 81 cases. Acta Psychiatr Neurol Scand 1960; 35:358–377.

26. Freed CR, Breeze RE, Rosenberg NL, Schneck SA, Kreik E, et al. Survival of implanted fetal dopamine cells and neurologic improvement 12 to 46 months after transplantation for Parkinson's disease. N Engl J Med 1992; 327(22):1549–1555.

27. Larson K, Ramig LO, Scherer RC. Acoustic and glottographic voice analysis during drug-related fluctuations in Parkinson's disease. J Med Speech-Lang Pathol 1994; 2:211–226.

28. Baker K, Ramig LO, Johnson A, Freed C. Preliminary speech and voice analysis following fetal dopamine transplants in 5 individuals with Parkinson disease. J Speech Hearing Res 1997; 40(3):615–626.

29. Yorkston KM. Treatment efficacy: dysarthria. J Speech Hearing Res 1996; 39:S46–S57.

30. Helm N. Management of palilalia with a pacing board. J Speech Hear Disord 1979; 44:350–353.

31. Ramig L, Countryman S, Thompson L, Horii Y. Comparison of two forms of intensive speech treatment for Parkinson disease. J Speech Hearing Res 1995; 38:1232–1251.

32. Ramig LO, Countryman S, O'Brien C, Hoehn M, Thompson L. Intensive speech treatment for patients with Parkinson's disease: short and long term comparison of two techniques. Neurology 1996; 47:1496–1504.

33. Leanderson R, Meyerson BA, Persson, A. Lip muscle function in parkinsonian dysarthria. Acta Otolaryngol 1972; 74:350–357.

34. Leanderson R, Meyerson BA, Persson, A. Effect of L-dopa on speech in parkinsonism an EMG study of labial articulatory function. J Neurol Neurosurg Psychiatry 1971; 43:679–681.

35. Moore CA, Scudder RR. Coordination of jaw muscle activity in parkinsonian movement: description and response to traditional treatment. In: Yorkston KM, Beukelman DR, eds. Recent Advances in Clinical Dysarthria. Boston: College-Hill Press, 1989.

36. Baker K, Ramig LO, Luschei E, Smith M. Thyroarytenoid muscle activity associated with hypophonia in Parkinson disease and aging. Neurology 1998; 51(6):1592–1598.

37. Hansen DG, Gerratt BR, Ward PH. Cinegraphic observations of laryngeal function in Parkinson's disease. Laryngoscope 1984; 94:348–353.

38. Estenne M, Hubert M, Troyer AD. Respiratory-muscle involvement in Parkinson's disease. N Engl J Med 1984; 311:1516.

39. Ackermann H, Ziegler W. Articulatory deficits in parkinsonian dysarthria. J Neurol Neurosurg Psychiatry 1991; 54:1093–1098.

40. Hoodin RB, Gilbert HR. Nasal airflows in Parkinsonian speakers. J Commun Disord 1989; 22:169–180.

41. Ho AK, Bradshaw JL, Iansek R, Alfredson R. Speech volume regulation in Parkinson's disease: effects of implicit cues and explicit instructions. Neuropsychologia 1999; 37:453–1460.

42. Ho AK, Bradshaw JL, Iansek T. Volume perception in parkinsonian speech. Mov Disord 2000; 15:1125–1131.

43. Darley FL, Aronson AE, Brown JR. Clusters of deviant speech dimensions in the dysarthrias. J Speech Hear Res 1969; 12:462–469.

44. Darley FL, Aronson A, Brown J. Differential diagnostic patterns of dysarthria. J Speech Hearing Res 1969; 12:246–269.
45. Logemann J, Boshes B, Fisher H. The steps in the degeneration of speech and voice control in Parkinson's disease. In: Siegfried J, ed. Parkinson's Diseases: Rigidity, Akinesia, Behavior. Vienna: Hans Huber, 1973.
46. Stewart C, Winfield L, Hunt A, Bressman SB, Fahn S, Blitzer A, Brin MF. Speech dysfunction in early Parkinson's disease. Mov Disord 1995; 10(5):562–565.
47. Ludlow CL, Bassich CJ. Relationships between perceptual ratings and acoustic measures of hypokinetic speech. In: McNeil MR, Rosenbek JC, Aronson AE, eds. The Dysarthrias: Physiology, Acoustics, Perception, Management. San Diego: College-Hill, 1984.
48. Canter GJ. Speech characteristics of patients with Parkinson's disease: I. Intensity, pitch and duration. J Speech Hear Disord 1963; 28:221–229.
49. Ludlow CL, Bassich CJ. Relationships between perceptual ratings and acoustic measures of hypokinetic speech. In: McNeil MR, Rosenbeck JC, Aronson AE, eds. Dysarthria of Speech: Physiology-Acoustics-Linguistics-Management. San Diego: College-Hill Press, 1983.
50. Metter EJ, Hanson WR. Clinical and acoustical variability in hypokinetic dysarthria. J Commun Disord 1986; 19:347–366.
51. Fox C, Ramig L. Vocal sound pressure level and self-perception of speech and voice in men and women with idiopathic Parkinson disease. Am J Speech-Lang Pathol 1997; 2:29–42.
52. Ho AK, Iansek R, Bradshaw JL. Motor instability in parkinsonian speech intensity. Neuropsychiatry Neuropsychol Behav Neurol 2001; 14:109–116.
53. King J, Ramig L, Lemke JH, Horii Y. Parkinson's disease: longitudinal changes in acoustic parameters of phonation. J Med Speech-Lang Pathol 1994; 2:29–42.
54. Zwirner P, Murry T, Woodson GE. Phonatory function of neurologically impaired patients. J Commun Disord 1991; 24:287–300.
55. Ramig L, Titze OR, Scherer R, Ringel, SP. Acoustic analysis of voices of patients with neurologic disease: rationale and preliminary data. Ann Otolaryngol Rhinol Laryngol 1988; 97:164–172.
56. Ramig LO, Shipp T. Comparative measures of vocal tremor and vocal vibrato. J Voice 1987; 1:62–167.
57. Ludlow CL, Bassich CJ, Connor NP, Coulter DC. Phonatory characteristics of vocal fold tremor. J Phonetics 1986; 14:509–515.
58. Philippbar SA, Robin DA, Luschei ES. Limb, jaw and vocal tremor in Parkinson's patients. In: Yorkston KM, Beukelman DR, eds. Recent Advances in Clinical Dysarthria. Boston: College-Hill Press, 1989.
59. Winholtz WS, Ramig LO. Vocal tremor analysis with the vocal demodulator. NCVS Status Prog Rep 1992; 2:119–137.
60. Smith M, Ramig LO, Dromey C, Perez K, Samandari R. Intensive voice treatment in Parkinson's disese: laryngostroboscopic findings. J Voice 1995; 9:453–459.
61. Perez K, Ramig LO, Smith M, Dromey C. The Parkinson larynx: tremor and videostroboscopic findings. J Voice 1996; 10:354–361.
62. Gerratt BR, Hansen DG, Berke GS. Glottographic measures of laryngeal function in individuals with abnormal motor control. In: Baer T, Sasaki C, Harris K, eds. Laryngeal Function in Phonation and Respiration. Boston: College-Hill Press, 1987.
63. Hirose H, Joshita Y. Laryngeal behavior in patients with disorders of the central nervous system. Hirano M, Kirchner JA, Bless DMNeurolaryngology: Recent Advances. Boston: Little, Brown, 1987.
64. Boecker H, Ceballos-Baumann A, Bartenstein P, Weindl A, Siebner HR, Fassbender T, Munz F, Schwaiger M, Conrad B. Sensory processing in Parkinson's and Huntington's disease: investigations with 3D H(2)(15)O-PET. Brain 1999; 122:1651–1665.
65. Luschei ES, Ramig LO, Baker KL, Smith M. Discharge characteristics of laryngeal single motor units during phonation in young and older adults and in persons with Parkinson disease. J Neurophysiol 1999; 81:2131–2139.
66. Cramer W. De spaak bij patienten met Parkinsonisme. Logop Phoniatr 1940; 22:17–23.
67. De la Torre R, Mier, M, Boshes B. Evaluation of respiratory function: preliminary observations. Q Bull Northwestern University Med School 1960; 34:332–336.
68. Laszewski Z. Role of the department of rehabilitation in preoperative evaluation of parkinsonian patients. J Am Geriatr Soc 1956; 4:1280–1284.
69. Mueller PB. Parkinson's disease: motor-speech behavior in a selected group of patients. Folia Phoniatr 1971; 23:333–346.

70. Marquardt TP. Characteristics of speech in Parkinson's disease: electromyographic, structural movement and aerodynamic measurements. Seattle: University of Washington, 1973.

71. Solomon NP, Hixon, TJ. Speech breathing in Parkinson's disease. J Speech Hear Res 1993; 36:294–310.

72. Schiffman PL. A "saw-tooth" pattern in Parkinson's disease. Chest 1985; 87:24–126.

73. Vincken WG, Gauthier SG, Dollfuss RE, Hanson RE, Parauay CM, Cosio MG. Involvement of upper-airway muscles in extrapyramidal disorders, a cause of airflow limitation. N Engl J Med 1984; 311(7):438–442.

74. Murdoch BE, Chenery HJ, Bowler S, Ingram, JCL. Respiratory function in Parkinson's subjects exhibiting a perceptible speech deficit: a kinematic and spirometric analysis. J Speech Hear Disord 1989; 54:610–626.

75. Hammen VL, Yorkston KM, Beukelman DR. Pausal and speech duration characteristics as a function of speaking rate in normal and parkinsonian dysarthric individuals. In: Yorkston KM, Beukelman DR, eds. Recent Advances in Clinical Dysarthria. Boston: College-Hill Press, 1989.

76. Hanson WR, Metter EJ. DAF Speech Rate Modification in Parkinson's disease: A report of two cases. In: Berry WR, ed. Clinical Dysarthria. San Diego: College-Hill Press, 1983.

77. Adams SG. Hypokinetic dysarthria in Parkinson's Disease. In: McNeil MR, ed. Clinical Management of Sensorimotor Speech Disorders. New York: Thieme, 1997.

78. Sapir S, Pawlas AA, Ramig LO, Countryman S, O'Brien C, Hoehn M, Thompson L. Voice and speech abnormalities in Parkinson disease: relation to severity of motor impairment, duration of disease, medication, depression, gender, and age. J Med Speech Lang Pathol 2001; 9(4):213–226.

79. Weismer G. Articulatory characteristics of parkinsonian dysarthria: segmental and phrase-level timing, spirantization and glottal-supraglottal coordination. In: McNeil MR, Rosenbeck J, Aronson AE, eds. The Dysarthrias: Physiology, Acoustics, Perception and Management. San Diego: College Hill Press, 1984.

80. Forrest K, Weismer G, Turner G. Kinematic, acoustic and perceptual analysis of connected speech produced by parkinsonian and normal geriatric adults. J Acoust Soc Am 1989; 85:2608–2622.

81. Ackermann H, Konczak J, Hertrich I. The temporal control of repetitive articulatory movements in Parkinson's disease. Brain Lang 1997; 56:312–319.

82. Caligiuiri MP. Labial kinematics during speech in patients with Parkinsonian rigidity. Brain 1987; 110:1033–1044.

83. Caligiuiri MP. The influence of speaking rate on articulatory hypokinesia in parkinsonian dysarthria. Brain Lang 1989; 36:493–502.

84. Caliguri MP. Short-term fluctuations in orofacial motor control in Parkinson's disease. In: Yorkson KM, Beukelman DR, eds. Recent Advances in Clinical Dysarthria. Boston: College Hill, 1989.

85. Conner NP, Abbs JH. Task-dependent variations in parkinsonian motor impairments. Brain 1991; 114:321–332.

86. Conner NP, Abbs JH, Cole KJ, Gracco VL. Parkinsonian deficits in serial mulitarticulate movements for speech. Brain 1989; 112(pt 4):997–1009.

87. Hirose H, Kiritan, S, Ushijima T, Yoshioka H, Sawashima M. Patterns of dysarthric movements in patients with parkinsonism. Fol Phoniatr 1981; 33(4):204–215.

88. Hirose H. Pathophysiology of motor speech disorders (dysarthria). Fol Phoniatr (Basel) 1986; 38:61–88.

89. Hunker CJ, Abbs JH, Barlow SM. The relationship between parkinsonian rigidity and hypokinesia in the orofacial system: a quantitative analysis. Neurology 1982; 32:749–754.

90. Dromey C. Articulatory kinematics in patients with Parkinson's disease using different speech treatment approaches. J Med Speech-Lang Pathol 2001; 8:155–161.

91. Gath I, Yair E. Analysis of vocal tract parameters in parkinsonian speech. J Acoust Soc Am 1988; 84:1628–1634.

92. Rosenfeld D. Parmacologic approaches to speech motor disorders. In: Vogel D, Cannito M, eds. Treating Disordered Speech Motor Control. Austin: Pro-ed, 1991:111–152.

93. Hunker CJ, Abbs JH. Physiological analyses of parkinsonian tremors in the orofacial system. In: McNeil MR, Rosenbek JC, Aronson AE The Dysarthrias: Physiology, Acoustics, Perception, Management. San Diego: College-Hill Press, 1984.

94. Netsell R, Daniel B, Celesia GG. Acceleration and weakness in parkinsonian dysarthria. J Speech Hear Disord 1975; 40:170–178.

95. Caligiuiri MP, Abbs JH. Response properties of the perioral reflex in Parkinson's disease. Exp Neurol 1987; 98:563–572.

96. Schneider JS, Diamond SG, Markham CH. Deficits in orofacial sensorimotor function in Parkinson's disease. Ann Neurol 1986; 19:275–282.

97. Schneider JS, Lidsky TI. Basal Ganglia and Behavior: Sensory Aspects of Motor Functioning. Toronto: Hans Huber, 1987.
98. Caligiuri MP. Labial kinematics during speech in patients with parkinsonian rigidity. Brain 1987; 110:1033–1044.
99. Connor NP, Abbs JH, Cole KJ, Gracco VL. Parkinsonian deficits in serial multiarticulate movements for speech. Brain 1989; 112:997–1009.
100. Connor NP, Abbs JH. Task-dependant variations in parkinsonian motor impairments. Brain 1991; 114:321–332.
101. Hoodin RB, Gilbert HR. Parkinsonian dysarthria: an aerodynamic and perceptual description of velopharyngeal closure for speech. Fol Phoniatr 1989; 41:249–258.
102. Koller WC. Sensory symptoms in PD. Neurology 1984; 34:957–959.
103. Tatton WG, Eastman MJ, Bedingham W, Verrier MC, Brucc IC. Defective utilization of sensory input as the basis for bradykinesia, rigidity and decreased movement repertoire in Parkinson's disease: a hypothesis. Can J Neurosci 1984; 11:136–143.
104. Diamond SG, Schneider JS, Markham CH. Oral sensorimotor defects in patients with Parkinson's disease. Adv Neurol 1987; 45:335–338.
105. Graber S, Hertrich I, Daum I, Spieker S, Ackermann H. Speech perception deficits in Parkinson's disease: underestimation of time intervals compromises identification of durational phonetic contrasts. Brain Lang 2002; 82:65–74.
106. Solomon NP, Robin DA, Lorell DM, Rodnitzky RL, Luschei ES. Tongue function testing in Parkinson's disease: indicators of fatigue. In: Till JA, Yorkston KM, Beukelman DR, eds. Motor Speech Disorders: Advances in Assessment and Treatment. Baltimore: Paul H. Brooks, 1994: 147–160.
107. Fox CM, Morrison CE, Ramig LO, Sapir S. Current perspectives on the Lee Silverman Voice Treatment (LSVT) for individuals with idiopathic Parkinson's disease. Am J Speech-Lang Pathol 2002; 11:111–123.
108. Ramig LO, Pawlas A, Countryman S. The Lee Silverman Voice Treatment (LSVT): A Practical Guide to Treating the Voice and Speech Disorders in Parkinson Disease. Iowa City, IA: National Center for Voice and Speech, 1995.
109. Ho AK, Iansek R, Bradshaw JL. Regulations of parkinsonian speech volume: the effect of interlocuter distance. J Neurol Neurosurg Psychiatry 1999; 67(2):199–202.
110. Curio G, Neuloh G, Numminen J, Jousmaki V, Hari R. Speaking modifies voice-evoked activity in the human auditory cortex. Human Brain Mapping 2000; 9:183–191.
111. Numminen J, Curio G. Differential effects of overt, covert and replayed speech on vowel-evoked responses of the human auditory cortex. Neurosci Lett 1999; 27:29–32.
112. Paus T, Perry DW, Zatorre RJ, Worsley KJ, Evans AC. Modulation of cerebral blood flow in the human auditory cortex during speech: role of motor-to-sensory discharges. Eur J Neurosci 1996; 8:2236–2246.
113. Albin RL, Young AB, Penny JB. The functional anatomy of basal ganglia disorders. Trends Neurosci 1989; 12:366–375.
114. Penny JB, Young AB. Speculations on the functional anatomy of basal ganglia disorders. Annu Rev Neurosci 1983; 6:73–94.
115. Berardelli A, Dick JP, Rothwell JC, Day BL, Marsden CD. Scaling of the size of the first agonist EMG burst during rapid wrist movements in patients with Parkinson's disease. J Neurol Neurosurg Psychiatry 1986; 49(11):1273–1279.
116. Demirci M, Grill, McShane, Hallet M. Impairment of kinesthesia in Parkinson's disease. Neurology 1995; 45:A218.
117. Nilsson H. Quantitative aspects of swallowing. Department of Neurology, Sweden, 1998.
118. Stroudley J, Walsh M. Radiographic assessment of dysphagia in Parkinson's disease. Br J Radiol 1991; 64:890–893.
119. Critchley EMR. Speech disorders of parkinsonism: a review. J Neurol Neurosurg Psychiatry 1981; 44:751–758.
120. Mawdsley C, Gamsu CV. Periodicity of speech in parkinsonism. Nature 1971; 231:315–316.
121. Mawdsley C. Speech and levodopa. Adv Neurol 1973; 3:33–47.
122. Nakano KK, Zubick H, Tyley HR. Speech defects of parkinsonian patients. Neurology 1973; 23(8):865–870.
123. Rigrodsky S, Morrison EB. Speech changes in parkinsonism during L-dopa therapy: preliminary findings. J Am Geriatr Soc 1970; 18:142–151.
124. Wolfe VI, Garvin JS, Bacon M, Waldrop W. Speech changes in Parkinson's disease during treatment with L-dopa. J Commun Disord 1975; 8(3):271–279.

125. Yaryura-Tobias JA, Diamond B, Merlis S. Verbal communication with L-dopa treatment. Nature 1971; 234:224–225.
126. Countryman S, Ramig LO. Effects of intensive voice therapy on speech deficits associated with bilateral thalamotomy in Parkinson's disease: a case study. J Med Speech-Lang Pathol 1993; 1(4):233–249.
127. Ghika J, Ghika-Schmid F, Fankhauser H, Assal G, Vingerhoets F, Albanese A, Bogousslavsky J, Favre J. Bilateral contemporaneous posteroventral pallidotomy for the treatment of Parkinson's disease: neuropsychological and neurological side effects. Report of four cases and review of the literature. J Neurosurg 1999; 91(2):313–321.
128. Schultz GM, Peterson T, Sapienza CM, Greer M, Friedman W. Voice and speech characteristics of persons with Parkinson's disease pre- and post-pallidotomy surgery: preliminary findings. J Speech Hear Res 1999; 42:1176–1194.
129. Weiner WJ, Lang AE. Movement Disorders; A Comprehensive Survey. Mount Kisko, NY: Futura, 1989.
130. Sarno MT. Speech impairment in Parkinson's disease. Arch Phys Med Rehabil 1968:269–275.
131. Allan CM. Treatment of non-fluent speech resulting from neurological disease: treatment of dysarthria. Br J Disord Commun 1970; 5:3–5.
132. Greene HCL. The Voice and Its Disorders. London: Pitman Medical, 1980.
133. Downie AW, Low JM, Lindsay DD. Speech disorders in parkinsonism: usefulness of delayed auditory feedback in selected cases. Br J Disord Commun 1981; 16:35–139.
134. Scott S, Caird FL. Speech therapy for Parkinson's disease. J Neurol Neurosurg Psychiatry 1983; 46:140–144.
135. Rubow RT, Swift E. A microcomputer-based wearable biofeedback device to improve transfer of treatment in parkinsonian dysarthria. J Speech Hearing Disord 1985; 50:178–185.
136. McNamara P, Obler LK, Au R, Durso R, Albert ML. Speech monitoring skills in Alzheimer's disease, Parkinson's disease and normal aging. Brain Lang 1992; 42:38–51.
137. Saint-Cyr JA, Taylor AE, Lang AE. Procedural learning and neostriatial dysfunction in man. Brain 1988; 111:941–959.
138. Stelmach GE. Basal ganglia impairment and force control. In: Requin J, Stelmach GE, eds. Tutorial in Motor Neuroscience. Netherlands: Kluwer Academic Publishers, 1991.
139. Schmidt RA. Motor Control and Learning. Champaign, Illinois: Human Kinetic Publishers, 1988.
140. Schmidt RA. A schema theory of discrete motor skill learning. Psychol Rev 1975; 82:225–260.
141. Astrand PO, Rodahl K. Textbook of Work Physiology. New York: McGraw-Hill, 1970.
142. Ramig LO, Bonitati C, Lemke J, Horii Y. Voice treatment for patients with Parkinson disease: development of an approach and preliminary efficacy data. J Med Speech-Lang Pathol 1994; 2:191–209.
143. Ramig LO. The role of phonation in speech intelligibility: a review and preliminary data from patients with Parkinson's disease. In: Kent RD, ed. Intelligibility in Speech Disorders: Theory, Measurement and Management. Amsterdam: John Benjamin, 1992.
144. Dromey C, Ramig LO, Johnson A. Phonatory and articulatory changes associated with increased vocal intensity in Parkinson disease: a case study. J Speech Hear Res 1995; 38:751–763.
145. Ramig LO, Sapir S, Countryman S, Pawlas AA, O'Brien C, Hoehn M, Thompson L. Intensive voice treatment (LSVT®) for individuals with Parkinson's disease: a 2 year follow-up. J Neurol Neurosurg Psychiatry 2001; 71:493–498.
146. Baumgartner C, Sapir S, Ramig LO. Voice quality changes following phonatory-respiratory effort treatment (LSVT®) versus respiratory effort treatment for individuals with parkinson disease. J Voice 2001; 15(1):105–114.
147. Sapir S, Ramig LO, Hoyt P, Countryman S, O'Brien C, Hoehn M. Phonatory-respiratory effort (LSVT®) vs. respiratory effort treatment for hypokinetic dysarthria: Comparing speech loudness and quality before and 12 months after treatment. Academy of Neurology, Vancouver, October 1999.
148. Ramig L, Sapir S, Fox C, Countryman S. Changes in vocal intensity following intensive voice treatment (LSVT®) in individuals with Parkinson disease: a comparison with untreated patients and with normal age-matched controls. Mov Disord 2001; 16:79–83.
149. Ramig LO, Dromey C. Aerodynamic mechanisms underlying treatment-related changes in SPL in patients with Parkinson disease. J Speech Hear Res 1996; 39:798–807.
150. Countryman S, Ramig LO, Pawlas AA. Speech and voice deficits in parkinsonian plus syndromes: Can they be treated? J Med Speech-Lang Pathol 1994; 2:211–225.
151. Schulman R. Articulatory dynamics of loud and normal speech. J Acoust Soc Am 1989; 85:295–312.

152. Ramig LO, Dromey C, Johnson A, Scherer R. The effects of phonatory, respiratory and articulatory effect treatment on speech and voice in Parkinson's disease. Motor Speech Conference, Sedona, AZ, April 1994.

153. Johnson A, Strand E, Ramig . The effect of intensive respiratory and laryngeal treatment on single word speech intelligibility and select articulatory acoustics in patients with Parkinson's disease. J Med Speech-Lang Pathol.

154. Liotti M, Ramig LO, Vogel D, New P, Cook C, Ingham RJ, Ingham JC, Fox P. Hypophonia in Parkinson's disease neural correlates of voice treatment revealed by PET. Neurology 2003; 60:432–440.

155. Yorkston KM, Miller RM, Strand EA. Management of Speech and Swallowing in Degenerative Diseases. Communication Skill Builders 1997.

156. De Angelis EC, Mourao LF, Ferraz HB, Behlau MS, Pontes PA, Andrade LA. Effect of voice rehabilitation on oral communication of Parkinson's disease patients. Acta Neurol Scand 1997; 96:199–205.

35

Physical and Occupational Therapy

Tanya Simuni, Katherine M. Martinez, and Mark W. Rogers

Feinberg School of Medicine, Northwestern University, Chicago, Illinois, U.S.A.

I. INTRODUCTION

Nonpharmacological therapy (physical, occupational, and speech therapies) plays a significant role in the multidisciplinary care of Parkinson's disease (PD) patients. Physical therapy (PT) and occupational therapy (OT) have traditionally constituted the mainstream treatment of postural instability, gait dysfunction, and range of motion (ROM) limitations in PD. Despite common use of PT/OT in PD, there are little objective data supporting their efficacy. There is a need for large randomized prospective studies to define the type, duration, and long-term implications of PT/OT in PD. This chapter will review available literature on the use of PT and OT in PD and outline an algorithmic approach to different PT strategies.

II. LITERATURE REVIEW

There are no data on the impact of PT/OT on the rate of PD progression. The majority of published studies focus on the role of PT as an adjunct intervention for the symptomatic management of PD. The studies that examine exercise and its role in PD vary significantly. The studies use different exercise types, intensities, and durations for various stages of PD. These variations make study comparisons challenging and provide minimal guidelines for the clinical use of PT. Some of the key randomized studies are reviewed below (Table 1). An in-depth review of published data can be found in the Cochrane database of systematic reviews (1,2).

There are few controlled studies examining the efficacy of PT in PD. Gibberd et al. (3) conducted a controlled crossover study of PT in PD. Twenty-four patients with stable medically treated PD were enrolled in the study. Subjects were assigned to active therapy versus inactive therapy groups (table games and crafts). Active therapy consisted of 3 months of outpatient PT, after which subjects received inactive therapy. The authors concluded that outpatient PT was not beneficial for patients with stable PD. The study

Table 1 Studies Comparing Modes of Therapy for Parkinson's Disease

Study (Ref.)	Type of intervention	Design	n	Duration	Follow-up
Gibberd, et al. 1981 (3)	PT vs. control	Crossover	24	3 months	None
Palmer, et al. 1986 (8)	PT vs. karate	Parallel group	14(7/7)	12 weeks	None
Gauthier, et al. 1987 (11)	OT vs. control	Parallel group	59(30/29)	5 weeks	12 months
Hurwitz 1989 (22)	PT vs. control	Parallel group	30(15/15)	8 months	None
Formisano, et al. 1992 (5)	PT vs. control	Parallel group	33 (16/17)	4 months	None
Comella, et al. 1994 (6)	PT vs. control	Crossover	16	4 weeks	6 months
Dam, et al. 1996 (19)	PT vs. sens PT	Parallel group	40 (20/20)	3×1-month sessions	9 months
Mohr, et al. 1996 (9)	PT vs. behavioral Tx	Parallel group	41 (20/21)	10 weeks	None
Thaut, et al. 1996 (27)	PT vs. rhythm PT vs. control	Parallel group	37 (15/11/11)	3 weeks	None
Schenkman, et al. 1998 (7)	PT vs. control	Parallel group	46 (23/23)	10 weeks	None
Marchese, et al. 2000 (20)	PT vs. sens PT	Parallel group	20 (10/10)	6 weeks	6 weeks
Miyai, et al. 2000 (10)	PT vs. treadmill	Crossover	10	4 weeks	None

PT = physical therapy; OT = occupational therapy; sens = sensory enhanced; TX = therapy.

was critiqued as to whether the selected outcome measures were optimal (4). Formisano et al. (5) studied the efficacy of a 4-month outpatient PT program compared to no therapy but equivalent staff attention time for the control group. Assessment was based on the Northwestern University Disability Scale. The PT group demonstrated improvement only in walking. Comella et al. (6) demonstrated a positive impact of PT on overall function of PD patients compared to controls based on improvements in the Unified Parkinson's Disease Rating Scale (UPDRS) motor and activities of daily living (ADL) subscores. The study was designed as a randomized prospective crossover study in which 16 subjects received 4 weeks of PT and had 4 weeks of normal activity separated by 6 months. However, the impact was transitory and subsided after the 6-month follow-up. Schenkman et al. (7) conducted a study in which 53 subjects were randomized to either a PT or placebo group. Patients in the PT group underwent an intensive exercise program aimed at improvement of spinal flexibility for 10 weeks. The study demonstrated a positive impact of PT on functional axial rotation and functional reach, a balance measure, and an indicator of the likelihood of falls. However, the duration of benefit was unclear, as the study did not have a long-term follow-up.

A number of studies focused on the comparative efficacy of different PT strategies. Palmer et al. (8) compared two types of physical therapy: stretching exercises versus karate training. Both groups received 12 weeks of outpatient group therapy with the assigned treatment modality. Both groups demonstrated improvement in tremor and bradykinesia but not rigidity. Timed walking improved in both groups but reached statistical significance only in the karate group. The study concluded that PT is beneficial independent of the specific modality. Mohr et al. (9) compared efficacy of standard PT versus behavioral therapy focused on relaxation stress reduction and social interaction training. Outcome was assessed based on the UPDRS and quality-of-life (QOL) measures. The authors demonstrated the beneficial effect of behavioral therapy on tremor reduction and QOL measures but no significant difference based on UPDRS. Miyai et al. (10) studied the impact of treadmill training with body weight support on functional disability in PD compared to conventional PT. Treadmill training resulted in greater improvement in UPDRS ADL and motor performance compared to conventional PT. The benefit was specifically noticed in speed of walking and gait initiation.

Gauthier et al. (11) studied the impact of OT on PD. Fifty-nine patients were randomly assigned to either 5 weeks of outpatient OT conducted twice a week in a group session or no therapy. Subjects were evaluated at the end of 5 weeks of therapy and 6 and 12 months later. The outcome measures included the Barthel Index of Activities of Daily Living, the Purdue Peg Board for dexterity evaluation, and items from an exptrapyramidal rating scale for assessment of PD signs. The study demonstrated clear benefit of OT at the end of the treatment phase that persisted at 6 months, and even at 12-month follow-up the active therapy group still demonstrated an improved degree of bradykinesia compared to baseline. This is the only long-term controlled study of efficacy of OT in PD management.

There is a paucity of data on the efficacy of PT/OT in the multidisciplinary management of PD. Little literature is available on therapeutic models for managing PD (12–14). Well-designed randomized controlled studies with long-term follow-up are necessary to establish the role of particular PT regimens in the treatment of PD. Meanwhile the choice of PT modality is based on the expertise and practice of the physical therapist involved in the care of the patient.

III. APPROACH TO PT INTERVENTION IN PD

PT intervention is important in the management of any condition associated with motor disability, specifically PD. Physical therapist knowledge of the pathology of movement disorders, strategies, and compensations for enhanced motor performance can improve PD disability by:

Minimizing secondary complications of PD (biomechanical, musculoskeletal, cardiovascular, respiratory, strength, balance, falls) through specific exercise and health-promotion strategies.

Enhancing motor performance of functional tasks with strategies to compensate for the basal ganglia pathology (visual and auditory cueing, task sequence, alignment, mental practice).

Educating and teaching adaptation for patient and caregiver (benefits of exercise, fall prevention, strategies for efficient movement, environmental changes, support groups).

Intervening during late stages when the PD patient is more dependent (positioning, bed mobility, skin care, equipment, caregiver training).

With advancements in the medical management of PD, patients are often not referred for PT until significant functional disability has occurred. However, an exercise regimen is important at any stage of the disease, even prior to the onset of functionally evident motor disability. Bridgewater and Sharpe (15) demonstrated changes in axial range of motion even in patients with early PD, which improved after 12 weeks of an aerobics-based exercise program. Optimizing performance at this early stage might minimize the overall rate of decline and the development of secondary complications of the disease.

A. Early PD

Patients should be educated as to the nature of motor disability in PD and potential functional limitations. Even in the absence of functional motor disability, it is beneficial to obtain a PT consultation to design an at-home exercise regimen. PD patients should be encouraged to continue their regular physical activities such as walking, house and yard chores, swimming, golf, yoga, tai chi, bowling, etc. If a patient does not engage in a specific physical activity, he or she should be encouraged to undertake a regular walking program. The patient's exercise habits and adherence to the scheduled routine should be reviewed regularly at physician visits. The routine should consist of a combination of stretching and aerobic exercises. Ideally the patient should exercise three times a week and perform aerobic exercises for a minimum of 30 minutes two to three times a week. An example of an exercise regimen for PD patients is shown in Table 2.

B. Moderately Advanced PD with Preserved Postural Stability

As the disease progresses, the PT regimen should be modified to develop appropriate compensatory strategies to maximize the current level of functional ability. Patients with later-stage PD have difficulty accomplishing complex sequences of movements. However, their motor performance can be enhanced by consciously focusing their attention on performing each component of a sequence separately.

1. Sensory Cues

Improvement of PD gait dysfunction with visual cues is a well-known, yet poorly understood phenomenon. PD patients can perform tasks better when they focus on the task at hand or rely on external cues (13,16). There are few studies that specifically address the value of various external cues (visual, auditory, and sensory) in PD PT regimens. Martin (17) examined the role of sensory cues in PD and demonstrated improvement in PD gait when visual cues were placed on the floor. Further studies supported the use of visual cues placed perpendicular to the direction of gait and spaced appropriately for the individual's step length for improving ambulation (18). Auditory cueing, most frequently reported as use of a metronome or a steady beat of music, is another form of external cueing used in PD. Dam et al. (19) compared a conventional PT regimen versus the same exercises performed with sensory enhancement including the use of a mirror, colored blocks, and other visual cues during exercise while listening to audio-cued tapes. There were no differences between the groups at the end of the active therapy phase, and both groups demonstrated benefit from PT. However, a month after completing therapy the conventional PT group was no different from baseline, while the sensory-cued group continued to demonstrate benefit based on the Northwestern University Disability Scale.

Table 2 Exercise Program for Patients with Early PD

I. Daily Stretching

Morning stretch: lie flat on your back without a pillow, bring arms overhead as far as you can and hold for 5 seconds. Repeat 10 times.

Lower trunk rotation: lie on your back roll your knees to one side and your arms and head to the other side.

Gastronemius stretch: stand about 2 feet away from the wall. Place hands on the wall and lean forward keeping your heels on the floor.

Evening stretch: prone lying with arms out to side or overhead for 1–2 minutes (work up to 5–10 minutes).

II. Strengthening/Balance/Posture/Functional Activities (three times per week)

From standing position take a large step forward and reach forward with the opposite arm.

Practice stand to sit from different height surfaces without upper extremity support (work toward lowest surface possible).

Practice stepping up and down a step or curb (vary speed and height of step). A metronome and/or music of various tempos could be used for auditory cues.

Practice stepping over an imaginary object. This will work on imagery, balance (single limb support), and foot clearance in stepping.

Trunk rotation and reaching: sit in a chair with the back of the chair against a table. Twist to the right and pretend to pick up an object off the table. Rotate as far as you can. Repeat in both directions.

III. Aerobic Exercise

Continue regular physical activities such as golf, yoga, bowling, swimming, jogging, house and yard chores.

Begin a walking program for a minimum of 30 minutes 2–3 times per week. Walking should emphasize long strides, adequate foot clearance, and walking at different speeds and terrain if possible. Walking can also be performed on a treadmill. A metronome and/or music of various tempos could be used for auditory cues.

Marchese et al. (20) demonstrated similar results. Visual cues are also useful in OT for PD. PD patients showed increased speed when reaching for a moving ball while maintaining accuracy of movement comparable to healthy individuals (21). Other studies have shown that lined paper can assist patients with PD while writing to utilize larger strokes and overcome micrography (13).

The mechanism of sensory cueing benefit in PD is poorly understood but is believed to be related to compensation of the defective internal trigger from the pallidum to the supplementary motor area. Alternatively, external cues may assist movement performance by engaging intact motor pathways involving the premotor cortex rather than impaired basal ganglia–supplementary motor area circuits. Sensory cueing is now routinely incorporated in PD PT exercise sessions and can be included in self-administered home PT programs by using video/audiotapes.

2. Home Versus Outpatient Physical Therapy

The majority of ambulatory PD patients receive PT in the outpatient setting, although there is a value of assessment of performance in the home environment (22). Some OT centers have settings that simulate the home environment and allow assessment of the patient's function in the kitchen, bathroom, etc. Nieuwboer et al. (23) addressed the issue of comparative efficacy of PT training performed in the home versus the hospital setting. The study population included patients with moderately advanced PD (12 years average disease duration), the majority of whom experienced motor fluctuations. Patients were randomly assigned to receive physical therapist–supervised PT either in the home or in the outpatient clinic. PT was aimed at improvement of specific functional limitations. Assessment was based on a functional activity scale and the UPDRS. Six weeks of PT resulted in significant improvement in the functional activities scale in both groups, although the benefit was more pronounced in the group treated in the home setting (21.5% improvement vs. 8.6%). The benefit declined after 3 months, but still persisted.

3. Group Versus Individual Physical Therapy

There are no studies comparing the efficacy of different PT settings for the same patient population. Individual therapy sessions are appropriate at initiation of therapy to address the particular individual's needs, but maintenance PT can be performed in a group setting. All studies have demonstrated declining benefit of PT within a short time after completion of the structured exercise program. There is poor compliance with the self-exercise regimens. Group exercise classes can improve compliance, allow patients to maintain the benefit gained with the initial individual PT program, and have a positive impact on the patients' quality of life. Such disease-oriented classes serve not only as exercise venues but also as effective support group sessions.

C. Advanced PD Associated with Postural Instability

The point in the disease process when patients report falling or near-falling events defines progression to advanced PD. At that time a formal structured PT program is imperative and should be geared to assessment of the need for ambulation assistance devices and balance training. PD patients should be routinely screened for the risk of falling. Physical therapists use the Berg balance scale, which has been validated for defining safe versus unsafe ambulators (24).

Though there is no effective PT modality that can control postural instability, there are exercise regimens that can improve freezing and difficulty with gait initiation (25). Enzensberger et al. (26) demonstrated the benefit of metronome therapy in improvement of gait initiation and freezing in PD patients. Marching music was less effective, and tactile stimulation produced a negative impact. Thaut and colleagues (27) also demonstrated a positive impact on gait with rhythmic auditory stimulation. Patients were assigned to standard gait training, the same gait training paradigm but with use of rhythmic auditory stimulation (RAS), musical rhythm, or no therapy. Subjects in the exercise groups demonstrated improvement in gait velocity compared to controls, but the degree of benefit was higher in the RAS group (24% vs. 7%).

Burleigh-Jacobs et al. (28) investigated the impact of cutaneous sensory cues on gait initiation in PD. The cutaneous cue, when used to trigger step initiation, showed improvements in anticipatory postural adjustments and step force production comparable to the level of controls. Patients can use visual cues (laser light or block design floor pattern) to overcome freezing phenomena. Other strategies that can be utilized include mental practice of a difficult task such as walking through a doorway or task specific visualization or imagery of the movement such as taking longer steps while walking.

Some patients use an inverted cane and step over the handle to overcome freezing. There was limited benefit of a modified "freezing" stick based on a controlled trial (29).

When making a referral for PT, physicians should specify the goal of therapy such as gait training to alert the physical therapist to the particular functional disability.

1. Risk for Falling

Elderly patients in general have multiple fall risk factors including musculoskeletal problems, declining visual acuity, impaired mental status, decreased reaction time, depression, and age-related decreased limits of stability (30). All of these factors can contribute to falling in PD in addition to the intrinsic PD-related impairment of postural control. The majority of PD patients (66–90%) will fall at some point, with recurrent falls occurring on an average of 10 years after the onset of the disease (31,32). Implementation of fall-prevention strategies depends on the cause of the fall. Information about the type of fall (trip, slip, fainting) is important. Patients should keep a fall diary with details of the date, time, and location of the fall, the task being performed, and their relation to PD medication status (33). Customized programs for minimizing the risk of falls can include rearranging the home environment, strategies for breaking down complex motor tasks into smaller components, implementation of attentional cues to focus on specific components of movements, or modifying the task to avoid multitask activities. If falls occur while rushing to the bathroom in the middle of the night, a bedside commode may decrease the distance a PD patient has to walk. Scheduling the most challenging postural task around peak medication effects is another alternative. Task-specific modifications such as standing with a wider base, practicing large steps during walking, and proper feet placement under the knees to facilitate standing up may be useful. Wide turns while walking or utilization of a "clock turn" strategy for turns in tight places can also be adopted (13). PD patients should be counseled on the risk of falling and falling precautions. Some PD centers have established "fall clinics," where patients are taught strategies to reduce fall risk and "safe" falling techniques.

2. Environmental Changes

Environmental changes can also enhance PD patients' mobility and decrease their risk of falls. Removing loose electrical cords and rugs and avoiding uneven sidewalks and other obstacles in the environment can decrease the risk for falls. Adequate lighting is essential; visual acuity and contract sensitivity decrease with age and can be maximized with good lighting (34). Handrails on stairs and in the bathrooms, stable chairs with supportive armrests, increasing elevation of seated surfaces such as the bed, couch, and chairs can make moving to and from standing and sitting more efficient. Lightweight bedding, and a combination of satin or silk sheets and nightwear may reduce friction and allow easier manipulation of covers and body positioning in bed. Assessment of the home and work environment will help to identify modifications that can enhance functional mobility, safety and efficiency of movement.

D. Advanced PD: Patients Confined to a Wheel Chair

In advanced PD, PT should be geared towards training of the patient and caregiver to accomplish safe mobility, use of a bedside commode, and use of assistance devices. Such an assessment is best performed by a home visiting physical/occupational therapist. The therapist can assess the home environment for safety and provide the family with recommendations for assistive or adaptive devices for the home. The occupational therapist can also provide information on the availability of home equipment like hospital beds and wheel chairs. It is also important to instruct caregivers as to proper body mechanics and techniques for lifting, turning, and transferring to prevent injury to the patient and caregiver and minimize energy expenditure. Training of the patient and caregiver on assisted standing and possibly walking are necessary to combat the complications of impaired mobility. Assessment and instruction in the use of equipment such as an adjustable bed that can be elevated or reclined, transfer aides such as mechanical lifts, wheelchairs, or commode chairs may be helpful in positioning and transfers.

Advanced PD patients are at high risk of aspiration pneumonias. Optimized positioning to maintain clear airways is important. Nutritional intake needs to be encouraged and monitored, as swallowing is often impaired. Patients should be regularly evaluated by a speech therapist. Immobility predisposes patients to skin breakdown and pressure areas. Frequent changes in position and proper support of high-risk areas are essential. The primary focus should be on maintenance of the maximum achievable activity level, comfort, and quality of life. In conclusion, PT/OT programs should be tailored to the needs of the particular patient based on the stage of the disease.

IV. ALTERNATIVE EXERCISE PROGRAMS

The word "alternative" is used in contrast to mainstream exercise regimens usually offered at PT centers. The preferred nomenclature for such nonconventional venues is complementary therapies. There has been greatly increased interest in nonconventional exercise regimens like yoga, tai chi, aquatherapy, and music therapy (35). The utility of these exercise venues is limited by the lack of published data.

A. PD and Yoga

In a recent survey of 201 PD patients, 40% used some kind of alternative therapy (AT) (36). Yoga and massage were among the three most common types of AT used. Despite the popularity of yoga among PD patients, there are no published data on its objective efficacy. Yoga, a complex discipline practiced in India for over 5000 years, has been embraced by western culture mainly because of its physical postures, called *asanas*. Yoga therapy combines effective stretching techniques with stress reduction and relaxation exercises. Yoga may be beneficial at any stage of PD, but more data on this issue are necessary.

B. PD and Acupuncture

There are some published data on the utility of acupuncture in the treatment of PD (35,37,38). Zhuang and Wang (38) published a report of acupuncture treatment in 29 PD patients, indicating improvement in PD disability, but there was no control group and the duration of benefit was not specified. Patients interested in acupuncture should be informed of the paucity of clinical evidence and warned of the potential risks of infection from the needle insertion.

C. Music Therapy in PD

Music therapy (MT) can be a powerful addition to conventional PT regimens. Even patients with fairly advanced PD appear to move much better with rhythmical music input. MT also contributes to the improvement of the emotional status of patients. Pacchetti et al. (39) examined the role of music therapy in improvement of PD disability. Thirty-two patients with stable medically treated PD were randomly assigned to 3 months of weekly sessions of either MT or standard PT. MT consisted of choral singing, voice exercises, and rhythmic body movements. PT sessions included stretching exercises, specific motor tasks, and strategies to improve balance and gait. Assessment measures included QOL and UPDRS. The study demonstrated a positive impact of MT on UPDRS motor and ADL scores, as well as QOL. Compared to PT, MT resulted in statistically significant benefit in reducing bradykinesia but not rigidity, and it was superior in improving, QOL scores. The benefit, however, subsided after 2 months without MT.

V. CONCLUSIONS

PT plays a significant role in the multidisciplinary management of PD (40). Although PT cannot change the natural course of PD, PT can have a positive impact on the functional limitations that develop with the progression of the disease and delay the onset of the physical disability. Despite wide use of PT in clinical practice, the data on its efficacy and the choice of particular PT regimens at different stages of PD are limited (40). Well-designed prospective studies are necessary to assess the impact of PT on the rate of PD progression and the prevention of motor disability. More research is needed to guide clinicians in the selecting the particular PT/OT modality for a given stage of PD and to evaluate the optimal frequency and duration. QOL measures should be incorporated in all studies that evaluate the efficacy of PT/OT in the management of PD.

REFERENCES

1. Deane KH, Jones D, Playford ED, Ben-Shlomo Y, Clarke CE. Physiotherapy for patients with Parkinson's disease: a comparison of techniques. Cochrane Database Syst Rev 2001; 3:CD002817.
2. Deane KH, Ellis-Hill C, Playford ED, Ben-Shlomo Y, Clarke CE. Occupational therapy for patients with Parkinson's disease. Cochrane Database Syst Rev 2001; 3:CD002813.
3. Gibberd FB, Page NG, Spencer KM, Kinnear E, Hawksworth JB. Controlled trial of physiotherapy and occupational therapy for Parkinson's disease. Br Med J (Clin Res Ed) 1981; 282(6271):1196.
4. Weiner WJ, Singer C. Parkinson's disease and nonpharmacologic treatment programs. J Am Geriatr Soc 1989; 37(4):359–363.
5. Formisano R, Pratesi L, Modarelli FT, Bonifati V, Meco G. Rehabilitation and Parkinson's disease. Scand J Rehabil Med 1992; 24(3):157–160.
6. Comella CL, Stebbins GT, Brown-Toms N, Guetz CG. Physical therapy and Parkinson's disease: a controlled clinical trial. Neurology 1994; 44(3 pt 1):376–378.
7. Schenkman M, Cutson TM, Kuchibhatla M, et al. Exercise to improve spinal flexibility and function for people with Parkinson's disease: a randomized, controlled trial. J Am Geriatr Soc 1998; 46(10):1207–1216.
8. Palmer SS, Mortimer JA, Webster DD, Bistevins R, Dickson GL. Exercise therapy for Parkinson's disease. Arch Phys Med Rehabil 1986; 67(10):741–745.
9. Mohr BV, Muller R, Mattes R, et al. Behavioral treatment of Parkinson's disease leads to improvement of motor skills and tremor reduction. Behavior therapy 1996; 27:235–255.
10. Miyai I, Iujmoto Y, Ueda Y, et al. Treadmill training with body weight support: its effect on Parkinson's disease. Arch Phys Med Rehabil 2000; 81(7):849–852.
11. Gauthier L, Dalziel S, Gauthier S. The benefits of group occupational therapy for patients with Parkinson's disease. Am J Occup Ther 1987; 41(6):360–365.
12. Schenkman M, Donovan J, Tsubota J, Kluss M, Stebbins P, Butler RJ. Management of individuals with Parkinson's disease: rationale and case studies. Phys Ther 1989; 69(11):944–955.
13. Morris ME. Movement disorders in people with Parkinson disease: a model for physical therapy. Phys Ther 2000; 80(6):578–597.
14. Rogers MW. Disorders of posture, balance, and gait in Parkinson's disease. Clin Geriatr Med 1996; 12(4):825–845.
15. Bridgewater KJ, Sharpe MH. Trunk muscle performance in early Parkinson's disease. Phys Ther 1998; 78(6):566–576.

16. Morris ME, Iansek R, Matyas TA, Summers JJ. Stride length regulation in Parkinson's disease. Normalization strategies and underlying mechanisms. Brain 1996; 119(pt 2):551–568.
17. Martin JP. The Basal Ganglia and Posture. London, Pitman Publishing Ltd., 1967.
18. Lewis GN, Byblow WD, Walt SE. Stride length regulation in Parkinson's disease: the use of extrinsic, visual cues. Brain 2000; 123(pt 10):2077–2090.
19. Dam M, Tonin P, Casson S, et al. Effects of conventional and sensory-enhanced physiotherapy on disability of Parkinson's disease patients. Adv Neurol 1996; 69:551–555.
20. Marchese R, Diverio M, Zucchi F, Lentino C, Abbruzzese G. The role of sensory cues in the rehabilitation of parkinsonian patients: a comparison of two physical therapy protocols. Mov Disord 2000; 15(5):879–883.
21. Majsak MJ, Kamunski T, Gentile AM, Flanagan JR. The reaching movements of patients with Parkinson's disease under self-determined maximal speed and visually cued conditions. Brain 1998; 121(pt 4):755–766.
22. Hurwitz A. The benefit of a home exercise regimen for ambulatory Parkinson's disease patients. J Neurosci Nurs 1989; 21(3):180–184.
23. Nieuwboer A, De Weerdt W, Dom R, Truyen M, Janssens L, Kamsma Y. The effect of a home physiotherapy program for persons with Parkinson's disease. J Rehabil Med 2001; 33(6):266–272.
24. Berg K, Wood-Dauphinee S, Williams JI. The balance scale: reliability assessment with elderly residents and patients with an acute stroke. Scand J Rehabil Med 1995; 27(1):27–36.
25. Kemoun G, Defebvre L. [Gait disorders in Parkinson disease. Gait freezing and falls: therapeutic management]. Presse Med 2001; 30(9):460–468.
26. Enzensberger W, Oberlander U, Stecker K. [Metronome therapy in patients with Parkinson disease]. Nervenarzt 1997; 68(12):972–977.
27. Thaut MH, McIntosh GC, Rice RR, Miller RA, Rathbun J, Brault JM. Rhythmic auditory stimulation in gait training for Parkinson's disease patients. Mov Disord 1996; 11(2):193–200.
28. Burleigh-Jacobs A, Horak FB, Nutt JG, Obeso JA. Step initiation in Parkinson's disease: influence of levodopa and external sensory triggers. Mov Disord 1997; 12(2):206–215.
29. Dietz MA, Goetz CG, Stebbins GT. Evaluation of a modified inverted walking stick as a treatment for parkinsonian freezing episodes. Mov Disord 1990; 5(3):243–247.
30. Lord SR. Instability and falls in elderly people. In: LaFont C, Baroni A, Allard M, Tidciksaar R, Vellas BJ, Garry PJ, Albarede JL, eds. Falls, Gait and Balance Disorders in the Elderly: From Successful Aging to Frailty, Facts Research and Intervention in Gerontology, 9(suppl). New York: Springer-Verlag, 1996:125–139.
31. Ashburn A, Stack E, Pickering RM, Ward CD. A community-dwelling sample of people with Parkinson's disease: characteristics of fallers and non-fallers. Age Ageing 2001; 30(1):47–52.
32. Bloem BR, Grimbergen YA, Cramer M, Willemsen M, Zwinderman AH. Prospective assessment of falls in Parkinson's disease. J Neurol 2001; 248(11):950–958.
33. Lord SR, Sherrington C, et al. Falls in Older People: Risk Factors and Strategies for Prevention. Cambridge, UK: Cambridge University Press, 2001.
34. Lord SR, Dayhew J. Visual risk factors for falls in older people. J Am Geriatr Soc 2001; 49(5): 508–515.
35. Manyam BV, Sanchez-Ramos JR. Traditional and complementary therapies in Parkinson's disease. Adv Neurol 1999; 80:565–574.
36. Rajendran PR, Thompson RE, Reich SG. The use of alternative therapies by patients with Parkinson's disease. Neurology 2001; 57(5):790–794.
37. Chen L. Clinical observations on forty cases of paralysis agitans treated by acupuncture. J Tradit Chin Med 1998; 18(1):23–26.
38. Zhuang X, Wang L. Acupuncture treatment of Parkinson's disease—a report of 29 cases. J Tradit Chin Med 2000; 20(4):265–267.
39. Pacchetti C, Mancini F, Aglieri R, Fundaro C, Martignoni E, Nappi G. Active music therapy in Parkinson's disease: an integrative method for motor and emotional rehabilitation. Psychosom Med 2000; 62(3):386–393.
40. The Movement Disorders Society Task Force. Physical and occupational therapy in Parkinson's disease. Movement disorders 2002; 17(suppl 4):S156–S159.

36

New and Experimental Drug Treatments

Peter A. LeWitt

*William Beaumont Hospital Research Institute and Clinical Neuroscience Center,
Wayne State University School of Medicine, Southfield, Michigan, U.S.A.*

I. INTRODUCTION

Although serendipity has enriched the therapeutics of Parkinson's disease (PD) with drugs like the antiviral compound amantadine, most of the important advances have followed the route of drug discovery based on rational pharmacology. Several important breakthroughs in modern neuroscience served to guide PD drug development. The finding with the greatest impact was Arvid Carlsson's recognition of dopamine's function as a transsynaptic neurotransmitter in the striatum and elsewhere in the central nervous system (CNS) (1). These laboratory observations subsequently led to levodopa's utilization as a precursor for correcting the PD brain's striatal dopamine deficiency. Another research contribution that helped to expand treatment options for PD was the discovery of specific dopamine receptor subtypes and the key role of the D2 receptor subtype in mediating the relief of parkinsonian features (2,3). Recognition of dual anatomical and functional circuits originating from the striatum (the direct and indirect outflow pathways) has sparked the search for neuromodulatory systems beyond the dopaminergic nigrostriatal pathway, which might be utilized for therapeutic advantage in PD. These systems involve glutamate, enkephalin, dynorphin, and adenosine, among other substances that act upon neuronal circuitry "downstream" from the dopaminergic nigrostriatal synapse (4). Serendipity has continued to play a role in finding new ways for treating PD, as shown by the recent demonstration that amantadine, beyond its symptomatic relief of primary parkinsonian features, can also act to suppress levodopa-induced dyskinesias (5).

Therapeutic options for PD now include several classes of drugs acting through and beyond the nigrostriatal dopaminergic system. For the majority of PD patients, these medications offer a means to control most of PD's motor disabilities. For those with declining medication benefits, several neurosurgical treatments have been developed from research into the functional characteristics of the brain pathways affected in PD. These interventions include applying high-frequency low-voltage electrical stimulation to various sites (6). Neurosurgical techniques are also being employed in several types of experimental approaches for restoring to the brain the type of cellular elements lost in PD (7).

For more than three decades, levodopa has been the most effective pharmacological means for managing PD. One of the greatest challenges for creating new PD therapeutics has been to match or improve upon levodopa's symptomatic effectiveness. Although this drug offers marked improvement in parkinsonian symptomatology, its propensity for adverse events has been a major limitation (8). Research for new PD therapies has been directed to avoid the dyskinesias and motor fluctuations affecting a large fraction of PD patients (9). In this chapter, the variety of medication trials currently underway will be discussed. These include not only symptomatic therapies, but also attempts at halting the development or progression of PD. Several clinical trials have been conducted or are underway to evaluate promising treatment options for neuroprotection (10).

The guiding points for PD drug development have been an expanding list of unmet needs posed by this chronic and often progressive disorder (Table 1). Optimizing symptomatic relief and better long-term outcomes are intermingled as goals of several recent clinical trials. The complexities of such studies are illustrated by recent long-term studies comparing the benefits and adverse effects from dopaminergic agonists versus levodopa. In one trial with ropinirole carried out for 5 years in 268 de novo PD patients (11), monotherapy with the dopaminergic agonist led to much lower incidence of dyskinesia than with levodopa alone, although ropinirole provided less symptomatic relief. Similar

Table 1 Major Unmet Needs in Parkinson's Disease

Symptomatic therapy comparable to the effectiveness of levodopa for the motor features of parkinsonism, but without long-term risks such as dyskinesia

Symptomatic relief for parkinsonian features sometimes unresponsive to dopaminergic, anticholinergic, or amantadine therapy (such as resting tremor, impaired posture, imbalance, diminished reflexes against falls, speech disturbance, and decreased dexterity)

Dystonia (as a primary feature, or related to the onset or wearing-off of dopaminergic effects)

Sensory disturbances associated with PD (such as dysesthesias and pain)

Optimal management for the various patterns of motor fluctuations:
    Wearing-off responses
    Unpredictable off states
    Situation-specific freezing
    Dyskinesia-improvement-dyskinesia pattern of levodopa response

Impaired cognitive function:
    Alterations in executive function, bradyphrenia, and other features of nondementing cognitive impairment in PD
    Progressive dementia (Alzheimer disease type and Lewy body disease type)

Fatigue and diminished motivation

Protection against progression of PD:
    Increasing loss of striatal dopaminergic projections
    Loss of compensatory responses maintaining a mild parkinsonian state
    Loss of long-duration responses to levodopa
    Neuronal damage associated with deposition of abnormal proteins, mitochondrial abnormalities, or other disease mechanisms
    Increasing disability due to loss of medication benefit

findings came from a comparison of monotherapy with either pramipexole or levodopa (12). Studies such as these emphasize the difficulties of even large, well-designed clinical investigations at determining what might be the best choice of therapy for all patients.

II. SYMPTOMATIC THERAPIES

A. Enhancing Dopaminergic Effect

Oral administration of antiparkinsonian medication presents a challenge for maintaining a uniform degree of symptomatic control, especially with respect to levodopa. Levodopa is absorbed in the upper small intestine by means of a facilitated L-neutral amino acid transport mechanism. As with the absorption of other amino acids, the uptake of levodopa is irregular and the variability in plasma drug concentrations underlies the most common category of motor fluctuation in advanced PD. A major limitation for achieving more continuous absorption is the drug's rapid passage through the relatively short territory where levodopa uptake can occur in the duodenum and jejunum. In the 1980s there was extensive research effort to create formulations with pharmacokinetic profiles extending beyond the marketed immediate-release tablets (13). Sustained-release products such as Madopar HBS and Sinemet CR (and its generic equivalents) provide, on average, a more extended plasma levodopa concentration profile than immediate-release forms. However, these products are generally unreliable in providing more consistent antiparkinsonian control. Delayed uptake and variable plasma levodopa concentrations occur even with closely spaced doses of the sustained-release preparations. For this reason, any future attempts at controlled-release formulations of levodopa may be limited. Recently, a new product was introduced in efforts to achieve more constancy in levodopa blood concentrations. This carbidopa/levodopa formulation is a tablet consisting of two connected wafers, each of which has different release properties (14,15). The net result is both immediate and delayed release of levodopa. This formulation likely provides the most extended release profile that can be achieved with oral administration of levodopa.

The most effective means for maintaining continuous and controlled delivery of levodopa, however, is by enteral infusion. A liquid suspension of levodopa can be administered directly into the duodenum or jejunum to achieve continuous uptake at a rate of infusion optimizing parkinsonian control. The constant infusion of the drug at a site beyond the stomach eliminates the major reason for irregularity in levodopa's effects. Conventional tablets of carbidopa/levodopa do not dissolve in water unless strongly acidified, and suspensions tend to settle out, producing variability in drug concentration. However, a microsuspension of carbidopa/levodopa can be created after fine pulverization and formulation with gelling agents (16). This product, Duodopa® (NeoPharma, Uppsala, Sweden), can be used chronically with a portable pump and a tube inserted through the stomach. Recent studies indicated that continuous delivery of Duodopa achieved near-constant blood levels of levodopa and excellent long-term control of wearing-off and dyskinesia (17).

Wearing-off is the most common type of motor fluctuation experienced by patients with long-standing PD. One pharmacological strategy has been slowing the eventual decline of effect from each dose of levodopa. Apart from the adjunctive use of the catechol-O-methyltransferase inhibitors tolcapone or entacapone (to block the peripheral diversion of levodopa to 3-O-methyldopa), the only other means for extending dopaminergic effect has been the use of centrally acting monoamine oxidase-B

(MAO-B) inhibitors (8,18). In addition to the currently marketed MAO-B inhibitor selegiline, an experimental MAO-B inhibitor currently in clinical trials, rasagiline, also has shown promise for helping patients with motor fluctuations (19). A recent trial found that 0.5–1.0 mg/day of this irreversible selective MAO-B inhibitor led to increased on time by a small but statistically significant amount (20). Rasagiline differs from selegiline in lacking amphetamine and methamphetamine metabolites that might contribute to selegiline's side effects.

B. Dopaminergic Agonists

Drugs that mimic the action of the natural neurotransmitter dopamine have been the predominant thrust of drug development in PD therapeutics. Termed dopaminergic agonists (DAs), these compounds have offered important alternatives to the limitations posed by chronic levodopa therapy. The search has continued for compounds with improved efficacy and selectivity at avoiding adverse effects. DAs comprise a number of chemical entities demonstrating that stimulating dopamine receptors by means other than the natural neurotransmitter can improve the cardinal features of PD. Listed in Table 2 are 27 dopaminergic compounds that have undergone clinical evaluation in PD. Ten of these are currently marketed, and two (rotigotine CDS and sumanirole) are undergoing clinical trials. Fourteen are ergot derivatives. Though their chemical structures vary greatly, DAs are screened for the common property of mimicking the effectiveness of the natural neurotransmitter at stimulating CNS receptors (2,3). The several known classes of dopamine receptors differ in their anatomical localization throughout the brain and in their activation properties (21). All of the DAs now in clinical use act predominantly at dopamine receptors that are not linked to adenylate cyclase mechanisms (the D2 receptor family). Most experience in working with DAs has suggested that activating the D2 receptor is necessary for achieving maximal relief of parkinsonism. Drug potency at D2 receptors seems to be the main determinant of differences among these drugs in clinical practice. There are two examples of DAs with just D1 (adenylate cyclase-linked) dopamine receptor activity that demonstrated effectiveness against PD in limited clinical trials. While one compound with activity limited to D1 receptors, SK & F 38393-A, did not exert antiparkinsonian effects (22), both the Sandoz compound CY 208–243 (23) and the Abbott compound ABT-431 (24,25) have shown effectiveness. The limited observations with each of these suggest that their actions do not differ from drugs with D2 agonism. One investigation found that the D1 agonist ABT-431 generated dyskinesias similar to those resulting from levodopa (25).

For the development of new DAs, the question of the ideal receptor stimulation profile has not been definitively answered. Some of the DAs in clinical use, including pergolide, pramipexole, and ropinirole, possess activity at stimulating the D3 and D4 receptors (26). The relationship between stimulating these receptors and clinical outcomes (including adverse effects such as dyskinesias or hallucinations) is not entirely clear. Each of the D2 receptor agonists differs in their affinities at the D3 and D4 receptors, and these pharmacological differences do not appear to translate into altered profiles of clinical effectiveness. Adverse effects of DAs are often the major limiting factors in their development. These problems include nausea and vomiting, hypotension, sedation, confusion, and hallucinations.

Because of their increased dopaminergic potency, DAs offer increased pharmacological versatility as to delivery systems that can be used. Unlike levodopa, these drugs do not

Table 2 Dopaminergic Agonists for Parkinson's Disease Currently Available or Having Undergone Clinical Trials

---

ABT-431
Apomorphine[ab]
Bromocriptine [Parlodel®][ac]
Cabergoline [Cabaser®][ac]
CF 35-397[c]
Ciladopa (AY27,110)
CI 201-678[c]
CQA 206-291 (and its active metabolite CQ 32-084)[c]
CQP 201-403[c]
CV 205-502[c]
CY 208-243[c]
α-Dihydroergocryptine [Almirid®][ac]
FCE 23884
Lergotrile[c]
Lisuride (Dopergin®)[ac]
Mesulergine (CU 32-085)[c]
Naxagolide (PHNO; MK-458)
N-Propyl-aporphine
Pergolide [Permax®][ac]
Piribedil [Trivastal®][a]
Pramipexole [Mirapex®][a]
Rotigotine CDS (N-0923, or SPM 962)[b]
Ropinirole [Requip®][a]
SK&F 38393-Λ
Sumanirole (PNU 95666)[b]
Talipexole[a]
Terguride[c]

---

[a]Currently marketed in one or more countries.
[b]Currently in clinical trials.
[c]Ergot structure compounds.

need facilitated transport uptake mechanisms. DAs are not subject to factors governing dopamine, such as metabolism by monoamine oxidase or other degradation pathways and in situ inactivation using reuptake mechanisms. Most DAs have been tested or marketed as oral medications. Apomorphine has a high first-pass metabolism and so needs to be administered by routes other than by the gastrointestinal system (27). In addition to subcutaneous injection, experimental delivery strategies for apomorphine have been tested using nasal, sublingual, rectal (suppository), and iontophoretic transdermal absorption routes (28).

Another dopamine agonist currently under development is rotigotine CDS (Schwarz Pharma). This drug, also designated as SPM 962, has the chemical structure (6S)-6-[propyl-[2-(2-thienyl) ethyl] amino-5,6,7,8-tetrahydro-1-naphthalenol. Rotigotine has high selectivity for the D2 dopamine receptor and is potent in animal models of parkinsonism. Because of high first-pass metabolism in the gastrointestinal tract, this drug has been developed exclusively for transdermal uptake using a silicone adhesive patch as a continuous delivery system (CDS). By this means, its pharmacokinetic profile offers near-constant dopaminergic stimulation. One multicenter study was reported in which rotigotine, in its earlier transdermal delivery form designated as N-0923, showed efficacy and good tolerability in advanced PD patients with motor fluctuations (29). Currently, several large-scale studies with rotigotine CDS are underway to evaluate its efficacy, safety, and tolerability. In one publication, a dose-related response rate of $\geq 20\%$ improvement in Unified Parkinson's Disease Rating Scale (UPDRS) motor section scores was found to be significantly greater than placebo responses using daily transdermal rotigotine doses of up to 18 mg (30). Other studies have also found rotigotine to exert actions against all features of PD (31).

Rotigotine has been studied as monotherapy in early PD (32). In a randomized placebo-controlled trial of transdermal rotigotine, the drug was well tolerated and resulted in significant, dose-related improvements on UPDRS activities of daily living and motor scores at the 13.5 and 18.0 mg/day doses (both p values < 0.001). Another large multi-center study investigated responses to rotigotine with daily patch drug contents of 9, 18, or 27 mg (33). While the two higher doses were associated with decreased daily "off" time (1.72 and 2.44 hours, respectively), the results were not statistically significant because of a marked placebo effect during the course of the study.

Sumanirole, also designated as PNU 95666-E, is currently under development by Pfizer (formerly, Pharmacia) (34). A potent full D2 dopamine receptor agonist, this compound lacks agonist activity at D1, D3, or D4 dopamine receptors. It has similar effectiveness to levodopa in reversing 1-methyl-4-phenyl-1,2,3,6-tetrahydropyridine (MPTP)–induced parkinsonism in rhesus monkeys but, unlike levodopa, does not produce dyskinesias (35). Sumanirole is currently in clinical trials as a monotherapy in PD and an adjunct to levodopa. In a double-blind, randomized, placebo-controlled study in levodopa-treated advanced PD patients, sumanirole was used from 1 to 48 mg/day and showed significant improvement in UPDRS scores, more on time in home diary evaluations, and permitted greater reduction in prior levodopa intake than placebo (36). This compound has a relatively short clearance half-life, and sustained-release formulations are under investigation.

III. NOVEL TREATMENTS FOR PARKINSON'S DISEASE

A. Antagonists of the Adenosine A$_{2A}$ Receptor

Drugs exerting selective inhibition of adenosine receptors constitute the newest class of antiparkinsonian drugs. The first of these compounds to be developed is istradefylline (KW-6002), a potent antagonist of the adenosine A$_{2A}$ receptor. This compound, whose chemical structure is (E)-1.3-diethyl-8-(3,4-dimethyoxystyryl)-7-methyl-3,7-dihydro-1H-purine-2,6-dione, was developed by Kyowa Pharmaceuticals, Inc. (37). Istradefylline is undergoing several large-scale clinical trials to evaluate its antiparkinsonian potential, following upon two promising studies conducted in patients with motor fluctuations and dyskinesias (38,39). The rationale for an adenosine antagonist is based on an expanding scientific literature highlighting the role of adenosine as a neuromodulator in the basal ganglia (40). This purine nucleoside acts through one of at least four subtypes of G-protein–coupled receptors. Of these, the A$_{2A}$ receptor is prominent in two basal ganglia structures, the caudate nucleus and globus pallidus. In the latter region, adenosine A$_{2A}$ receptors are located primarily on medium-sized spiny output neurons that are GABAergic, express enkephalin, and are colocalized with D2 dopamine receptors (41). The medium-sized spiny neuron appears to regulate much of the phenomenology in response to antiparkinsonian medications (4). Adenosine in the striatum interacts with both the indirect (striato-pallidal) and direct (striato-globus pallidus interna/nigral) efferent pathways. Elsewhere in the CNS, adenosine inhibits the release of acetylcholine (42) and interacts with the effects of other neuroactive substances including dopamine, dynorphin, substance P, and enkephalin. Adenosine's major influence in the basal ganglia, however, appears to be complex interactions exerted in the globus pallidus on GABA release as well as presynaptic modulation of this neurotransmitter's inhibitory actions (43,44). When the GABAergic pathways mediated by adenosine A_{2A} receptors are blocked, there is decreased stimulation of striato-pallidal output neurons. The net effect is apparently a compensatory response for the diminished regulation of this circuitry by dopaminergic nigrostriatal innervation.

Like another adenosine A_{2A} antagonist, KF17837, istradefylline increased rotations in an animal model of parkinsonism, the 6-hydroxydopamine-(6-OHDA)-hemilesioned rat (45). Administration of istradefylline reversed motor impairments even in D2 dopamine receptor knockout mice, demonstrating the independence of adenosine antagonism from interactions with the dopaminergic system. Antiparkinsonian effects from istradefylline have also been observed for MPTP-lesioned cynomolgus monkeys (46). The unique feature of istradefylline is that, despite its ability to reverse the motor features of parkinsonism, it did not produce dyskinesias even in nonhuman primates primed to generate these involuntary movements from dopaminergic drugs (47–49).

The two published studies with istradefylline have confirmed its potential for contributing to PD therapeutics. In one double-blind, placebo-controlled randomized clinical trial, istradefylline was administered in daily doses of either 40 or 80 mg to 15 subjects (38). The study was designed to investigate whether this drug might potentiate levodopa's antiparkinsonian effects or substitute for levodopa. A steady-state levodopa infusion was used to assess the effects of istradefylline as an adjunctive therapy. When the infusion rate was suboptimal for antiparkinsonian control, the 80 mg/day doses enhanced the effects of the levodopa regimen. Supplementary istradefylline reduced all features of parkinsonism, especially resting tremor. These benefits occurred without causing the same degree of dyskinesia that a steady-state levodopa infusion produced when adjusted to produce optimal antiparkinsonian control. When the experimental levodopa infusion was discontinued, subjects receiving istradefylline experienced continuing on time for an average of 47 minutes more than those receiving placebo. There were no significant adverse effects reported from istradefylline. Since the benefits of 40 mg/day doses were less than those of the 80 mg/day doses, the authors concluded that the optimal dose of istradefylline might be in excess of 80 mg/day.

Another proof-of-concept study evaluated istradefylline as an adjunct therapy for 83 levodopa-treated PD patients with motor fluctuations and peak-dose dyskinesias (39). In this double-blind, placebo-controlled randomized trial, subjects received up to 20 or 40 mg/day. Home diary ratings of "off," "on," or "on" with dyskinesia states indicated a beneficial effect of the istradefylline regimens. The adjunctive adenosine antagonist led to a mean decrease in "off" time of 1.2 hours, as compared to a 0.5-hour increase in "off" time in the placebo treatment group ($p = 0.004$). Eight-hour clinic observations of "off" and "on" time showed a similar benefit for istradefylline versus placebo. Istradefylline was also associated with an increase in dyskinesia, reported as both an adverse event and as time spent in a state of "on with dyskinesia" ($p = 0.001$). Adverse effects of the drug were generally mild and included nausea, dizziness, vomiting, and insomnia.

Istradefylline continues to be studied in the United States and Canada and has been joined in an international series of clinical trials by another selective antagonist of the adenosine A_{2A} receptor, SCH 420814 (Schering-Plough Pharmaceuticals).

B. Antidyskinesia Therapies

The control of involuntary movements of a dyskinetic or dystonic nature has been a major challenge in PD therapeutics. Especially since these involuntary movements are generally linked to the peak benefit (or, rarely, onset and wearing-off) of dopaminergic therapies, the means for blocking these problems without detracting from antiparkinsonian effect have been the target of several experimental approaches. In some instances, dyskinesias occurring in animal models of parkinsonism have helped to predict the usefulness of anti-dyskinetic drugs. For example, in monkeys with parkinsonism generated by prior MPTP treatment, administration of clonidine, physostigmine, the N-methyl-D-aspartate antagonist MK-801, or methysergide could attenuate levodopa-induced dyskinesias (50). The drugs in this study that can be safely administered to humans have not been found in clinical trial experience to be useful at controlling dyskinesias. As mentioned above, the promise in animal studies shown by the selective adenosine antagonist istradefylline (48) has not translated into experience from clinical investigation (39). However, other investigations with available drugs such as propranolol (51), amantadine (5), and dextromethorphan (52) have given positive results at lessening levodopa-induced dyskinesias by mechanisms other than blocking dopamine receptors.

In recent studies, two novel compounds with blocking effects against levodopa-induced dyskinesias in animal models of parkinsonism have gone on to clinical trials. In each instance, the antidyskinetic effects reported were not associated with exacerbation of parkinsonian motor features. Idazoxan, an α_2 antagonist, was effective in a randomized, placebo-controlled clinical trial in 18 PD patients using 10–40 mg of the drug (53). The threshold dose for benefit was 20 mg, and no significant adverse effects occurred. Sarizotan (EMD 62225), a selective full agonist at the serotonin $5HT_{1A}$ receptor, has prominent anti-dyskinetic properties demonstrated in both rodent and monkey models of parkinsonism-associated dyskinesias (54). This compound also blocks the D4 subclass of dopamine receptors, though it is not clear if this property confers the antidyskinetic effect. Sarizotan is under development by Merck KGaA and is currently being studied in clinical trials to determine if dyskinesias can be suppressed without detracting from the antiparkinsonian effect of levodopa. In a 6-month open-label study using a maximum of 10 mg twice daily, a reduction in dyskinesia was found without a loss of antiparkinsonian control (55).

C. Neuroprotective Therapies

Increasing inquiry into the pathogenesis of PD identified other possible disease mechanisms beyond oxidative stress, such as impaired mitochondrial respiration, excitotoxicity (glutamate and others), intrinsic and extrinsic neurotoxins, immune system activation, and failure of neurotrophin support. A discussion of these topics is beyond the scope of this chapter, though analogies from studies in cell culture systems and animal models of parkinsonism have led directly to some of the clinical trials described below. One of the key questions underlying some of the latest pharmacological approaches to neuroprotection is whether neuronal loss in PD proceeds by apoptosis or necrosis (or combinations of these mechanisms) (56a). Since apoptosis can be initiated by a number of different insults, intervention with its cascade of cellular processes leading to neuronal death has opened a number of pharmacological targets.

A trial was conducted by the Parkinson Study Group investigating the possible neuroprotective actions of the reversible MAO-B inhibitor lazabemide (Roche Pharmaceuticals). Lazabemide, which, unlike selegiline, is not converted to amphetamine metabolites, is rapidly cleared and thus provided an opportunity to differentiate the persistence of MAO-B inhibitor as a means for continued symptomatic effect versus neuroprotection. Results of the lazabemide trial indicated less progression of parkinsonian disability over the course of one year, as compared to the placebo group (56b). Rasagiline is, like selegiline, a propylpargyline and an irreversible inhibitor of MAO-B, but it also possesses other properties that might confer neuroprotective effects. It antagonizes three cellular processes that promote apoptosis: intranuclear translocation of glyceraldehyde-3-phosphate-dehydrogenase (GADPH), induction of Bcl-2, and activation of mitochondrial permeability transition (57,58). Rasagiline also induces glial-derived neurotrophic factor, another factor that antagonizes apoptosis. In the MPTP model of striatal dopaminergic lesioning, rasagiline treatment has shown enhanced recovery even after the toxin was administered. From clinical trials currently underway, it may be possible to learn if the increased potency of rasagiline, as compared to selegiline, will offer a means to decreasing disease progression. Clinical studies with lazabemide were halted, but rasagiline is planned for marketing on the basis of its dopaminergic enhancing properties and so may be available for use as a neuroprotective agent if clinical trials demonstrate effectiveness.

The first attempts at neuroprotection in PD focused upon the possibility that oxidative stress or defective antioxidant mechanisms were responsible for the start or progression of the disease. The range of etiological options has expanded greatly (10,57). Besides the MAO-B inhibitors, several other neuroprotective trials have been undertaken in the past 10 years. In several instances these studies have been conducted with drugs exerting neurotrophic-like effects in animal models of neurodegeneration. For example, these compounds enhanced motor recovery in mice previously administered MPTP. One clinical trial was carried out with AMG-474 (Amgen), an orally administered compound classified as a neuroimmunophyllin. AMG-474 (also designated as NIL-A), administered at 200 or 1000 mg 4 times per day, was given to 300 PD patients enrolled in a randomized, placebo-controlled study lasting 24 weeks. While the results of this investigation have not been reported formally, a press release from its sponsor stated that the study was negative. In all likelihood the study's short duration was inadequate for testing a possible neuroprotective action.

Other studies have been undertaken to learn if the progression of PD might be arrested with substances that enhanced the vitality of neurons. Peptides structurally and functionally related to neurotrophic factor have been under consideration since their delivery to the brain in animal models of neurodegeneration has produced marked improvements. One study investigated repeated administration of glial cell line–derived neurotrophic factor (GDNF), administered by an implanted intracerebroventricular catheter and access port on a monthly basis (59). This randomized placebo-controlled trial in 50 advanced PD patients used GDNF doses ranging from 25 to 4000 μg. After 8 months for all subjects (and a 20-month extension for some), no improvements in clinical ratings were detected. Several types of adverse effect were reported, including paresthesias, weight loss, and hyponatremia. The failure of drug effect could have been due to failure of the peptide to penetrate from the cerebrospinal fluid compartment into affected brain regions. Another approach to the neurotrophic question has investigated direct delivery of GDNF into the putamen using an implanted catheter. Five patients with advanced PD treated in this manner over one year showed no significant adverse effects and promising clinical results (60a). UPDRS assessments revealed that GDNF treatment produced a 39% reduction in off-medication motor ratings and 61% improvement in the UPDRS activities of daily living. Furthermore, dyskinesias on medication were decreased by 64%. The participants in this study were also assessed by ^{18}F-DOPA positron emission tomography (PET) studies to assess the integrity of the presynaptic nigrostriatal dopaminergic projects. At 18 months, as compared to baseline status, subjects receiving intraputaminal GDNF evolved an average of 28% increase in putaminal dopamine storage.

Studies are currently underway testing the effects of CEP-1347 (also designated as KT7515). CEP-1347 (Cephalon, Inc.) is a small molecule that acts as an inhibitor of mixed lineage kinase-3, a major component in the transcription factor c-Jun–mediated terminal kinase signaling pathway in apoptotic neuronal death. The cascade of events using this pathway has been hypothesized to be one mechanism by which substantia nigra neurons are lost in PD. With CEP-1347, several pathways leading to experimental loss of neuronal PC12 cells, sympathetic neurons, and various in vivo models of neurodegeneration can be blocked (60b–66). In MPTP-induced parkinsonism, for example, this compound has improved survival of neurons in the substantia nigra. A randomized, placebo-controlled study of CEP-1347 was carried out to demonstrate its safety and tolerability using 50 mg twice daily (67). No symptomatic effects against PD were observed. This compound is undergoing more extensive testing by the Parkinson Study Group in North America for its potential as a neuroprotective agent.

TCH346 (also designated in laboratory research reports as CGP3466 or CGP3466B) is a novel compound under development by Novartis Pharma and currently in clinical trials assessing whether it might be a neuroprotective agent in PD. Although it has some structural similarities with the MAO-B inhibitor deprenyl, TCH346 is not an inhibitor of this enzyme. Its presumed mechanism as a neuroprotective agent is binding to the glycolytic enzyme GAPDH. There is considerable evidence that GAPDH is a key step in age-induced neuronal apoptosis (68,69). Since the loss of neurons in PD has some evidence to suggest a mechanism involving programmed cell death, an antiapoptotic therapeutic strategy has had considerable impetus. The effects of TCH346 have been studied in cultured PC12 cells (which share with dopaminergic neurons the properties of dopamine synthesis and metabolism). With the presence of TCH346 in culture medium, this compound showed binding to GAPDH in partially differentiated PC12 cells. The result was reduction of an increase in GAPDH concentrations and its nuclear translocation that occurred when apoptosis was induced (70). In other experiments using a human neuroblastoma cell line (PAJU cells) forced into apoptosis by rotenone treatment, TCH346 increased their survival, even in cells manipulated to overexpress GAPDH (71).

TCH346 has also been tested in vivo in rhesus monkeys rendered parkinsonian by two systemic injections of MPTP. With subcutaneous administration of TCH346 2 hours following the second MPTP treatment and continuing twice daily for 2 weeks (0.0142 mg/kg), this compound almost completely blocked the development of parkinsonian features (72). The basis for improved outcomes was studied in the striatal and substantia nigra regions, using staining for tyrosine hydroxylase and glial fibrillary acidic protein immunoreactivity. The TCH346 treatment resulted in sparing of the usual loss caused by MPTP in substantia nigra neurons and their dopaminergic projections to the striatum. Taken together with the cell culture findings, these findings with respect to

MPTP-induced parkinsonism suggested that TCH346 might be effective at slowing (or possibly reversing) the worsening of PD. Completion of a large-scale randomized double-blind placebo-controlled trial with TCH346 is anticipated soon.

Beyond the notion of neuroprotective or neurorestorative approaches using neurotrophic substances, another trial has targeted a metabolic abnormality detected in the PD brain and systemically. A reduction in activity of complex I in the mitochondrial chain of electron transport prompted a trial of coenzyme Q10, an antioxidant and the electron acceptor for complex I. Oral administration of coenzyme Q10 with 1200 mg per day (but not less) resulted in improvements and no adverse effects (73). In this randomized placebo-controlled double-blind study in 80 otherwise untreated PD subjects, coenzyme Q10 resulted in less disability over the planned 16 months of the study ($p = 0.0416$) for the 6.69 point improvement in the adjusted mean score for total UPDRS in the 1200 mg/day treatment group. No improvement was seen at the lower doses of 300 and 600 mg/day. Analysis of the results indicated that most of the benefit from 1200 mg/day was attributable to less functional decline in activities of daily living rather than amelioration of clinical signs on examination. While this study does not establish the complex I mitochondrial defect in PD as the mechanism for disease progression, these results open the door for another means for intervening in PD. A further trial to evaluate higher doses of coenzyme Q10 is planned.

IV. CONCLUSIONS

New treatments for PD are emerging simultaneously on several fronts. Beyond refinements in established drug therapeutics, such as dopaminergics, anticholinergics, and extenders of levodopa effect, several new therapeutic classes are under active investigation. This research may lead to new options for symptomatic therapy beyond the current limitations posed by declining efficacy and side effects. Discovery of novel chemical entities and new therapeutic targets has been the predominant source of progress in improving the therapy of PD. However, utilizing an old drug to solve some of the most challenging problems of PD is the legacy of apomorphine. First used in PD in 1951, apomorphine was rediscovered to be useful for managing off states and other aspects of motor fluctuations because of its options for continuous delivery and administration as a rescue therapy. Apomorphine also has been explored for its potential for administration in a number of alternative routes (28). As with apomorphine, delivery systems offering optimized pharmacokinetic profiles or better penetration to the CNS may be critical for progress in controlling the unsolved problems of PD (13). Novel concepts for delivery of complex biological molecules created from genetic transcription and translation have been devised for using viral vectors to deliver into the brain recombinant L-aromatic amino acid decarboxylase or neurotrophic factors (74).

Avoiding adverse outcomes from chronic therapy is a challenge for future drug development. The best way to manage PD may involve the combined use of drugs whose symptomatic actions are redundant with the high effectiveness of levodopa. Support for this notion has already been provided by long-term studies with dopaminergic agonists, which both lessen the risk for dyskinesias and appear to slow progression of the disease (11,12,75). Although levodopa does not appear to be intrinsically toxic (76), its propensity to induce dyskinesias may go beyond its short pharmacokinetic half-life (77). For this reason, the evaluation of improvements over levodopa may require studies lasting 5 years or longer to assess long-term outcomes.

The options for using neuroprotective strategies to halt the progression of PD are also taking exciting directions. The neuroprotection initiative of the National Institutes of Health (10) joins the concerted efforts of several pharmaceutical firms in developing and testing new ways for blocking the disease process. There has already been considerable experience with the methods and pitfalls of such studies. The evaluation of motor impairments and disabilities has been augmented in recent years by the promise of neuroimaging with PET and single photon emission computed tomography (SPECT) scans as surrogate markers of the underlying disease (78).

REFERENCES

1. Carlsson A. Treatment of Parkinson's with L-DOPA. The early discovery phase, and a comment on current problems. J Neural Transm 2002; 109:777–787.
2. Newman-Tancredi A, Cussac D, Audinot V, Nicolas JP, De Ceuninck F, Boutin JA, Millan MJ. Differential actions of antiparkinson agents at multiple classes of monoaminergic receptor. II. Agonist and antagonist properties at subtypes of dopamine D_2-like receptor and alpha$_1$/alpha$_2$-adrenoceptor. J Pharmacol Exp Ther 2002a; 303:805–814.
3. Newman-Tancredi A, Cussac D, Quentric Y, Touzard M, Verriele L, Carpentier N, Millan MJ. Differential actions of antiparkinson agents at multiple classes of monoaminergic receptor. III. Agonist and antagonist properties at serotonin, 5-HT$_1$ and 5-HT$_2$ receptor subtypes. J Pharmacol Exp Ther 2002; 303:815–822.
4. Chase TN, Oh JD. Striatal mechanisms and pathogenesis of parkinsonian signs and motor complications. Ann Neurol 2000; 47(suppl 4):S122–S129.
5. Verhagen Metman L, Del Dotto P, van den Munckhof P, Fang J, Mouradian MM, Chase TN. Amantadine as treatment for dyskinesias and motor fluctuations in Parkinson's disease. Neurology 1998a; 50:1323–1326.
6. Kumar R, Lozano AM, Montgomery E, Lang AE. Pallidotomy and deep brain stimulation of the pallidum and subthalamic nucleus in advanced Parkinson's disease. Mov Disord 1998; 13:73–82.
7. Bjorklund A, Lindvall O. Cell replacement therapies for central nervous system disorders. Nat Neurosci 2000; 6:537–544.
8. LeWitt PA. Extending the action of levodopa's effects. In: LeWitt PA, Oertel WH, eds. Parkinson's Disease: The Treatment Options. London: Martin Dunitz Publishers, 1999:141–158.
9. Parkinson Study Group. Impact of deprenyl and tocopherol treatment on Parkinson's disease in DATATOP subjects requiring levodopa. Ann Neurol 1996; 39:37–45.
10. Ravina BM, Fagan SC, Hart RG, Hovinga CA, Murphy DD, Dawson TM, Marler JR. Neuroprotective agents for clinical trials in Parkinson's disease: A systematic assessment. Neurology 2003; 60:1234–1240.
11. Rascol O, Brooks D, Korczyn A, De Deyn PP, Clarke CE, Lang AE. A five-year study of the incidence of dyskinesia in patients with early Parkinson's disease who were treated with ropinirole or levodopa. N Engl J Med 2000; 342:1484–1491.
12. Parkinson Study Group. Pramipexole vs. levodopa as initial treatment for Parkinson disease. JAMA 2000; 284:1931–1938.
13. LeWitt PA, Albanese A. New delivery systems for anti-parkinsonian drugs. Adv Neurol 1999; 80:549–554.
14. Crevoisier C, Monreal A, Metzger B, Nilsen. Comparative single- and multiple-dose pharmacokinetics of levodopa and 3-O-methyldopa following a new dual-release and a conventional slow-release formulation of levodopa and benserazide in healthy volunteers. Eur Neurol 2003; 49:39–44.
15. Crevoisier C, Zerr P, Calvi-Gries F, Nilsen T. Effects of food on the pharmacokinetics of levodopa in a dual-release formulation. Eur J Pharm Biopharm 2003; 55:71–76.
16. Nyholm D, Askmark H, Gomes-Trolin C, Knutson T, Lennernas H, Nystrom C, Aquilonius SM. Optimizing levodopa pharmacokinetics: intestinal infusion versus oral sustained-release tablets. Clin Neuropharmacol 2003; 26:156–163.
17. Nilsson D, Nyholm D, Aquilonius SM. Duodenal levodopa infusion in Parkinson's disease—long-term experience. Acta Neurol Scand 2001; 104:343–348.
18. Rascol O. Monoamine oxidase inhibitors: is it time to up the TEMPO? Lancet Neurol 2003; 2:142–143.

19. Akao Y, Youdim MB, Davis BA, Naoi M, Rabey JM. Rasagiline mesylate, a new MAO-B inhibitor for the treatment of Parkinson's disease: a double-blind study as adjunctive therapy to levodopa. J Neurochem 2001; 78:727–735.

20. Parkinson Study Group. A controlled trial of rasagiline in early Parkinson disease. The TEMPO study. Arch Neurol 2002; 59:1937–1943.

21. Missale C, Russel SN, Robinson SW, et al. Dopamine receptor: from structure to function. Physiol Rev 1998; 78:189–225.

22. LeWitt PA, Galloway MP. Implications for D-1 agonism in anti-parkinsonian therapeutics. In: Calne DB, Fahn S, Marsden CD, Goldstein M, eds. Vol. II. Recent Developments in Parkinson's Disease. Florham Park, NJ: Macmillan, 1987:75–89.

23. Emre M, Rinne UK, Rascol O, et al. Effects of a selective partial D1 agonist, CY208-243, in de novo patients with Parkinson's disease. Mov Disord 1992; 7:239–243.

24. Rascol O, Blin O, Thomas C, et al. ABT-431, a D1 receptor agonist has efficacy in Parkinson's disease. Ann Neurol 1999; 45:736–741.

25. Rascol O, Nutt JG, Blin O, et al. Induction by a dopamine D1 receptor agonist ABT-431 of dyskinesia similar to levodopa in patients with Parkinson's disease. Arch Neurol 2001; 58:249–254.

26. Perachon S, Schwartz JC, Sokoloff P. Functional properties of new antiparkinsonian drugs at recombinant human dopamine D1, D2, and D3 receptors. Eur J Pharmacol 1999; 366:293–300.

27. Dewey RB Jr., Hutton JT, LeWitt PA, Factor SA. A randomized double-blind placebo-controlled trial of subcutaneously injected apomorphine for parkinsonian "off" states. Arch Neurol 2001; 58:1385–1392.

28. Neef C, van Laar T. Pharmacokinetic-pharmacodynamic relationships of apomorphine in patients with Parkinson's disease. Clin Pharmacokinet 1999; 37:257–171.

29. Hutton JT, Chase TN, Verhagen L, Juncos JL, Koller WC, Pahwa R, LeWitt PA, Calne DB, Tsui JKC, Waters CH, Calabrese VP, Bennett JP, Barrett R, Morris JL. Transdermal dopamine D_2 receptor agonist therapy in Parkinson's disease with N-0923 TDS: a double blind, placebo-controlled study. Mov Disord 2001; 16:459–463.

30. Bianchine J, Poole K, Woltering F. Efficacy and dose response of the novel transdermally applied dopamine agonist rotigotine CDS in early Parkinson's disease. Neurology 2002; 58(suppl 3): A162–A163.

31. Verhagen Metman L, Gillespie M, Farmer C, Bibbiani F, Konitsiotis S, Morris M, Shill H, Bara-Jimenez W, Mouradian MM, Chase TN. Continuous transdermal dopaminergic stimulation in advanced Parkinson's disease. Clin Neuropharmacol 2001:163–169.

32. Fahn S, Parkinson Study Group. Rotigotine transdermal system (SPM-962) is safe and effective as monotherapy in early Parkinson's disease (PD). Poster presentation at the XIVth International Congress on Parkinson's disease, Helsinki, Finland, 2001; July 28–August 1.

33. Quinn N, SP 511 Investigators. Rotigotine transdermal delivery system (TDS) (SPM 962)— a multicenter double-blind, randomized, placebo-controlled trial to assess the safety and efficacy of rotigotine TDS in patients with advanced Parkinson's disease. Presentation at the XIVth International Congress on Parkinson's disease, Helsinki, Finland, 2001; July 28–August 1.

34. de Paulis T. Sumanirole Pharmacia. Curr Opin Invest Drugs 2003; 4:77–82.

35. McCall RB, Nichols NF, Svensson KA, Meglasson MD, Huff RM. Sumanirole: the first highly D2 selective dopamine receptor agonist intended for the treatment of Parkinson's disease. Presented at the 7th International Congress of Parkinson's Disease and Movement Disorders, Miami, Florida, November 2002; 10–14.

36. Gomez-Mancilla B, Sumanirole Study Group, Kelzer KA, Chapman K, Wang M, Simpson S. Sumanirole is a promising new agent in the treatment of Parkinson's disease. Presented at the 7th International Congress of Parkinson's Disease and Movement Disorders, Miami, Florida, November 2002; 10–14.

37. Knutsen LJ, Weiss SM. KW-6002 (Kyowa Hakko Kogyo). Curr Opin Invest Drugs 2001; 2: 668–673.

38. Bara-Jimenez W, Sherzai A, Dimitrova T, Favit A, Bibbiani F, Gillespie M, Morris MJ, Mouradian MM, Chase TN. Adenosine A_{2A} receptor antagonist treatment of Parkinson's disease. Neurology 2003; 61:293–296.

39. Hauser RA, Hubble JP, Truong DD. Randomized trial of the adenosine A_{2A} receptor antagonist istradefylline in advanced PD. Neurology 2003; 61:297–303.

40. Kase H, Richardson PJ, Jenner P (eds). Adenosine receptors and Parkinson's disease. San Diego: Academic Press, 2000: 1–275.

41. Hettinger BD, Lee A, Linden J, Rosin DL. Ultatrstructural localization of adenosine A_{2A} receptors suggests multiple cellular sites for modulation of GABAergic neurons in rat striatum. J Comp Neurol 2001; 431:331–346.

42. Kirk I, Richardson PJ. Adenosine A_{2A} receptor-mediated modulation of striatal [^{3}H]GABA and [^{3}H]acetylcholine release. J Neurochem 1994; 62:960–966.

43. Mori A, Shindou T, Ichimura M, Nonaka H, Kase H. The role of adenosine A_{2A} receptors in regulating GABAergic synaptic transmission in striatal medium spiny neurons. J Neurosci 1996; 16:605–611.

44. Shindou T, Mori A, Kase H, Ichimura M. Adenosine A_{2A} receptor enhances $GABA_A$-mediated IPSCs in the rat globus pallidus. J Physiol 2001; 532:423–434.

45. Koga K, Kurokawa M, Ochi M, Nakamura J, Kuwana Y. Adenosine A(2A) receptor antagonists KF17837 and KW-6002 potentiate rotation induced by dopaminergic drugs in hemi-Parkinsonian rats. Eur J Pharmacol 2000; 408:249 255.

46. Grondin R, Bedard PJ, Hadj Tahar A, Gregoire L, Mori A, Kase H. Antiparkinsonian effect of a new selective adenosine A2A receptor antagonist in MPTP-treated monkeys. Neurology 1999; 52:1673–1677.

47. Kanda T, Tashiro T, Kuwana Y, Jenner P. Adenosine A2A receptors modify motor function in MPTP-treated common marmosets. Neuroreport 1998; 9:2857–2860.

48. Kanda T, Jackson MJ, Smith LA, Pearce RK, Nakamura J, Kase H, Kuwana Y, Jenner P. Adenosine A2A antagonist: a novel antiparkinsonian agent that does not provoke dyskinesia in parkinsonian monkeys. Ann Neurol 1998; 43:507–513.

49. Kanda T, Jackson MJ, Smith LA, Pearce RK, Nakamura J, Kase H, Kuwana Y, Jenner P. Combined use of the adenosine A(2A) antagonist KW-6002 with L-DOPA or with selective D1 or D2 dopamine agonists increases antiparkinsonian activity but not dyskinesia in MPTP-treated monkeys. Exp Neurol 2000; 162:321–327.

50. Gomez-Mancilla B, Bédard P. Effects of nondopaminergic drugs on L-dopa-induced dyskinesias in MPTP-treated monkeys. Clin Neuropharmacol 1993; 16:418–427.

51. Carpentier AF, Bonnet AM, Vidailhet M, Agid Y. Improvement of levodopa induced dyskinesia by propranolol in Parkinson's disease. Neurology 1996; 46:1548–1551.

52. Verhagen Metman L, Del Dotto P, Natte R, et al. Dextromethorphan improves levodopa-induced dyskinesias in Parkinson's disease. Neurology 1998b; 51:203–206.

53. Rascol O, Arnulf I, Peyro-Saint Paul H, Brefel-Courbon C, Vidailhet M, Thalamas C, Bonnet AM, Descombes S, Bejjani B, Fabre N, Montastruc JL, Agid Y. Idazoxan, an alpha-2 antagonist, and L-DOPA-induced dyskinesias in patients with Parkinson's disease. Mov Disord 2001; 16:708–713.

54. Bibbiani F, Oh JD, Chase TN. Serotonin 5-HT1A agonist improves motor complications in rodent and primate parkinsonian models. Neurology 2001; 57:1829–1834.

55. Olanow CW, Goetz C, Mueller T, Nutt J, Rascol O, Russ H. A prospective, 6-month multicenter, open label dose-rising study of the effect of Sarizotan on dyskinesia in Parkinson's disease. Presented at the 7th International Congress of Parkinson's Disease and Movement Disorders, Miami, Flordia, November 2002; 10–14.

56a. Jellinger KA. Cell death mechanism in Parkinson's disease. J Neural Transm 2000; 107:1–27.

56b. Parkinson Study Group. A controlled trial of lazabemide (Ro 19-6327) in levodopa-treated Parkinson's disease. Arch Neurol 1994; 51:342–347.

57. Maruyama W, Akao Y, Carrillo MC, Kitani K, Youdim MBH, Naoi M. Neuroprotection by propylargylamines in Parkinson's disease. Suppression of apoptosis and induction of prosurvival genes. Neurotoxicol Teratol 2002; 24:675–682.

58. Youdim MB, Amit T, Bar-Am O, Weinstock M, Yogev-Falach M. Amyloid processing and signal transduction properties of antiparkinson-antialzheimer neuroprotective drugs rasagiline and TV3326. Ann NY Acad Sci 2003; 993:378–386.

59. Nutt JG, Burchiel KJ, Comella CL, Jankovic J, Lang AE, Laws ER Jr., Lozano AM, Penn RD, Simpson RK Jr., Stacy M, Wooten GF, ICV GDNF Study Group. Randomized double-blind trial of glial cell line-derived neurotrophic factor (GDNF) in PD. Neurology 2003; 60:69–73.

60a. Gill SS, Patel NK, Hotton GR, O'Sullivan K, McCarter R, Bunnage M, Brooks DJ, Svendsen CN, Heywood P. Direct brain infusion of glial derived neurotrophic factor (GDNF) in Parkinson's disease. Nat Med 2003; 9:589–595.

60b. Maroney AC, Glicksman MC, Basma AN, Walton KM, Knight E, Murphy CA, Bartlett BA, Finn JP, Angeles T, Matsuda Y, Neff NT, Dionne CA. Motoneuron apoptosis is blocked by CEP-1347 (KT 7515), a novel inhibitor of the JNK signaling pathway. J Neurosci 1998; 18:104–111.

61. Maroney AC, Finn JP, Bozyczko-Coyne D, O'Kane T, Neff NT, Tolkovsky AM, Park DS, Yan CYI, Troy CM, Greene LA. CEP-1347 (KT 7515), an inhibitor of JNK activation, rescues

sympathetic neurons and neuronally differentiated PC12 cells from death evoked by three distinct insults. J Neurochem 1999; 73:1–12.

62. Saporito MS, Brown EM, Miller MS, Carswell S. CEP-1347/KT-7515, an inhibitor of c-jun N-terminal kinase activation, attenuates the 1-methyl-4-phenyl tetrahydropyridine-mediated loss of nigrostriatal dopaminergic neurons in vivo. J Pharmacol Exp Ther 1999; 288:421–427.

63. Saporito MS, Thomas BA, Scott RW. MPTP activates c-Jun NH(2)-terminal kinase (JNK) and its upstream regulatory kinase MKK4 in nigrostriatal neurons in vivo. J Neurochem 2000; 75:1200–1208.

64. Saporito MS, Hudkins RL, Maroney AC. Discovery of CEP-1347/KT-7515, an inhibitor of the JNK/SAPK pathway for the treatment of neurodegenerative diseases. Prog Med Chem 2002; 40:23–62.

65. Harris CA, Deshmukh M, Tsui-Pierchala B, Maroney AC, Johnson EM Jr., Ylikoski J. Inhibition of the c-Jun N-terminal kinase signaling pathway by the mixed lineage kinase inhibitor CEP-1347 (KT7515) preserves metabolism and growth of trophic factor-deprived neurons. J Neurosci 2002; 22:103–113.

66. Bilsland JG, Harper SJ. CEP-1347 promotes survival of NGF responsive neurones in primary DRG explants. Neuroreport 2003; 14:995–999.

67. Schwid SR, Parkinson Study Group. CEP-1347 in Parkinson's disease: a pilot study. Presented at the 7th International Congress of Parkinson's disease and Movement Disorders, Miami, Florida, November 2002; 10–14.

68. Ishitani R, Kimura M, Sunaga K, Katsube N, Tanaka M, Chuang DM. An antisense oligonucleotide to glyceraldehyde-3-phosphate-dehydrogenase blocks age-induced apoptosis of mature cerebro-cortical neurons in culture. J Pharmacol Exp Ther 1996; 278:447–454.

69. Ishitani R, Sunaga K, Hirano A, Saunders P, Katsube N, Chuang DM. Evidence that glyceraldehyde-3-phosphate-dehydrogenase is involved in age-induced apoptosis in mature cerebellar neurons in culture. J Neurochem 1996; 66:928–935.

70. Carlile GW, Chalmers-Redman RME, Tatton NA, Pong A, Borden KE, Tatton WG. Reduced apoptosis after nerve growth factor and serum withdrawal: conversion of tetrameric gluteraldehyde-3-phosphate dehydrogenase to a dimer. Mol Pharmacol 2000; 57:2–12.

71. Kragten E, Lalande I, Zimmerman K, Roggo S, Schindler P, Muller D, van OJ, Waldmeier P, Furst P. Glyceraldehyde-3-phosphate dehydrogenase, the putative target of the antiapoptotic compounds CGP 3466 and R-(-)-deprenyl. J Biol Chem 1998; 273:5821–5828.

72. Andringa G, Cools AR. The neuroprotective effects of CGP 3466B in the best in vivo model of Parkinson's disease, the bilaterally MPTP-treated rhesus monkey. J Neural Transm Suppl 2000; 60:215–225.

73. Shults CW, Oakes D, Kieburtz K, Beal MF, Hass R, Plumb S, Juncos JL, Nutt J, Shoulson I, Carter J, Kompliti K, Perlmutter JS, Reich S, Stern M, Watts RL, Kurlan R, Mohlo, Harrison M, Lew M. Parkinson Study Group. Effects of coenzyme Q10 in early Parkinson's disease: evidence for slowing of the functional decline. Arch Neurol 2002; 59:1541–1550.

74. Latchman DS, Coffin RS. Viral vectors in the treatment of Parkinson's disease. Mov Disord 2000; 15:9–17.

75. Parkinson Study Group. Dopamine transporter brain imaging to assess the effects of pramipexole vs levodopa on Parkinson disease progression. JAMA 2002; 287:1653–1661.

76. Agid Y, Ahlskog E, Albanese A, et al. Levodopa in the treatment of Parkinson's disease: a consensus meeting. Mov Disord 1999; 14:911–913.

77. Maratos EC, Jackson MJ, Pearce RK, Cannizzaro C, Jenner P. Both short- and long-acting D-1/D-2 dopamine agonists induce less dyskinesia than L-DOPA in the MPTP-lesioned common marmoset (*Callithrix jacchus*). Exp Neurol 2003; 179:90–102.

78. Marek K, Jennings D, Seibyl J. Do dopamine agonists or levodopa modify Parkinson's disease progression? Eur J Neurol 2002; 9(suppl 3):15–22.

37

Mitochondrial Dysfunction and Therapies

Clifford W. Shults

*University of California, San Diego, School of Medicine, La Jolla,
and VA San Diego Healthcare System, San Diego, California, U.S.A.*

I. INTRODUCTION

The discovery that 1-methyl-4-phenyl-1,2,3,6-tetrahydropyridine (MPTP), which causes a parkinsonian syndrome in humans, nonhuman primates, and mice (1,2), acts through inhibition of complex I of the mitochondrial electron transport chain (ETC) (3,4) stimulated investigation of a possible role for mitochondrial dysfunction in Parkinson's disease (PD) (5).

II. ROLE OF MITOCHONDRIA IN OXIDATIVE PHOSPHORYLATION

Mitochondria, which are present in nearly all eukaryotic cells, are hypothesized to have developed from the symbiotic association between glycolytic proto-eukaryotic cells and oxidative bacteria (6). Mammalian mitochondria have retained a small, circular genome of approximately 16,500 base pairs, which encode 13 proteins involved in oxidative phosphorylation, 22 transfer ribonucleic acids (RNAs) and 12S and 16S ribosomal RNAs. The remaining components of mitochondria are encoded in the nucleus.

Mitochondria are composed of an outer membrane, an intermembrane space, an inner membrane, and a matrix. Pyruvate, which is generated largely by glycolysis in the cytosol, is metabolized to acetyl CoA on the inner membrane. Acetyl CoA, which is also a product of fatty acid oxidation, is in turn metabolized via the citric acid cycle to CO_2 and high-energy electrons, which are carried by the activated carrier molecules nicotinamide adenine dinucleotide (NADH) and flavin adenine dinucleotide ($FADH_2$). The high-energy electrons are transferred into the ETC by NADH to complex I and succinate via $FADH_2$ to complex II. The ETC, which is located in the inner membrane, is composed of five complexes: complex I (NADH:ubiquinone oxidoreductase), complex II (succinate:ubiquinone oxidoreductase), complex III (ubiquinol:cytochrome *c* oxidoreductase), complex IV (cytochrome c oxidase), and complex V [H^+-translocating adenosine triphosphate (ATP) synthase]. The transport of electrons down the ETC is energetically favorable, and the energy released is used by complexes I, III, and IV to transport protons from the matrix to the intermembrane space. The transport of protons creates a proton and electrochemical gradient across the inner membrane; the pH in the matrix is about 8 and the pH in the intermembrane space is about 7, similar to that in the cytosol. The energy stored in the electrochemical proton gradient is used to drive complex V (ATP synthase) to form ATP.

Transport of high-energy electrons through the ETC can also be a source not only of ATP but also of reactive oxygen species (ROS), as the high-energy electrons can react with O_2 to form superoxide (7). It has been estimated that up to 2% of the O_2 consumed by healthy mitochondria is converted to superoxide, and this amount is higher in damaged and aged mitochondria. Manganese superoxide dismutase (SOD2) in the matrix converts the superoxide to hydrogen peroxide (H_2O_2), and H_2O_2 is typically detoxified by glutathione peroxidase, thioredoxin, and catalase (levels of catalase are low in most regions of the brain). However, in the presence of transition metals, H_2O_2 can be converted by the Fenton reaction to the highly reactive hydroxyl radical. Production of ROS can damage components of the mitochondria, including the mitochondrial deoxyribonucleic acid (DNA), lipids, and protein.

III. ROLE OF MITOCHONDRIA IN APOPTOSIS

In addition to its role in the bioenergetics of the cell or perhaps because of its central position in the energetics of the cell, the mitochondrion has evolved to play a central role in apoptosis or programmed cell death.

The mechanisms that lead to death of the nigral, dopaminergic neurons in PD are not fully understood. Evidence has accumulated to suggest that apoptosis is involved in this process, but this is debated (8,9). Apoptosis is a part of the normal function of multicellular organisms (10) and plays a role in normal processes such as elimination of cells during development, removal of cells infected by viruses, and homeostasis in tissues in which production of new cells is balanced by elimination of older cells. Apoptosis is defined morphologically, and the characteristics of apoptosis include chromatin condensation, nuclear fragmentation, condensation of cell contents, and formation of small membrane-bound vesicles, which are phagocytosed by nearby cells without accompanying inflammation (11,12).

Apoptosis can be triggered by both external and internal pathways, which act through activation of cysteine aspartyl-specific proteases (caspases) (10). The external pathways are activated through ligation of death receptors, such as tumor necrosis factor receptor-1, and the internal pathway works through mitochondria and release of proapoptotic factors, such as cytochrome c, which activate the caspase pathways. In addition, some proapoptotic factors released from mitochondria act in a caspase-independent fashion, by acting as nucleases (e.g., endonuclease G), nuclease activators [e.g., apoptosis-inducing factor (AIF)], sequesterers of inhibitors of apoptosis proteins (IAPs) (Smac/DIABLO) or serine proteases (e.g., Omi/HtrA2, which also interact with IAPs) (13).

Members of the Bcl-2 family serve as proapoptotic or antiapoptotic factors (13,14) typically through interactions in the mitochondria. The proapoptotic members of the Bcl-2 family are classified into two groups; the multidomain members, e.g., Bax and Bak, and BH3-only members, e.g., Bad, Bid, and Bim (14). Apoptotic signals can cause Bax and Bak to form complexes in the mitochondrial outer membrane and allow release of cytochrome c and other proapoptotic molecules. The BH3-only members of the Bcl-2 family serve as sensors of cellular integrity; Bad for growth factor withdrawal, Bid for external pathway signals, and Bim for cytoskeletal integrity. The BH3-only proteins can stimulate Bax and Bak to form multimer complexes in the mitochondrial membrane by mechanisms that are not fully understood.

Mitochondria are considered to influence apoptosis at a number of levels: (a) maintenance of ATP levels, (b) maintenance of the mitochondrial membrane potential, and (c) release of proapoptotic factors. The mitochondrial permeability transition pore (PTP) has been demonstrated to play an important role in certain models of apoptosis. The molecules comprising the PTP are not fully defined, but it is thought to be composed of the outer membrane voltage-dependent anion channel (VDAC), the inner membrane adenine nucleotide translocase (ANT), the mitochondrial benzodiazepine receptor, and cyclophilin D (15). The permeability transition is described as a sudden increase in the permeability of the mitochondrial membrane to solutes with a mass of less than 1.5 kDa. Opening of the PTP leads to entry of K^+, Mg^{+2}, and Ca^{+2} and water, which results in swelling of the matrix, rupture of the outer membrane, and leakage of the proteins, including the proapoptotic proteins. Inhibitors of PTP, such as the cyclophilin D inhibitor cyclosporin A and the ANT inhibitor bongkrekic acid, block apoptosis in some systems, supporting the involvement of the PTP in apoptosis in some systems. Opening of the PTP is controlled by the transmembrane potential ($\Delta\Psi_m$) (the probability of opening increasing with decreasing $\Delta\Psi_m$) and the pH of the matrix (the probability of opening decreasing with acidification of the matrix if the pH drops below 7.0). Elevated cytosolic Ca^{2+} also induces PTP. A number of models of PTP opening have been proposed. In the PTP-induced mitochondrial swelling model there is rapid depolarization of the mitochondria, swelling, and rupture of the outer membrane with release of proapoptotic molecules. However, in some situations cytochrome c can be released without swelling of the matrix and rupture of the outer membrane, and mechanisms other than PTP-induced swelling may occur in these situations (13). Proapoptotic members of the Bcl-2 family, such as Bax and Bak, may form channels with or without interaction with components of the PTP and allow release of cytochrome c and other proapoptotic molecules.

Similarly, the role of reduction in $\Delta\Psi_m$ in release of cytochrome c and other proapoptotic molecules from the mitochondria is not fully defined. In some models of apoptosis, cells with lowered $\Delta\Psi_m$ appear destined for apoptosis (16,17). Although cells with disrupted $\Delta\Psi_m$ appear to be doomed to cell death, in some models of apoptosis reduction in $\Delta\Psi_m$ occurs late and may be a subsequent event, and dissipation of $\Delta\Psi_m$ cannot be considered as a prerequisite for apoptosis. In some instances, dissipation of $\Delta\Psi_m$ may serve to amplify the apoptotic signaling.

The evidence reviewed above indicates that the central role that mitochondria play in cellular bioenergetics positions them as an index of the viability of the cell and mitochondria can initiate or amplify proapoptotic signals in the cell.

Development of antiapoptotic drugs is an active area of research (10), but developers of antiapoptotic therapies for PD will need to be mindful of the possibility of neoplasia, and treatments will optimally be selectively directed toward cells that degenerate in PD. Although the degenerative process affects both nigral and extranigral neurons (18), one would expect that the first target for antiapoptotic therapies in PD would be the nigral dopaminergic neurons.

IV. EVIDENCE FOR MITOCHONDRIAL DYSFUNCTION IN PD

Insights into the mechanisms through which MPTP is toxic to the ETC led investigators to study mitochondrial function in PD. Schapira et al. (19) studied mitochondrial function in various regions in brains from patients with PD and multiple system atrophy (MSA) and normal control subjects. They found a selective reduction in the activity of complex I in the substantia nigra (SN) in PD brains. The finding of reduced complex I activity in the SN has been confirmed by Janetzky et al. (20). At approximately the same time Parker et al. (21) reported a significant reduction in complex I activity in platelets from patients with relatively advanced PD, and this observation has been confirmed (22–24). These studies were typically carried out in tissue from patients with advanced disease, and the possibility remained that the reduction in complex I activity could have been due to medication used to treat PD and/or the debilitation that occurs with advanced disease. Haas et al. (25) postulated that if mitochondrial impairment is involved in the pathogenesis of PD, it should occur in patients with early, unmedicated disease. They carried out a study in which mitochondrial function was evaluated in platelets in patients with early, untreated PD, age- and gender-matched control subjects, and spouses, who served as a control for the home environment. They found a significant reduction in complex I activity in the PD patients compared to both control groups and a significant reduction in the activity of complex I/III in the PD subjects compared to the age- and gender-matched control subjects (25). They also found that treatment of the PD subjects with carbidopa/levodopa for one month and carbidopa/levodopa with selegiline for a second month did not affect mitochondrial function (26). These findings indicate that the impairment in mitochondrial activity found in PD patients is not the result of debilitation or drugs and suggest that mitochondrial dysfunction plays a role in the development of the illness.

The etiology of the mitochondrial dysfunction remains uncertain; it could be the result of genetic factors (in either mitochondrial or nuclear DNA) and/or acquired injury to the mitochondria (either endogenous or exogenous toxins). A number of mutations in the nuclear genome have been associated with PD, but none to date have occurred in genes encoding mitochondrial proteins (27,28). Swerdlow et al. (29) have used cybrids in which mitochondria from PD patients have replaced the normal mitochondria in cultured neuroblastoma cells and found that the resultant cell lines had a 20% reduction in complex I activity, increased oxygen free radical production, and increased sensitivity to 1-methyl-4-phenylpyridinium (MPP+). Schapira's group replicated this finding (30), but Schon and Manfredi (28) reported that not all groups could reproduce this abnormality in cybrids with mitochondrial DNA from PD patients. One concern about cybrid studies is the possibility for clonal selection. Studies in which the mitochondrial genome has been examined have not revealed common mutations in PD patients. However, because of heteroplasmy in the mitochondrial genome, such studies could fail to detect mutations that occur in a minority of the mitochondria. Only three mutations in mitochondrial DNA have been associated with parkinsonism, and in none of the three was there classical PD (28).

Circumstantial evidence supports the hypothesis that oxidative damage in mitochondria can lead to mutations in mitochondrial DNA and that such damage may set up a vicious cycle of damage to the mitochondrial DNA leading to further oxidative stress (27). It is of interest that highest levels of the "common" 5 kb deletion in the aged brain occur in the substantia nigra, caudate, and putamen.

The impairment in mitochondrial function could be due to injury by toxins, either endogenous or exogenous. A number of possible exogenous toxins have been identified, including MPTP (1), rotenone (31), and paraquat (32). Nakai et al. (33) have reported that infusion of MPP+, the active metabolite of MPTP, into the rat striatum resulted in reduction in both redox activity and mitochondrial membrane potential in striatal synaptosomes. Bywood and Johnson (34) also found a relative vulnerability of nigral dopaminergic neurons to rotenone, as well as MPP+ and antimycin, in slice preparations from the rat midbrain. Of note, epidemiological studies have consistently found an association between PD and exposure to pesticides (35).

Endogenous toxins may impair mitochondrial function. As mentioned above, the mitochondria are the major but not the only source of ROS in dopaminergic neurons (36). It is plausible that impairment of mitochondrial function could result in an increase in the production of oxygen free radicals and further injury to the mitochondria. Other endogenous mitochondrial toxins have been reported, such as isoquinolines (37). Isoquinolines and MPP+ have also been shown to inhibit α-ketoglutarate dehydrogenase (38). N-Methyl(R)salsolinol, which is found in the cerebrospinal fluid in patients with PD, causes apoptosis of dopaminergic neurons through reduction of the mitochondrial membrane potential (39).

α-Synuclein is a major component of Lewy bodies, and mutations in the gene for α-synuclein are very rare causes of PD (40). A connection between α-synuclein and mitochondrial dysfunction has been reported by Hsu et al. (41) in which cells genetically engineered to overexpress α-synuclein were found to have impaired mitochondrial function.

V. DEVELOPMENT OF THERAPIES TARGETED TO MITOCHONDRIAL FUNCTION

The observation of reduced activity of both complexes I and II/III in platelet mitochondria from patients with early untreated PD prompted Shults and colleagues to examine the levels of coenzyme Q_{10} in the mitochondria (25). Coenzyme Q_{10} is the electron acceptor for both complex I and complex II. They reported a significant reduction (33%) in the levels of coenzyme Q_{10} in mitochondria in PD patients compared to control subjects (42). Matsubara et al. (43) reported that the serum level of coenzyme Q_{10} in parkinsonian patients $(0.57 \pm 0.26 \,\mu g/mL)$ was significantly lower than that in patients with stroke of similar age $(0.77 \pm 0.29 \,\mu g/mL)$. This group had previously found patients without neurological disease to have higher levels of coenzyme Q_{10} $(0.85 \pm 0.28 \,\mu g/mL)$ than those found in PD patients (44). Similarly, Molina et al. (45) reported that the serum level of coenzyme Q_{10}, but not the coenzyme Q_{10}/cholesterol ratio, was reduced in patients with Lewy body disease. However, Jiménez-Jiménez et al. (46) did not find a reduction in the serum level of coenzyme Q_{10} in PD.

Beal et al. subsequently reported that oral supplementation with coenzyme Q_{10} in one-year-old mice reduced the damage to the nigrostriatal dopaminergic system caused by treatment with MPTP (47). This led Shults and colleagues to carry out a phase II study of the effects of coenzyme Q_{10} in patients with early PD (48). Eighty subjects were randomly assigned to receive either placebo or coenzyme Q_{10} at dosages of 300, 600, or

1200 mg/d, and all subjects also received α-tocopherol (vitamin E) at a dosage of 1200 IU/d. The subjects were evaluated with the Unified Parkinson's Disease Rating Scale (UPDRS) at baseline and months 1, 4, 8, 12, and 16 and were followed until the subject had developed disability requiring treatment with levodopa or for a maximum of 16 months. The primary response variable was the change in the total score on the UPDRS at baseline compared to that at the last visit. The adjusted mean total UPDRS changes were placebo, +11.99; 300 mg/d, +8.81; 600 mg/d, +10.82; and 1200 mg/d, +6.69 (+ indicates worsening). The p-value for the primary analysis, test for a linear trend between dosage and the mean change in the total UPDRS score, was 0.0855, which met the study's prespecified criteria for a positive trend for the trial. A prespecified secondary analysis comparing each treatment group to the placebo group found a significant difference between the 1200 mg/d and placebo groups ($p = 0.04$, uncorrected for multiple comparisons). This group also studied mitochondrial function in platelets taken from the patients at baseline and last visit. They determined the activity of the ETC from NADH to cytochrome c (complexes I and III; this assay is dependent on the endogenous coenzyme Q_{10}) and found a significant increase in the activity of the ETC with coenzyme Q_{10}. Although these results are encouraging, Shults and colleagues have advised that it would be premature for patients with PD to take high doses of coenzyme Q_{10} until a larger, definitive study has confirmed the findings of the phase II study.

Horvath et al. (49) reported that 10 days of oral supplementation with coenzyme Q_{10} (15–22 mg/kg) prior to treatment with MPTP in primates significantly attenuated the loss of nigral dopaminergic neurons. This dosage range is similar to that used in the phase II trial in patients with PD. Horvath et al. presented data to support the hypothesis that the mechanism of action of coenzyme Q_{10} was through activation of uncoupling protein 2 (UCP2). Another possible mechanism is through inhibition of the mitochondrial PTP (50).

Other therapies directed at mitochondrial function have been shown in animal models of PD to ameliorate damage to the nigrostriatal dopaminergic system. Beal's group demonstrated that creatine can attenuate damage to the nigrostriatal dopaminergic system in MPTP-treated mice (51). Moussaoui et al. (52) showed that ebeselen can be beneficial in MPTP-treated monkeys. Seaton et al. (53) reported that cyclosporine, which modulates the mitochondrial transition pore, could attenuate rotenone, MPP+, and tetrahydroisoquinoline-induced damage in PC12 cells, but cyclosporin A is too toxic to be used in PD.

VI. CONCLUSION

Mitochondria are crucial not only to the bioenergetics of the cell but also to the process of cell death. Substantial data indicate impaired mitochondrial function, particularly of complex I of the ETC, in some patients with PD, and it appears likely that mitochondria contribute to the pathogenic processes that occur in many PD patients. Therapies targeted at mitochondrial function hold promise to slow the progression of PD.

REFERENCES

1. Langston JW, Ballard P, Tetrud JW, Irwin I. Chronic parkinsonism in humans due to a produce of meperidine-analog synthesis. Science 1983; 219:979–980.
2. Beal MF. Experimental models of Parkinson's disease. Nat Rev Neurosci 2001; 2(5):325–334.

3. Singer TP, Castagnoli N Jr., Ramsay RR, Trevor AJ. Biochemical events in the development of parkinsonism induced by 1-methyl-4-phenyl-1,2,3,6-tetrahydropyridine. J Neurochem 1987; 49:1–8.

4. Przedborski S, Jackson-Lewis V, Djaldetti R, Liberatore G, Vila M, Vukosavic S, Almer G. The parkinsonian toxin MPTP: action and mechanism. Restor Neurol Neurosci 2000; 16(2): 135–142.

5. Greenamyre JT, Sherer TB, Betarbet R, Panov AV. Complex I and Parkinson's disease. IUBMB Life 2001; 52(3–5):135–141.

6. Wallace DC. Mitochondrial diseases in man and mouse. Science 1999; 283(5407):1482–1488.

7. Halliwell B. Role of free radicals in the neurodegenerative diseases: therapeutic implications for antioxidant treatment. Drugs Aging 2001; 18(9):685–716.

8. Kingsbury AE, Mardsen CD, Foster OJ. DNA fragmentation in human substantia nigra: apoptosis or perimortem effect? Mov Disord 1998; 13(6):877–884.

9. Andersen, JK. Does neuronal loss in Parkinson's disease involve programmed cell death? Bioessays 2001; 23(7):640–646.

10. Reed JC. Apoptosis-based therapies. Nat Rev Drug Discov 2002; 1(2):111–121.

11. Zimmermann KC, Bonzon C, Green DR. The machinery of programmed cell death. Pharmacol Ther 2001; 92(1):57–70.

12. Nijhawan D, Honarpour N, Wang X. Apoptosis in neural development and disease. Ann Rev Neurosci 2000; 23:73–87.

13. van Gurp M, Festjens N, van Loo G, Saelens X, Vandenabeele P. Mitochondrial intermembrane proteins in cell death. Biochem Biophys Res Commun 2003; 304(3):487–497.

14. Tsujimoto Y. Cell death regulation by the Bcl-2 protein family in the mitochondria. J Cell Physiol 2003; 195(2):158–167.

15. Ly JD, Grubb DR, Lawen. The mitochondrial membrane potential ($\Delta\Psi$m) in apoptosis; an update. Apoptosis 2003; 8:115–128.

16. Zamzami N, Marchetti P, Castedo M, Decaudin D, Macho A, Hirsch T, Susin SA, Petit PX, Mignotte B, Kroemer G. Sequential reduction of mitochondrial transmembrane potential and generation of reactive oxygen species in early programmed cell death. J Exp Med 1995; 182: 367–377.

17. Kroemer G. Mitochondrial control of apoptosis: an introduction. Biochem Biophys Res Commun 2003; 304(3):433–435.

18. Braak H, Braak E. Pathoanatomy of Parkinson's disease. J Neurol 2000; 247(2).II3–110.

19. Schapira AH, Mann VM, Cooper JM, Dexter D, Daniel SE, Jenner P, Clark JB, Marsden CD. Anatomic and disease specificity of NADH CoQ1 reductase complex I) deficiency in parkinson's disease. J Neurochem 1990; 55:2142–2145.

20. Janetzky B, Hauck S, Youdim MBH, Riederer P, Jellinger K, Pantucek F, Zochling R, Boissl KW, Reichmann H. Unaltered aconitase activity, but decreased complex I activity in substantia nigra pars compacta of patients with Parkinson's disease. Neurosci Lett 1994; 169:126–128.

21. Parker WD Jr, Boyson SJ, Parks JK. Abnormalities of the electron transport chain in idiopathic Parkinson's disease. Ann Neurol 1989; 26:719–723.

22. Krige D, Carroll MT, Cooper JM, Marsden CD, Schapira AHV. Platelet mitochondrial function in Parkinson's disease. Ann Neurol 1992; 32:782–788.

23. Yoshino H, Nakagawa-Hattori Y, Kondo T, Mizuno Y. Mitochondrial complex I and II activities of lymphocytes and platelets in Parkinson's disease. J Neural Transm 1992; 4:27–34.

24. Benecke R, Strümper P, Weiss H. Electron transfer complexes I and IV of platelets are abnormal in Parkinson's disease but normal in Parkinson-plus syndromes. Brain 1993; 116:1451–1463.

25. Haas R, Nasirian F, Nakano K, Ward D, Pay M, Hill R, Shults CW. Low platelet mitochondrial Complex I and Complex II/III activity in early untreated Parkinson's disease. Ann Neurol 1995; 37:714–722.

26. Shults CW, Nasirian F, Ward DM, Nakano K, Pay M, Hill LR, Haas RH. Carbidopa/levodopa and selegiline do not affect platelet mitochondrial function in early parkinsonism. Neurology 1995; 45:344–348.

27. Chomyn A, Attardi G. MtDNA mutations in aging and apoptosis. Biochem Biophys Res Commun 2003 9; 304(3):519–529.

28. Schon EA, Manfredi G. Neuronal degeneration and mitochondrial dysfunction. J Clin Invest 2003; 111(3):303–312.

29. Swerdlow RH, Parks JK, Miller SW, Tuttle JB, Trimmer PA, Sheehan JP, Bennett JP Jr., Davis RE, Parker WD Jr. Origin and functional consequences of the complex I defect in Parkinson's disease. Ann Neurol 1996; 40(4):663–671.

30. Gu M, Cooper JM, Taanman JW, Schapira AH. Mitochondrial DNA transmission of the mitochondrial defect in Parkinson's disease. Ann Neurol 1998; 44(2):177–186.

31. Betarbet R, Sherer TB, MacKenzie G, Garcia-Osuna M, Panov AV, Greenamyre JT. Chronic systemic pesticide exposure reproduces features of Parkinson's disease. Nat Neurosci 2000; 3(12):1301–1306.

32. McCormack AL, Thiruchelvam M, Manning-Bog AB, Thiffault C, Langston JW, Cory-Slechta DA, Di Monte DA. Environmental risk factors and Parkinson's disease: selective degeneration of nigral dopaminergic neurons caused by the herbicide paraquat. Neurobiol Dis 2002; 10(2):119–127.

33. Nakai M, Mori A, Watanabe A, Mitsumoto Y. 1-Methyl-4-phenylpyridinium (MPP+) decreases mitochondrial oxidation-reduction (REDOX) activity and membrane potential (Deltapsi(m)) in rat striatum. Exp Neurol 2003; 179(1):103–110.

34. Bywood PT, Johnson SM. Mitochondrial complex inhibitors preferentially damage substantia nigra dopamine neurons in rat brain slices. Exp Neurol 2003; 179(1):47–59.

35. Tanner CM, Aston DA. Epidemiology of Parkinson's disease and akinetic syndromes. Curr Opin Neurol 2000; 13(4):427–430.

36. Adams JD Jr., Chang ML, Klaidman L. Parkinson's disease: redox mechanisms. Curr Med Chem 2001; 8(7):809–814.

37. Nagatsu T. Isoquinoline neurotoxins in the brain and Parkinson's disease. Neurosci Res 1997; 29(2):99–111.

38. McNaught KS, Carrupt PA, Altomare C, Cellamare S, Carotti A, Testa B, Jenner P, Marsden CD. Isoquinoline derivatives as endogenous neurotoxins in the aetiology of Parkinson's disease. Biochem Pharmacol 1998; 56(8):921–933.

39. Akao Y, Maruyama W, Shimizu S, Yi H, Nakagawa Y, Shamoto-Nagai M, Youdim MB, Tsujimoto Y, Naoi M. Mitochondrial permeability transition mediates apoptosis induced by N-methyl(R)salsolinol, an endogenous neurotoxin, and is inhibited by Bcl-2 and rasagiline, N-propargyl-1(R)-aminoindan. J Neurochem 2002; 82(4):913–923.

40. Goedert M. Alpha-synuclein and neurodegenerative diseases. Nat Rev Neurosci 2001; 2:492–501.

41. Hsu LJ, Sagara Y, Arroyo A, Rockenstein E, Sisk A, Mallory M, Wong J, Takenouchi T, Hashimoto M, Masliah E. Alpha-synuclein promotes mitochondrial deficit and oxidative stress. Am J Pathol 2000; 157(2):401–410.

42. Shults CW, Haas RH, Passov D, Beal MF. Coenzyme Q10 levels correlate with the activities of complexes I and II/III in mitochondria from parkinsonian and nonparkinsonian subjects. Ann Neurol 1997; 42:261–264.

43. Matsubara T, Azuma T, Yoshida S, Yamagami T. Serum coenzyme Q-10 level in Parkinson syndrome. In: Folkers K, Littarru P, Yamagami T, eds. Biomedical and Clinical Aspects of Coenzyme Q. Amsterdam: Elsevier Science Publishers BV, 1991:159–166.

44. Yamagami T, Okishio T, Toyama S, Kishi T. Correlation of serum coenzyme Q10 level and leukocute complex II activity in normal and cardiovascular patients. In: Folkers K, Yamagami T, eds. Biomedical and Clinical Aspects of Coenzyme Q. Amsterdam: Elsevier Science Publishers BV, 1991:79–89.

45. Molina JA, de Bustos F, Ortiz S, Del Ser T, Seijo M, Benito-Léon J, Oliva JM, Pérez S, Manzanares J. Serum levels of coenzyme Q in patients with Lewy body disease. J Neural Transm 2002; 109(9):1195–1201.

46. Jiménez-Jiménez FJ, Molina JA, de Bustos F, García-Redondo A, Gómez-Escalonilla C, Martínez-Salio A, Berbel A, Camacho A, Zurdo M, Barcenilla B, Enríquez de Salamanca R, Arenas J. Serum levels of coenzyme Q10 in patients with Parkinson's disease. J Neural Transm 2000; 107:177–181.

47. Beal MF, Matthews RT, Tieleman A, Shults CW. Coenzyme Q_{10} attenuates the 1-methyl-4-phenyl-1,2,3,6-tetrahydropyridine (MPTP) induced loss of striatal dopamine and dopaminergic axons in aged mice. Brain Res 1998; 783:109–114.

48. Shults CW, Oakes D, Kieburtz K, Beal MF, Haas R, Plumb S, Juncos JL, Nutt J, Shoulson I, Carter J, Kompoliti K, Perlmutter JS, Reich S, Stern M, Watts RL, Kurlan R, Molho E, Harrison M, Lew M. Parkinson Study Group. Effects of coenzyme Q10 in early Parkinson disease—evidence of slowing of the functional decline. Arch Neurol 2002; 59:1541–1550.

49. Horvath TL, Diano S, Leranth C, Garcia-Segura LM, Cowley MA, Shanabrough M, Elsworth JD, Sotonyi P, Roth RH, Dietrich EH, Matthews RT, Barnstable CJ, Redmond DE Jr. Coenzyme Q induces nigral mitochondrial uncoupling and prevents dopamine cell loss in a primate model of Parkinson's disease. Endocrinology 2003; 144(7):2757–2760.

50. Walter L, Nogueira V, Leverve X, Heitz MP, Bernardi P, Fontaine E. Three classes of ubiquinone analogs regulate the mitochondrial permeability transition pore through a common site. J Biol Chem 2000; 275(38):29521–29527.
51. Matthews RT, Ferrante RJ, Klivenyi P, Yang L, Klein AM, Mueller G, Kaddurah-Daouk R, Beal MF. Creatine and cyclocreatine attenuate MPTP neurotoxicity. Exp Neurol 1999; 157(1):142–149.
52. Moussaoui S, Obinu MC, Daniel N, Reibaud M, Blanchard V, Imperato A. The antioxidant ebselen prevents neurotoxicity and clinical symptoms in a primate model of Parkinson's disease. Exp Neurol 2000; 166(2):235–245.
53. Seaton TA, Cooper JM, Schapira AH. Cyclosporin inhibition of apoptosis induced by mitochondrial complex I toxins. Brain Res 1998; 809(1):12–17.

38

Trophic Factors: Potential Therapies

Greg A. Gerhardt and Don M. Gash

University of Kentucky, Chandler Medical Center, Lexington, Kentucky, U.S.A.

I. INTRODUCTION

Parkinson's disease (PD) is a neurodegenerative disease that involves the loss of dopamine neurons in the pars compacta region of the substantia nigra (1,2). These neurons send out fibers, which extensively innervate neurons in the basal ganglia, especially in the caudate and putamen, and modulate basal ganglia activity via synaptic release of the neurotransmitter dopamine. Extensive loss of dopamine innervation in the caudate and putamen is required before the cardinal features of PD are observed; these include bradykinesia, rigidity, postural instability, and disturbances in balance and tremor (2). Thus, an effective treatment for PD should involve an approach to prevent and/or slow degeneration of dopamine neurons and their processes. In addition, drug treatments that promote the restoration and regeneration of damaged or dying dopamine neurons would be of significant benefit.

Trophic factors are endogenous proteins capable of promoting the development, growth, and/or survival of neurons. Many are highly expressed during development to promote growth and differentiation of neurons. These proteins are highly potent molecules, binding to receptors and eliciting biological effects at concentrations in the femtomolar to nanomolar range. More than 20 trophic factors have been identified, showing potential for use in a variety of neurodegenerative diseases including PD (3,4). Although there is little evidence that deficiencies of trophic factors are associated with the etiology of PD (5), several factors have been shown to produce significant beneficial effects on dopamine neurons in culture and a few in animal models (for review, see Ref. 3). Those producing effects on dopamine neurons in vitro include, but are not limited to, fibroblast growth factor (FGF), epidermal growth factor (EGF), transforming growth factor-α (TGF-α), ciliary neurotrophic factor (CNTF), platelet-derived growth factor (PDGF), brain-derived neurotrophic factor (BDNF), and glial cell line–derived neurotrophic factor (GDNF) (3,4). Because of their striking effects in vitro and in vivo many investigators have proposed the use of trophic factors in the treatment of PD (6–12).

517

However, of all the factors investigated, GDNF is the only trophic factor shown to dramatically protect and enhance dopamine neuron function in vivo in rats and monkeys (13–21). GDNF produces behavioral changes, which are consistent with protection, restoration, and/or enhanced function of dopamine neurons in animal models. In addition, GDNF has recently shown promise in a phase I clinical trial (22) in advanced PD patients. This chapter will focus on some basic properties of trophic factors and more specifically the preclinical and clinical data that support the potential use of GDNF in patients with PD. Other potential growth factors have been delineated in several excellent recent reviews for use in PD and other neurodegenerative diseases (3,4).

II. NEUROTROPHIC FACTORS

The potential benefits from the use of neurotrophic factors in PD are fourfold. First, delivery of a trophic factor to the basal ganglia may slow the degeneration of dopamine neurons during the disease state. This could "arrest" or slow the progression of the illness, perhaps allowing for extended use of drug therapies in PD patients and decreased side effects. In general, a long-held view since the discovery of growth factors is that early intervention into the brain of a PD patient with growth factors may be beneficial in stopping the further progression of PD. Second, the neurotrophic factor may, with its inherent capabilities, improve the function of the remaining dopamine neurons. It is also possible that some neurotrophic factors may stimulate inherent regenerative capabilities in injured neurons and, in fact, restore function to the damaged dopamine neurons. Third, it is quite possible that these proteins may enhance the function of residual dopamine neurons, thus improving the capacity of the normal dopamine system to function in patients with PD. Fourth, it has been shown in animal models that trophic factors may enhance the growth and function of fetal tissue grafts (23,24) and in the future perhaps stem cells. Thus, the use of neurotrophic factors may some day be combined with cell-replacement therapies to improve the reinnervation of the brain by these tissues (25).

III. GDNF

Cloning of GDNF from rat B49 cells supports the idea that this factor is a distant member of the transforming growth factor-β (TGF-β) superfamily (3, 26–28). The purification and cloning of the new trophic factors neurturin (27), persephin (30), and artemin (31), all structurally related to GDNF, has established the existence of this new family of neurotrophic factors. GDNF is a heparin-binding protein and acts as a disulfide-bonded dimer. Each portion of the mature protein consists of 134 amino acid residues, with 93% identity between the human and rat sequences. The naturally occurring dimer has a molecular weight of ~30 kDa and is glycosylated.

GDNF is widely expressed throughout the body during development and in adults in many neuronal (e.g., striatum, cerebellum, cortex) (see Refs. 32–34) and nonneuronal tissues (e.g., kidney, gut) (see Refs. 32,35,36). GDNF uses a multisubunit receptor system, which consists of a glycosyl-phosphatidylinositol (GPI)–anchored membrane protein, termed GFRα-1, ("β" subunit) that can bind GDNF and facilitate its interaction with the tyrosine kinase Ret receptor ("α" subunit) (see Refs. 26,37,38). Three other GPI-anchored membrane proteins are now known, namely GFRα-2, 3, and 4 (39–43). Mechanistically, little is known at the present time about the intracellular phosphorylation signaling mechanisms that occur acutely and chronically following activation of Ret via GDNF or the related factors neurturin, persephin, and artemin.

IV. MORPHOLOGICAL AND FUNCTIONAL EFFECTS OF INTRANIGRALLY ADMINISTERED GDNF IN NORMAL RHESUS MONKEYS

Studies involving GDNF treatment in rat models (19,44) are limited in their relevance to humans. Rodents have a much smaller nervous system, which differs significantly in numerous neuroanatomical and neurochemical parameters from that of humans. In contrast, nonhuman primates possess a central nervous system and behavioral repertoire much closer to the human than the rodent.

Normal monkeys were evaluated prior to and then for 3–4 weeks following a single injection of 150 µg rhGDNF into the right substantia nigra using magnetic resonance imaging (MRI)–guided stereotaxic procedures (45). The behavioral effects over the 3-week observation period following GDNF treatment were small, with blinded observers unable to distinguish between GDNF- and vehicle-treated animals (45). The most consistent behavioral response to GDNF treatment was weight loss, which averaged about 7% of total body weight over the 3-week period after trophic factor administration; conversely, vehicle-treated animals averaged 3% weight gain over the same period. None of the other behavioral responses that might be expected from stimulating central dopamine pathways, such as nausea, dyskinesia, or stereotypic behavior, were observed in the monkeys. Even though the GDNF injections were into the right nigral region, no unilateral effects on motor behavior were observed. Amplitudes of K^+-evoked dopamine release, measured by in vivo voltammetric techniques, were significantly increased after the single 150 µg intranigral administration of GDNF (45). The GDNF-induced increase in K^+-stimulated dopamine overflow parallels that observed in rats (18). The signals recorded from the striatum of GDNF-treated monkeys were almost twofold greater than those measured in vehicle-treated primates (45). The GDNF-enhanced dopamine release cannot be related to alterations in the storage or synthesis of dopamine within the striatum. In fact, dopamine levels within the ipsilateral substantia nigra and ventral tegmental area of rhesus monkeys treated with GDNF were approximately twofold greater than those in the contralateral region and in control animals. Homovanillic acid (HVA), the major dopamine metabolite in the rhesus monkey, was found to be significantly elevated in the substantia nigra, ventral tegmental area, and striatum, with a trend toward increased HVA levels in the putamen. The HVA/dopamine turnover ratios were not significantly different between vehicle and GDNF recipients. Tyrosine hydroxylase (TH) immunoreactivity suggested that GDNF treatment leads to increases in dopamine cell size and number in the ipsilateral mesencephalon, similar to those observed in culture (27) and adult rodent dopamine neurons in vivo (44,46,47). An observation unique to the nonhuman primate studies was that GDNF can sufficiently diffuse to stimulate TH-positive axons and dendrites over at least a 2 mm rostral-caudal gradient (45). Histological data suggested that there was some tissue damage resulting from the intranigral injections of 150 µg of GDNF, but dopamine neurons appeared relatively unaffected by the injections, probably due to the neuroprotective and neurorestorative effects of GDNF reported for rodent midbrain dopamine neurons (46–50). The results indicate that, in the adult rhesus monkey, a single intranigral

GDNF injection induces a significant upregulation of mesencephalic dopamine neurons lasting for weeks. Thus, GDNF can produce prolonged effects after a single injection into the brain of rhesus monkeys.

V. GDNF ATTENUATION OF SYMPTOMS IN ANIMAL MODELS OF PARKINSON'S DISEASE

A. Functional Recovery in Parkinsonian Monkeys Treated with Acute Injections of GDNF

The effects of GDNF administered to rhesus monkeys with hemiparkinsonian features induced by the infusion of 1-methyl-4-phenyl-1,2,3,6-tetrahydropyridine (MPTP) through the right cartoid artery have been studied (14,15,51). In humans and nonhuman primates, MPTP induces neurochemical, neuropathological, and behavioral features, with numerous similarities to those found in idiopathic PD (52–54). MPTP-treated nonhuman primates display the cardinal symptomology of PD: bradykinesia, rigidity, postural instability and tremor (51,55–57). Histological and neurochemical alterations in the brain induced by MPTP administration also resemble those found in PD.

Three routes of GDNF delivery into unilateral MPTP-treated monkeys were tested: intranigral, intracaudate, and intracerebroventricular (ICV). GDNF was not administered until the animals were at least 3 months post–MPTP treatment and displayed stable parkinsonian symptoms. Prior to and following GDNF administration the animals were analyzed for changes in behavior, using a nonhuman primate hemiparkinsonian rating scale (58). While no significant behavioral changes were observed in the control group, the GDNF recipients showed functional improvements, which lasted throughout the 4-week test period. The ICV-treated animals were also assessed for the ability to respond to repeated dosing of GDNF. In both ICV GDNF treatment groups, the effects of trophic factor administration were very striking by the third week following an intra-cerebral injection. Bradykinesia, rigidity, and postural instability were significantly improved by intracerebral injections of GDNF in MPTP-lesioned monkeys. Neuronal size was found to be significantly larger in the GDNF recipients. Multiple tissue punches were also taken from the basal ganglia and midbrain of ICV-treated monkeys for high-performance liquid chromatography–electrochemical (HPLC-EC) determinations of dopamine and its metabolites. Significant increases in dopamine were measured in the substantia nigra, ventral tegmental area, and globus pallidus, but 3,4-dihydroxyphenylacetic acid (DOPAC) and HVA levels within the striatum were not significantly affected (14).

In another series of experiments the effects of intracerebrally administered GDNF were carried out in MPTP-treated common marmosets (59). In these studies, marmosets received parenteral administration of MPTP, which produced bilateral degeneration of the nigrostriatal pathway. Intraventricular injections of GDNF (10, 100, or 500 µg) were administered 9 and 13 weeks post–MPTP treatment. This produced a dose-related improvement in locomotor activity and motor disabilities, which were significant following the 100 and 500 µg doses of GDNF.

The findings from unilateral and bilateral MPTP-lesioned monkeys demonstrate that intracerebrally administered GDNF partially restores dopamine levels in the midbrain, stimulates the growth of surviving dopamine neurons, and significantly improves motor functions.

B. Studies of the Effects of Chronic Intracerebral GDNF in Advanced Parkinsonian Monkeys

A recent series of studies was carried out to determine the effects of chronic infusions of 5 or 15 µg/day GDNF into either the lateral ventricle or the striatum, using programmable pumps, in rhesus monkeys with neural deficits modeling the terminal stages of PD (15). The infusions of GDNF produced functional improvements, which were associated with a pronounced upregulation and regeneration of nigral dopamine neurons and their processes innervating the striatum. When compared to vehicle recipients, these functional improvements were associated with many changes. First, there was a greater than 30% bilateral increase in nigral dopamine neuron cell size with a greater than 20% bilateral increase in the number of TH-positive nigral cells. Second, there were greater than 70% and greater than 50% bilateral increases in dopamine metabolite (HVA) levels in the striatum and the globus pallidus. Third, there were 233% and 155% increases in dopamine levels in the periventricular striatal region and in the globus pallidus, respectively, on the lesioned side. Finally, a fivefold increase in TH positive fiber density was observed in the periventricular striatal region on the lesioned side. All of these effects from chronic administration of GDNF are greater than those previously seen from single injections of GDNF (14).

Kordower and colleagues (20) carried out another series of studies to determine the effects of chronic GDNF administered by a lentiviral delivery approach (lenti-GDNF). Lenti-GDNF was injected into the striatum and substantia nigra of young adult rhesus monkeys treated one week prior with MPTP. Extensive GDNF expression with retrograde and anterograde transport was observed in the animals, with GDNF gene expression lasting for 8 months. Chronic GDNF treatment reversed motor deficits seen in a hand reach task. In addition, nigrostriatal degeneration was prevented in the lenti-GDNF treated monkeys that received MPTP.

These data support that chronic delivery of GDNF can have both neurorestorative and neuroprotective effects on dopamine neuronal systems in MPTP-treated rhesus monkeys. Clearly, the sustained delivery of GDNF, by infusion or viral delivery approaches, greatly enhances the effects of this protein on MPTP-induced damage to the nigrostriatal dopamine system in nonhuman primates.

C. Effects of Chronic Delivery of GDNF in Aged Rhesus Monkeys

The effects of GDNF on stimulus-evoked release of dopamine and motor speed (16) in aged rhesus monkeys (21–27 years old, $n = 10$) have been studied as a possible "early-stage" animal model of PD. While no changes were observed in the vehicle controls ($n = 5$), chronic infusions of 7.5 µg GDNF/day into the right lateral ventricle initially increased upper limb movement speed up to 40% on an automated hand-reach task. These effects were maintained for at least 2 months after replacing GDNF with vehicle and further increased up to 50% following reinstatement of GDNF treatment for one month. The extent of the improvements are shown by the fact that, upper limb motor performance times of the aged GDNF-treated animals ($n = 5$) recorded at the end of the study were similar to those of five young adult monkeys (8–12 years old). Stimulus-evoked release of dopamine was significantly increased up to 130% in the right caudate nucleus and putamen and up to 116% in both the right and left substantia nigra of the aged GDNF recipients compared to vehicle controls. Also, basal extracellular levels of dopamine were bilaterally increased up to 163% in the substantia nigra of the aged GDNF-treated animals.

These studies suggest that the effects of GDNF on the release of dopamine in the basal ganglia may be responsible for improvements in motor function and support the hypothesis that functional changes in dopamine release may contribute to motoric dysfunctions characterizing senescence. Aging nonhuman primates may represent an early-stage model of PD, supporting that early intervention in PD patients may result in enhanced repair of dopamine neurons.

VI. SITE-SPECIFIC DELIVERY: A FAILED CLINICAL TRIAL INVOLVING INTRAVENTRICULAR DELIVERY OF GDNF IN 50 PATIENTS WITH PD

Based on the promising studies of the effects of GDNF in animal models of PD, a clinical trial testing GDNF by ventricular delivery using an indwelling reservoir in 50 PD patients was done (60). While the doses of GDNF (25–4000 µg/month) were in excess of those employed for nonhuman primate studies, little therapeutic efficacy was observed in these PD patients. In fact, one patient that came to autopsy showed no significant effects of the GDNF on dopamine neurons (61). The problem may have been with the site and method of delivery—monthly injections of the trophic factor into the lateral ventricle. Sufficient titers of GDNF may not have diffused through the ventricular wall and brain parenchyma to the targeted neuronal population: dopamine neurons in the substantia nigra and their afferent projections to the putamen. Studies have demonstrated the limited penetration of GDNF through the ventricular wall as compared to the adequate diffusion of GDNF observed with intraparenchymal infusion into the striatum of nonhuman primates (62).

VII. INTRAPARENCHYMAL GDNF DELIVERY: THE KEY TO SUCCESS?

GDNF does not cross the blood-brain barrier and cannot be taken orally. GDNF is not a dopamine neuron-specific factor, as its expression is found in a number of neuronal systems. Even if it could be taken orally, its high potency at GDNF receptors would likely result in side effects, precluding its clinical use. One of the current challenges is to better define delivery systems for GDNF to optimize its actions. These may require continuous or timed infusion of low-dose GDNF into specific brain sites, which may produce the best effects. Novel methods for chronic delivery or prolonged release of GDNF into the nigrostriatal pathway already have been reported in rodents and monkeys using biodegradable biomaterials (63), viral vectors (11,20,21), encapsulated cells genetically engineered to produce GDNF (64,65), and computer-controlled infusion pumps (15,16,66). Along these lines, the safety and efficacy of chronically infusing a low dose of GDNF using a SynchroMed[TM] implantable pump (Model 8616-10, Medtronic Inc., Minneapolis, MN) attached by tubing to a catheter implanted into the right lateral ventricle or into the putamen of monkeys with MPTP-induced parkinsonism has been tested (15). The excellent control achieved by the pumps and infusion catheters has made this approach the best for initial trials in humans.

VIII.   INTRAPARENCHYMAL DELIVERY: A PROMISING PHASE I TRIAL IN PATIENTS WITH LATER STAGE PD

In a pilot study (22), advanced PD patients with a previous history of good response to levodopa underwent unilateral or bilateral insertion of drug infusion cannulae into the dorsal putamen. Human recombinant GDNF was chronically infused via indwelling SynchroMed pumps. Patients were assessed pre- and postoperatively according to the Core Assessment Program for Intracerebral Transplantations (CAPIT) (67) in order to document changes in disease severity and medication requirements. The patients had 18^F-dopa positron emission tomography (PET) scans at baseline, 6, and 12 months after GDNF infusion to assess putamen dopamine terminal function and correlate this with any symptomatic benefits.

Chronic GDNF infusion resulted in improved motor function in all patients, reduction in off-time duration and severity, reduction in dyskinesia duration and severity, and a corresponding increase in on-time duration. In four out of five patients reviewed at 12 months of drug administration, motor [Unified Parkinson's Disease Rating Scale (UPDRS) III] and activities of daily living (UPDRS II) scores improved by 49% and 65%, respectively, in the off-medication state, and by 33% and 43%, respectively, in the on-medication state. Off-medication timed motor tests improved to preoperative best on-medication times in the four cases, with a composite of the timed motor tests at 12 months showing improvements of 50% and 23% in the off- and on-medication states, respectively. Chronic GDNF infusion was tolerated well in all patients, and limited side effects were observed.

IX.   CONCLUSIONS

It has been over 50 years since the discovery of the first prototypical nerve growth factor (NGF) by Stanley Cohen, Rita Levy-Montalcini, and Viktor Hamburger (68,69), and yet the use of these factors for potential repair of damaged brain systems has yet to be carried out. GDNF produces effects on damaged and dying dopamine neurons and on dopamine neurons in aged rats and monkeys with motor deficits (14–16,19,48,66). Studies demonstrate from acute and chronic infusions of GDNF that there appear to be both short-term and long-term effects of GDNF on dopamine neurons. Thus, GDNF does not appear to be just a support factor, but also may transform the dopamine neurons into a modified functional state (16). While data from the intraparenchymal clinical trial in humans looks encouraging (22), extensive blinded efficacy trials will need to be conducted before it can be determined if GDNF or other trophic molecules will prove useful in treating patients with PD. Their use remains of great interest, due to the hope of using some agent to produce regeneration or restoration of dopamine neurons to slow or stop the progression of PD.

ACKNOWLEDGMENTS

This work was supported by USPHS grants MH01245, AG06434, NS39787, and AG13494. In addition, much of the work could not have been carried out without support from Amgen, Inc. and Medtronic, Inc.

REFERENCES

1. Bernheimer H, Birkmayer W, Hornykiewicz O, Jellinger K, Seitelberger F. Brain dopamine and the syndromes of Parkinson and Huntington. Clinical, morphological and neurochemical correlations. J Neurol Sci 1973; 20:415–455.
2. Hornykiewicz O, Kish S. Biochemical pathology of Parkinson's disease. Adv Neurol 1987; 45: 19–34.
3. Collier TJ, Sortwell CE. Therapeutic potential of nerve growth factors in Parkinson's disease. Drugs Aging 1999; 14(4):261–287.
4. Thorne RG, Frey WH II. Delivery of neurotrophic factors to the central nervous system, pharmacokinetic considerations. Clin Pharmacokinet 2001; 40(12):907–946.
5. Hornykiewicz O. Parkinson's disease and the adaptive capacity of the nigrostriatal dopamine system: possible neurochemical mechanisms. Adv Neurol 1993; 60:140–147.
6. Lindsay RM, Altar CA, Cedarbaum JM, Hyman C, Wiegand SJ. The therapeutic potential of neurotrophic factors in the treatment of Parkinson's disease. Exp Neurol 1993; 124:103–118.
7. Magal E, Burnham P, Varon S, Louis J-C. Convergent regulation by ciliary neurotrophic factor and dopamine of tyrosine hydroxylase expression in cultures of rat substantia nigra. Neuroscience 1993; 52:867–881.
8. Hyman C, Juhasz M, Jackson C, Wright P, Ip NY, Lindsay RM. Overlapping and distinct actions of the neurotrophins BDNF, NT-3 and NT-4/5 on cultured dopaminergic and GABAergic neurons of the ventral mesencephalon. J Neurosci 1994; 4(1):335–347.
9. Olson L. Neurotrophins in neurodegenerative disease: theoretical issues and clinical trials. Neurochem Int 1994; 25(1):1–3.
10. Olson L, Backman L, Ebendal T, Eriksdotter-Jonhagen M, Hoffer B, Humpel C, Freedman R, Giacobini M, Meyerson B, Nordberg A. Role of growth factors in degeneration and regeneration in the CNS: clinical experiences with NGF in Parkinson's and Alzheimer's diseases. J Neurol 1994; 242(1 suppl 1):S12–S15.
11. Bjorklund A, Kirik D, Rosenblad C, Georgievska B, Lundberg C, Mandel RJ. Towards a neuroprotective gene therapy for Parkinson's disease: use of adenovirus, AAV and lentivirus vectors for gene transfer of GDNF to the nigrostriatal system in the rat Parkinson model. Brain Res 2000; 886:82–98.
12. Brundin P. GDNF treatment in Parkinson's disease: time for controlled clinical trials? Brain 2002; 125(pt 10):2149–2151.
13. Beck KD, Valverde J, Alexi T, Poulsen K, Moffat B, Vandlen RA, Rosenthal A, Hefti F. Mesencephalic dopaminergic neurons protected by GDNF from axotomy-induced degeneration in the adult brain. Nature 1995; 373:339–341.
14. Gash DM, Zhang Z, Ovadia A, Cass WA, Yi A, Simmerman L, Russell D, Martin D, Lapchak PA, Collins F, Hoffer BJ, Gerhardt GA. Functional recovery in parkinsonian monkeys treated with GDNF. Nature 1996; 380:252–255.
15. Grondin R, Zhang Z, Yi A, Maswood N, Cass WA, Andersen AH, Elsberry DD, Klein MC, Gerhardt GA, Gash DM. Striatal GDNF infusion promotes structural and functional recovery in advanced parkinsonian monkeys. Brain 2002; 125(10):2191–2201.
16. Grondin R, Cass WA, Zhang Z, Stanford JA, Gash DM and Gerhardt, GA. GDNF increases stimulus-evoked dopamine release and motor speed in aged rhesus monkeys. J Neurosci 2003; 23(5):1974–1980.
17. Hou JGG, Lin LFH, Mytilineou C. Glial cell line-derived neurotrophic factor exerts neurotrophic effects on dopaminergic neurons in vitro and promotes their survival and regrowth after damage by 1-methyl-4-phenylpyridinium. J Neurochem 1996; 66:74–82.
18. Hebert MA, van Horne CG, Hoffer BJ, Gerhardt GA. Functional effects of GDNF in normal rat striatum: presynaptic studies using in vivo electrochemistry and microdialysis. J Pharmacol Exp Ther 1996; 279(3):1181–1190.
19. Hebert MA, Gerhardt GA. Behavioral and neurochemical effects of intranigral GDNF administration on aged Fischer 344 rats. J Pharmacol Exp Therapeut 1997; 282:760–768.
20. Kordower JH, Emborg ME, Bloch J, Ma SY, Chu Y, Leventhal L, McBride J, Chen EY, Palfi S, Roitberg BZ, Brown WD, Holden JE, Pyzalski R, Taylor MD, Carvey P, Ling Z, Trono D, Hantraye P, Deglon N, Aebischer P. Neurodegeneration prevented by lentiviral vector delivery of GDNF in primate models of Parkinson's disease. Science 2000; 290:767–773.
21. Palfi S, Leventhal L, Chu Y, Ma SY, Emborg M, Bakay R, Deglon N, Hantraye P, Aebischer P, Kordower JH. Lentivirally delivered glial cell line-derived neurotrophic factor increases the number

of striatal dopaminergic neurons in primate models of nigrostriatal degeneration. J Neurosci 2002; 22(12):4942–4954.

22. Gill SS, Patel NK, O'Sullivan K, Brooks DJ, Hotton GR, Svendsen CN. Intraparenchymal putamenal administration of glial-derived neurotrophic factor in the treatment of advanced Parkinson's disease. Neurology 2002; 58(3):A241.

23. Clarkson ED, Zawada WM, Freed CR. GDNF improves survival and reduces apoptosis in human embryonic dopaminergic neurons in vitro. Cell Tissue Res 1997; 289(2):207–210.

24. Granholm AC, Helt C, Srivastava N, Backman C, Gerhardt GA. Effects of age and GDNF on noradrenergic innervation of the hippocampal formation: studies from intraocular grafts. Microsc Res Tech 2001; 54(5):298–308.

25. Freed CR, Greene PE, Breeze RE, Tsai WY, DuMouchel W, Kao R, Dillon S, Winfield H, Culver S, Trojanowski JQ, Eidelberg D, Fahn S. Transplantation of embryonic dopamine neurons for severe Parkinson's disease. N Engl J Med 2001; 344(10):710–719.

26. Airaksinen MS, Saarma M. The GDNF family: signaling, biological functions and therapeutic value. Nat Rev Neurosci 2002; 3(5):383–394.

27. Lin L-FH, Doherty DH, Lile JD, Bektesh S, Collins F. GDNF: A glial cell line-derived neurotrophic factor for midbrain dopaminergic neurons. Science 1993; 260:1130–1132.

28. Lin L-FH, Zhang TJ, Collins F, Armes LG. Purification and initial characterization of rat B49 glial cell line-derived neurotrophic factor. J Neurochem 1994; 63:58–768.

29. Kotzbauer, PT, Lampe, PA, Heuckeroth, RO, Golden, JP, Creedon, DJ, Johnson Jr., EM, Milbrandt J. Neurturin, a relative of glial cell line-derived neurotrophic factor. Nature 1996; 384:467–470.

30. Milbrandt J, de Sauvage, FJ, Fahrner TJ, Baloh RH, Leitner ML, Tansey MG, Lampe PA, Heuckeroth RO, Kotzbauer, PT, Simburger, KS, Golden, JP, Davies, JA, Vejsada, R, Kato, AC, Hynes, M, Sherman, D, Nishimura, M, Wang, L-C, Vandlen, R, Moffat, B, Klein, RD, Poulsen, K, Gray, C, Graces, A, Henderson, CE, Phillips, HS, Johnson Jr., EM. Persephin, a novel neurotrophic factor related to GDNF and neurturin. Neuron 1998; 20:245–253.

31. Baloh RH, Tansey MG, Lampe PA, Fahrner TJ, Enomoto H, Simburger KS, Leitner ML, Araki T, Johnson EM Jr., Milbrant J. Artemin a novel member of the GDNF ligand family, supports peripheral and central neurons and signals through the GFRα3-RET receptor complex. Neuron 1998; 21:1291–1302.

32. Choi Lundberg DL, Bohn MC. Ontogeny and distribution of glial cell line-derived neurotrophic factor (GDNF) mRNA in rat. Dev Brain Res 1995; 85:80 88.

33. Springer JE, Mu X, Bergmann LW, Trojanoski JQ. Expression of GDNF mRNA in rat and human nervous tissue. Exp Neurol 1994; 127:67–170.

34. Strömberg I, Bjorklund L, Johansson M, Tomac A, Collins F, Olson L, Hoffer B, Humpel C. Glial cell line-derived neurotrophic factor is expressed in the developing but not adult striatum and stimulates developing dopamine neurons in vivo. Exp Neurol 1993; 124:401–412.

35. Suter-Crazzolara C, Unsicker K. GDNF is expressed in two forms in many tissues outside the CNS. NeuroReport 1994; 5:2486–2488.

36. Trupp M, Rydén M, Jörnavall C, Funakoshi H, Timmusk T, Arenas E, Ibanez CF. Peripheral expression and biological activities of GDNF, a new neurotrophic factor for avian and mammalian peripheral neurons. J Cell Biol 1995; 130:137–148.

37. Jing S, Wen D, Yu Y, Holst PL, Luo Y, Fang M, Tamir R, Antonio L, Hu Z, Cupples R, Louis J-C, Hu S, Altrock BW, Fox GM. GDNF-induced activation of the Ret protein tyrosine kinase is mediated by GDNFR-α, a novel receptor for GDNF. Cell 1996; 85:1113–1124.

38. Treanor JJS, Goodman L, de Sauvage F, Stone DM, Poulsen KT, Beck CD, Gray C, Armanini MP, Pollock RA, Hefti F, Phillips HS, Goddard A, Moore MW, Buj-Bello A, Davies AM, Asai N, Takahashi M, Vandlen R, Henderson CE, Rosenthal A. Characterization of a multicomponent receptor for GDNF. Nature 1996; 382:80–83.

39. Baloh RH, Tansey MG, Golden JP, Creedon DJ, Heuckeroth RO, Keck CL, Zimonjic DB, Popescu NC, Johnson EM Jr., Milbrandt J. TrnR2, a novel receptor that mediates neurturin and GDNF signaling through Ret. Neuron 1997; 18:793–802.

40. Buj-Bello A, Adu J, Pinon LGP, Horton A, Thompson J, Rosenthal A, Chinchetru M, Buchman V, Davies AM. Neurturin responsiveness requires a GPI-linked receptor and the ret receptor tyrosine kinase. Nature 1997; 387:721–724.

41. Naveilhan P, Baudet C, Mikaels A, Shen L, Westphal H, Ernfors P. Expression and regulation of GFRα-3, a glial cell line-derived neurotrophic factor family receptor. Proc Natl Acad Sci USA 1998; 95:1295–1300.

42. Worby CA, Vega QC, Chao HH, Seasholtz AF, Thompson RC, Dixon JE. Identification and characterization of GFRalpha-3, a novel Co-receptor belonging to the glial cell line-derived neurotrophic receptor family. J Biol Chem 1998; 273(6):3502–3508.

43. Thompson SA, Doxakis E, Pinon LGP, Strachan P, Buj-Bello A, Wyatt S, Buchman VL, Davies AM. GFRα-4, a new GDNF family receptor. Mol Cell Neurosci 1998; 11:117–126.

44. Hoffer BJ, Hoffman A, Bowenkamp K, Huettl P, Hudson J, Martin D, Lin L-FH, Gerhardt G. Glial cell line-derived neurotrophic factor reverses toxin-induced injury to midbrain dopaminergic neurons in vivo. Neurosci Lett 1994; 182:107–111.

45. Gash DM, Zhang Z, Cass WA, Ovadia A, Simmerman L, Martin D, Russell D, Collins F, Hoffer BJ, Gerhardt GA. Morphological and functional effects of intranigrally administered GDNF in normal rhesus monkeys. J Comp Neurol 1995; 363:345–358.

46. Bowenkamp KE, Hoffman AF, Gerhardt GA, Henry MA, Biddle PT, Hoffer BJ, Granholm A-C. Glial cell line-derived neurotrophic factor supports survival of injured midbrain dopaminergic neurons. J Comp Neurol 1995; 355:479–489.

47. Hudson J, Granholm A-C, Gerhardt GA, Henry MA, Hoffman A, Biddle P, Leela NS, Mackerlova L, Lile JD, Collins F, Hoffer BJ. Glial cell line-derived neurotrophic factor augments midbrain dopaminergic circuits in vivo. Brain Res Bull 1995; 36:425–432.

48. Beck K, Knusel B, Hefti F. The nature of the trophic action of brain-derived neurotrophic factor, des(1-3)-insulin-like growth factor-1, and basic fibroblast growth factor on mesencephalic dopaminergic neurons developing in culture. Neuroscience 1993; 52:855–866.

49. Kearns CM, Gash DM. GDNF protects nigral dopamine neurons against 6-hydroxydopamine in vivo. Brain Res 1995; 672:104–111.

50. Tomac A, Lindquist E, Lin L-FH, Orgen SO, Young D, Hoffer BJ, Olson L. Protection and repair of the nigrostriatal dopaminergic system by GDNF in vivo. Nature 1995; 373:335–339.

51. Smith RD, Zhang Z, Kurlan R, McDermott M, Gash DM. Developing a stable bilateral model of parkinsonism in rhesus monkeys. Neuroscience 1993; 52:7–16.

52. Brooks BA, Eidelberg E, Morgan WW. Behavioral and biochemical studies in monkeys made hemiparkinsonian by MPTP. Brain Res 1987; 419:329–332.

53. Langston JW, Ballard P, Tetrud JW, Irwin I. Chronic parkinsonism in humans due to a product of meperidine-analog synthesis. Science 1983; 219:979–980.

54. Langston JW, Langston EB, Irwin I. MPTP-induced parkinsonism in human and non-human promotes—clinical and experimental aspects. Acta Neurol Scand 1984; 100:49–54.

55. Bankiewicz KS, Oldfield EH, Chiueh CC, Doppman JL, Jacobowitz DM, Kopin IJ. Hemiparkinsonism in monkeys after unilateral internal cartoid artery infusion of 1-methyl-4-phenyl-1,2,3,6-tetrahydropyridine (MPTP). Life Sci 1986; 39:7–16.

56. Kurlan R, Kim MH, Gash DM. The time course and magnitude of spontaneous recovery of parkinsonism produced by intracarotid administration of 1-methyl-4-phenyl-1,2,3,6-tetrahydropyridine to monkeys. Ann Neurol 1991a; 29:677–679.

57. Kurlan R, Kim MH, Gash DM. Oral levodopa dose-response study in MPTP-induced hemiparkinsonian monkeys: assessment with a new rating scale for monkey parkinsonism. Mov Disord 1991b; 6:111–118.

58. Ovadia A, Zhang Z, Gash DM. Increased susceptibility to MPTP toxicity in middle-aged rhesus monkeys. Neurobiol Aging 1995; 16:931–937.

59. Costa S, Iravani MM, Pearce RK, Jenner P. Glial cell line-derived neurotrophic factor concentration dependently improves disability and motor activity in MPTP-treated common marmosets. Eur J Pharmacol 2001; 412:45–50.

60. Nutt JG, Bronstein JM, Carter JH, Comella CL, Cravets M, Davis TL, Jankovic J, Klein M, Koller WC, Lang AE, Lee DR, O'Brien CF, Pahwa R, Schultz B. Intraventricular administration of GDNF in the treatment of Parkinson's disease. Neurology 2001; 56(3):A375.

61. Kordower JH, Palfi S, Chen EY, Ma SY, Sendera T, Cochran EJ, Cochran EJ, Mufson EJ, Penn R, Goetz CG, Comella CD. Clinicopathological findings following intraventricular glial-derived neurotrophic factor treatment in a patient with Parkinson's disease. Ann Neurol 1999; 46(3):419–424.

62. Ai Y, Markesbery W, Zhang Z, Grondin R, Elseberry D, Gerhardt GA, Gash DM. Intraputamenal infusion of GDNF in aged rhesus monkeys: distribution and dopaminergic effects. J Comp Neurol 2003; 461:250–261.

63. Tornqvist N, Bjorklund L, Almqvist P, Wahlberg L, Stromberg I. Implantation of bioactive growth factor-secreting rods enhances fetal dopaminergic graft survival, outgrowth density, and functional recovery in a rat model of Parkinson's disease. Exp Neurol 2000; 164(1):130–138.

64. Zurn AD, Widmer HR, Aebischer P. Sustained delivery of GDNF: towards a treatment for Parkinson's disease. Brain Res Brain Res Rev 2001; 36(2–3):222–229.
65. Ostenfeld T, Tai YT, Martin P, Deglon N, Aebischer P, Svendsen CN. Neurospheres modified to produce glial cell line-derived neurotrophic factor increase the survival of transplanted dopamine neurons. Neurosci Res 2002; 69(6):955–965.
66. Maswood N, Grondin R, Zhang Z, Stanford JA, Surgener SP, Gash DM, Gerhardt GA. Effects of chronic intraputamenal infusion of glial cell line-derived neurotrophic factor (GDNF) in aged rhesus monkeys. Neurobiol Aging 2002; 23:881–889.
67. Langston JW, Widner H, Goetz CG, Brooks D, Fahn S, Freeman T, Watts R. Core assessment program for intracerebral transplantations (CAPIT). Mov Disord 1992; 7(1):2–13.
68. Cohen S, Levi-Montalcini R, Hamburger V. A nerve growth-stimulating factor isolated from sarcomas 37 and 180. Proc Natl Acad Sci 1954; 40:1014–1018.
69. Levi-Montalcini R. The nerve growth factor 35 years later. Science 1987; 237(4819):1154–1162.

39
Neural Stem Cell Therapy

Robert E. Gross

Emory University School of Medicine, Atlanta, Georgia, U.S.A.

I. INTRODUCTION

Cell therapy offers the possibility of restoring the degenerated nigrostriatal pathway and thereby improving the symptoms of Parkinson's disease (PD) (1,2). Neural stem cells have the potential to provide a limitless source of cells for this purpose, eliminating the need for human fetal cells with its associated supply limitations and ethical concerns. However, mixed results in two prospective, randomized, sham-controlled trials of fetal cell replacement in advanced PD patients have tempered the enthusiasm for cell therapy and mitigated the need for such an unlimited supply of cells (3,4). Yet neural stem cells may offer several advantages over human fetal cells. This chapter will address some fundamental aspects of stem cell biology that pertain to their use in neural restorative approaches and review the progress in generating dopaminergic (DA) neurons in vitro and the results of cell replacement in animal models of PD. Finally, other possible roles for stem cells in neural restoration will be discussed.

II. THE BIOLOGY OF NEURAL STEM CELLS

Through the process of cell proliferation and differentiation, the one-celled zygote gives rise to the mature organism, with billions of differentiated cells performing multitudinous disparate functions (Fig. 1) (5). Most, if not all, cells of the mature animal are the differentiated progeny of stem cells, which are functionally defined by their capacity for self-renewal (i.e., one of the products of its cell division is identical to itself) as well as the production of multipotent progenitor cells (which may themselves be stem cells, but more restricted in their developmental repertoire) (6–8). Within the inner cell mass of the blastocyst, early in development, reside embryonic stem (ES) cells (9,10). ES cells are capable of unlimited, undifferentiated proliferation and are pluripotent, able to give rise to every differentiated cell type of the mature organism. Totipotency, a characteristic of the fertilized egg, implies the capability of forming the entire organism, including

529

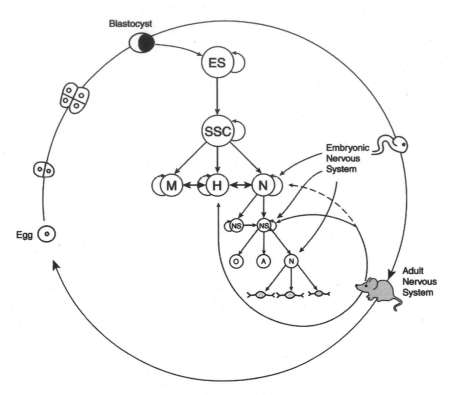

Figure 1 Life cycle of the stem cell. The totipotent egg gives rise to stem cells through a process of cellular division and developmental fate restriction. Embryonic stem (ES) cells are derived from the inner cell mass of the blastocyst. They self-renew (backwards arrow) and are pluripotent, giving rise to somatic stem cells (SSC) of various tissues, such as hematopoietic (H), muscle (M), or neural (N). The latter, also self-renewing, may be capable of transdifferentiation (sidewards arrows). They give rise to more restricted stem cells. Neural stem cells (NS), for example, can only generate cells committed to differentiation along neural lineages: astroglial (A), oligodendroglial (O), and neuronal (N). More restricted stem and progenitor cells may also be isolated from the embryonic and adult nervous systems.

trophoblastic tissue, which ES cells do not have. In contrast, the mature neurons of the central nervous system (CNS) are highly differentiated and nonproliferative. The developmental processes that unfurl between ES cells and the most differentiated cells proceed through the generation of transitory progenitor cells that have progressively decreasing proliferative capacity and progressively increasing developmental restrictions (5).

CNS neural stem cells are tissue-specific transitory cells that reside within the CNS and give rise to all of the neural cell types: neurons, astrocytes, and oligodendrocytes. The intermediary cells, which have not been well characterized, may include neuronal restricted progenitors and glial restricted progenitors, although this view has been questioned (11,12). Neural stem cells were thought to be restricted to producing only neural lineages (13). Evidence has been presented that neural stem cells can "transdifferentiate" to give rise to nonneural cell types (14,15), and that other tissue-specific stem cells (e.g., hematopoetic and mesenchymal) can generate neurons (16–18). Although this is highly controversial (19,20), it is conceivable that tissue-specific stem cells can dedifferentiate one or two steps and redifferentiate down a different tissue-specific pathway.

In several adult tissues that are exposed to environmental stress and associated high rates of cell turnover, as in the hematopoietic and gastrointestinal systems, there is a constant need for new cells which are supplied by more or less well-characterized tissue-specific stem cells that persist into adulthood (21). The CNS was not thought to be one of those systems, and dogma held that no new neurons were produced in adult brains (22–24). However, Reynolds and Weiss (25) discovered cells in the adult CNS with neural stem cell characteristics. Subsequent research revealed that there is ongoing neurogenesis in at least two regions of the adult CNS: the anterior subventricular zone (SVZ), which gives rise to new interneurons in the olfactory bulb, and the subgranular zone of the dentate gyrus of the hippocampus (6,7,26,27). SVZ neural stem cells and hippocampal progenitor cells (they are not in fact stem cells) have been well characterized. Whether there are other populations of stem cells in the adult CNS is unclear.

Since all differentiated cells of the mature CNS are probably produced by neural stem cells, it stands to reason that a stem cell could be identified that is capable of generating the DA neurons of the substantia nigra. Since the first discovery of neural stem cells, the search for such a cell has been the focus of cell-replacement efforts for PD. The cells that have been used in most fetal transplant experiments and clinical trials are not neural stem cells, but rather nigral neurons undergoing terminal differentiation (2). Proliferative neuroblasts that produce a high proportion of DA neurons upon differentiation have also been characterized, but their proliferative capacity is very limited in comparison to neural stem cells (28,29). Efforts to produce DA neurons from stem cells of various sources are beginning to yield encouraging results.

III. TYPES OF NEURAL STEM CELLS

It would be ideal if, as in the hematopoietic system, a particular neural stem cell could be isolated from the developing (or adult) CNS based on the profile of antigens it expresses on its cell surface (e.g., through a technique such as fluorescence activated cell sorting, FACS), cloned as an individual cell, and expanded in cell culture through the use of one or more mitogenic factors (30). In this way the precise developmental repertoire of a uniquely identified cell could be established both in vitro and in vivo following transplantation into the developing or adult CNS (6–8). Unfortunately, with few exceptions this has yet to be achieved (31–33), and the result is that the precise identification of most neural stem cells characterized is not known. Most of the neural stem cells that have been described fall into one of four categories (Table 1).

A. Mitogen-Dependent Neural Stem/Progenitor Cells

These are cell populations obtained from the developing or adult CNS that proliferate (most often in suspension culture as "neurospheres") in the presence of one or more mitogens, usually epidermal growth factor (EGF) or fibroblast growth factor 2 (FGF2), formerly basic FGF (bFGF). Upon removal of the mitogen and exposure to adherent substrates, the undifferentiated cells cease proliferating and begin to differentiate. They are capable of generating all three lineages, but the proportion may vary depending on the origin of the cells, culture conditions, and/or exposure to various factors (7). Mitogen-dependent neural stem cells are appealing because they are nonproliferative in the absence of mitogen,

Table 1 Types of Neural Stem and Progenitor Cells

Type of stem/progenitor cell	Examples	Pros	Cons
Mitogen-dependent neural stem/progenitor cells	Species: mouse, rat, human Regions: forebrain, midbrain, neural tube Ages: fetal, adult Mitogens: EGF, FGF2, LIF	Normal karyotype No oncogenic gene expression Mitogen-dependent proliferation Capable of advanced phenotypic differentiation Adult sources available	Heterogeneous cell population Difficult to generate clonal population Difficult to transfect Ethical issues surrounding fetal sources
Embryonic stem (ES) cell–derived neural progenitor cells	Species: mouse, nonhuman primate, human Protocol for neural induction: embryoid bodies + factors PA6 stromal feeder layer + factors	Normal karyotype No oncogenic gene expression Endless, undifferentiated proliferation of parent ES lines Ease of cloning homogeneous cell populations Ease of transgene expression Access to earlier neural lineages	Difficult to maintain and manipulate in culture Potential for teratomas Ethical issues surrounding use of human embryos
Immortalized neural stem/progenitor cells	C17.2: mouse PN cerebellum RN33B: rat E13 medullary raphe HNSC.100: human embryonic forebrain	Clonal homogeneous cell population Ease of transfection	Limitations in mature phenotypic differentiation Oncogene expression with potential for transformed growth Difficulties in maintaining transgene expression
Teratocarcinoma–derived neural progenitor cells	Human NTera2 cells	Homogeneous cell population	Derived from teratocarcinoma Potential for neoplastic growth

Abbreviations: EGF, epidermal growth factor; FGF2, fibroblast growth factor 2; LIF, leukemia growth factor; E, embryonic.

and thus may be considerably safer for cell transplantation paradigms. Moreover, they seem to have substantial capacity for advanced phenotypic differentiation.

B. Embryonic Stem Cells

Extensive work has been done with mouse ES cells, which have been used to study countless genes in chimeric progeny derived from introduction of transfected ES cells into early embryos. Only recently, however, have human ES cells been successfully cultured and maintained (34,35). Both mouse and human ES cells give rise to neural progenitor populations under various protocols (36), and included within these progenitors are cells that differentiate along a DA lineage. Although significant ethical and political issues surround the use of human ES cells, recent progress suggests that from a biological perspective cell transplantation is feasible with ES cell–derived neural progenitor cells.

C. Immortalized Neural Stem Cells

Neural stem cells that are able to proliferate in the absence of mitogens have been produced by transfecting mitogen-dependent cells with an immortalizing oncogene (e.g., v-myc) (37,38). This helps in maintaining certain cells with more limited proliferative capacity in long-term continuous cell culture and may aide in attempts to clone a homogeneous cell line that is derived from a single neural stem cell, and therefore more amenable to in-depth characterization. Alternatively, immortalized lines have been produced by exposing primary cell mixtures to an immortalizing oncogene in an effort to clone rare novel stem or progenitor cell lines from cells of the CNS whose response to mitogens is not known.

Several interesting cell lines have been produced in this way, but they vary in their ability to differentiate in vitro and in vivo following transplantation. Although some lines are able to integrate into many different tissues of the CNS and differentiate in a region-specific fashion that is apparently identical to endogenous neighboring neurons (39–44), other lines seem incapable of even generating mature-appearing neurons under various culture conditions (45,46). It may be that the presence of the immortalizing oncogene limits the differentiation capabilities of some cell lines (even when a temperature sensitive allele is used) (7), or that cell lines immortalized at earlier stages are less capable of generating mature appearing neurons than those from later stage cells (8,39).

Most of the cell lines have been generated by stable transfection with a temperature-sensitive mutant of an immortalizing gene [e.g., simian virus 40 (SV40) large T antigen], and as a result these cell lines cease to proliferate and begin to differentiate when the temperature is raised above 37°C (either in vitro or in vivo). Nevertheless, the potential for producing a neoplasm upon transplantation is a potential drawback of the use of immortalized neural stem cells in cell therapy paradigms, although the cell lines have not exhibited transformed behavior either in vitro or in vivo (38). On the other hand, cell lines may be ideal for use in ex vivo gene therapy strategies in the nervous system.

D. Teratocarcinoma-Derived Cells

Human embryonal carcinoma cell lines (ECCs) have been derived from a teratocarcinoma and are capable of generating cells from each of the three germ layers (37). Although these cells are neoplastic and therefore proliferate without mitogens, both in vitro and following transplantation, upon extended culture in the presence of retinoic acid they generate nonproliferative cells that differentiate into neurons (hNTera2 cells) (37,47–49). These cells have been used in many animal models for cell therapeutic paradigms (50) and have even been transplanted into patients with basal ganglia strokes in clinical trials (51). Despite the absence of neoplasms developing in animals and patients, their potential for this complication limits the usefulness of hNT2 cells.

IV. GENERATION OF DOPAMINE NEURONS FROM NEURAL STEM CELLS IN VITRO

This section discusses the results of attempts to produce DA neurons from each of the types of neural stem/progenitor cells (Fig. 2); the results of transplantation of these cells in animal models of PD will be examined in the subsequent section.

A. Mitogen-Dependent Neural Stem/Progenitor Cells

1. Forebrain-Derived Neural Stem/Progenitor Cells

The forebrain contains the developing cortical mantle, which is derived from the ventricular zone (VZ), but also the subependymal or SVZ. Other structures include the striatum (derived from the lateral and medial ganglionic eminences) and thalamus, which may contain their own stem cell populations. Often it is not clear from which region stem

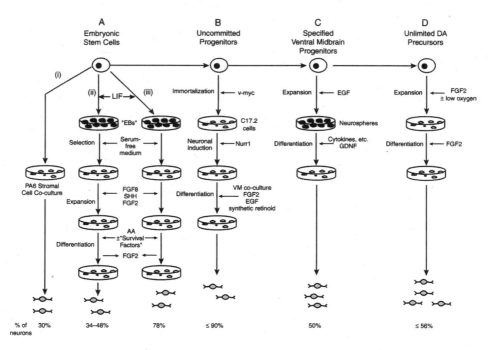

Figure 2 Methods used to generate dopamine (DA) neurons from embryonic stem cells and their progeny. Various methods have been used to generate DA neurons, and their efficiency is indicated by the "percent of neurons" that are DA neurons from each method. Most methods involve an expansion phase and a differentiation phase. Abbreviations: EB, embryoid bodies; LIF, leukemia inhibitory factors; FGF, fibroblast growth factor; SHH, sonic hedgehog protein; AA, ascorbic acid; VM, ventral mesencephalon; EGF, epidermal growth factor; GDNF, glial cell line–derived neurotrophic factor. See text for further explanation.

cells that are proliferating in cell cultures actually arose. For example, the neural stem cells produced in so-called striatal cultures are most likely from the SVZ.

Subventricular Zone Neural Stem Cells

SVZ neural stem cells from the adult forebrain were the first CNS cells characterized that had the properties of stem cells (25), but the existence of a similar population with essentially identical properties in the embryonic CNS was subsequently described (52). In the presence of EGF, these cells proliferate endlessly as neurospheres in suspension cell culture and differentiate into neurons, astrocytes, and oligodendrocytes on adherent substrates upon removal of EGF. Among differentiated progeny of SVZ cells, astrocytes predominate, neurons comprise approximately 20%, and oligodendrocytes are rare, but all three lineages can be selectively induced with epigenetic factors (53–55). Neurons derived from SVZ neural stem cells express appropriate neuron-specific markers [e.g., type III β-tubulin, microtubule-associated proteins (MAPs),] and manifest evoked action potentials in vitro (56–58). SVZ neural stem cells give rise in vivo to the rostral migratory stream (RMS), comprising astrocytes and neuroblasts that tangentially migrate to the olfactory bulb where the neurons take up residence as interneurons (in contrast to the predominant radial migration of neuroblasts that populate the cortical mantle) (26,27). Whether SVZ neural stem cells give rise to other populations of neurons is not clear, although some work suggests that these cells are identical to cells derived from the VZ throughout the neuraxis (59–61). The principal cell of origin of SVZ neural stem cells has been a matter of some debate (12). It appears that astrocytes within the ependyma or SVZ (33,62–64), radial glia (65–68), or even ependymal cells themselves (64,69) behave as neural stem cells in vitro and in vivo. The more extensive SVZ of the embryo remains as the anterior SVZ in the adult, continuing to give rise to the RMS throughout adult life (26,70,71).

The predominant neurotransmitter phenotype of SVZ neural stem cells is gamma-amino butyric acid (GABA), and only rarely and in small numbers have dopaminergic neurons been generated in SVZ cultures in vitro. Svendsen et al. (72) found no tyrosine hydroxylase–positive (TH+) neurons generated from EGF-expanded embryonic rat striatal cultures. In the presence of FGF2 and glial-conditioned medium, however, 10–20% of the neurons derived from forebrain neural stem cells expressed TH (73,74), but GABA remained the predominant phenotype even under these conditions. SVZ cells also have been successfully cultured from adult human tissue adjacent to the lateral ventricle in the presence of EGF (75,76). There is no evidence of significant numbers of DA neurons in these cultures.

Human Embryonic Forebrain Progenitor Cells

Cells with properties similar to SVZ neural stem cells have been cultured, in some instances continuously for long periods, from the telencephalic region of 5- to 12-week embryonic human brain, in the presence of EGF and bFGF with or without leukemia inhibitory factor (LIF) (57,72,77–81). As with SVZ cells, the minority of differentiated cells produced by these cultures are neurons, although Caldwell et al. (56) increased the yield of neurons to greater than 60% by manipulating culture conditions and trophic factor (especially NT-4) support to increase neuronal survival. In general, the majority of neurons generated are GABAergic or glutamatergic (56,80–82). TH+ neurons comprise less than 0.1% in most cases and are not increased by treatment with a wide range of neurotrophic factors (56,82), although Piper et al. (83) generated 2% of neuronal cells (80% of total cells) expressing TH immunoreactivity (IR).

Adult Hippocampal Progenitor Cells

The subgranular region of the dentate gyrus in the hippocampal formation is neurogenic in adult mammals, including humans (84,85). Adult hippocampal neural progenitor (AHNP) cells have been successfully cultured and upon grafting to the adult brain survive, integrate, and differentiate in a region-specific manner in neurogenic regions. In particular, when transplanted to the RMS, AHNP cells migrate to the olfactory bulb where they express TH, a property of bulb neurons but not of hippocampal neurons (84,86). When cultured in vitro, these cells produce a small number of TH+ neurons, along with other transmitter phenotypes. However, when Nurr1, a regulatory locus for TH gene expression (87), is overexpressed in these cells, the TH phenotype is further induced, but not other proteins that define midbrain DA neurons (88).

Cortical Stem/Progenitor Cells

In contrast to the stem cells of the SVZ, which give rise to tangentially migrating cells, the VZ generates neuroblasts that migrate radially to the cortical mantle. Cells satisfying the criteria for being stem cells have been cultured from embryonic cortex (89,90), but there is no evidence for generation of DA neurons from these progenitors in vitro.

2. Ventral Midbrain-Derived Neural Stem/Progenitor Cells

Following the description of SVZ neural stem cells derived from the forebrain, there was a push to identify similar precursor cells in the region of the midbrain that might give rise to the DA neurons of the substantia nigra. Although the cell of origin of these neurons has not been elucidated, concurrent work has begun to elucidate the epigenetic and genetic factors that regulate the generation of the dopaminergic phenotype. For example, it is known that the generation of DA neurons in the ventral midbrain requires the presence of sonic hedgehog protein (Shh) and FGF8 (91–93) and the expression within DA precursors of the Nurr1 (87,94), En-1 (95), and Lmx1b and Ptx3 genes (96,97). Subsequent work has incorporated these findings into strategies for increasing the production of DA neurons from stem cell cultures.

FGF2-Expanded Ventral Midbrain Precursor Cells

DA neurons in the ventral mesencephalon (VM) appear as early as embryonic day 13 in the rat. Studer and colleagues (28) dissected day 12 VM, prior to the appearance of any TH+ neurons, and described conditions for the 30-fold expansion of proliferating cells in the presence of FGF2 (Fig. 2D). Upon removal of FGF2, cells differentiated into TH-IR neurons (18.4%), also immunoreactive for DA and the dopamine transporter (DAT). Cultivation under low-oxygen conditions led to a further increase in the proliferation and differentiation and an inhibition of apoptosis of DA precursors from the rat VM (29). In 3% O_2 56% of neurons were TH+ in contrast to 18% under 20% O_2, an effect that was partially mimicked by addition of erythropoietin. However, it must be noted that these cells are not stem cells and have limited proliferative capacity.

Mitogen-Expanded Ventral Midbrain Neural Stem cells

Some success has been obtained with the generation of neural stem cells from the VM. Ling et al. (98) cultured rat embryonic mesencephalic stem cells with EGF for extended periods (Fig. 2C). Further treatment of the cells with interleukins(IL)-1 and -11, LIF, and glial-derived neurotrophic factor (GDNF), and exposure to striatal and mesencephalic membrane fragments led to morphologically mature TH- and DAT-immunoreactive neurons, with yields of 20–25% of the overall cells (50% of neurons overall). Subsequently, a clonal line of nonimmortalized midbrain-derived neurospheres (EGF-expanded) was isolated, which upon treatment with IL-1α produced 98% of the total cells as TH+ (99).

Sawamoto and colleagues (100) used a unique approach to isolate DA precursor cells from the ventral midbrain. They dissected the midbrain VZ from transgenic rats and mice expressing green fluorescent protein (GFP) from a neural precursor-specific promoter (nestin). Following FACS for GFP+ cells, they were expanded as neurospheres with EGF/FGF2, and characterized. The GFP+ spheres from the VM yielded all three neural lineages including TH- and DAT-IR neurons, whereas spheres produced from the striatal region did not give rise to TH+ cells.

Human Ventral Midbrain Stem/Progenitor Cells

Some of these techniques have been used to culture and expand human VM precursor and neural stem cells. Using the techniques of Studer et al. (28), human primary VM precursors were expanded in the presence of FGF2 for 7 days and differentiated with cyclic adenosine monophosphate (cAMP) and ascorbic acid (101). Sixty-two percent of cells were neuronal, of which 21% were TH-IR, and yielded DA by high-performance liquid chromatography. Neural stem cells have also been induced to differentiate into DA neurons using the cytokine approach. Although insignificant numbers of TH+ cells were produced from VM neurospheres grown in EGF and FGF2, despite culturing them in low oxygen, the addition of cytokines and GDNF in the presence of striatal co-cultures produced 1% DA neurons (102). Other conditions have been described [brain-derived neurotrophic factor (BDNF), dopamine, forskolin] that led to 80% of neurons expressing the DA phenotype (103).

3. Hindbrain/Spinal Cord Neural Stem/Progenitor Cells

Embryonic spinal cord contains a population of cells called neuroepithelial precursors (NEPs) that can be purified using immunological techniques (FACS, immunopanning) and give rise to more restricted progenitors that exclusively produce neurons [neuron restricted progenitors (NRPs)] or glial cells [glial restricted progenitors (GRPs)] (104,105). There is no evidence that spinal cord NRPs are capable of producing DA neurons.

B. Embryonic Stem Cell–Derived Neural Stem Cells

Conditions have been described for the generation of neural progenitor cells from both mouse and human ES cell lines in vitro (Fig. 2A) (36,106–115). ES cells will permit the isolation of earlier neural stem cells than can be isolated from older fetal or adult animals, including dopaminergic lineages which are generated early in development. However, little is known regarding the molecular controls governing the generation of specific lineages either in vivo or in vitro, and the specific generation of DA neurons from ES cells remains a challenge.

1. Mouse Embryonic Stem Cells

Methods have been pioneered to generate increased numbers of DA neurons from neural restricted progeny of ES cells in vitro. Kawasaki et al. (116) described a method for generating a high percentage of neurons from mouse ES cells by cultivating them upon a layer of PA6 stromal cells, which provided a stromal-derived inducing activity (SDIA) (Fig. 2Ai). Thirty percent of neurons were TH+ (16% of total cells), whereas the GABAergic, cholinergic, and serotonergic phenotypes represented 18, 9, and 2% of neurons. The TH-IR neurons also expressed other markers of DA neurons (Nurr1, Ptx3), and released significant amounts of DA in response to depolarization. This work was extended to primate ES cells, where similar efficiency of DA neuron generation was observed (117).

Lee et al. (114) used a multistep procedure involving the harvesting and treatment with FGF2 of embryoid bodies (EB), cell aggregates that bud off of ES cultures followed by exposure to FGF8, Shh, and ascorbic acid (Fig. 2Aii). This yielded 34% of neurons expressing the DA phenotype. Addition of a cocktail of survival factors including IL-1β, GDNF, and others yielded 43% TH+ neurons (118). When a plasmid expressing Nurr1 was introduced and the ES cells subjected to a similar multistage procedure, 78% of neurons were DA (Fig. 2Aiii) (119). Depolarization-dependent DA release was demonstrated, as was the expression of various gene products particular to normal DA neurons. The authors estimate that two to three DA neurons can be generated per ES cell, leading to the potential to produce nearly unlimited numbers of DA neurons for neural restorative approaches (114). Finally, Ying et al. (112) described a simple monolayer culture system for the neural differentiation of mouse ES cells, relying on the knock-in expression of GFP from a very early neural promoter, *sox1*, that is downregulated in differentiated neural tissue. They were able to follow and then purify neural progenitors and subsequently study conditions to maximize their production, and, with addition of FGF8 and Shh, they generated significant numbers of TH+ neurons.

2. Human Embryonic Stem Cells

Zhang et al. (113) used the embryoid body technique with human ES cell lines and generated neural tube structures that could be isolated and differentiated following withdrawal of FGF2 to yield all three neural lineages. The lines used had to be propagated on mouse fibroblast feeder layers. They subsequently isolated neural progenitors propagated as suspension cultures similar to neurospheres. The majority of neurons generated were glutamatergic, with some GABA, but a small number expressed TH. Reubinoff et al. (35,36) confirmed the above, generating neurons expressing markers for GABA and glutamate (35% and 15%, respectively, of neurons) and rarely (< 1%) TH and 5-HT, following differentiation of EGF/FGF2 expanded ES cell–derived neurospheres. Carpenter and colleagues (107,120) treated EBs with retinoic acid and differentiated them in medium containing growth factors and neurotrophic factors. Various neurotransmitter phenotypes of neurons were produced, 3% of which expressed TH. Additional work is needed to generate significant numbers of DA neurons from human ES cells.

Each of the previous studies required culturing of ES cells on mouse fibroblast feeder layers to maintain their pluripotency, or the use of mouse fibroblast conditioned medium, which could contaminate human cells with mouse cells and compromise any attempt to introduce these cells into patients. Others have now successfully derived and maintained human ES cells on human feeder cell layers (121,122). This opens the way for producing neuronal cells, DA neurons in particular, from human ES cells never exposed to animal cells, a safer product for transplantation clinical trials.

C. Immortalized Neural Stem/Progenitor Cell Lines

The C17.2 cell line was produced by immortalizing cerebellar precursor cells with the *v-myc* oncogene (40). These cells are capable of integrating widely in the embryonic nervous system and of region-specific differentiation (123). Wagner et al. (124) induced a TH phenotype by transfecting C17.2 cells with the Nurr1 gene (Fig. 2B). Most of the Nurr1-expressing clones generated a large proportion of βIII-tubulin immunoreactive cells, in contrast to 30–40% from the parental clone. These neurons, however, did not express TH until they were exposed to FGF2 and EGF, co-cultured with primary embryonic VM, and treated with a synthetic retinoid analog, whereupon a yield of up to 90% TH+ neurons was achieved. The inductive activity of VM cultures was determined to emanate from Type 1 astrocytes and seemed to be soluble, highly labile, and region-specific, but not identical to GDNF. Other immortalized cell lines have been examined, including some derived from EGF-dependent neurospheres, but little progress has been made in producing significant numbers of DA neurons from them (41,125).

D. Teratocarcinoma-Derived Cells

Human NTera2 cells, when cultured for short periods of time (126) or with lithium chloride (127), generate up to 60% of neurons expressing immunoreactivity for TH and other DA markers.

V. RESULTS OF NEURAL STEM CELL TRANSPLANTS

Most of the stem cell populations described have been grafted into the ventricles of neonatal or embryonic animals to explore their integration and differentiation in the normal developmental milieu (6,7). Most are able to survive, integrate, and produce neurons in neurogenic regions, whereas in nonneurogenic regions mostly astrocytes are produced. More apropos to the question of their utility in the treatment of PD, a number of the above-described cells have been grafted into the striatum of rodents treated with 6-hydroxydopamine (6-OHDA) to destroy the DA nigral neurons and their striatal projections. The ability of the cells to survive, differentiate into DA neurons, and ameliorate pharmacologically induced rotational behavior has been examined (Table 2). There are no reports of the results of neural stem cell implantations into the brains of nonhuman primates, much less the brains of PD patients.

A. Mitogen-Dependent Neural Stem Cells

1. Forebrain-Derived Neural Stem/Progenitor Cells

The few DA neurons that are found within forebrain-derived progenitor cells have been incapable of suppressing rotational behavior in the rodent 6-OHDA model of PD. Svendsen et al. (72) grafted rat striatal and VM, EGF-expanded cells into 6-OHDA rats. The grafts tended to be very thin, in contrast to robust grafts typically observed following transplantation of primary VM tissue, and no effect on rotational behavior was observed.

Human progenitor/stem cells have also been grafted into the rodent striatum. Ostenfeld et al. (128) expanded human embryonic forebrain tissue 100-fold with EGF and FGF2 and then implanted various numbers of cells into the 6-OHDA–lesioned striatum. Although fiber outgrowth was robust, TH+ cells were only transiently seen in a few of the animals, and no effect on rotational behavior was observed. When cells that were satisfactorily characterized as stem cells were expanded from the human forebrain (10^7-fold in the presence of EGF, FGF2, and LIF) and implanted into the adult (nonlesioned) striatum, generally glial cells were generated that migrated into the striatum. The neurons that were generated tended to remain near the implantation site and did not differentiate into TH+ neurons (60). Denervation of the striatum led to a slight increase in the number of DA neurons found within grafts of forebrain progenitor cells (129).

Table 2 Results from Transplantation of Neural Stem/Progenitor Cells in Animal Models of Parkinson's Disease

Study (Ref.)	Cell source[a]	Host	TH + cells in graft	Effects on rotational behavior	Teratomas
Forebrain Stem/Progenitor Cells					
Svendsen et al., 1996 (72)	Rat EGF—SVZ NS cells	Rat 6-OHDA	−	No change	
Ostenfeld et al., 2000 (128)	Human EGF/FGF2 - forebrain NP cells	Rat 6-OHDA	+/−	No change	
Fricker et al., 1999 (60)	Human EGF/FGF2/LIF - forebrain NP cells	Adult rat	−	NA	
Midbrain Stem/Progenitor/Precursor Cells					
Svendsen et al., 1996 (72)	Rat EGF - VM NS cells	Rat 6-OHDA	+	No change	
	Human EGF - VM NS cells	Rat 6-OHDA	+	NA	
Carvey et al., 2001 (99)	Rat EGF–VM clonal NS cells: cytokines	Rat 6-OHDA	+/−	No change	
	Rat EGF – VM clonal NS cells: + cytokines	Rat 6-OHDA	++	88% ↓	
Nishino et al., 2000 (129)	Rat EGF or FGF2 - VM NS cells	Rat 6-OHDA	++	↓ in 1/2	
Studer et al., 1998 (28)	Rat FGF2–VM precursor cells	Rat 6-OHDA	+++	75% ↓ ($p < 0.05$)	
Sawamoto et al., 2001 (100)	Rat EGF+FGF2-nestin-GFP + VZ NS cells	Rat 6-OHDA	++	65% ↓ ($p < 0.01$)	
Sanchez-Pernaute et al., 2001 (101)	Human FGF2 – VM precursor cells	Rat 6-OHDA	+++	35% ↓ (n.s.)	
	Human FGF2 – cortex precursor cells	Rat 6-OHDA	−	13% ↑ (n.s.)	
Embryonic Stem Cells					
Deacon et al., 1998 (131)	Mouse ES cells (embryoid bodies)	Rat 6-OHDA	+++	NR	Some
Kim et al., 2002 (119)	Mouse ES-wild-type cells	Rat 6-OHDA	++	50% ↓ ($p < 0.05$)	No
	Mouse ES-Nurr1 cells	Rat 6-OHDA	++	>100% ↓ ($p < 0.001$)	No
Bjorklund et al., 2002 (132)	Mouse ES cells (embryoid bodies)	Rat 6-OHDA	+++	55% ↓ ($p < 0.001$)	5/25
Kawasaki et al., 2000 (116)	Mouse ES cells (SDIA induced)	Mouse 6-OHDA	++	NA	No
Kawasaki et al., 2002 (117)	Primate ES cells (SDIA induced)	Mouse 6-OHDA	++	NA	No

[a] All embryonic donors.

Abbreviations: EGF, epidermal growth factor; SVZ, subventricular zone; FGF, fibroblast growth factor; LIF, leukemia inhibitory factor; VM, ventral mesencephalon; GFP, green fluorescent protein; VZ, ventricular zone; SDIA, stromal-derived inducing activity; 6-OHDA, 6-hydroxydopamine; ES, embryonic stem; NS cells, neural stem cells; NP cells, neural progenitor cells; NA, not assessed; NR, not reported; n.s., not significant.

2. Midbrain-Derived Neural Stem/Progenitor Cells

Studer and colleagues used expanded rat VM precursors in the presence of FGF2, reaggregated and differentiated them into TH+ neurons by withdrawing FGF2 in the presence of serum, and transplanted them into 6-OHDA–lesioned rats (28). Although these experiments used amplified neuroblasts rather than true stem cells, they demonstrated a 75% decrease in rotational behavior in five animals, but less response in two other animals. Grafts were similar in size and morphology to primary grafted neurons (Fig. 3A). Similar results were obtained from FGF2-expanded human VM precursors (101).

Early work with progenitor/stem cells expanded from the rodent ventral midbrain in the presence of EGF and/or FGF2 did not yield significant numbers of TH+ neurons, and the results of grafting these preparations to the striatum of 6-OHDA rats was unsatisfactory (72) (Table 2). Human cells expanded from the VM did produce some TH+ neurons (possibly carried over from the initial primary culture), but rotational behavior was not assessed in these animals. However, the results of transplanting the expanded and cloned rat VM lines of Carvey and colleagues (98,99), which produced high percentages of DA neurons in the presence of cytokines and other factors, were more encouraging. Following grafting into 6-OHDA–lesioned rats (Fig. 3B), a decrease in rotational behavior of 88% was observed, whereas untreated cells were ineffective. The FACS sorted nestin-GFP expressing cells of Sawamato and colleagues (100) were also able to ameliorate rotational behavior significantly. Histological analysis confirmed the survival of significant numbers of TH+ neurons within the lesioned striatum (Fig. 3C), some of which were labeled with bromodeoxyuridine to mark newly generated cells. Moreover, rotational reduction correlated highly with the number of TH-IR neurons in the striatum.

B. Embryonic Stem Cell–Derived Neural Stem/Progenitor Cells

When grafted into the ventricles of developing mice, both mouse and human ES cells yield cells of all three neural lineages that integrate and participate in the development of the entire brain (31,36,113,130). Initial work with ES cells in the parkinsonian model involved grafting of untreated embryoid bodies directly into the striatum. Within these cultures are not only neural cells (of each lineage) but nonneural cells as well. Moreover, the number of DA neurons may be expected to be small. Deacon et al. (131) implanted mouse embryoid bodies into the striatum of nondenervated and 6-OHDA denervated rats. Graft size was variable and included evidence of cell proliferation in situ. A large proportion of grafts included TH+ neurons, in addition to 5-HT+ neurons, as well as large numbers of astroglial cells and nonneural cells. Putative DA neurons (which were nonimmunoreactive for dopamine-β-hydroxylase) elaborated axons which projected into the host striatal tissue, avoiding white matter fascicles reminiscent of host innervation patterns. However, no change in rotational behavior was observed, and the growth of teratomas derived from proliferating nonneural precursors occurred. Subsequent experiments used lower numbers of dissociated ES cells to minimize possible autocrine and paracrine mitogenic effects of ES cells and maximize host-graft effects on differentiation (132). Numerous TH+ neurons were seen in all animals with viable grafts at 14–16 weeks survival (Fig. 3D), but 5HT neurons (2:1 DA:5HT) and some other neurotransmitter phenotypes were seen as well Other DA markers were co-expressed, such as DAT. Numerous graft-derived astrocytes were also present, as were markers from other cell layers (e.g., keratin) in occasional grafts. Animals with DA neuron–containing grafts manifested decreased amphetamine-induced rotations as compared to sham-operated animals. Functional imaging biomarkers also

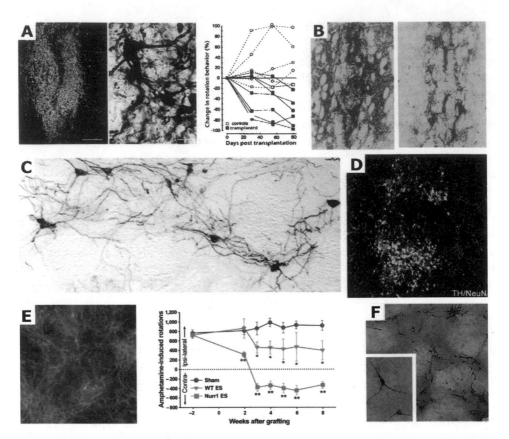

Figure 3 Transplantation of neural stem cells in the 6-OHDA rat model of Parkinson's disease. (A) FGF2-expanded mesencephalic precursors following transplantation showing TH immunoreactivity in low power of graft (left) and at higher power showing differentiated DA neurons (center). Effect on amphetamine-induced rotational response is shown at right. (From Ref. 28.) (B) Cytokine-treated mesencephalic progenitor cells in transplant immunoreactive for TH (right) as compared to typical results seen after grafting of embryonic VM Tissue (left) (From Ref. 99.) (C) Flow-sorted nestin-GFP[+] mesencephalic progenitors immunoreactive for TH following grafting. (From Ref. 100.) (D) Embryonic stem cells 16 weeks following grafting demonstrating co-expression of TH and the nuclear neuronal marker NeuN. (From Ref. 132.) (E) Nurrl-transfected embryonic stem cells–derived neural precursors expressing TH immunoreactivity (mostly) as well as serotonin immunoreactivity following in vitro differentiation procedure (left). Grafting led to marked amelioration of amphetamine-induced rotational behavior compared to wild-type ES cells (right). (From Ref. 119.) (F) TGFα–induced endogenous neural stem cells were found to migrate and differentiate into TH-immunoreactive neurons (shown at higher power, inset) in the striatum. (From Ref. 138.)

showed evidence of increased DA activity in the grafted animals. Although 20% of the animals developed fatal teratomas, in the animals without teratomas markers of cell proliferation were absent, consistent with terminal differentiation.

In vitro techniques have led to the production of higher numbers of DA neurons from mouse, primate, and human ES cell cultures using specific and nonspecific inducers of the DA phenotype. Moreover, these cultures provide some isolation of neural progenitors from other non-neural tissue, decreasing the likelihood of teratoma formation. Results of their engraftment have been encouraging. Using SDIA-induced ES cells, 22% of mouse (116) and 8% of primate (117) TH+ cells survived engraftment and integrated into the 6-OHDA–lesioned mouse striatum without generating teratomas. Rotational behavior, could not be addressed in the mouse model. Impressive results were obtained, however, from grafting the FGF2/Shh-treated Nurr1-transfected ES cells into the rat 6-OHDA– lesioned striatum (119). Robust engraftment was observed, where the vast majority of neurons were TH+. Markers of cell proliferation (e.g., Ki-67) were absent, and no teratomas were observed. Grafted neurons showed electrophysiological traits similar to mesencephalic neurons. Finally, whereas wild-type ES cells produced a slight recovery of amphetamine-induced rotation, Nurr1-ES cells yielded a marked change leading to contralateral, as opposed to ipsilateral rotation (Fig. 3E). Improvements were also seen in a battery of nonpharmacologically induced behaviors akin to those seen in human PD.

Despite the cautionary approach mandated by the possibility of inducing neoplasms with ES cell grafts, the results with in vitro generated DA neurons are encouraging. Results from similar experiments with primate models of PD are anticipated; the success with generating SDIA-induced primate ES cell–derived DA neurons has set the stage for these experiments (117).

C. Immortalized Neural Stem Cells

The Nurr1-transfected C17.2 cells were differentiated in vitro prior to being injected into the adult mouse (nonlesioned) striatum. Twelve days later survival of the cells was poor, but a few differentiated DA neurons were visualized. The cells have yet to be implanted in the 6-OHDA rat model.

D. Teratocarcinoma-Derived Neural Progenitor Cells

When hNT2 cells were cultured under optimized conditions for generating DA neurons and then grafted to the 6-OHDA–lesioned striatum, they either failed to produce (47) or produced insufficient numbers of DA neurons (133) to ameliorate rotational behavior.

VI. STIMULATION OF ENDOGENOUS NEURAL STEM CELLS

Another ramification of the discovery of adult stem/progenitor cells is the possibility of stimulating the proliferation and differentiation of endogenous progenitors to replace lost neurons, such as in PD. Neurodegeneration might itself provoke an environment that is conducive to the proliferation and differentiation of such progenitors (134–136), for example, through the release of cytokines (98) or neurotrophins (137) in response to inflammation. However, 6-OHDA lesions alone were unable to induce neurogenesis in the adult substantia nigra (138). Alternatively, infusion of growth factors or transfection of endogenous cells with vectors encoding trophic factors (in vivo gene therapy) may be necessary (139–141). For example, Fallon et al. (138) showed that infusion of transforming growth factor-alpha (TGF-α) into the lateral ventricles leads to massive proliferation and migration of stem cells into the striatum in animals with 6-OHDA lesions. Beginning 14 days after the infusion, βIII-tubulin–positive cells were seen in the striatum, as well as astrocytic cells. After 3-4 weeks, increasing numbers of TH+ cells were seen in the striatum (Fig. 3F), associated with a 31% reduction in rotational behavior. The nature and source of these striatal DA neurons is not known.

The stimulation of endogenous stem cells to replace midbrain substantia nigra DA neurons would require a population of cells that have the potential to generate this phenotype in the adult. Lie et al. (142) found actively dividing cells in the adult nigra which in situ generated new glial but not neuronal cells. Cultured in vitro, these progenitors could generate neurons, as well as after transplantation into the hippocampus (a neurogenic region in the adult), but only glial cells when grafted into the nigra (which is non-neurogenic).

VII.   EX VIVO GENE THERAPY USING NEURAL STEM CELLS

The previously discussed contexts required neural stem cells to differentiate into DA neurons and integrate into the existing neuronal circuitry in a physiologically functional manner. An alternative approach to ameliorating the DA deficits of PD is ex vivo gene therapy, in which a cellular vector is used to deliver biochemicals (e.g., neurotransmitters such as DA), trophic factors, or other gene products that modify the structure, function, or survival of endogenous neurons (38). In this context, neural stem cells may offer certain advantages over other cells (Table 1). First, they are genetically normal, i.e., have normal karyotype and do not express immortalizing oncogenes, adding a measure of safety over immortalized cell lines. Second, neural stem cells migrate and integrate well into the adult nervous system, in contrast to other cellular vectors such as fibroblasts or myoblasts. Third, their propensity towards astroglial differentiation in nonneurogenic regions is acceptable, or perhaps even advantageous (143). Towards this end, the availability of a clonal population of well-characterized neural stem cells that can be easily transfected and characterized in vitro is an advantage (144,145).

Neural stem cells have been engineered to produce trophic factors to support DA neurons. Both GDNF and the related molecule persephin have been expressed in C17.2 stem-like cells (146,147). When grafted to the striatum of wild-type mice, they integrated, differentiated (to neurons, astrocytes, and oligodendrocytes) and expressed the trophic factors for short periods of time before being rejected. Each graft was able to mitigate the loss of endogenous DA neurons in the substantia nigra following 6-OHDA administration and partially ameliorate rotational behavior following the lesions. In nude mice the grafts survived for long periods. Using a lentiviral vector, GDNF has also been expressed in rat forebrain-derived neurospheres, which were then implanted into the striatum of 6-OHDA–lesioned rats prior to grafting of primary VM tissue (148). Although the GDNF–neural stem cells increased the number of surviving DA neurons in the VM cografts, there was no additional effect on rotational behavior compared to VM grafts alone, and GDNF–neural stem cells had no effects in the absence of the co-grafts. As with the C17.2 cells, expression of GDNF was poor at 2 months, indicating downregulation of the transgene or graft rejection. Similar results have been produced with efforts to express TH (and related enzymes in the DA biosynthetic pathway) in neural stem cell lines (e.g., C17.2), where rapid downregulation of the transgenes was observed (38).

Issues that need to be addressed with regard to ex vivo gene therapy include variability of expression based on integration site, downregulation of expression, and graft rejection. It is possible that grafting unaltered neural stem cells can provide some measure of trophic support that can "rescue" endogenous DA neurons in 1-methyl-4-phenyl-1,2,3,6-tetrahydropyridine (MPTP)–treated mice, with associated improvements in rotational behavior (149).

VIII. CONCLUDING COMMENTS

Two seemingly conflicting developments have dominated the field of cell therapy for PD. The first is the discovery and continued development of techniques for the isolation and manipulation of neural stem cells. The ability to generate seemingly endless quantities of neurons that express DA markers and seem to function appropriately has raised the specter that cell therapy using stem cell–derived DA neurons is close at hand. Against this backdrop have been the sobering results of the clinical trials of fetal tissue implantation for PD. These results would appear to significantly dampen the promise of neural stem cells for PD.

There may in fact be ways in which stem cell–derived DA neurons provide advantages over fetal DA neurons, which may reignite the promise of this technology. First, stem cells will allow the generation of large numbers of well-characterized, and possibly even pure, DA neurons. While it is not necessarily the case that pure neuronal implantations are the correct approach, we certainly will be in a better position to predetermine exactly what we want contained in the grafts. Particular ratios of neurons and glial cells may be achievable. Second, by being able to define the composition of grafts, we may be able to eliminate components that in fetal grafts may contribute to rejection, such as blood vessels and related elements. Third, rejection may be further avoided by developing the ability to generate autografts from patients' own stem cells, by developing a bank of stem cells with large variations in histotypes, or by removing antigenic histocompatibility loci (77,150). Conceivably, stem cells can be tailor-generated for a patient from his or her own nuclei by nuclear transplantation (see Fig. 1) (77). Fourth, we are already capable of engineering stem cell–derived cells to express genes that may be important for the generation of DA neurons (e.g., Nurr1) and for modification of survival, engraftment, differentiation, process outgrowth, synaptogenesis, and physiological function. Thus, neural stem cells may eventually become a source of DA neurons superior to fetal tissue and lead to improved results in future cell therapy trials for PD.

REFERENCES

1. Olanow CW, Freeman T, Kordower J. Transplantation of embryonic dopamine neurons for severe Parkinson's disease. N Engl J Med 2001; 345:146–147.
2. Bjorklund A, Lindvall O. Cell replacement therapies for central nervous system disorders. Nat Neurosci 2000; 3:537–544.
3. Freed CR, Greene PE, Breeze RE, et al. Transplantation of embryonic dopamine neurons for severe Parkinson's disease. N Engl J Med 2001; 344:710–719.
4. Freeman TB, Goetz, CG, Kordower, JH, Stoessel, AJ, Brin, MF, Shannon, KM, Perl, D, Godbold, J, Olanow, CW. Double blind control trial of bilateral fetal nigral transplantation in Parkinson's disease. 6th International Congress of the Cell Transplant Society, Atlanta, GA, 2003:91.
5. Slack JMW. From Egg to Embryo. Cambridge, U.K.: Cambridge University Press, 1985.
6. McKay R. Stem cells in the central nervous system. Science 1997; 276:66–71.
7. Gage FH. Mammalian neural stem cells. Science 2000; 287:1433–1438.
8. Temple S. Stem cell plasticity—building the brain of our dreams. Nat Rev Neurosci 2001; 2:513–520.
9. Martin GR. Isolation of a pluripotent cell line from early mouse embryos cultured in medium conditioned by teratocarcinoma stem cells. Proc Natl Acad Sci USA 1981; 78:7634–7638.
10. Evans MJ, Kaufman MH. Establishment in culture of pluripotential cells from mouse embryos. Nature 1981; 292:154–156.
11. Morrison SJ, Shah NM, Anderson DJ. Regulatory mechanisms in stem cell biology. Cell 1997; 88:287–298.

12. Alvarez-Buylla A, Garcia-Verdugo JM, Tramontin AD. A unified hypothesis on the lineage of neural stem cells. Nat Rev Neurosci 2001; 2:287–293.
13. McKay R. Mammalian deconstruction for stem cell reconstruction. Nat Med 2000; 6:747–748.
14. Clarke DL, Johansson CB, Wilbertz J, et al. Generalized potential of adult neural stem cells. Science 2000; 288:1660–1663.
15. Bjornson CR, Rietze RL, Reynolds BA, Magli MC, Vescovi AL. Turning brain into blood: a hematopoietic fate adopted by adult neural stem cells in vivo. Science 1999; 283:534–537.
16. Woodbury D, Schwarz EJ, Prockop DJ, Black IB. Adult rat and human bone marrow stromal cells differentiate into neurons. J Neurosci Res 2000; 61:364–370.
17. Mezey E, Chandross KJ, Harta G, Maki RA, McKercher SR. Turning blood into brain: cells bearing neuronal antigens generated in vivo from bone marrow. Science 2000; 290:1779–1782.
18. Brazelton TR, Rossi FM, Keshet GI, Blau HM. From marrow to brain: expression of neuronal phenotypes in adult mice. Science 2000; 290:1775–1779.
19. Morshead CM, Benveniste P, Iscove NN, van der Kooy D. Hematopoietic competence is a rare property of neural stem cells that may depend on genetic and epigenetic alterations. Nat Med 2002; 8:268–273.
20. Wagers AJ, Sherwood RI, Christensen JL, Weissman IL. Little evidence for developmental plasticity of adult hematopoietic stem cells. Science 2002; 297:2256–2259.
21. Weissman IL. Stem cells: units of development, units of regeneration, and units in evolution. Cell 2000; 100:157–168.
22. Gross CG. Neurogenesis in the adult brain: death of a dogma. Nat Rev Neurosci 2000; 1:67–73.
23. Rakic P. DNA synthesis and cell division in the adult primate brain. Ann NY Acad Sci 1985; 457:193–211.
24. Ramon y Cajal S. Degeneration and Regeneration of the Nervous System (Trans Day, R.M., from the 1913 Spanish ed.). London: Oxford University Press, 1928.
25. Reynolds BA, Weiss S. Generation of neurons and astrocytes from isolated cells of the adult mammalian central nervous system. Science 1992; 255:1707–1710.
26. Alvarez-Buylla A, Lois C. Neuronal stem cells in the brain of adult vertebrates. Stem Cells 1995; 13:263–272.
27. Luskin MB. Restricted proliferation and migration of postnatally generated neurons derived from the forebrain subventricular zone. Neuron 1993; 11:173–189.
28. Studer L, Tabar V, McKay RD. Transplantation of expanded mesencephalic precursors leads to recovery in parkinsonian rats. Nat Neurosci 1998; 1:290–295.
29. Studer L, Csete M, Lee SH, et al. Enhanced proliferation, survival, and dopaminergic differentiation of CNS precursors in lowered oxygen. J Neurosci 2000; 20:7377–7383.
30. Weissman IL. Translating stem and progenitor cell biology to the clinic: barriers and opportunities. Science 2000; 287:1442–1446.
31. Uchida N, Buck DW, He D, et al. Direct isolation of human central nervous system stem cells. Proc Natl Acad Sci USA 2000; 97:14720–14725.
32. Tamaki S, Eckert K, He D, et al. Engraftment of sorted/expanded human central nervous system stem cells from fetal brain. J Neurosci Res 2002; 69:976–986.
33. Rietze RL, Valcanis H, Brooker GF, Thomas T, Voss AK, Bartlett PF. Purification of a pluripotent neural stem cell from the adult mouse brain. Nature 2001; 412:736–739.
34. Thomson JA, Itskovitz-Eldor J, Shapiro SS, et al. Embryonic stem cell lines derived from human blastocysts. Science 1998; 282:1145–1147.
35. Reubinoff BE, Pera MF, Fong CY, Trounson A, Bongso A. Embryonic stem cell lines from human blastocysts: somatic differentiation in vitro. Nat Biotechnol 2000; 18:399–404.
36. Reubinoff BE, Itsykson P, Turetsky T, et al. Neural progenitors from human embryonic stem cells. Nat Biotechnol 2001; 19:1134–1140.
37. Gottlieb DI. Large-scale sources of neural stem cells. Annu Rev Neurosci 2002; 25:381–407.
38. Martinez-Serrano A, Bjorklund A. Immortalized neural progenitor cells for CNS gene transfer and repair. Trends Neurosci 1997; 20:530–538.
39. Whittemore SR, Onifer SM. Immortalized neural cell lines for CNS transplantation. Prog Brain Res 2000; 127:49–65.
40. Snyder EY, Deitcher DL, Walsh C, Arnold-Aldea S, Hartwieg EA, Cepko CL. Multipotent neural cell lines can engraft and participate in development of mouse cerebellum. Cell 1992; 68:33–51.
41. Renfranz PJ, Cunningham MG, McKay RD. Region-specific differentiation of the hippocampal stem cell line HiB5 upon implantation into the developing mammalian brain. Cell 1991; 66:713–729.

42. Lundberg C, Field PM, Ajayi YO, Raisman G, Bjorklund A. Conditionally immortalized neural progenitor cell lines integrate and differentiate after grafting to the adult rat striatum. A combined autoradiographic and electron microscopic study. Brain Res 1996; 737:295–300.

43. Catapano LA, Sheen VL, Leavitt BR, Macklis JD. Differentiation of transplanted neural precursors varies regionally in adults striatum. Neuroreport 1999; 10:3971–3977.

44. Martinez-Serrano A, Hantzopoulos PA, Bjorklund A. Ex vivo gene transfer of brain-derived neurotrophic factor to the intact rat forebrain: neurotrophic effects on cholinergic neurons. Eur J Neurosci 1996; 8:727–735.

45. Son JH, Chun HS, Joh TH, Cho S, Conti B, Lee JW. Neuroprotection and neuronal differentiation studies using substantia nigra dopaminergic cells derived from transgenic mouse embryos. J Neurosci 1999; 19:10–20.

46. Prasad KN, Carvalho E, Kentroti S, Edwards-Prasad J, Freed C, Vernadakis A. Establishment and characterization of immortalized clonal cell lines from fetal rat mesencephalic tissue. In Vitro Cell Dev Biol Anim 1994; 30A:596–603.

47. Saporta S, Willing AE, Colina LO, et al. In vitro and in vivo characterization of hNT neuron neurotransmitter phenotypes. Brain Res Bull 2000; 53:263–268.

48. Andrews PW. Retinoic acid induces neuronal differentiation of a cloned human embryonal carcinoma cell line in vitro. Dev Biol 1984; 103:285–293.

49. Pleasure SJ, Lee VM. NTera 2 cells: a human cell line which displays characteristics expected of a human committed neuronal progenitor cell. J Neurosci Res 1993; 35:585–602.

50. Philips MF, Muir JK, Saatman KE, et al. Survival and integration of transplanted postmitotic human neurons following experimental brain injury in immunocompetent rats. J Neurosurg 1999; 90:116–124.

51. Nelson PT, Kondziolka D, Wechsler L, et al. Clonal human (hNT) neuron grafts for stroke therapy: neuropathology in a patient 27 months after implantation. Am J Pathol 2002; 160:1201–1206.

52. Reynolds BA, Tetzlaff W, Weiss S. A multipotent EGF-responsive striatal embryonic progenitor cell produces neurons and astrocytes. J Neurosci 1992; 12:4565–4574.

53. Gross RE, Mehler MF, Mabie PC, Zang Z, Santschi L, Kessler JA. Bone morphogenetic proteins promote astroglial lineage commitment by mammalian subventricular zone progenitor cells. Neuron 1996; 17:595–606.

54. Cohen RI, Marmur R, Norton WT, Mehler MF, Kessler JA. Nerve growth factor and neurotrophin-3 differentially regulate the proliferation and survival of developing rat brain oligodendrocytes. J Neurosci 1996; 16:6433–6442.

55. Michaelson MD, Mehler MF, Xu H, Gross RE, Kessler JA. Interleukin-7 is trophic for embryonic neurons and is expressed in developing brain. Dev Biol 1996; 179:251–263.

56. Caldwell MA, He X, Wilkie N, et al. Growth factors regulate the survival and fate of cells derived from human neurospheres. Nat Biotechnol 2001; 19:475–479.

57. Piper DR, Mujtaba T, Rao MS, Lucero MT. Immunocytochemical and physiological characterization of a population of cultured human neural precursors. J Neurophysiol 2000; 84:534–548.

58. Vescovi AL, Parati EA, Gritti A, et al. Isolation and cloning of multipotential stem cells from the embryonic human CNS and establishment of transplantable human neural stem cell lines by epigenetic stimulation. Exp Neurol 1999; 156:71–83.

59. Winkler C, Fricker RA, Gates MA, et al. Incorporation and glial differentiation of mouse EGF-responsive neural progenitor cells after transplantation into the embryonic rat brain. Mol Cell Neurosci 1998; 11:99–116.

60. Fricker RA, Carpenter MK, Winkler C, Greco C, Gates MA, Bjorklund A. Site-specific migration and neuronal differentiation of human neural progenitor cells after transplantation in the adult rat brain. J Neurosci 1999; 19:5990–6005.

61. Tropepe V, Sibilia M, Ciruna BG, Rossant J, Wagner EF, van der Kooy D. Distinct neural stem cells proliferate in response to EGF and FGF in the developing mouse telencephalon. Dev Biol 1999; 208:166–188.

62. Doetsch F, Caille I, Lim DA, Garcia-Verdugo JM, Alvarez-Buylla A. Subventricular zone astrocytes are neural stem cells in the adult mammalian brain. Cell 1999; 97:703–716.

63. Laywell ED, Rakic P, Kukekov VG, Holland EC, Steindler DA. Identification of a multipotent astrocytic stem cell in the immature and adult mouse brain. Proc Natl Acad Sci USA 2000; 97:13883–13888.

64. Chiasson BJ, Tropepe V, Morshead CM, van der Kooy D. Adult mammalian forebrain ependymal and subependymal cells demonstrate proliferative potential, but only subependymal cells have neural stem cell characteristics. J Neurosci 1999; 19:4462–4471.

65. Noctor SC, Flint AC, Weissman TA, Dammerman RS, Kriegstein AR. Neurons derived from radial glial cells establish radial units in neocortex. Nature 2001; 409:714–720.
66. Noctor SC, Flint AC, Weissman TA, Wong WS, Clinton BK, Kriegstein AR. Dividing precursor cells of the embryonic cortical ventricular zone have morphological and molecular characteristics of radial glia. J Neurosci 2002; 22:3161–3173.
67. Malatesta P, Hartfuss E, Gotz M. Isolation of radial glial cells by fluorescent-activated cell sorting reveals a neuronal lineage. Development 2000; 127:5253–5263.
68. Malatesta P, Hack MA, Hartfuss E, et al. Neuronal or glial progeny. Regional differences in radial glia fate. Neuron 2003; 37:751–764.
69. Johansson CB, Momma S, Clarke DL, Risling M, Lendahl U, Frisen J. Identification of a neural stem cell in the adult mammalian central nervous system. Cell 1999; 96:25–34.
70. Luskin MB, McDermott K. Divergent lineages for oligodendrocytes and astrocytes originating in the neonatal forebrain subventricular zone. Glia 1994; 11:211–226.
71. Luskin MB, Parnavelas JG, Barfield JA. Neurons, astrocytes, and oligodendrocytes of the rat cerebral cortex originate from separate progenitor cells: an ultrastructural analysis of clonally related cells. J Neurosci 1993; 13:1730–1750.
72. Svendsen CN, Clarke DJ, Rosser AE, Dunnett SB. Survival and differentiation of rat and human epidermal growth factor-responsive precursor cells following grafting into the lesioned adult central nervous system. Exp Neurol 1996; 137:376–388.
73. Daadi M, Arcellana-Panlilio MY, Weiss S. Activin co-operates with fibroblast growth factor 2 to regulate tyrosine hydroxylase expression in the basal forebrain ventricular zone progenitors. Neuroscience 1998; 86:867–880.
74. Daadi MM, Weiss S. Generation of tyrosine hydroxylase-producing neurons from precursors of the embryonic and adult forebrain. J Neurosci 1999; 19:4484–4497.
75. Roy NS, Wang S, Jiang L, et al. In vitro neurogenesis by progenitor cells isolated from the adult human hippocampus. Nat Med 2000; 6:271–277.
76. Kirschenbaum B, Nedergaard M, Preuss A, Barami K, Fraser RA, Goldman SA. In vitro neuronal production and differentiation by precursor cells derived from the adult human forebrain. Cereb Cortex 1994; 4:576–589.
77. Svendsen CN, Smith AG. New prospects for human stem-cell therapy in the nervous system. Trends Neurosci 1999; 22:357–364.
78. Svendsen CN, Caldwell MA, Shen J, et al. Long-term survival of human central nervous system progenitor cells transplanted into a rat model of Parkinson's disease. Exp Neurol 1997; 148:135–146.
79. Svendsen CN, Caldwell MA, Ostenfeld T. Human neural stem cells: isolation, expansion and transplantation. Brain Pathol 1999; 9:499–513.
80. Chalmers-Redman RM, Priestley T, Kemp JA, Fine A. In vitro propagation and inducible differentiation of multipotential progenitor cells from human fetal brain. Neuroscience 1997; 76:1121–1128.
81. Carpenter MK, Cui X, Hu ZY, et al. In vitro expansion of a multipotent population of human neural progenitor cells. Exp Neurol 1999; 158:265–278.
82. Ostenfeld T, Joly E, Tai YT, et al. Regional specification of rodent and human neurospheres. Brain Res Dev Brain Res 2002; 134:43–55.
83. Piper DR, Mujtaba T, Keyoung H, et al. Identification and characterization of neuronal precursors and their progeny from human fetal tissue. J Neurosci Res 2001; 66:356–368.
84. Suhonen JO, Peterson DA, Ray J, Gage FH. Differentiation of adult hippocampus-derived progenitors into olfactory neurons in vivo. Nature 1996; 383:624–627.
85. Gage FH, Ray J, Fisher LJ. Isolation, characterization, and use of stem cells from the CNS. Annu Rev Neurosci 1995; 18:159–192.
86. Gage FH, Coates PW, Palmer TD, et al. Survival and differentiation of adult neuronal progenitor cells transplanted to the adult brain. Proc Natl Acad Sci USA 1995; 92:11879–11883.
87. Zetterstrom RH, Williams R, Perlmann T, Olson L. Cellular expression of the immediate early transcription factors Nurr1 and NGFI-B suggests a gene regulatory role in several brain regions including the nigrostriatal dopamine system. Brain Res Mol Brain Res 1996; 41:111–120.
88. Sakurada K, Ohshima-Sakurada M, Palmer TD, Gage FH. Nurr1, an orphan nuclear receptor, is a transcriptional activator of endogenous tyrosine hydroxylase in neural progenitor cells derived from the adult brain. Development 1999; 126:4017–4026.
89. Davis AA, Temple S. A self-renewing multipotential stem cell in embryonic rat cerebral cortex. Nature 1994; 372:263–266.

90. Tsai RY, McKay RD. Cell contact regulates fate choice by cortical stem cells. J Neurosci 2000; 20:3725–3735.

91. Ye W, Shimamura K, Rubenstein JL, Hynes MA, Rosenthal A. FGF and Shh signals control dopaminergic and serotonergic cell fate in the anterior neural plate. Cell 1998; 93:755–766.

92. Hynes M, Rosenthal A. Specification of dopaminergic and serotonergic neurons in the vertebrate CNS. Curr Opin Neurobiol 1999; 9:26–36.

93. Perrone-Capano C, Di Porzio U. Genetic and epigenetic control of midbrain dopaminergic neuron development. Int J Dev Biol 2000; 44:679–687.

94. Witta J, Baffi JS, Palkovits M, Mezey E, Castillo SO, Nikodem VM. Nigrostriatal innervation is preserved in Nurr1-null mice, although dopaminergic neuron precursors are arrested from terminal differentiation. Brain Res Mol Brain Res 2000; 84:67–78.

95. Simon HH, Saueressig H, Wurst W, Goulding MD, O'Leary DD. Fate of midbrain dopaminergic neurons controlled by the engrailed genes. J Neurosci 2001; 21:3126–3134.

96. Smidt MP, Asbreuk CH, Cox JJ, Chen H, Johnson RL, Burbach JP. A second independent pathway for development of mesencephalic dopaminergic neurons requires Lmx1b. Nat Neurosci 2000; 3:337–341.

97. Smidt MP, van Schaick HS, Lanctot C, et al. A homeodomain gene Ptx3 has highly restricted brain expression in mesencephalic dopaminergic neurons. Proc Natl Acad Sci USA 1997; 94:13305–13310.

98. Ling ZD, Potter ED, Lipton JW, Carvey PM. Differentiation of mesencephalic progenitor cells into dopaminergic neurons by cytokines. Exp Neurol 1998; 149:411–423.

99. Carvey PM, Ling ZD, Sortwell CE, et al. A clonal line of mesencephalic progenitor cells converted to dopamine neurons by hematopoietic cytokines: a source of cells for transplantation in Parkinson's disease. Exp Neurol 2001; 171:98–108.

100. Sawamoto K, Nakao N, Kakishita K, et al. Generation of dopaminergic neurons in the adult brain from mesencephalic precursor cells labeled with a nestin-GFP transgene. J Neurosci 2001; 21:3895–3903.

101. Sanchez-Pernaute R, Studer L, Bankiewicz KS, Major EO, McKay RD. In vitro generation and transplantation of precursor-derived human dopamine neurons. J Neurosci Res 2001; 65:284–288.

102. Storch A, Paul G, Csete M, et al. Long-term proliferation and dopaminergic differentiation of human mesencephalic neural precursor cells. Exp Neurol 2001; 170:317–325.

103. Riaz SS, Jauniaux E, Stern GM, Bradford HF. The controlled conversion of human neural progenitor cells derived from foetal ventral mesencephalon into dopaminergic neurons in vitro. Brain Res Dev Brain Res 2002; 136:27–34.

104. Rao MS, Mayer-Proschel M. Glial-restricted precursors are derived from multipotent neuroepithelial stem cells. Dev Biol 1997; 188:48–63.

105. Mayer-Proschel M, Kalyani AJ, Mujtaba T, Rao MS. Isolation of lineage-restricted neuronal precursors from multipotent neuroepithelial stem cells. Neuron 1997; 19:773–785.

106. Bain G, Kitchens D, Yao M, Huettner JE, Gottlieb DI. Embryonic stem cells express neuronal properties in vitro. Dev Biol 1995; 168:342–357.

107. Carpenter MK, Inokuma MS, Denham J, Mujtaba T, Chiu CP, Rao MS. Enrichment of neurons and neural precursors from human embryonic stem cells. Exp Neurol 2001; 172:383–397.

108. Kuo HC, Pau KY, Yeoman RR, Mitalipov SM, Okano H, Wolf DP. Differentiation of monkey embryonic stem cells into neural lineages. Biol Reprod 2003; 68:1727–1735.

109. Li M, Pevny L, Lovell-Badge R, Smith A. Generation of purified neural precursors from embryonic stem cells by lineage selection. Curr Biol 1998; 8:971–974.

110. Okabe S, Forsberg-Nilsson K, Spiro AC, Segal M, McKay RD. Development of neuronal precursor cells and functional postmitotic neurons from embryonic stem cells in vitro. Mech Dev 1996; 59:89–102.

111. Schuldiner M, Eiges R, Eden A, et al. Induced neuronal differentiation of human embryonic stem cells. Brain Res 2001; 913:201–205.

112. Ying QL, Stavridis M, Griffiths D, Li M, Smith A. Conversion of embryonic stem cells into neuroectodermal precursors in adherent monoculture. Nat Biotechnol 2003; 21:183–186.

113. Zhang SC, Wernig M, Duncan ID, Brustle O, Thomson JA. In vitro differentiation of transplantable neural precursors from human embryonic stem cells. Nat Biotechnol 2001; 19:1129–1133.

114. Lee SH, Lumelsky N, Studer L, Auerbach JM, McKay RD. Efficient generation of midbrain and hindbrain neurons from mouse embryonic stem cells. Nat Biotechnol 2000; 18: 675–679.

115. Dinsmore J, Ratliff J, Deacon T, et al. Embryonic stem cells differentiated in vitro as a novel source of cells for transplantation. Cell Transplant 1996; 5:131–143.

116. Kawasaki H, Mizuseki K, Nishikawa S, et al. Induction of midbrain dopaminergic neurons from ES cells by stromal cell-derived inducing activity. Neuron 2000; 28:31–40.

117. Kawasaki H, Suemori H, Mizuseki K, et al. Generation of dopaminergic neurons and pigmented epithelia from primate ES cells by stromal cell-derived inducing activity. Proc Natl Acad Sci USA 2002; 99:1580–1585.

118. Rolletschek A, Chang H, Guan K, Czyz J, Meyer M, Wobus AM. Differentiation of embryonic stem cell-derived dopaminergic neurons is enhanced by survival-promoting factors. Mech Dev 2001; 105:93–104.

119. Kim JH, Auerbach JM, Rodriguez-Gomez JA, et al. Dopamine neurons derived from embryonic stem cells function in an animal model of Parkinson's disease. Nature 2002; 418:50–56.

120. Xu C, Inokuma MS, Denham J, et al. Feeder-free growth of undifferentiated human embryonic stem cells. Nat Biotechnol 2001; 19:971–974.

121. Amit M, Margulets V, Segev H, et al. Human feeder layers for human embryonic stem cells. Biol Reprod 2003; 68:2150–2156.

122. Richards M, Fong CY, Chan WK, Wong PC, Bongso A. Human feeders support prolonged undifferentiated growth of human inner cell masses and embryonic stem cells. Nat Biotechnol 2002; 20:933–936.

123. Taylor RM, Snyder EY. Widespread engraftment of neural progenitor and stem-like cells throughout the mouse brain. Transplant Proc 1997; 29:845–847.

124. Wagner J, Akerud P, Castro DS, et al. Induction of a midbrain dopaminergic phenotype in Nurr1-overexpressing neural stem cells by type 1 astrocytes. Nat Biotechnol 1999; 17:653–659.

125. Shihabuddin LS, Brunschwig JP, Holets VR, Bunge MB, Whittemore SR. Induction of mature neuronal properties in immortalized neuronal precursor cells following grafting into the neonatal CNS. J Neurocytol 1996; 25:101–111.

126. Zigova T, Barroso LF, Willing AE, et al. Dopaminergic phenotype of hNT cells in vitro. Brain Res Dev Brain Res 2000; 122:87–90.

127. Zigova T, Willing AE, Tedesco EM, et al. Lithium chloride induces the expression of tyrosine hydroxylase in hNT neurons. Exp Neurol 1999; 157:251–258.

128. Ostenfeld T, Caldwell MA, Prowse KR, Linskens MH, Jauniaux E, Svendsen CN. Human neural precursor cells express low levels of telomerase in vitro and show diminishing cell proliferation with extensive axonal outgrowth following transplantation. Exp Neurol 2000; 164:215–226.

129. Nishino H, Hida H, Takei N, Kumazaki M, Nakajima K, Baba H. Mesencephalic neural stem (progenitor) cells develop to dopaminergic neurons more strongly in dopamine-depleted striatum than in intact striatum. Exp Neurol 2000; 164:209–214.

130. Brustle O, Spiro AC, Karram K, Choudhary K, Okabe S, McKay RD. In vitro-generated neural precursors participate in mammalian brain development. Proc Natl Acad Sci USA 1997; 94:14809–14814.

131. Deacon T, Dinsmore J, Costantini LC, Ratliff J, Isacson O. Blastula-stage stem cells can differentiate into dopaminergic and serotonergic neurons after transplantation. Exp Neurol 1998; 149:28–41.

132. Bjorklund LM, Sanchez-Pernaute R, Chung S, et al. Embryonic stem cells develop into functional dopaminergic neurons after transplantation in a Parkinson rat model. Proc Natl Acad Sci USA 2002; 99:2344–2349.

133. Baker KA, Hong M, Sadi D, Mendez I. Intrastriatal and intranigral grafting of hNT neurons in the 6-OHDA rat model of Parkinson's disease. Exp Neurol 2000; 162:350–360.

134. Snyder EY, Yoon C, Flax JD, Macklis JD. Multipotent neural precursors can differentiate toward replacement of neurons undergoing targeted apoptotic degeneration in adult mouse neocortex. Proc Natl Acad Sci USA 1997; 94:11663–11668.

135. Sheen VL, Macklis JD. Targeted neocortical cell death in adult mice guides migration and differentiation of transplanted embryonic neurons. J Neurosci 1995; 15:8378–8392.

136. Macklis JD. Transplanted neocortical neurons migrate selectively into regions of neuronal degeneration produced by chromophore-targeted laser photolysis. J Neurosci 1993; 13:3848–3863.

137. Wang Y, Sheen VL, Macklis JD. Cortical interneurons upregulate neurotrophins in vivo in response to targeted apoptotic degeneration of neighboring pyramidal neurons. Exp Neurol 1998; 154:389–402.

138. Fallon J, Reid S, Kinyamu R, et al. In vivo induction of massive proliferation, directed migration, and differentiation of neural cells in the adult mammalian brain. Proc Natl Acad Sci USA 2000; 97:14686–14691.

139. Benraiss A, Chmielnicki E, Lerner K, Roh D, Goldman SA. Adenoviral brain-derived neurotrophic factor induces both neostriatal and olfactory neuronal recruitment from endogenous progenitor cells in the adult forebrain. J Neurosci 2001; 21:6718–6731.
140. Zigova T, Pencea V, Wiegand SJ, Luskin MB. Intraventricular administration of BDNF increases the number of newly generated neurons in the adult olfactory bulb. Mol Cell Neurosci 1998; 11: 234–245.
141. Craig CG, Tropepe V, Morshead CM, Reynolds BA, Weiss S, van der Kooy D. In vivo growth factor expansion of endogenous subependymal neural precursor cell populations in the adult mouse brain. J Neurosci 1996; 16:2649–2658.
142. Lie DC, Dziewczapolski G, Willhoite AR, Kaspar BK, Shults CW, Gage FH. The adult substantia nigra contains progenitor cells with neurogenic potential. J Neurosci 2002; 22:6639–6649.
143. Ericson C, Wictorin K, Lundberg C. Ex vivo and in vitro studies of transgene expression in rat astrocytes transduced with lentiviral vectors. Exp Neurol 2002; 173:22–30.
144. Rubio FJ, Bueno C, Villa A, Navarro B, Martinez-Serrano A. Genetically perpetuated human neural stem cells engraft and differentiate into the adult mammalian brain. Mol Cell Neurosci 2000; 16:1–13.
145. Villa A, Snyder EY, Vescovi A, Martinez-Serrano A. Establishment and properties of a growth factor-dependent, perpetual neural stem cell line from the human CNS. Exp Neurol 2000; 161:67–84.
146. Akerud P, Holm PC, Castelo-Branco G, Sousa K, Rodriguez FJ, Arenas E. Persephin-overexpressing neural stem cells regulate the function of nigral dopaminergic neurons and prevent their degeneration in a model of Parkinson's disease. Mol Cell Neurosci 2002; 21:205–222.
147. Akerud P, Canals JM, Snyder EY, Arenas E. Neuroprotection through delivery of glial cell line-derived neurotrophic factor by neural stem cells in a mouse model of Parkinson's disease. J Neurosci 2001; 21:8108–8118.
148. Ostenfeld T, Tai YT, Martin P, Deglon N, Aebischer P, Svendsen CN. Neurospheres modified to produce glial cell line-derived neurotrophic factor increase the survival of transplanted dopamine neurons. J Neurosci Res 2002; 69:955–965.
149. Ourednik J, Ourednik V, Lynch WP, Schachner M, Snyder EY. Neural stem cells display an inherent mechanism for rescuing dysfunctional neurons. Nat Biotechnol 2002; 20:1103–1110.
150. Smith AJ, De Sousa MA, Kwabi-Addo B, Heppell-Parton A, Impey H, Rabbitts P. A site-directed chromosomal translocation induced in embryonic stem cells by Cre-loxP recombination. Nat Genet 1995; 9:376–385.

Index

About the Editors

RAJESH PAHWA is Associate Professor of Neurology and Director of the Parkinson's Disease and Movement Disorder Center, University of Kansas Medical Center, Kansas City, Kansas. The author or coauthor of numerous journal articles and professional publications, he is the coeditor of the *Handbook of Parkinson's Disease, Third Edition* (Marcel Dekker, Inc.). Dr. Pahwa received the M.D. degree (1983) from the University of Bombay, India.

KELLY E. LYONS is Research Associate Professor of Neurology and Director of Research at the Parkinson's Disease and Movement Disorder Center, University of Kansas Medical Center, Kansas City, Kansas. The coeditor of the *Handbook of Parkinson's Disease, Third Edition* (Marcel Dekker, Inc.) and author or coauthor of numerous articles and professional publications, Dr. Lyons received the M.A. (1991) and Ph.D. (1993) degrees in cognitive and experimental psychology from the University of Kansas, Lawrence, Kansas.

WILLIAM C. KOLLER is Professor of Neurology at Mount Sinai School of Medicine, New York, New York. Serving on the editorial board for the Neurological Disease and Therapy series (Marcel Dekker, Inc.), he is the author, coauthor, editor, or coeditor of numerous journal articles and several books including the *Handbook of Parkinson's Disease, Third Edition; Etiology of Parkinson's Disease*; the *Handbook of Tremor Disorders*; and *Parkinsonian Syndromes* (all titles, Marcel Dekker, Inc.). Dr. Koller received the M.S. (1971) and Ph.D. (1974) degrees in pharmacology and the M.D. degree (1976) from Northwestern University Medical School, Chicago, Illinois.

ISBN 0-8247-5455-7

90000